Lecture Notes in Computer Science   8515

Commenced Publication in 1973
Founding and Former Series Editors:
Gerhard Goos, Juris Hartmanis, and Jan van Leeuwen

Constantine Stephanidis   Margherita Antona (Eds.)

Universal Access in Human-Computer Interaction

Aging and Assistive Environments

8th International Conference, UAHCI 2014
Held as Part of HCI International 2014
Heraklion, Crete, Greece, June 22-27, 2014
Proceedings, Part III

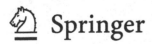 Springer

Volume Editors

Constantine Stephanidis
Foundation for Research and Technology - Hellas (FORTH)
Institute of Computer Science
N. Plastira 100, Vassilika Vouton, 70013 Heraklion, Crete, Greece
and University of Crete, Department of Computer Science
Heraklion, Crete, Greece
E-mail: cs@ics.forth.gr

Margherita Antona
Foundation for Research and Technology - Hellas (FORTH)
Institute of Computer Science
N. Plastira 100, Vassilika Vouton, 70013 Heraklion, Crete, Greece
E-mail: antona@ics.forth.gr

ISSN 0302-9743   e-ISSN 1611-3349
ISBN 978-3-319-07445-0   e-ISBN 978-3-319-07446-7
DOI 10.1007/978-3-319-07446-7
Springer Cham Heidelberg New York Dordrecht London

Library of Congress Control Number: 2014939292

LNCS Sublibrary: SL 3 – Information Systems and Application, incl. Internet/Web and HCI

Typesetting: Camera-ready by author, data conversion by Scientific Publishing Services, Chennai, India

Printed on acid-free paper

Springer is part of Springer Science+Business Media (www.springer.com)

Foreword

The 16th International Conference on Human–Computer Interaction, HCI International 2014, was held in Heraklion, Crete, Greece, during June 22–27, 2014, incorporating 14 conferences/thematic areas:

Thematic areas:

- Human–Computer Interaction
- Human Interface and the Management of Information

Affiliated conferences:

- 11th International Conference on Engineering Psychology and Cognitive Ergonomics
- 8th International Conference on Universal Access in Human–Computer Interaction
- 6th International Conference on Virtual, Augmented and Mixed Reality
- 6th International Conference on Cross-Cultural Design
- 6th International Conference on Social Computing and Social Media
- 8th International Conference on Augmented Cognition
- 5th International Conference on Digital Human Modeling and Applications in Health, Safety, Ergonomics and Risk Management
- Third International Conference on Design, User Experience and Usability
- Second International Conference on Distributed, Ambient and Pervasive Interactions
- Second International Conference on Human Aspects of Information Security, Privacy and Trust
- First International Conference on HCI in Business
- First International Conference on Learning and Collaboration Technologies

A total of 4,766 individuals from academia, research institutes, industry, and governmental agencies from 78 countries submitted contributions, and 1,476 papers and 225 posters were included in the proceedings. These papers address the latest research and development efforts and highlight the human aspects of design and use of computing systems. The papers thoroughly cover the entire field of human–computer interaction, addressing major advances in knowledge and effective use of computers in a variety of application areas.

This volume, edited by Constantine Stephanidis and Margherita Anton, contains papers focusing on the thematic area of Universal Access in Human-Computer Interaction, addressing the following major topics:

- Design for aging
- Health and rehabilitation applications

- Accessible smart and assistive environments
- Assistive robots
- Mobility, navigation, and safety

The remaining volumes of the HCI International 2014 proceedings are:

- Volume 1, LNCS 8510, Human–Computer Interaction: HCI Theories, Methods and Tools (Part I), edited by Masaaki Kurosu
- Volume 2, LNCS 8511, Human–Computer Interaction: Advanced Interaction Modalities and Techniques (Part II), edited by Masaaki Kurosu
- Volume 3, LNCS 8512, Human–Computer Interaction: Applications and Services (Part III), edited by Masaaki Kurosu
- Volume 4, LNCS 8513, Universal Access in Human–Computer Interaction: Design and Development Methods for Universal Access (Part I), edited by Constantine Stephanidis and Margherita Antona
- Volume 5, LNCS 8514, Universal Access in Human–Computer Interaction: Universal Access to Information and Knowledge (Part II), edited by Constantine Stephanidis and Margherita Antona
- Volume 7, LNCS 8516, Universal Access in Human–Computer Interaction: Design for All and Accessibility Practice (Part IV), edited by Constantine Stephanidis and Margherita Antona
- Volume 8, LNCS 8517, Design, User Experience, and Usability: Theories, Methods and Tools for Designing the User Experience (Part I), edited by Aaron Marcus
- Volume 9, LNCS 8518, Design, User Experience, and Usability: User Experience Design for Diverse Interaction Platforms and Environments (Part II), edited by Aaron Marcus
- Volume 10, LNCS 8519, Design, User Experience, and Usability: User Experience Design for Everyday Life Applications and Services (Part III), edited by Aaron Marcus
- Volume 11, LNCS 8520, Design, User Experience, and Usability: User Experience Design Practice (Part IV), edited by Aaron Marcus
- Volume 12, LNCS 8521, Human Interface and the Management of Information: Information and Knowledge Design and Evaluation (Part I), edited by Sakae Yamamoto
- Volume 13, LNCS 8522, Human Interface and the Management of Information: Information and Knowledge in Applications and Services (Part II), edited by Sakae Yamamoto
- Volume 14, LNCS 8523, Learning and Collaboration Technologies: Designing and Developing Novel Learning Experiences (Part I), edited by Panayiotis Zaphiris and Andri Ioannou
- Volume 15, LNCS 8524, Learning and Collaboration Technologies: Technology-rich Environments for Learning and Collaboration (Part II), edited by Panayiotis Zaphiris and Andri Ioannou
- Volume 16, LNCS 8525, Virtual, Augmented and Mixed Reality: Designing and Developing Virtual and Augmented Environments (Part I), edited by Randall Shumaker and Stephanie Lackey

I would like to thank the Program Chairs and the members of the Program Boards of all affiliated conferences and thematic areas, listed below, for their contribution to the highest scientific quality and the overall success of the HCI International 2014 Conference.

This conference could not have been possible without the continuous support and advice of the founding chair and conference scientific advisor, Prof. Gavriel Salvendy, as well as the dedicated work and outstanding efforts of the communications chair and editor of *HCI International News*, Dr. Abbas Moallem.

I would also like to thank for their contribution towards the smooth organization of the HCI International 2014 Conference the members of the Human–Computer Interaction Laboratory of ICS-FORTH, and in particular George Paparoulis, Maria Pitsoulaki, Maria Bouhli, and George Kapnas.

April 2014   Constantine Stephanidis
                                                 General Chair, HCI International 2014

Organization

Human–Computer Interaction

Program Chair: Masaaki Kurosu, Japan

Jose Abdelnour-Nocera, UK
Sebastiano Bagnara, Italy
Simone Barbosa, Brazil
Adriana Betiol, Brazil
Simone Borsci, UK
Henry Duh, Australia
Xiaowen Fang, USA
Vicki Hanson, UK
Wonil Hwang, Korea
Minna Isomursu, Finland
Yong Gu Ji, Korea
Anirudha Joshi, India
Esther Jun, USA
Kyungdoh Kim, Korea

Heidi Krömker, Germany
Chen Ling, USA
Chang S. Nam, USA
Naoko Okuizumi, Japan
Philippe Palanque, France
Ling Rothrock, USA
Naoki Sakakibara, Japan
Dominique Scapin, France
Guangfeng Song, USA
Sanjay Tripathi, India
Chui Yin Wong, Malaysia
Toshiki Yamaoka, Japan
Kazuhiko Yamazaki, Japan
Ryoji Yoshitake, Japan

Human Interface and the Management of Information

Program Chair: Sakae Yamamoto, Japan

Alan Chan, Hong Kong
Denis A. Coelho, Portugal
Linda Elliott, USA
Shin'ichi Fukuzumi, Japan
Michitaka Hirose, Japan
Makoto Itoh, Japan
Yen-Yu Kang, Taiwan
Koji Kimita, Japan
Daiji Kobayashi, Japan

Hiroyuki Miki, Japan
Shogo Nishida, Japan
Robert Proctor, USA
Youngho Rhee, Korea
Ryosuke Saga, Japan
Katsunori Shimohara, Japan
Kim-Phuong Vu, USA
Tomio Watanabe, Japan

Engineering Psychology and Cognitive Ergonomics

Program Chair: Don Harris, UK

Guy Andre Boy, USA
Shan Fu, P.R. China
Hung-Sying Jing, Taiwan
Wen-Chin Li, Taiwan
Mark Neerincx, The Netherlands
Jan Noyes, UK
Paul Salmon, Australia

Axel Schulte, Germany
Siraj Shaikh, UK
Sarah Sharples, UK
Anthony Smoker, UK
Neville Stanton, UK
Alex Stedmon, UK
Andrew Thatcher, South Africa

Universal Access in Human–Computer Interaction

Program Chairs: Constantine Stephanidis, Greece, and Margherita Antona, Greece

Julio Abascal, Spain
Gisela Susanne Bahr, USA
João Barroso, Portugal
Margrit Betke, USA
Anthony Brooks, Denmark
Christian Bühler, Germany
Stefan Carmien, Spain
Hua Dong, P.R. China
Carlos Duarte, Portugal
Pier Luigi Emiliani, Italy
Qin Gao, P.R. China
Andrina Granić, Croatia
Andreas Holzinger, Austria
Josette Jones, USA
Simeon Keates, UK

Georgios Kouroupetroglou, Greece
Patrick Langdon, UK
Barbara Leporini, Italy
Eugene Loos, The Netherlands
Ana Isabel Paraguay, Brazil
Helen Petrie, UK
Michael Pieper, Germany
Enrico Pontelli, USA
Jaime Sanchez, Chile
Alberto Sanna, Italy
Anthony Savidis, Greece
Christian Stary, Austria
Hirotada Ueda, Japan
Gerhard Weber, Germany
Harald Weber, Germany

Virtual, Augmented and Mixed Reality

Program Chairs: Randall Shumaker, USA, and Stephanie Lackey, USA

Roland Blach, Germany
Sheryl Brahnam, USA
Juan Cendan, USA
Jessie Chen, USA
Panagiotis D. Kaklis, UK

Hirokazu Kato, Japan
Denis Laurendeau, Canada
Fotis Liarokapis, UK
Michael Macedonia, USA
Gordon Mair, UK

Jose San Martin, Spain
Tabitha Peck, USA
Christian Sandor, Australia

Christopher Stapleton, USA
Gregory Welch, USA

Cross-Cultural Design

Program Chair: P.L. Patrick Rau, P.R. China

Yee-Yin Choong, USA
Paul Fu, USA
Zhiyong Fu, P.R. China
Pin-Chao Liao, P.R. China
Dyi-Yih Michael Lin, Taiwan
Rungtai Lin, Taiwan
Ta-Ping (Robert) Lu, Taiwan
Liang Ma, P.R. China
Alexander Mädche, Germany

Sheau-Farn Max Liang, Taiwan
Katsuhiko Ogawa, Japan
Tom Plocher, USA
Huatong Sun, USA
Emil Tso, P.R. China
Hsiu-Ping Yueh, Taiwan
Liang (Leon) Zeng, USA
Jia Zhou, P.R. China

Online Communities and Social Media

Program Chair: Gabriele Meiselwitz, USA

Leonelo Almeida, Brazil
Chee Siang Ang, UK
Aneesha Bakharia, Australia
Ania Bobrowicz, UK
James Braman, USA
Farzin Deravi, UK
Carsten Kleiner, Germany
Niki Lambropoulos, Greece
Soo Ling Lim, UK

Anthony Norcio, USA
Portia Pusey, USA
Panote Siriaraya, UK
Stefan Stieglitz, Germany
Giovanni Vincenti, USA
Yuanqiong (Kathy) Wang, USA
June Wei, USA
Brian Wentz, USA

Augmented Cognition

**Program Chairs: Dylan D. Schmorrow, USA,
and Cali M. Fidopiastis, USA**

Ahmed Abdelkhalek, USA
Robert Atkinson, USA
Monique Beaudoin, USA
John Blitch, USA
Alenka Brown, USA

Rosario Cannavò, Italy
Joseph Cohn, USA
Andrew J. Cowell, USA
Martha Crosby, USA
Wai-Tat Fu, USA

Rodolphe Gentili, USA
Frederick Gregory, USA
Michael W. Hail, USA
Monte Hancock, USA
Fei Hu, USA
Ion Juvina, USA
Joe Keebler, USA
Philip Mangos, USA
Rao Mannepalli, USA
David Martinez, USA
Yvonne R. Masakowski, USA
Santosh Mathan, USA
Ranjeev Mittu, USA

Keith Niall, USA
Tatana Olson, USA
Debra Patton, USA
June Pilcher, USA
Robinson Pino, USA
Tiffany Poeppelman, USA
Victoria Romero, USA
Amela Sadagic, USA
Anna Skinner, USA
Ann Speed, USA
Robert Sottilare, USA
Peter Walker, USA

Digital Human Modeling and Applications in Health, Safety, Ergonomics and Risk Management

Program Chair: Vincent G. Duffy, USA

Giuseppe Andreoni, Italy
Daniel Carruth, USA
Elsbeth De Korte, The Netherlands
Afzal A. Godil, USA
Ravindra Goonetilleke, Hong Kong
Noriaki Kuwahara, Japan
Kang Li, USA
Zhizhong Li, P.R. China

Tim Marler, USA
Jianwei Niu, P.R. China
Michelle Robertson, USA
Matthias Rötting, Germany
Mao-Jiun Wang, Taiwan
Xuguang Wang, France
James Yang, USA

Design, User Experience, and Usability

Program Chair: Aaron Marcus, USA

Sisira Adikari, Australia
Claire Ancient, USA
Arne Berger, Germany
Jamie Blustein, Canada
Ana Boa-Ventura, USA
Jan Brejcha, Czech Republic
Lorenzo Cantoni, Switzerland
Marc Fabri, UK
Luciane Maria Fadel, Brazil
Tricia Flanagan, Hong Kong
Jorge Frascara, Mexico

Federico Gobbo, Italy
Emilie Gould, USA
Rüdiger Heimgärtner, Germany
Brigitte Herrmann, Germany
Steffen Hess, Germany
Nouf Khashman, Canada
Fabiola Guillermina Noël, Mexico
Francisco Rebelo, Portugal
Kerem Rızvanoğlu, Turkey
Marcelo Soares, Brazil
Carla Spinillo, Brazil

Distributed, Ambient and Pervasive Interactions

**Program Chairs: Norbert Streitz, Germany,
and Panos Markopoulos, The Netherlands**

Juan Carlos Augusto, UK
Jose Bravo, Spain
Adrian Cheok, UK
Boris de Ruyter, The Netherlands
Anind Dey, USA
Dimitris Grammenos, Greece
Nuno Guimaraes, Portugal
Achilles Kameas, Greece
Javed Vassilis Khan, The Netherlands
Shin'ichi Konomi, Japan
Carsten Magerkurth, Switzerland

Ingrid Mulder, The Netherlands
Anton Nijholt, The Netherlands
Fabio Paternó, Italy
Carsten Röcker, Germany
Teresa Romao, Portugal
Albert Ali Salah, Turkey
Manfred Tscheligi, Austria
Reiner Wichert, Germany
Woontack Woo, Korea
Xenophon Zabulis, Greece

Human Aspects of Information Security, Privacy and Trust

**Program Chairs: Theo Tryfonas, UK,
and Ioannis Askoxylakis, Greece**

Claudio Agostino Ardagna, Italy
Zinaida Benenson, Germany
Daniele Catteddu, Italy
Raoul Chiesa, Italy
Bryan Cline, USA
Sadie Creese, UK
Jorge Cuellar, Germany
Marc Dacier, USA
Dieter Gollmann, Germany
Kirstie Hawkey, Canada
Jaap-Henk Hoepman, The Netherlands
Cagatay Karabat, Turkey
Angelos Keromytis, USA
Ayako Komatsu, Japan
Ronald Leenes, The Netherlands
Javier Lopez, Spain
Steve Marsh, Canada

Gregorio Martinez, Spain
Emilio Mordini, Italy
Yuko Murayama, Japan
Masakatsu Nishigaki, Japan
Aljosa Pasic, Spain
Milan Petković, The Netherlands
Joachim Posegga, Germany
Jean-Jacques Quisquater, Belgium
Damien Sauveron, France
George Spanoudakis, UK
Kerry-Lynn Thomson, South Africa
Julien Touzeau, France
Theo Tryfonas, UK
João Vilela, Portugal
Claire Vishik, UK
Melanie Volkamer, Germany

HCI in Business

Program Chair: Fiona Fui-Hoon Nah, USA

Andreas Auinger, Austria
Michel Avital, Denmark
Traci Carte, USA
Hock Chuan Chan, Singapore
Constantinos Coursaris, USA
Soussan Djamasbi, USA
Brenda Eschenbrenner, USA
Nobuyuki Fukawa, USA
Khaled Hassanein, Canada
Milena Head, Canada
Susanna (Shuk Ying) Ho, Australia
Jack Zhenhui Jiang, Singapore
Jinwoo Kim, Korea
Zoonky Lee, Korea
Honglei Li, UK
Nicholas Lockwood, USA
Eleanor T. Loiacono, USA
Mei Lu, USA

Scott McCoy, USA
Brian Mennecke, USA
Robin Poston, USA
Lingyun Qiu, P.R. China
Rene Riedl, Austria
Matti Rossi, Finland
April Savoy, USA
Shu Schiller, USA
Hong Sheng, USA
Choon Ling Sia, Hong Kong
Chee-Wee Tan, Denmark
Chuan Hoo Tan, Hong Kong
Noam Tractinsky, Israel
Horst Treiblmaier, Austria
Virpi Tuunainen, Finland
Dezhi Wu, USA
I-Chin Wu, Taiwan

Learning and Collaboration Technologies

Program Chairs: Panayiotis Zaphiris, Cyprus, and Andri Ioannou, Cyprus

Ruthi Aladjem, Israel
Abdulaziz Aldaej, UK
John M. Carroll, USA
Maka Eradze, Estonia
Mikhail Fominykh, Norway
Denis Gillet, Switzerland
Mustafa Murat Inceoglu, Turkey
Pernilla Josefsson, Sweden
Marie Joubert, UK
Sauli Kiviranta, Finland
Tomaž Klobučar, Slovenia
Elena Kyza, Cyprus
Maarten de Laat, The Netherlands
David Lamas, Estonia

Edmund Laugasson, Estonia
Ana Loureiro, Portugal
Katherine Maillet, France
Nadia Pantidi, UK
Antigoni Parmaxi, Cyprus
Borzoo Pourabdollahian, Italy
Janet C. Read, UK
Christophe Reffay, France
Nicos Souleles, Cyprus
Ana Luísa Torres, Portugal
Stefan Trausan-Matu, Romania
Aimilia Tzanavari, Cyprus
Johnny Yuen, Hong Kong
Carmen Zahn, Switzerland

External Reviewers

Ilia Adami, Greece
Iosif Klironomos, Greece
Maria Korozi, Greece
Vassilis Kouroumalis, Greece

Asterios Leonidis, Greece
George Margetis, Greece
Stavroula Ntoa, Greece
Nikolaos Partarakis, Greece

HCI International 2015

The 15th International Conference on Human–Computer Interaction, HCI International 2015, will be held jointly with the affiliated conferences in Los Angeles, CA, USA, in the Westin Bonaventure Hotel, August 2–7, 2015. It will cover a broad spectrum of themes related to HCI, including theoretical issues, methods, tools, processes, and case studies in HCI design, as well as novel interaction techniques, interfaces, and applications. The proceedings will be published by Springer. More information will be available on the conference website: http://www.hcii2015.org/

General Chair
Professor Constantine Stephanidis
University of Crete and ICS-FORTH
Heraklion, Crete, Greece
E-mail: cs@ics.forth.gr

Table of Contents – Part III

Design for Aging

Health and Rehabilitation Applications

Accessible Smart and Assistive Environments

Assistive Robots

Mobility, Navigation and Safety

Design for Aging

MobileQuiz: A Serious Game for Enhancing the Physical and Cognitive Abilities of Older Adults

Thomas Birn, Clemens Holzmann, and Walter Stech

Universitiy of Applied Sciences Upper Austria
Department of Mobile Computing
Softwarepark 11, 4232 Hagenberg, Austria
http://www.fh-hagenberg.at

Abstract. The ageing process involves physical and cognitive challenges. It is a known fact that (outdoor) physical activity can help to counter these issues and improve the quality of life. One way to motivate older adults doing exercises are serious games. They embody the concept of game-based learning and exercising, and they are designed to solve a problem along with providing and engaging training experience. Based on recent research, we have developed a concept of an outdoor serious game, which has been designed to keep older adults mobile and enhance their cognitive abilities at the same time. We have developed a prototype and evaluated it in a user study with elderly participants. The results show a high acceptance by the test participants, indicating that this kind of game is interesting for the target group. The usability of the prototype has also been evaluated and shows good average scores.

Keywords: Serious games, accessible games, design for aging.

1 Introduction

The great increase of the old population and the increasing social costs are urgent issues society should address with proper plans [1]. By 2060, the US population of adults over 65 is expected to increase from 43 to 92 million [2]. This increase has direct and severe implications for society and individuals as well. It is therefore in the society's best interest to find solutions that will keep people healthy and mobile at low cost. With age come certain changes to the human body resulting in various difficulties and challenges. These can be either of physical nature (affecting hearing, vision and motor skills) or of mental nature (including difficulties in perception, attention and memory) [3]. It is a known fact that next to purely mental training, frequent physical activity can help to counter not only the physical challenges, but also positively influences the mental apparatus [4]. Investigations showed, that especially outdoor physical activity has potential to improve the mental health [5,6]. Based on recent research, we conclude that regular, combined physical and mental training has the potential to improve the quality of life of older adults.

An important success factor in getting elderly to perform exercises on a regular basis is their motivation. This motivation can be increased by the help of

C. Stephanidis and M. Antona (Eds.): UAHCI/HCII 2014, Part III, LNCS 8515, pp. 3–14, 2014.
© Springer International Publishing Switzerland 2014

serious games, which offer concepts for motivating their players. They embody game-based learning and exercising, and they are designed to solve a problem along with providing and engaging training experience [7]. In contrast to games for pure entertainment, the focus of serious games lies on the training aspect. A higher motivation can be achieved by using a set of well known gratification and motivation techniques, like for example a scoring system [8] or the implementation of a social component, as suggested by Planic et al. [8] and Brox et al. [9].

The goal of the presented work was to develop a location-based, serious game for elderly people, which combines physical and mental training in a way that keeps them motivated to play on a regular basis. From a technical viewpoint, the ideal computing platform for this purpose are state-of-the-art smartphones, which are equipped with a sophisticated set of sensors and considerable processing power. In particular, features such as included GPS, digital compass and inertial sensors as well as a big screens make them attractive for mobile location-based games. Moreover, a representative survey targeting the elderly of five EU countries has concluded that the age-divide for mobile phone usage is narrowing faster than for regular computer use [10]. However, although more and more older adults are familiar with smartphones, existing interface designs may not be suitable for the majority of them [11]. This requires a special consideration of universal access in the design phase of mobile applications for the elderly.

In this paper, we propose a serious game called MobileQuiz that combines the above mentioned aspects: The physical and mental training in a game context that is both accessible and usable for older adults, and which will motivate them to play. In the following section we will present the related concepts. We will then proceed with a detailed description of our game concept, the technical approach and a prototypical implementation for Android phones. Afterwards, we will present a first evaluation of the prototype which has been carried out with 8 participants.

2   Related Work

Recent research showed a huge number of game concepts designed to foster the physical strength of its players. Kyung-Sik et al. [12] studied a game design in which the player is prompted to control an avatar with a foot board and hand-held controllers. The study "Exergames for Elderly" investigated the use of the Nintendo Wii Fit[1] platform to enhance physical fitness [9]. Burke et al. investigated a game, in which the player has to catch oranges with a physical basket [13]. Games, that are played with mobile devices for enhancing the physical strength are e.g. "Penguin Toss" and "Bowling" as developed by Sunwoo et al. [14]. In contrast to our concept however, these games are not optimized for older adults and their key purpose is limited to physical training.

A serious game for enhancing the mental fitness is "ElderGames", a memory-like game played on a table [15]. Another example is the serious game described

---

[1] http://wiifit.com/

in [16], which should stimulate the cognitive abilities of Altzheimer's patients by letting them resemble daily life activities in a game. These games are designed for older adults with the aim to improve their cognitive abilities, physical training aspect are not included though.

Besides stationary games as mentioned above, recent work investigated location-based games that are played outdoors and on mobile devices. In the mobile fitness game "SmartRabbit" for example, the goal is to run a certain distance in the shortest time possible [17]. Another example is the "Business Consultant" game [18], which guides the player through a set of nearby locations, who has to conduct virtual interviews at each target location. The difference of such games to our concept lies in the lack of optimization for older adults.

As summarized in Table 1, the majority of these works make use of one single training aspect or focus on the technical game development, but they lack an optimization for older adults. Because little has been done to address the issue of digital game design for older adults with the focus on physical exertion together with mental training [3], our approach combines those two concepts with a focus on user experience for older adults and the motivation aspect.

Table 1. A summary of the training and game aspects of the related concepts

	[9]	[12]	[13]	[14]	[15]	[16]	[17]	[18]
Designed for seniors					⊗	⊗		
Physical training	⊗	⊗	⊗	⊗			⊗	⊗
Mental training					⊗	⊗		⊗
Mobile device				⊗			⊗	⊗

3   MobileQuiz Concept and Characteristics

MobileQuiz is a serious game where the player has to conduct an outdoor challenge based on the principles of geocaching. The goal is to find and reach predefined locations based on spatial cues. Once a location has been reached, the player has to answer questions in order to get points and unlock the information about how to reach the next location. The game design aims to (i) be elder friendly, (ii) enhance the player's physical mobility, (iii) strengthen the player's mental ability and (iv) orientation, while (v) motivating him or her to play the game again. In order to achieve those aims, the concept includes different components that cover the respective areas as shown in Table 2 and explained in the following concept description.

The key aspect of the game is the wayfinding (WF) the users have to perform while playing the game. It combines the physical workout when walking from destination to destination with mental training when looking for the right way

Table 2. The overall aims are mapped to the concept components: Wayfinding (WF), Map (MA), Quiz (QZ), User Interface (UI) and Personalization (PE)

	WF	MA	QZ	UI	PE
(i) Senior friendly				⊗	
(ii) Physical fitness	⊗				
(iii) Mental fitness	⊗		⊗		
(iv) Orientation training	⊗	⊗			
(v) Motivation			⊗		⊗

to go. The wayfinding forces the players to orientate themselves. A map (MA) visualization and directions also add up to the orientation training aspect. The gaming component of the concept - the quiz - will train the mental fitness of the players while giving additional motivation to them when receiving points for right answers (QZ). A specifically adapted user interface makes sure that the game suits the needs of older adults when it comes to the interface design. The game can be personalized (PE) in terms of two game modes. This ensures additional motivation as the game has a wider application.

The game is entirely played outdoors. At the beginning of each game, the player can choose between two different game modes. Both will provide different settings and advantages as described in Section 3.1. However, the basic game principles stay the same. After the selection of a mode, the current game setting includes a set of at least two different locations the player has to visit successively by foot. An analog compass, together with the distance to the next location (see Figure 1a), is shown at the display of the mobile device and helps the player to reach the destination. If the player is not able to find the location, a navigation function is included, which shows the shortest path to the destination on a map and gives turn-by-turn directions if desired. How locations are added to the game will be explained in more detail in the following sections.

The access to the game questions is triggered by the GPS module of the mobile device whenever the next destination has been reached. At this point, the player has to answer questions that are either related to the location or to the region surrounding that location. A screenshot with an example question is shown in Figure 1b. The player gets points once a destination has been reached and when answering a question correctly. Once all the questions for the location are answered, the compass that shows the direction to the next location is unlocked and shown on the display. This cycle repeats until all locations have been visited. At the end of the game, a summary of the finished game is shown to the player. Since all game runs are stored on the device, the player can revise the played games at any time including a map of the actual path the player travelled and the list of questions that have been answered. The correct and chosen answers are highlighted in different colors.

3.1 Game Modes

The proposed game has two modes, an automatic and a manual one:

- **Automatic Mode:** The automatic mode uses nearby points of interest to generate a game run. The player has the option to specify the minimum and maximum number of locations to be added to the game, which allows for an approximate estimation of the game duration.
- **Manual Mode:** In this mode, the player is able to use custom locations in the game. A search function provides a category-based search of nearby points of interest. After a successful search, certain points of interest can be added as new location to the game. Previously found and selected locations can always be re-selected for future game runs.

Providing a manual in addition to an automatic game modes is mainly for two reasons. First, the game can be better personalized to the needs of the player by supporting custom locations. Second, it provides the opportunity to alter the game in a way that allows for a better integration into everyday life, which in turn adds to the motivation aspect. This combination of modes allows for different usage scenarios, ranging from the integration of the game with simple daily routines to the exploration of unknown cities.

Each mode will guide the player back to the starting location when the last location of a game has been reached. This allows the user to get back to the starting point, which is assumed to be a well known location. Otherwise, the player may find himself in an unfamiliar area once the game has been finishes.

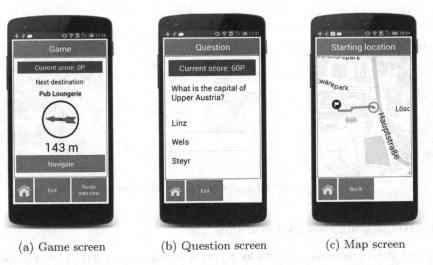

(a) Game screen	(b) Question screen	(c) Map screen

Fig. 1. The game screen (a) shows the direction and distance to the next destination. After the destination is reached, the player receives points and has to answer a question (b). A map screen (c) provides guidance to the next destination when the "navigate" button is pressed.

3.2   User Interface Design

The user interface of the game has been designed according to several guidelines for graphical building user interfaces for older adults [5, 8, 11]. It has been kept simple while showing task-relevant information only. The use of big fonts and a high contrast color scheme additionally adds to the accessibility for older adults. The basic layout of the game stays the same for all views. In order to be more consistent throughout the service, the layout of all screens includes buttons with a positive-negative-semantic. The left ("negative") button will always undo the last action or exit the current state. The right ("positive") button will trigger the most reasonable action (for example: saving a location, starting a game, etc.); it is disabled if no action is available. The design is depicted in Figure 1.

4   Technical Approach

A fully functional prototype implementation of the service has been built following the described concept. One major challenge was to retrieve nearby locations as well as questions that are related to these locations. Our approach to generate a quiz route includes three main steps that are shown in Figure 2. At first, the searching and processing of nearby points of interest is needed. As we are not aware of any existing toolkits or public APIs for generating location-based questions, this is a key aspect of the technical implementation we had to face. The third step is the combination of generated locations and questions to a reasonable quiz route.

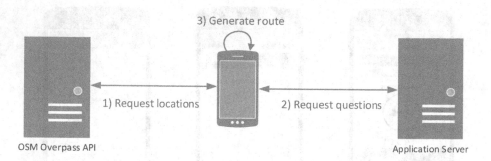

Fig. 2. Generating a quiz route includes three steps

4.1   Requesting Nearby Locations

The first step of requesting nearby locations is only necessary if the player chooses the *automatic mode*, since the *manual mode* already includes self-defined locations. Once the player hits the "Start Game" button, the device will conduct a search for nearby locations. For the prototype implementation, the surrounding search diameter has been limited to 800 meters, which has shown to be a reasonable distance in initial tests. In order to get publicly available points of interest, we used the Overpass API of the OpenStreetMap[2] (OSM) project. The API request can be parameterized with the following metrics:

- The center of the search that will be conducted,
- the diameter of the search area, and
- the types of points of interest.

The result is a list of nearby points of interest fitting the parameters. The types of the requested points of interest were limited to a subset of most reasonable types. Instead of including arbitrary location types like toilets, we focused on noteworthy places like common sights, places of worship and parks, but also supermarkets, restaurants and banks.

4.2   Requesting Quiz Questions

The automatic generation of location-based quiz questions is a complex task and would require huge efforts to implement. For the prototype implementation, the quiz questions were therefore provided manually via a web interface on the application server. A question can be defined by setting the following parameters:

- The coordinates of its center,
- a radius defining the validity of the question,
- the question itself,
- and a set of answer possibilities where the correct one is marked.

The specified radius defines a diameter around the center of the question, defining its area of validity. This allows for a generic and flexible way to create questions as they can be set to be valid for a relatively small area (for example a building or a park) or for wide areas (like country regions or even whole districts). It is important to note, that this approach could be improved by adding the option to use polygons for defining areas. This would allow for a more detailed level of definition.

4.3   Generating a Quiz Route

Generating a quiz route on the mobile device includes the previously mentioned fetching of locations and retrieving of quiz questions from the application server. The locations and questions are then merged to a game route. The process consists of the following steps:

1. Fetching of surrounding points of interest from OSM data for the *automatic mode* or fetching all surrounding custom locations in *manual mode*.
2. Calculating the diameter that is formed by all fetched nearby locations.
3. This diameter and the user's location are sent to the application server in order to request suitable questions. The server returns all questions whose diameters overlap with that of the nearby locations.

---

[2] http://www.openstreetmap.org

4. The fetched points of interest and questions are then merged on the mobile device by assigning each question the closest point of interest (if it has not been assigned to another question yet). This is done under the assumption that spatial proximity is a good indicator for the relation between a certain question and a geographic location.

5. The last step in the process uses methods of heuristic optimization to calculate the "best" route that includes all selected locations. We define the best route as a connection between all points of interest so that no cycles and no double visits of sub-paths occur. For the route generation, just points of interest which have been assigned to a question are considered. For the prototype implementation, we solved this travelling salesman problem with the techniques of simulated annealing, what provides good results in a reasonable time for our prototype implementation. Because of already stated reasons, the starting location is added to the game as the fixed destination before the calculation begins.

Once the game route has been generated, the player can navigate to the first location.

5   Evaluation

The prototype has been evaluated with user tests. The main purpose was to assess the usability and acceptance of the concept in an initial study. The questions of interest are whether such a game is accepted by the target group or not, and if the provided concept is sufficiently usable. An assessment of specific physical and mental improvements has not been made. The evaluation of this would need long-term studies in an controlled environment. Therefore, the focus was on

1. the assessment of the usability of the concept and the user interface,
2. the observation how intuitive the prototype was to use for the participants,
3. the identification of potential design flaws, and
4. the assessment if this kind of game will be accepted by the target group.

5.1   Methodology and Setup

The tests were performed by eight participants, 3 male and 5 female, between the age of 60 and 71 (M=65.8, SD=3.9). The small sample size should be sufficient to gain insights into the most common usability problems [19] and to get an estimate about the user satisfaction. Four of the participants are using a feature phone regularly for making telephone calls. Two of the participants had already used a smart phone before, the rest had not have used either a smart phone or a feature phone before. The participants had to perform tasks using the prototype, which included one actual game run and some tasks to configure the game as well as reviewing played games. Overall, there were four different assignments:

1. Start an automatic game and play it to the end.
2. Add a place to a manual game.
3. View the location properties of an already defined location.
4. Review the previously played game and look at your answers to the questions.

For the test run, we created a set of questions in the surrounding areas of the test participants via the web interface. The questions were related to the area and some nearby points of interest. During the execution of the tasks, we gathered the times it took to complete them as well as data from observations by the study instructor. We also advised the participants to think aloud during the tests. The sequence of the tasks had to be performed three times in order to assess the learning curve of the game. After finishing all scenarios, the participants were asked to fill out the System Usability Scale (SUS) [21] questionnaire to assess the overall system usability.

5.2   Timing Results

All participants were able to finish all tasks. The first task included the navigation from one location to another in different settings. To compensate for the resulting differences in task times, only the duration for starting the application and for configuring and starting the game has been taken into account for task one. Figure 3a shows how much time it took the participants in average to perform the task sequence for each run. The lowest time for the first run was 213 seconds for the slowest participant and 196 seconds for the fastest with a mean of 216.13 (SD=15.71) seconds. The second run was faster with the slowest time of 168 seconds, the fastest time of 154 seconds and a mean of 159.63 seconds (SD=4.98). In the third run, the slowest time was 161 seconds, the fastest time was 141 seconds and the mean time was 151.38 seconds (SD=6.99).

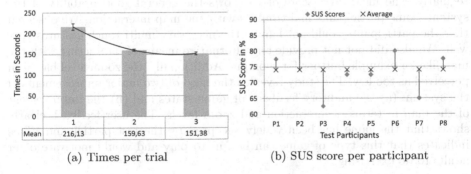

(a) Times per trial   (b) SUS score per participant

Fig. 3. The mean task times (a) show an improvement of 30% for the third run compared to the first run. The SUS scores per participants (b) show an overall good usability.

5.3   User Feedback

After finishing all test scenarios, the participants were asked to give feedback and some ideas of potential design flaws and potential for improvement. Some participants mentioned the usefulness of an additional audio feedback when approaching a destination. This way, the visual focus would not lie on the display of the mobile device all the time. During the execution of task two, some participants had a hard time when picking a point of interest from the map. They claimed that the zoom level is too low. In general, the participants had troubles when interacting with the map. When asked for their opinion about the tasks, some participants stressed that they would prefer a simpler user interface for task two, the adding of a new location to the manual game. The remaining tasks were perceived as positive and usable by the participants. When asked if the participants had fun playing the game, all but one of them totally agreed. All but one participants would also recommend the game to friends. Additionally, the participants were asked to fill out the SUS questionnaire; the aggregated result shows an overall SUS score of 75 (SD=7.55) on a scale from 1 to 100. Figure 3b shows the SUS score per participant with the lowest value of 63 and a highest value of 85.

5.4   Discussion

The results of the eight individual test runs can be seen as outcome of an initial study and are not significant due to the small sample size. They allow, however, the drawing of conclusions concerning the user satisfaction of the evaluated game and the overall experience of such kind of games. The gathered quantitative data show a clear learning curve with a mean improvement of 30% (min=23.3%,max=34.1%) for the third trial compared to the first run (see Fig. 3a). This indicates that the participants, which had little to non experience with smart phones, are able to learn the used procedures in the game when playing regularly. The mean SUS score of 75 shows the general good usability of the system. Some participants had troubles with the map interaction. We observed that the participants could not handle the necessary multi touch gestures very well. We also did not not provide any alternative means of interacting with the map like for example buttons for zooming. Additionally, the zoom level has been perceived as too low. The study revealed the need of two major improvements of the system: (a) the auditory feedback of game states and (b) the improvement of the map in terms of interaction and zoom levels. The user feedback clearly shows that the game has been widely accepted by the test participants. This indicates that this type of game can be fun to play and would motivate older adults to do exercising.

6   Conclusion and Future Work

The introduced concept combines physical exertion and cognitive training to one outdoor game. The design of the concept defines different components in order to reach the concept aims. A prototype has been implemented following a profound technical approach and evaluated in a user study. The main purpose of the study was to show how this kind of games will be accepted by the target group and if the presented concept implementation is usable. We showed that the majority of the test participants are satisfied with the usefulness of the concept and the provided usability. The participants had fun playing the game and the majority would recommend it to friends. We see potential for future investigation in the visualization and interaction of maps in mobile, location-based serious games, as well as in the automatic generation of context based quiz questions. Another future development could be the introduction of a social component to share game results in order to motivate the player further, as suggested by Planic et al. [8] and Brox et al. [9].

Acknowledgement. The MobileQuiz game has been developed as a part of the MOBILE.OLD project. The project MOBILE.OLD acknowledges the financial support within the Ambient Assisted Living (AAL) programme funded by the European Union and the respective "National Research Promotion Programmes" of the federal ministries of the partner countries Austria, Germany, Spain, Romania, UK and The Netherlands.

References

1. Nehmer, J., Becker, M., Karshmer, A., Lamm, R.: Living assistance systems: an ambient intelligence approach. In: 28th International Conference on Software Engineering, pp. 43–50 (2006)
2. United States Census Bureau (2014), http://www.census.gov/ (accessed January 2014)
3. Gerling, K.M., Schild, J., Masuch, M.: Exergame design for elderly users: the case study of SilverBalance. In: 7th International Conference on Advances in Computer Entertainment, pp. 66–69 (2010)
4. Center for Desease Control and Prevention (2013), http://www.cdc.gov/physicalactivity/everyone/health/index.html (accessed September 2013)
5. Zajicek, M.: Interface Design for Older Adults. In: EC/NSF Workshop on Universal Accessibility of Ubiquitous Computing, pp. 60–65 (2001)
6. Pretty, J., Peacock, J., Sellens, M., Griften, M.: The mental and physical health outcomes of green exercise. International Journal of Environmental Health Research 15(5), 319–337 (2005)
7. Tan, C.T., Soh, D.: Augmented Reality Games: A Review. In: Proc. GAMEON-ARABI. European Multidiscilinary Society for Modelling and Simulation Technology (2010)
8. Planic, R., Isabella, N., Kampel, M.: Exergame Design Guidelines for Enhancing Elderly's Physical and Social Activities. In: 3rd International Conference on Ambient Computing, Applications, Services and Technologies, pp. 58–63 (2013)
9. Brox, E., Luque, L.F., Evertsen, G.J., Hernandez, J.E.G.: Exergames for elderly: Social exergames to persuade seniors to increase physical activity. In: 5th International Conference on Pervasive Computing Technologies for Healthcare, pp. 546–549 (2011)

10. European Commission: Seniorwatch 2 - Assessment of the Senior Market for ICT Progress and Developments (2008),
    http://ec.europa.eu/information_society/newsroom/cf/
    document.cfm?action=display&doc_id=526 (accessed January 30, 2014)
11. Kurniawan, S.: Older people and mobile phones: A multi-method investigation. In: Human-Computer Studies, vol. 66, pp. 889–901 (2008)
12. Kyung-Sik, K., Seong-Suk, O., Jin-Ho, A., Sun-Hyung, L.: Development of a walking game for the elderly using controllers of hand buttons and foot boards. In: 17th International Conference on Computer Games, pp. 158–161 (2012)
13. Burke, J.W., McNeill, M.D.J., Charles, D.K., Morrow, P.J., Crosbie, J.H., McDonough, S.M.: Serious Games for Upper Limb Rehabilitation Following Stroke. In: Games and Virtual Worlds for Serious Applications, pp. 103–110 (2009)
14. Sunwoo, J., Wallace, Y., Lutteroth, C., Wünsche, B.: Mobile games for elderly healthcare. In: 11th International Conference of the NZ Chapter of the ACM Special Interest Group on Human-Computer Interaction, pp. 73–76 (2010)
15. Gamberini, L., Fabregat, M., Spagnolli, A., Prontu, L., Seragila, B., Alcaniz, M., Zimmermann, A., Rontti, T., Grant, J., Jensen, R., Gonzales, A.L.: Eldergames: Videogames for empowering, training and monitoring elderly cognitive capabilities. In: 6th International Conference of the International Society for Gerontechnology, vol. 7(2), p. 111 (2008)
16. Imbeault, F., Bouchard, B., Bouzouane, A.: Serious games in cognitive training for Alzheimers patients. In: 1st International Conference on Serious Games and Applications for Health, pp. 1–8 (2011)
17. Marins, D.R., de Justo, M.O.D., de Chavec, B.A.M., D'Ipolitto, C.: SmartRabbit: A Mobile Exergame Using Geolocation. In: 2011 Symposium on Games and Digital Entertainment, pp. 232–240 (2011)
18. Parsons, D., Petrova, K., Hokyoung, R.: Mobile Gaming - A Serious Business! In: 7th International Conference on Wireless, Mobile and Ubiquitous Technology in Education, pp. 17–24 (2012)
19. Nielsen, J.: Estimating the number of subjects needed for thinking aloud test. International Journal of Human-Computer Studies, 385–397 (1994)
20. Lewis, J.R.: IBM Computer Usability Satisfaction Questionnaires. Phsychometric Evaluation and Instructions for Use. International Journal of Human-Computer Interaction, 57–78 (1995)
21. Brooke, J.: SUS - A quick and dirty usability scale. Usablity Evaluation in Industry 1, 189–194 (1996)

Does Web Design Matter?
Examining Older Adults' Attention to Cognitive and Affective Illustrations on Cancer-Related Websites through Eye Tracking

Nadine Bol[1], Jennifer C. Romano Bergstrom[2], Ellen M.A. Smets[3], Eugène F. Loos[1], Jonathan Strohl[2], and Julia C.M. van Weert[1]

[1] Amsterdam School of Communication Research / ASCoR, University of Amsterdam, Amsterdam, The Netherlands
{n.bol,e.f.loos,j.c.m.vanweert}@uva.nl
[2] Fors Marsh Group, Arlington, Virginia, USA
{jbergstrom,jstrohl}@forsmarshgroup.com
[3] Department of Medical Psychology, Academic Medical Center / AMC, University of Amsterdam, Amsterdam, The Netherlands
e.m.smets@amc.uva.nl

Abstract. This study examines how adults pay attention to cognitive and affective illustrations on a cancer-related webpage and explores age-related differences in the attention to these cognitive and affective webpages. Results of an eye-tracking experiment ($n = 20$) showed that adults spent more time attending to the illustrations on the cognitive webpage than the illustrations on the affective webpage. Furthermore, older adults spent about 65% less time fixating the webpages than younger adults. Whereas older adults had less attention for illustrations on the cognitive webpage then younger adults, they spent equal time viewing the illustrations on the affective webpage as younger adults.

Keywords: eye tracking, aging, attention, fixation duration, cancer-related information, cognitive and affective illustrations, e-health.

1 Introduction

The Internet offers a viable source for disseminating cancer information and is increasingly used by cancer patients. Many hospitals also refer their patients to information on the Web, such as patient portals and hospital websites. Hence, a lot of cancer-related information is presented online and sometimes even exclusively online [1]. Even though older adults use the Internet progressively more [2], including for health information [3], this does not necessarily mean that they understand online cancer information. The ability to seek, find, and understand cancer information from electronic sources is markedly lower among older adults [4]. This might be a result of, among other things, declines in older adults' basic abilities, such as cognitive (e.g., decreased working memory) and sensory (e.g., decreased visual acuity) modalities [5].

C. Stephanidis and M. Antona (Eds.): UAHCI/HCII 2014, Part III, LNCS 8515, pp. 15–23, 2014.

To make online cancer information more understandable for older adults, illustrations can be added with the aim to expand cognitive capacity. Older adults often have a smaller total cognitive capacity than younger adults and would therefore benefit more from having online information presented in multiple formats, such as text and illustrations [6]. However, we currently lack knowledge on how older adults use illustrations on cancer-related websites and whether different types of illustrations are differently used. We distinguish between cognitive illustrations (i.e., images that complement text and help people to understand it) and affective illustrations (i.e., images that mainly aim to evoke positive feelings and to generate positive emotions). Whereas cognitive illustrations are expected to increase understanding and recall of information through expanding people's cognitive capacity, affective illustrations might increase these outcomes in a different way. According to the socioemotional selectivity theory, older adults have more emotion-related goals and use these goals to encode and memorize information [7]. As a result, older adults are expected to spend more time to affective illustrations and consequently recall this information better. This is called the positivity effect and might explain a greater attentional focus of older adults on affective information [8].

Previous empirical research has shown both positive effects (e.g., increased website satisfaction and recall of information) of adding cognitive and affective illustrations to text information [9], [10] as well as no or mixed effects of adding such illustrations (e.g., increased recall of information but only for younger adults) [11], [12]. More insight into how older adults use cognitive and affective illustrations can help to understand these differences. Using eye-tracking data, we therefore aim to (a) examine how adults pay attention to cognitive and affective cancer-related webpages and (b) explore possible age-related differences in attention to cognitive and affective webpages.

2   Method

2.1   Stimulus Material

We created two English versions of a cancer-related webpage that modeled the website of the Netherlands Cancer Institute (NKI). The Dutch version of the webpage was used in previous studies [11], [12]. This specific webpage contained information on Radio Frequency Ablation (RFA) treatment, which is a minimally invasive treatment to treat metastases in the lung. The content of the text information was kept constant across the two versions of the webpage. The only difference between the webpages was the figures: In one version, two cognitive illustrations were included on the webpage and in the other version, two affective illustrations were included on the webpage. Illustrations were extensively pre-tested in two previous studies in order to choose the most appropriate cognitive and affective illustrations [11], [12]. The webpages used in this study are presented in Figures 1 and 2 respectively.

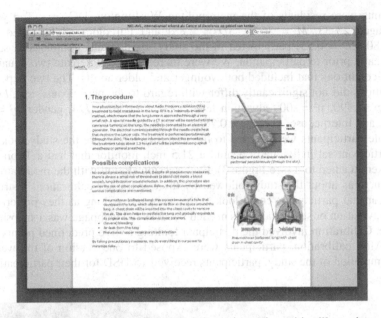

Fig. 1. The webpage containing RFA information and cognitive illustrations

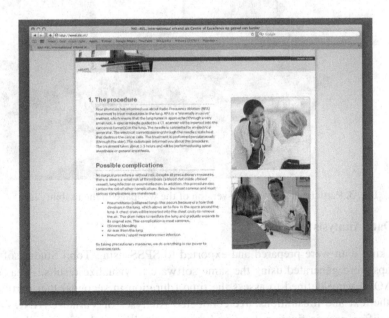

Fig. 2. The webpage containing RFA information and affective illustrations

2.2   Participants and Procedure

Participants were residents of the metropolitan Washington, DC area. Ten younger adults (aged 23-33, $M = 26.50$, $SD = 2.88$) and ten older adults (aged 51-70, $M = 58.80$, $SD = 6.55$) participated in the study. Participants completed a screener questionnaire prior to participation. We were therefore able to create two equal experimental conditions that included both younger and older adults. The two experimental conditions did not significantly differ with regard to the participants' age, $F(1, 18) = 0.00$, $p = .990$, $\eta^2 = .00$, education level, $\chi^2 = 1.11$, $p = .774$, gender, $\chi^2 = 0.20$, $p = .655$, and Internet use, $F(1, 18) = 0.26$, $p = .616$, $\eta^2 = .01$.

Eligible participants were invited to the usability lab where the study took place. Each participant sat individually behind a 21.5 inch monitor that had a Tobii X2-60 eye tracker attached to it (see Figure 3). Each session started with the moderator reading instructions about the study followed by the eye-tracker calibration. Instructions made clear that participants could look at the webpage as long as they preferred and that no navigation or search task was needed because the webpage was a snapshot of a webpage. Calibration involved the participant looking at five predefined points on the screen. After calibration, participants were exposed to one version of the webpage. Upon completion of the study, participants received 15 USD for their participation.

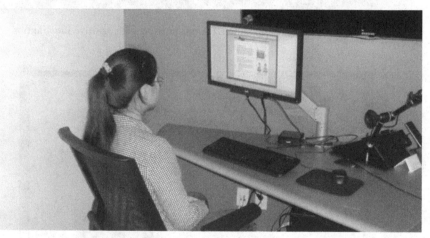

Fig. 3. Participant viewing one version of the webpage in the usability lab

2.3   Data Analysis

Eye-tracking data were prepared and exported to SPSS using Tobii Studio software. Heat maps were generated using the same software to visualize results. Areas of Interest (AOIs) were defined to assess the time (duration in seconds) that participants fixated the text and illustrations. We conducted Analyses of Variance (ANOVAs) to measure differences in fixation duration between cognitive and affective illustrations, to explore differences between the younger and older age group, and to examine age-related differences within the two experimental conditions.

3 Results

3.1 Attention to the Webpage

The eye-tracking data were analyzed to determine how much time participants fixated the cognitive webpage and the affective webpage, overall. Participants spent on average 63.65 seconds viewing the full webpage (SD = 41.85). We examined the illustrations AOI for the cognitive webpage and the affective webpage and found that across all participants, there were significant differences in fixation duration between the cognitive and affective illustrations, $F(1, 16)$ = 23.46, p < .001, η^2 = .59, such that people spent more time on the cognitive illustrations (M = 12.12, SD = 9.24) than the affective illustrations (M = 1.25, SD = 1.38). No differences were found in fixation duration for the text when comparing the cognitive webpage and the affective webpage, $F(1, 16)$ = 0.04, p = .838, η^2 = .00.

3.2 Age-Related Differences in Attention to the Webpage

Next we examined age-related differences in attention to the webpage and found that older adults spent significantly less time fixating the webpages compared to younger adults, $F(1, 16)$ = 22.09, p < .001, η^2 = .58. Whereas younger adults spent on average 93.83 seconds viewing the webpages (SD = 36.47), older adults only spent 33.47 seconds on average viewing the webpages (SD = 18.55), indicating that older adults spent almost 65% less time viewing the webpages than younger adults (Table 1).

Table 1. Fixation duration (in seconds) stratified by condition and age group (n = 20)

		Fixation duration on the webpage		Fixation duration on the text		Fixation duration on the illustrations	
	n	M	SD	M	SD	M	SD
Cognitive illustrations	10	70.72	46.67	57.24	36.06	12.12	9.24
Younger adults	5	107.49	30.78	87.85	26.45	18.26	8.84
Older adults	5	33.96	19.13	26.63	14.75	5.98 [b*]	4.46
Affective illustrations	10	56.57	38.75	54.70	38.42	1.25 [c***]	1.38
Younger adults	5	80.17	39.72	77.34	40.50	2.06 [d***]	1.57
Older adults	5	32.97	20.20	32.07	20.02	0.44	0.41
Total	20	63.65	41.85	55.97	37.25	6.69	8.51
Younger adults	10	93.83	36.47	82.59	32.72	10.16	10.42
Older adults	10	33.47[a***]	18.55	29.35[a***]	16.82	3.21[a**]	4.18

Note. The higher the fixation duration the more attention was paid to (elements of) the webpage. M = Mean; SD = Standard Deviation.
[a]Mean differs significantly compared to younger adults. [b]Mean differs significantly compared to younger adults in the cognitive illustrations condition. [c]Mean differs significantly compared to the cognitive illustrations condition. [d]Mean differs significantly from younger adults in the cognitive illustrations condition. * p < .05. ** p < .01. *** p < .001.

Next we examined age-related differences to the AOIs (text and illustrations). We found that older adults spent significantly less time fixating the text information ($M = 29.35$, $SD = 16.82$) than younger adults ($M = 82.59$, $SD = 32.72$), $F(1, 16) = 19.16$, $p < .001$, $\eta^2 = .55$, across both webpages, $F(1, 16) = 19.16$, $p < .001$, $\eta^2 = .55$. This is depicted in the mean fixation duration heat maps shown in Figure 4 (cognitive webpage) and Figure 5 (affective webpage). We also found a significant webpage × age interaction, $F(1, 16) = 5.64$, $p = .030$, $\eta^2 = .26$, such that younger adults attended to the cognitive illustrations more than older adults, $F(1, 17) = 6.45$, $p = .021$, but there was no difference in attention to the illustrations for older adults (shown in Figure 6). Moreover, younger adults attended more to the illustrations on the cognitive website than to the illustrations on the affective website, $F(1, 17) = 17.31$, $p = .001$ (shown in Figures 4 and 5). Fixation duration results are shown in Table 1 and Figure 7.

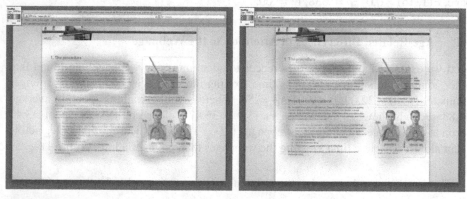

Fig. 4. Mean fixation duration heat maps for the cognitive website for younger (left) and older (right) participants

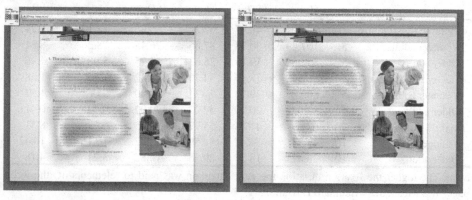

Fig. 5. Mean fixation duration heat maps for the affective website for younger (left) and older (right) participants

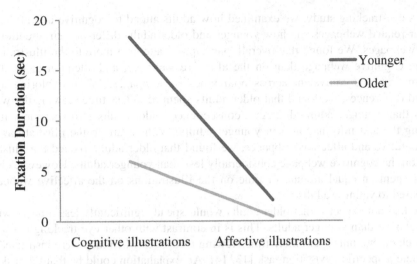

Fig. 6. The interaction effect between type of webpage and age on fixation duration to the illustrations on the cognitive and affective webpage

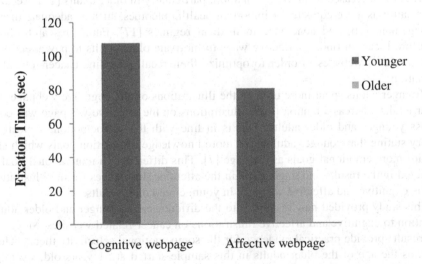

Fig. 7. Mean fixation duration for viewing the cognitive and affective webpages stratified by age group

4   Conclusion and Discussion

In this eye-tracking study, we examined how adults attend to cognitive and affective cancer-related webpages and how younger and older adults differ in their attention to such webpages. We found that overall, participants attended more to the illustrations on the cognitive webpage than on the affective webpage, and attention to the text information was equivalent across both types of webpages. When exploring age-related differences, we found that older adults spent 65% less time viewing the web-pages than younger adults did. As a consequence, older adults also spent less time reading the text information than younger adults. With regard to the illustrations on the cognitive and affective webpages, we found that older adults fixated the illustra-tions on the cognitive webpage considerably less than younger adults. However, older adults spent an equal amount of time on the illustrations on the affective webpage compared to younger adults.

We had not expected that older adults would spend significantly less time viewing the webpage than younger adults. This is in contrast with other eye-tracking research in which older adults spent more time viewing webpages when they were instructed to complete a specific navigation task [13, 14]. An explanation could be that the task of this particular study was to view a snapshot of the webpage as long as the participant preferred rather than completing a navigation task. In our study, Internet experience might have played a less important role but might be a predictor of navigation task completion time [14], [15]. This low attention score among the older age group should however be considered as a related study revealed that attention to the text information increased recall of information, particularly in older adults [12]. Recall of information is a prerequisite for important health outcomes, such as adequate disease management [16] and adherence to medical regimes [17]. Future research should therefore focus on finding effective ways to motivate older adults to pay attention to cancer-related websites in order to optimize their recall of online cancer-related in-formation.

Younger adults spent more time on the illustrations on the cognitive webpage than older adults whereas attention to the illustrations on the affective webpage was equal across younger and older adults. This is in line with the socioemotional selectivity theory stating that younger adults hold more knowledge acquisition goals which shift toward more emotional goals as they age [7]. This difference in motivational goals is reflected in the results and might explain the attention differences for the illustrations on the cognitive and affective webpage in younger and older adults.

This study provided new insights into the differences in younger and older adults' attention to cognitive and affective illustrations on cancer-related websites. Moreover, our results provide practical evidence for the socioemotional selectivity theory. How-ever, as the age of the older adults in this sample started at 51 years old, we might have underestimated the attention to emotional information (i.e., the affective web-page in older age) since attention to emotional material increases even more after the age of 70 [7]. Nevertheless, this study shows that websites may need to be designed differently when older adults are the primary user group.

References

1. Lippincott, G.: Gray Matters: Where Are the Technical Communicators in Research and Design for Aging Audiences? IEEE Transactions on Professional Communication 47, 157–170 (2004)
2. Zickuhr, K.: Generations (2010),
   http://pewinternet.org/Reports/2010/Generations-2010.aspx
3. Cresci, M.K., Jarosz, P.A., Templin, T.N.: Are Health Answers Online for Older Adults? Educ. Gerontol. 38, 10–19 (2012)
4. Xie, B.: Older Adults, Health Information, and the Internet. Interactions 15, 44–46 (2008)
5. Becker, S.A.: A Study of Web Usability for Older Adults Seeking Online Health Resources. ACM Trans. Comput. Hum. Interact. 11, 357–406 (2004)
6. Van Gerven, P.W.M., Paas, F.G.W.C., Van Merriënboer, J.J.G., Schmidt, H.G.: Cognitive Load Theory and the Acquisition of Complex Cognitive Skills in the Elderly: Towards an Integrative Framework. Educ. Gerontol. 26, 503–521 (2000)
7. Carstensen, L.L., Isaacowitz, D.M., Charles, S.T.: Taking Time Seriously: A Theory of Socioemotional Selectivity. Am. Psychol. 54, 165–181 (1999)
8. Mather, M., Carstensen, L.L.: Aging and Motivated Cognition: The Positivity Effect in Attention and Memory. Trends Cogn. Sci. 9, 496–502 (2005)
9. Van Weert, J., Van Noort, G., Bol, N., Van Dijk, L., Tates, K., Jansen, J.: Tailored Informa-tion for Cancer Patients on the Internet: Effects of Visual Cues and Language Complexity on Information Recall and Satisfaction. Patient Educ. Couns. 84, 368–378 (2011)
10. Park, S., Lim, J.: The Effect of Graphical Representation on Learner's Learning Interest and Achievement in Multimedia Learning. Association for Educational Communications and Technology, Chicago (2004)
11. Bol, N., Van Weert, J.C.M., De Haes, J.C.J.M., Loos, E.F., De Heer, S., Sikkel, D., Smets, E.M.A.: Using Cognitive and Affective Illustrations to Enhance Older Adults' Website Satisfaction and Recall of Online Cancer-Related Information. Health Commun. 29, 678–688 (2013)
12. Bol, N., Van Weert, J.C.M., Loos, E.F., Romano Bergstrom, J.C., Bolle, S., Smets, E.M.A.: Are Illustrations Worth a Thousand Words? Using Eye Tracking to Predict Older Adults' Recall of Online Cancer-Related Information. In: Production (2014)
13. Tullis, T.S.: Older Adults and the Web: Lessons Learned from Eye-Tracking. In: Stephanidis, C. (ed.) HCI 2007. LNCS, vol. 4554, pp. 1030–1039. Springer, Heidelberg (2007)
14. Loos, E.F.: In Search of Information on Websites: A Question of Age? In: Stephanidis, C. (ed.) Universal Access in HCI, Part II, HCII 2011. LNCS, vol. 6766, pp. 196–204. Springer, Heidelberg (2011)
15. Hill, R.L., Dickinson, A., Arnott, J.L., Gregor, P., McIver, L.: Older Users' Eye Movements: Experience Counts. In: Proceedings of the SIGCHI Conference on Human Factors in Computing Systems, CHI 2011, Vancouver, BC, Canada, pp. 1151–1160.
16. Kravitz, R.L., Hays, R.D., Sherbourne, C.D., DiMatteo, M.R., Rogers, W.H., Ordway, L., Greenfield, S.: Recall of Recommendations and Adherence to Advice Among Patients With Chronic Medical Conditions. Arch. Intern. Med. 153, 1869–1878 (1993)
17. Linn, A.J., Van Dijk, L., Smit, E.G., Jansen, J., Van Weert, J.C.M.: You Never Forget What is Worth Remembering: The Relation Between Recall of Medical Information and Medication Adherence in Patients With Inflammatory Bowel Disease. J. Crohns Coli-tis 550, e543–e550 (2013)

Heuristics in Ergonomic Design
of Portable Control Devices for the Elderly

Marcin Butlewski[1], Edwin Tytyk[1], Kamil Wróbel[2], and Sławomir Miedziarek[3]

[1] Poznan University of Technology, Chair of Ergonomics and Quality Management
11 Strzelecka St., Poznan, Poland
{marcin.butlewski,edwin.tytyk}@put.poznan.pl
[2] Poznan University of Technology, Poland
kamil.wrobel@doctorate.put.poznan.pl
[3] Komenski State School of Higher Education in Leszno, Poland
s.miedziarek@pwsz.edu.pl

Abstract. The prolonging life expectancy and, as a result of it, the growing number of people of elderly age means that more attention should be devoted to the design of ergonomic equipment which includes the needs of this group of customers. Elderly people often suffer due to poorly designed technical facilities, which discourages them from using equipment to improve the quality of their lives. The article summarizes the identified needs of elderly people in relation to control devices along with the general guidelines for the ergonomic design and design approaches for people with disabilities including: universal design, inclusive design, design-for-all, barrier-free design, and accessible design. Among the most important limitations of elderly people are included: reduced psychomotor and sensory efficiency and range of motion, decreased strength, and a decreased ability to remember. In this way a checklist is comprised of criteria such as anthropometric compatibility, ease of use and handling, transparency and visibility, tolerance for error, sensory substitution, and palpability and feelings. The list of identified criteria is evaluated by users resulting in a quantification of individual requirements. Based on interviews with users, an identification and classification is also made of the basic groups of control devices used by the elderly. As a result of these measures checklists are obtained to evaluate each group of the control devices, which examine the typical and commonly used devices in the Polish market. Some selected devices have also been subjected to an evaluation during arranged performance situations involving elderly persons. The information obtained during this is discussed within the article.

Keywords: ergonomic design, heuristic methods, design, ergonomics, devices for the elderly.

1 Introduction

Thanks to advances in medicine and improvement of the quality of life, its average length is constantly growing, now reaching in the EU an average level of 76.7 years

C. Stephanidis and M. Antona (Eds.): UAHCI/HCII 2014, Part III, LNCS 8515, pp. 24–33, 2014.

for men and 82.6 for women. This is not the final value as it is estimated that the average life time will be extended for the next 5-9 years in the first half of the twenty-first century, and the age limit achieved by women in the future may reach values between 120 and 130 years [12]. This gas an impact, among other demographic changes, on the effect called aging. A clear effect of this trend is discernible in the Population median age index, which in 2011 amounted to 41.3 years in 27 EU countries, and over the next 40 years it is likely to reach the level of 48 [14].This means that there is a need for addressing the needs of elderly people in the designed products, services, architectural environment, and even workplaces in a better way. The products will not only have to meet the safety requirements in the currently understood criteria [15], but also take into account the cumulative aspects of user groups, which are the elderly, that are susceptible to certain factors. [7]. The ergonomic design also allows for achievement of such product parameters, which make it resistant to the occurrence of some abnormalities in the manufacturing process itself, which obtains a minimal loss of quality, with the planned cost of production [31].Thus, ergonomic approach allows to keep a balanced development in all areas of human functioning. [22] Hence, it appears that there is no alternative to ergonomic design in the context of an aging society. We need to be better prepared for a number of socio-economic changes because the current pension solutions cease to be effective, and the period of professional activity will increase significantly [6].

One of the important issues in the design for the elderly is the difficulty in defining the characteristics of the general population and an indication of their actual needs. This is due to the large variation of the design characteristics of the elderly, their low representation among decision-makers and the difficulty in obtaining data regarding their needs. This last factor arises from the fact that an aging period is a natural time when all kinds of activities are associated with an increasing effort and in a way it gives permission to exclude these users from certain groups of solutions (attempts to sanction the right age to drive a vehicle, etc.). Leaving aside the moral issues of such considerations into the safety of a group of users at the expense of an exemption of others, it should be noted that there are a number of solutions where the lack of adaptation to the needs of elderly users is not justified by any rational reason. Enabling elderly people to use modern technical equipment will ensure the maintenance of health and safety [30] and also will allow to create a proactive environment [20]. What is more, a suitable and ergonomic design of equipment for the elderly will be connected with obtaining high efficiency of the anthro-technical system [8], as well as with facilitating the implementation of useful social functions for a long time [21]. An example of a group of objects which low or high ergonomic quality may significantly affect the quality of life of elderly people are portable control devices. Appropriate adjustment of these devices to the psychomotor needs of the elderly will be crucial in their independence or self-sufficiency.

The purpose of this article is to present pilot studies undertaken by their authors to identify the ergonomic features of portable control devices for example, remote controls, and to build a model of ergonomic quality of these devices for later verification. Due to the chosen target study, the notion of the precision regarding control motion while using the device was not included. The only function that was taken into account was only the precision of the selection and activation of individual control segments.

2   Ergonomic Features of Portable Control Devices

Ergonomic design criteria for the control devices can be found in the Directive on machinery [11], which states that they should meet the following requirements: to be clearly visible and identifiable, ought to use pictograms where appropriate, positioned in such a way as to be safely operated without hesitation or loss of time and without ambiguity, designed in such a way that the movement of the control device is consistent with its effect, positioned in such a way that their operation cannot cause additional risk, designed or protected in such a way that the desired effect, where a hazard is involved, can only be achieved by a deliberate action, made in such a way as to withstand foreseeable forces; particular attention must be paid to emergency stop devices liable to be subjected to considerable forces. Under ergonomics the norm gives that under intended conditions of use, the discomfort, fatigue, physical and psychological stress faced by the operator must be reduced to the minimum possible, taking into account some ergonomic principles for example: allowing for the variability of the operator's physical dimensions, strength and stamina.

Among the identified ergonomic criteria principles one should also indicate the optimum layout of control devices due to their importance, frequency, order of use, and the grouping of functionally related equipment [28]. It is significant however how the information will be entered [18], what is the length of steering movements affecting their accuracy as described by Fitt's law [13, 16], non-visual support [29]. Devices ergonomics also should be considered in terms of compatibility, and hence the possibility to use multiple devices in the same way [25].

Ergonomics of portable control devices is not as simple as it might seem to be and the sole rules citation that are formulated by various authors is only a resulting fragment of a problem. It should be noted that the functional quality of the equipment is influenced by the quality of the realized interaction in the perceptual-motor process [9].The quality of implementing the interaction can also be described from the intangible assets point of view, and as a result it may be subject to requirements such as usability, learnability, flexibility, customizability, observability and robustness [32, 36].The design principles developed for people with disabilities are also not without significance [5].

To sum up, it can be observed that there is a large variety of sources and levels of ergonomic requirements in regard with portable control devices. It should be also noted that most of these will result in the range of functionality of the implemented remote control devices.

3   Senior Needs in Portable Control Devices Design

Studies indicate that the needs of the elderly are mainly due to perceptual deficits and the weakening of psychomotor function [38, 39]. This relationship reflects the needs of those who use portable control devices, which has been proven by the studies on Latin American community. Design suggestions from older adults included making the numbers and buttons larger and installing auto-shut off timers on remote control devices [34].

Elderly people certainly feel more discomfort associated with the need to perform forced and repetitive movements which only aggravate part of the musculoskeletal system. Slight movements performed during control operations cause the movements of the muscles in the shoulder, upper arm, forearm and index finger to be activated. Research that was made on touch screens showed that after longer periods, a significant arm fatigue occurs, what is ergonomically critical especially for older users [1].This means that the mapping of manipulative abilities requires a model of dysfunction [4] which appears at the specified user with age.

Another important factor in the process of designing portable control devices while taking into account the needs of elderly people is required strength, accuracy and speed of movement. These are the factors which affect the size of the required parameters initiating various device functions. The variation in this field results from different functionality of the elderly, as well as relations between the grip, the direction of a force and the speed of implementing steering motion [35].The authors suggest that grip strength decreases with age, but at least in the initial period of an old age rather slightly [24] greater declines are observed after the age of 70 years [41, 42]. A slip force is another analyzed parameter, which indicates the strength that is used in order to prevent an item from slipping from the hand. This force is only slightly greater than the weight of the item and in the case of the elderly it is higher than in younger people. It translates to less coordination when lifting [27], as well as the reduced level of sweating, which affects greatly the coefficient of friction. [10]. In turn, analogically, in the case of equipment initiated by voice, an input parameter will be an adequate strength and a clarity of voice. This type of signal modality is of the utmost importance for people with significant psychomotor dysfunction. However, due to the specificity of an issue as well as a significant level of error diagnosis [37] it was not included in the present model of ergonomic quality.

With age, the ability to perform multiple functions simultaneously (divisibility), the ability to remember and distinguish is declining. This usually results in reduced demand for the number of used features. [23] Thus it may be desirable to reduce unnecessary or rarely used features by hiding or inactivating them. Besides, too many functions made it difficult to distinguish the desired function from others [26].

4   Method Description

The procedure of the findings consisted in collecting the identified in literature needs of the elderly in the field of portable control devices. The needs were assigned design criteria using QFD method. This step allowed the determination of the final list of requirements. The research group was 6 people (3 women and 3 men) aged 65 to 84 years. The study uses the approach of ethnography design [40] which process was recorded using a video camera. Test procedure consisted in assessing the validity of the previously identified features of the portable control devices through the test person, who then was shown 3 universal remote controls (these can be programmed to control different devices), two of which are laid down as devices for seniors. By using these devices a subject's task was to perform 3 sequences of action:

- following the steps of battery replacement (removing previously inserted battery and inserting the new batteries),
- programming remote controls on the basis of the information contained in the user's manual instructions, (in view of the methodological difficulties of separating the issue of control from the characteristics of the manual instruction, the evaluation of this step occurred in a total way, the instructions have been translated, and then presented in a unified form),
- making an identical control sequence by using each of the remote controls.

During the process of carrying out the tasks, the tested person was not forced to keep a certain pace to perform the activities. There was not also any interference in the way the activities were performed even if it was wrong. After doing the above activities, the tested person assessed the workload when using NASA TLX devices [17], and then evaluated the fulfillment of the requirements that have been previously accepted for validity. NASA TLX scale was chosen due to the factors described in the literature such as it is more acceptable to participants [19] and it is more sensitive to mental workload differences than the second widely used method - SWAT [33]. In order to assess the validity as well as to check whether it complies with all the requirements, a 3-point scale was used, due to the fact that the tests that have been previously carried out with much smaller precision, caused confusion and the subjects chose   values from the beginning, middle and end of the scale.

All the persons prior to study, filled in a questionnaire regarding their health. None of them showed an impaired hand function to a considerable or moderate degree, and the previously mentioned health problems, according to the respondents, did not affect the possibility to use the equipment.

5   Results

The features of ergonomic portable control devices, which representative can be a universal TV remote control, that are presented to evaluate older remote controls are:

1. grabability - proper shaping of the user's hand,
2. buttons availability - the ability to select key accurately,
3. ease to recognize the application of a key - distinguishability, size of the keys and their signs,
4. recognition of the device from other devices – the faciliation of device search,
5. visibility of the function regardless of the lighting conditions - backlighting,
6. resistance to the user's errors and the possibility to correct them,
7. safe use and technical maintenance of equipment,
8. appropriate weight of the device and its balancing,

9. ease of use - intuitive controlling - predictability - compliance with practice
10. the logic of a device - coherence,
11. easy cleaning of all surfaces,
12. ease of use – battery replacement,
13. mechanical resistance of a device,
14. durability of the printed symbols and text,
15. feedback – confirmation of the control element activation,
16. reduced squeeze strength of the device with your hand (appropriate level of force to the coefficient of friction),
17. reducing the forces necessary to activate the button of the device,
18. alternative service in the event of the inability to use the default hand,
19. stability to place the device on the surface when running the function by selecting keys on the resting remote control,
20. stability of buttons that are in contact with a finger,
21. ability to use the device in conditions limiting the precision of the movement such as wearing gloves.

The presented criteria constitute only some that were considered during the selection of ergonomic features of portable control devices. Their full listing would exceed the permissible volume of the article.

Prior to the experiment, according to respondents, the most important requirements for the comfort of use were the requirements of the following numbers: 3, 4, 5, 7, 10, 13, 14, 15 This means that the greatest significance were such features as: function recognition, keys visibility, logic, and durability.

This article did not present an assessment of compliance with the requirements for individual remote controls, because they proved to be correlated with actual users' sensations only to a small extent - the criterion was very well or well evaluated : ease of use – replacement of the battery, whereby it was observed that these individuals had considerable difficulty in performing this activity. It was also observed in some cases that the test persons were inclined to show appreciation for the rated products by arguing that they do so in order for the manufacturer to be more satisfied, or because they find themselves guilty of the result in performing a particular activity.

In verbal assessment, not confirmed by results of assessments, the least appreciated device was the one with LCD touch panel. Despite backlight, the lack of palpable keys was assessed by all respondents negatively. The ambiguity of buttons was also considered as something negative in most cases, which appeared in one of the remote controls as a result of the button marked with a 0/10. This button was confused with pressing 0 (zero) and hampered its search. The applied backlighting did not compensate for a small color contrast, particularly in the case of periodic operation of the backlight that was manually actuated. The application of NASA TLX tool allowed to state a greater implementation of the Temporal Demand and Frustration level, especially when performing maintenance activities - battery replacement and programming the device. Clearly, the tool showed a very large scale of differences between the noticeable components of the load among respondents. The problem among respondents when testing was a poor distinguishability of the analyzed components such as: Performance and Effort. It has been eventually decided that before continuing the use of this device for the evaluation of workload for the elderly it should be thoroughly verified in terms of applicability.

An important limitation during the process of studies was a number of compared devices - the tested subjects got quickly bored with repetitive tasks. Thus, in the future the usability of devices for the elderly need to also take into account this aspect. A general methodological note is that despite the lack of time constraints of tasks, the subjects felt intense stress and pressure caused by "The influence of the observer". They commented several times that the observation while performing tasks exerts a strong level of stress, which was also reflected in the results of the NASA TLX. The effectiveness of the work is dependent on many degradator (environmental hazards) of which stress plays a very significant role [2].

6   Conclusion

The conducted study had a pilot character and aimed to validate the research tools, hence the obtained results are only an estimate. Without a doubt, the identified criteria have important influence on shaping the ergonomic quality of control portable devices. The implementation of ethnographic design approach was very successful [3]. It revealed discrepancies between verbal assessment of the user and the real way of task implementation.

It should be noted that the devices that were specially adapted for the elderly did not fulfill part of its function – they were supplied with an unreadable and intricate manual, without drawings. The decrease in the number of function keys that was desired by older people in simple control tasks produced a significant impediment to nonstandard actions that needed to be performed using a combination of a few buttons. At the same time, it revealed the conflict between ergonomic quality of use, technical support, the programming and the exchange of power source.

References

1. Ahlstrom, B., Lehman, S., Marmolin, T.: Over-coming touch screen user fatigue by workplace design. In: Bauersfeld, P., Bennett, J., Lynch, G. (eds.) Conference on Human Factors in Computing Systems, Monterey, California, May 3-7, pp. 101–102. ACM, New York (1992)
2. Bajda, A., Wrażeń, M., Laskowski, D.: Diagnostics the quality of data transfer in the management of crisis situation. Electrical Review 87(9A), 72–78 (2011)
3. Bichard, J.-A., Greene, C., Ramster, G., Staples, T.: Designing ethnographic encounters for enriched HCI. In: Stephanidis, C., Antona, M. (eds.) UAHCI 2013, Part I. LNCS, vol. 8009, pp. 3–12. Springer, Heidelberg (2013)
4. Branowski, B., Pohl, P., Rychlik, M., Zablocki, M.: Integral Model of the Area of Reaches and Forces of a Disabled Person with Dysfunction of Lower Limbs as a Tool in Virtual Assessment of Manipulation Possibilities in Selected Work Environments. In: Stephanidis, C. (ed.) Universal Access in HCI, Part II, HCII 2011. LNCS, vol. 6766, pp. 12–21. Springer, Heidelberg (2011)

5. Branowski, B., Zabłocki, M.: Kreacja i kontaminacja zasad projektowania i zasad konstrukcji w projektowaniu dla osób niepełnosprawnych, Creation and blending of the design and construction principles for people with disabilities. Ergonomia produktu. Ergonomiczne zasady projektowania produktów, Product ergonomics. Ergonomic principles of products design (red.) Jan Jabłoński, Wyd. Politechniki Poznańskiej (2006) ISBN: 83-7143-238-0
6. Butlewski, M.: Extension of working time in Poland as a challenge for ergonomic design. Machines, Technologies, Materials, International Virtual Journal, Publisher Scientific Technical Union of Mechanical Engineering (Year VII issue November 2013) ISSN 1313-0226
7. Butlewski, M.: The issue of product safety in contemporary design. In: Safety of the System, Technical, Organizational and Human Work Safety Determinants. Red. Szymon Salamon. Wyd. PCzęst. Częstochowa, pp. 1428–1600 (2012) ISBN 978-83-63500-13-9, ISSN 1428-1600
8. Butlewski, M., Tytyk, E.: The assessment criteria of the ergonomic quality of anthropotechnical mega-systems. In: Vink, P. (ed.) Advances in Social and Organizational Factors, pp. 298–306. CRC Press, Taylor and Francis Group, Boca Raton, London (2012) ISBN 978-1-4398-8
9. Card, S., Moran, T., Newell, A.: The Psychology of Human-Computer Interaction. Lawrence Erlbaum Associates Inc., Hillsdale (1983)
10. Comaish, S., Botoms, E.: The skin and friction: Deviations from Amonton's laws and the effects of hydration and lubrication. British Journal of Dermatology 8, 37–43 (1971)
11. Directive 2006/42/EC of the European Parliament and of the Council of 17 May 2006 on machinery, and amending Directive 95/16/EC
12. Duda, K.: The aging process. In: Marchewka, A., Dąbrowski, Z., Żołądź, J.A. (eds.) Physiology of Aging: Prevention and Rehabilitation/Red. Nauk., p. 15. Publishing House PWN, Warszawa (2013) (in Polish)
13. Epps, B.W.: Comparison of six cursor control devices based on Fitts' law models. In: Proceedings of the 30th Annual Meeting of the Human Factors Society, Dayton, Ohio, September 29–3 October, vol. 29, pp. 327–313. Human Factors & Ergonomics Society, Santa Monica, CA (1986)
14. European Demographic Data Sheet (2012), http://www.iiasa.ac.at/
15. Adam, G.: Assessment of compliance with minimum safety requirements in machine operation: a case of assessing the control devices of a press. In: Arezes, P.M. (ed.) Occupational Safety and Hygiene, pp. s.497–s.501. Taylor and Francis Group, London (2013) ISBN: 978-1-138-00047-6
16. Grobelny, J., Karwowski, W., Drury, C.: Usability of Graphical Icons in the Design of Human-Computer Interfaces. International Journal of Human-Computer Interaction 18(2), 167–182 (2005) DOI: 10.1207/s15327590ijhc1802_3
17. Hart, S.G., Staveland, L.E.: Development of NASA-TLX (Task Load Index): results of empirical and theoretical research. In: Hancock, P.A., Meshkati, N. (eds.) Human Mental Workload, pp. 5–39. Elsevier, New York (1988)
18. Harvey, C., Stanton, N., Pickering, C., McDonald, M., Zheng, P.: To twist or poke? A method for identifying usability issues with the rotary controller and touch screen for control of in-vehicle information systems. Ergonomics 54(7), 609–625 (2011)
19. Hill, S.G., Iavecchia, H.P., Byers, J.C., Bittner, A.C., Zaklad, A.L., Christ, R.E.: Comparison of four subjective workload rating scales. Hum. Factors 34, 429–439 (1992)
20. McLoughlin, I., Maniatopoulos, G., Wilson, R., Martin, M.: Hope to Die Before You Get Old? Public Management Review 11(6), 857–880 (2009), doi:10.1080/14719030903319002

21. Jasiak, A., Misztal, A.: Ergonomic problems of an aging rural population. In: Solecki, L. (ed.) Problems of the Elderly and the Disabled in Agriculture, pp. 314–321. Institute of Agricultural Medicine, Lublin (2004) ISBN 83-7090-091-7

22. Jasiulewicz-Kaczmarek, M.: The role of ergonomics in implementation of the social aspect of sustainability, illustrated with the example of maintenance. In: Arezes, P., Baptista, J.S., Barroso, M., Carneiro, P., Lamb, P., Costa, N., Melo, R., Miguel, A.S., Perestrelo, G. (eds.) Occupational Safety and Hygiene, pp. 47–52. CRC Press, Taylor & Francis, London (2013) ISBN 978-1-138-00047-6

23. Zhou, J., Rau, P.-L.P., Salvendy, G.: Use and Design of Handheld Computers for Older Adults: A Review and Appraisal. International Journal of Human-Computer Interaction 28(12), 799–826 (2012), doi:10.1080/10447318.2012.668129

24. Yanand John, J.H., Downing, H.: Effects of Aging, Grip Span, and Grip Style on Hand Strength. Research Quarterly for Exercise and Sport 72(1), 71–77 (2001), doi:10.1080/02701367.2001.10608935

25. Juliszewski, T., Kiełbasa, P., Trzyniec, K.: Procedury obsługi urządzeń sygnalizacyjnych i sterowniczych wybranych maszyn rolniczych. In: Rolnicza, I. (ed.) Procedures for Handling Signal and Control Devices of Selected Agricultural Machinery, Agricultural Engineering ISSN 1429-7264, R. 16, nr 4, t. 1

26. Kang, N.E., Yoon, W.C.: Age- and experience-related user behavior differences in the use of complicated electronic devices. International Journal of Human–Computer Studies 66, 425–437 (2008)

27. Gilles, M.A., Wing, A.M.: Age-Related Changes in Grip Force and Dynamics of Hand Movement. Journal of Motor Behavior 35(1), 79–85 (2003)

28. McCormick, E.: Antropotechnika WNT Warszawa (1964)

29. McCormick, E.J.: Human Factors in Engineering and Design. McGraw-Hill, New York (1976)

30. Meyer, B., Bouhuis, D.G., Czaja, S.J., Roger, W.A., Schneider-Hufschmidt, M., Fozard, J.L.: How can we make technology ÃÄelder friendlyÃÄ? In: Altom, M.W., Williams, M.G. (eds.) CHI 1999 Human Factors in Computing Systems, pp. 81–82. ACM SIGCHI, New York (1999)

31. Mrugalska, B., Kawecka-Endler, A.: Practical application of product design method robust to disturbances. Human Factors and Ergonomics in Manufacturing and Service Industries 22(2), s.121–s.129 (2012)

32. Nielsen, J.: Heuristic evaluation. In: Nielsen, J., Mack, R.L. (eds.) Usability Inspection Methods. John Wiley & Sons, New York (1994)

33. Nygren, T.E.: Psychometric properties of subjective workload measurement techniques: implications for their use in the assessment of perceived mental workload. Hum. Factors 33, 17–33 (1991)

34. Pennathur, P.R., Contreras, L.R., Dowling, W.: Perceived technology needs among older Mexican Americans. Gerontechnology 7(1), 58–61 (2008), doi:http://dx.doi.org/10.4017/gt.2008.07.01.006.00

35. Biswas, P., Langdon, P.: Developing Multimodal Adaptation Algorithm for Mobility Impaired Users by Evaluating Their Hand Strength. International Journal of Human-Computer Interaction 28(9), 576–596 (2012), doi:10.1080/10447318.2011.636294

36. Prussak, W.: Ergonomiczne zasady projektowania oprogramowania komputerowego. In: Jabłoński, J. (ed.) Eronomic Design Principles of Software, Szczegółowe Ergonomiczne zasady Projektowania, Detailed Ergonomic Design Principles, w: J. Jabłoński (red.), Ergonomia produktu. Ergonomiczne zasady projektowania produktów, Product ergonomics. Ergonomic principles of products design, Wydawnictwo Politechniki Poznańskiej, Poznań (2006)

37. San-Segundo, R., Cordoba, R., Ferreiros, J., Macias-Guarasa, J., Montero, J.M., Fernández, F., D'haro, L.F., Barra, R., Barra, R.: Speech Technology at Home: Enhanced Interfaces for People with Disabilities. Intelligent Automation & Soft Computing 15(4), 647–666 (2009)
38. Schaie, K.W.: Cognitive aging. In: Pew, R., van Hemmel, S. (eds.) Technology for Adaptive Aging: Report and Papers. National Research Council. The National Academies Press, Washington, DC (2004)
39. Schieber, F.: Human factors and aging: Identifying and compensating for age-related deficits in sensory and cognitive function. In: Schaie, K.W., Charness, N. (eds.) Influences of Technological Change on Individual Aging. Springer Publishing Company, New York (2003)
40. Vinck, D.: Everyday engineering: an ethnography of design and innovation. Taylor and Francis (2003) ISBN 0-262-22065-2
41. Nagasawa, Y., Demura, S.: Age and Sex Differences in Controlled Force Exertion Measured by a Computing Bar Chart Target-Pursuit System. Measurement in Physical Education and Exercise Science 13(3), 140–150 (2009)
42. Żołądź, J.A., Majerczak, J., Duda, K.: Aging and human physical performance. In: Gorski, J. (ed.) Physiology of Exercise and Physical Training. PZWL Medical Publishing (2011)

Efficiency of a Video and a Tutorial
in Teaching Older Adults to Interact with Smartphones

Jorge Ribeiro and Ana Correia de Barros

Fraunhofer Portugal AICOS, Porto, Portugal
{jorge.ribeiro,ana.barros}@fraunhofer.pt

Abstract. While smartphones and tablets increasingly offer the possibility to act as healthcare devices, older adults, who may benefit from these new technologies, might be left behind due to technological illiteracy and lack of proper instructions. This study documents an experiment to evaluate and compare different instructional methods to teach older adults to perform a task on a smartphone. Although we did find that older adults were able to learn, no significant differences between instructional methods were found, and retention period is not known. The qualitative analysis suggests some influence of the users' initial perception of task difficulty over task performance.

Keywords: Older adults, learning, smartphone, instructional materials.

1 Introduction

Information and Communication Technology (ICT) is becoming increasingly prevalent, namely within healthcare [1]. Disruptive services allow people to monitor their health at home and at their own pace [2]. Specifically, smartphones are being widely used as health monitoring devices. However, a number of older adults may be left out of these new possibilities due to technological illiteracy or inefficient instructions.

Guidelines on how to design for older adults may be found in the literature; however, there is a lack of studies focusing on whether or not older adults are able to learn certain aspects of interaction with ICT and what techniques may be used to enhance the learning process. Previous studies have examined older adults' preferences and needs for learning to use technology [3] and mobile devices [4], or have explored novel interfaces to improve learnability [5]. Other studies have assessed the efficiency of different instructional materials on older adults' ability to learn to use technological devices. Mykityshyn et al. focused on a blood glucose meter [2], Rogers et al. on Automatic Teller Machines [6], and Struve and Wandke on ticket vending machines [7], but to our knowledge, there are no studies focusing on smartphone applications. The goal of this study was two-fold: 1) understand how older adults learn to use touchscreen enabled interfaces and 2) assess the effectiveness of 2 different learning methods and compare their perceived ease of use by older adults. Ultimately, the results of this study aim to inform the design of solutions that support older adults in the process of learning novel interactions.

C. Stephanidis and M. Antona (Eds.): UAHCI/HCII 2014, Part III, LNCS 8515, pp. 34–45, 2014.
© Springer International Publishing Switzerland 2014

2   Methods

The study was structured in two complementary phases that took place approximately two months apart. In the first phase we explored the effectiveness of an instructional video as a learning method with a control group; in the second phase we introduced an interactive tutorial. The protocol for each condition included two sessions that took place at different points in time – between 8 and 14 days apart (M = 11.45 days) – in order to understand short-term and long-term effects of the different learning methods (retention). Sessions took around five to thirty minutes and were video recorded.

Participants of the first phase were randomly assigned to either the instructional video or the control group; participants of the second phase were directly assigned to the tutorial condition. A demographic questionnaire was administered at the beginning of the experiment to gather information regarding participants' technological and educational background. In the first session participants were introduced to the smart-phone and were taught the basics of the touchscreen interaction in order to provide a common ground among participants. The application and tasks were then described to all participants and additional instructions were given according to participants' assigned conditions. During the test participants did not have access to the instructional material. Before the beginning of each test participants were asked to rate their confidence; after the test they were asked to rate the task ease of use [8]. After the first test, participants in the two learning conditions were also asked two questions regarding the learning material.

The test consisted of two tasks: Task 1 required participants to turn off an alarm, and Task 2 involved participants adding a new alarm. Participants were required to complete two trials per session.

2.1   Materials

All tests were conducted with an HTC Titan with a 4.7' screen, running Windows Phone 7.5, and configured with the "dark" theme. The application used in the experiment consisted of the alarm clock that comes by default with the Windows Phone 7 (WP7). This application was chosen because 1) older adults are most likely familiar with a traditional alarm clock; 2) since it takes advantage of previous knowledge and experience of older adults with traditional alarm clocks, it was easier to devise and explain tasks to participants; 3) the task addresses a potential need of older adults, so they are more likely to be motivated and engaged; 4) it is not overly complex; and 5) it comes by default with WP7.

2.2   Instructional Materials

Instructional Video. The video used in the experiment guided participants step-by-step through the tasks. The video portrayed a person using the device form the user's point of view and was shown to participants through the device, given that on a realistic scenario the video would likely be used to assist older adults within the application. The video was also accompanied by the narration of the steps being performed.

The instructional video was 34 seconds in length and participants watched it between 1 and 6 times (M = 3.00).

Interactive Tutorial. The tutorial allowed participants to have a first contact with the application before the actual test. The goal of this learning method was to provide seniors with a hands-on experience and to explore a common learning pattern: learn by doing. Most participants chose to carry out the tutorial only once; only two participants completed the tutorial twice.

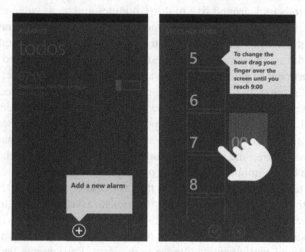

Fig. 1. Add a new alarm (left); Change the hour (right)

The tutorial consisted of a simulated interface of the alarm clock that included additional information to guide participants through the steps. In the interactive tutorial provided to participants steps were separated into discrete units, each one shown on a different screen. Each step required participants to complete a single action, which could be a tap or a swipe. To teach participants what were the trigger elements, screens were dimmed down, except for the areas relevant to the task (Fig. 1. , left). Based on a successful previous experience [9], a box with an arrow pointing to the trigger element was used to describe the action that had to be performed. To teach participants to swipe, an illustration of a hand pointing to the swipe area and with an animation of the correct gesture was used (Fig. 1. , right). While visually the tutorial was identical to the alarm clock, the interaction of was somehow different and stricter than the original time picker.

2.3   Participants

The study was conducted with thirty-three older adults with ages between 61 and 92 (M = 74.79, SD = 6.84), recruited from local day-care centers. Details of the participants may be found on Table 1. No formal screening was used to assess older adults' cognitive abilities or visual acuity. Participants were only required to be able to read.

Seniors' educational background varied greatly, ranging from no complete primary education to a doctoral degree. Nevertheless, the majority of participants only finished primary school or less (n = 21, 64%), seven participants (21%) went to middle school, and five (15%) achieved some sort of higher education. On average participants completed 6.56 years of education (SD = 3.82).

Most participants did not own a computer, nor had experience with computers or related technology. Only five participants owned a computer, and one participant was used to use one at work (this senior retired recently and did not use a computer since then). In contrast with computer usage, the majority of participants owned a mobile phone (90.9%, n = 30); only three participants did not own one, and in the tutorial group all participants owned a mobile phone. Of those participants who own a mobile phone, 70% use it every day. Although most participants stated that they use their phone on a daily basis, the usage that they give to the device is rather limited. From the feedback gathered, a large number of seniors would only use the phone to receive calls from their family. Frequently, the phone was a gift from their children or grandchildren. Older adults would recurrently comment that they did not know how to send or reply to messages or how to perform other more complicated tasks, and that they needed to ask their sons, granddaughters or nieces for help.

Of all thirty-three participants in the study only one owned a touchscreen device – this mobile device was not what it is ordinarily defined as a smartphone, but rather a feature phone with a resistive touch screen. However, sixteen participants (48%) had previous contact with smartphones through usability tests. While 71% (n = 5) of seniors had taken part in previous usability tests with smartphones, three of them had participated in those tests more than a year ago.

Table 1. Participant categorization

	Control (n = 13)	Video (n = 13)	Tutorial (n = 7)
Age (years)	73.23 (6.78)	75.92 (4.48)	75.57 (10.08)
Gender	8 F, 5 M	9 F, 4 M	6 F, 1 M
Education (years)	7.08 (4.03)	5.23 (4.51)	6.57 (3.82)
Computer	23%	7%	29%
Mobile phone	84%	92%	100%
Familiarity w/ smartphones	46%	38%	71%
Retention (days)	12.55 (1.58)	12.00 (1.67)	8.86 (1.07)

3   Results

3.1   Instructional Materials

In the end of the first session participants in the learning conditions were asked to evaluate on an 8-point scale how clear the instructional material was, and how easy it was to learn to use the application. Participants in the video condition attributed an average rate of 4.15 to the first question and 4.23 to the second one. Participants in the tutorial condition attributed an average rate of 5.20 to the first question, and an average rate of 5.00 to the second one. When compared to the instructional video, these results may suggest that the tutorial has better acceptance among older adults, but with only five data points in the tutorial condition, a confident conclusion cannot be offered.

Nevertheless, when we consider that test subjects in general, but older adults in particular, tend to praise the material that they are being presented [10] and blame themselves for the difficulties experienced [11],the results obtained are rather low and seem to indicate that participants had real trouble understanding the instructional material. In sum, it seems that in both cases the overall learning experience was not as positive as desired.

3.2   Confidence Ratings

Confidence ratings were collected on an 8-point scale before each trial. The average scores for each trial are presented in Fig. 2. Participants in the learning condition began the experiment less confident than those in the control group. There was also an overall increase in participants' confidence ratings between trials within the same session, with the exception of participants in learning conditions in the first session. After the retention interval there were no substantial differences between groups in terms of participants' confidence ratings. Moreover, in the learning conditions, the decline in confidence after the first trial of the session was not observed.

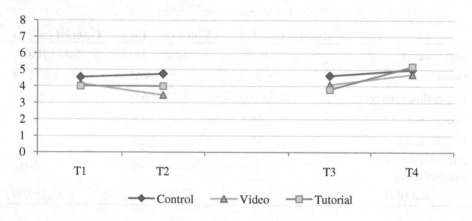

Fig. 2. Confidence ratings

3.3   Ease of Use Ratings

After each trial participants were asked to rate on an 8-point scale how easy they considered the tasks they had performed. The average scores for each trial are presented in Fig. 3. In the first session the average rates of participants in the video condition were lower than the other two conditions, but similar to the control group in the second session. There was also a consistent increase on participants' ratings between trials, though stronger in the first session.

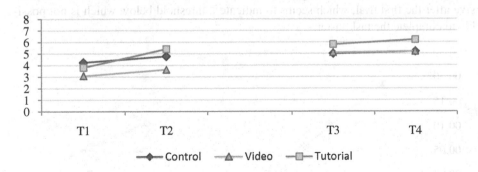

— Control — Video — Tutorial

Fig. 3. Ease of use ratings

3.4   Performance

To evaluate participants' performance between groups we measured the completion rate, the completion time, and the number of errors. A task was considered completed with success when all subtasks were completed. No specific order was enforced, and subtasks were not required to be completed in a single run. The time for Task 1 was counted from the moment the phone was handed to participants, or as soon as participants finished reading the instructions (for those who chose to read the task instructions again), until the instant they turned off the alarm. The completion time for Task 2 was considered from the moment participants completed Task 1, or as soon as they finished rereading the instructions, until the moment they saved the alarm. Only participants who completed the task were considered in the completion time analysis.

	T1		T2		T3		T4	
	TC	T	TC	T	TC	T	TC	T
Task 1: Turn off the alarm								
Control	92%	00:19	92%	00:06	73%	00:11	91%	00:04
Video	100%	00:05	85%	00:05	100%	00:08	100%	00:06
Tutorial	100%	00:03	100%	00:02	86%	00:05	100%	00:05
Task 2: Add a new alarm								
Control	58%	02:09	58%	01:16	64%	02:29	73%	01:21
Video	69%	01:39	62%	01:34	82%	01:45	91%	01:15
Tutorial	86%	04:51	86%	02:27	71%	02:40	71%	01:29

T1-T4: Trials; TC: Task completion; T: Task completion time (mm:ss).

3.5   Task 1: Turn Off the Alarm

In the first trial participants in the learning conditions were more successful and faster than participants in the control group. Differences between conditions are less expressive after the first trial, which seems to indicate a threshold below which is not possible to complete the task faster.

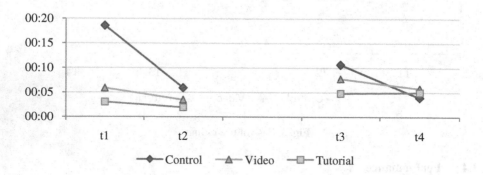

Fig. 4. Task completion time (geometric mean)

3.6   Task 2: Add a New Alarm

Compared to the results from Task 1, participants in the tutorial condition were slower than participants in the other conditions. On the other hand, these participants achieved a higher success rate. There were also considerable improvements between trials within the same session.

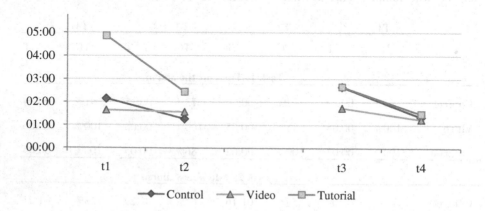

Fig. 5. Task completion time (geometric mean)

3.7   Gestures

To understand the influence of each condition in the teaching of new gestures, we looked into how seniors interacted with the time picker, since that was the only control that could be manipulated by tapping or swiping. This analysis took into account data from the first trial and included participants who had been excluded from the main analysis because they had not completed all sessions. As a result, the analysis included 12 participants from the control group, 13 from the video condition, and 9 from the tutorial. In the case of the tutorial condition, we excluded participants who were not able to swipe during the training stage, for the reason that they would not be able to transfer a gesture they did not have an opportunity to learn.

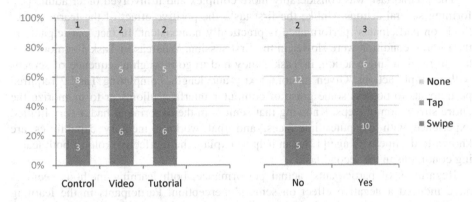

Fig. 6. Types of gestures performed by participants according to condition (left) and familiarity with smartphones (right)

The results suggest a positive effect of both learning conditions in coaching older adults the swipe gesture. That is, participants in the learning conditions were more likely to swipe while using the time picker. When we take into account familiarity with smartphones, the results also suggest a relation between familiarity with smartphone and swipe incidence.

4   Discussion

In this study we aimed to assess the effectiveness of an instructional video in teaching older adults to use a smartphone interface. We were not able to find consistent and significant differences between conditions in terms of seniors' learning, but we observed some differences worth analyzing. Furthermore, while this study pertains to a different domain and the methods are somehow distinct, these results are not consistent with findings from previous studies that found a positive effect of an instructional video [2] and a hands-on experience [6] in teaching older adults to use an interface.

We observed some noteworthy differences between conditions in some metrics. The first distinction that ought to be made is in the length and complexity of tasks.

The first task in the experiment was rather simple and only required participants to tap a simple button, so the burden on seniors' memory was minimal. Participants only had to recall where to tap and both learning conditions were effective in teaching older adults how to turn off the alarm: older adults were faster and more efficient. While most participants were able to turn off the alarm, seniors in the learning conditions were faster, and to our understanding, more certain of their actions. This does not mean that seniors in the learning conditions had a deep understanding of workings of the system or that they were fully aware of their actions, but indicates nonetheless that they were able to replicate what they had experienced moments before. While it is just a part of the learning process, mimicking some procedure can be a valuable step towards learning how a system works.

The second task was considerably more complex and it involved older adults performing several actions. Unlike the first task, the positive effect of the learning methods on participants' performance is practically nonexistent. In fact, participants in the tutorial condition were slower in the first session. Whereas in Task 1 seniors only had to recall a single action, in Task 2 they had to go through a sequence of screens with multiple actions. Given its complexity and length, completing Task 2 required participants to possess some grasp of computer interface idioms or to memorize the entire succession of steps. Knowing that seniors in the experiment had a very limited experience with computer interfaces, and that working memory capabilities are known to decline with age [12], can help to explain the ineffective role of both learning conditions in the second task.

Regardless of participants' actual performance, both learning methods seem to have induced a negative effect on seniors' perception. Participants in the learning conditions began the experiment less confident than seniors in the control group who only had a vague idea of the tasks. In short, knowing in advance the content of the experiment did not help making seniors more at ease; in fact, it might have done the opposite. Moreover, by the second trial participants' confidence had declined or stayed the same, an effect that was not observed in the control group or in the second session. Regarding the video, the origin for the conflict between participants' performance and perception pertains perhaps to the reference point that the video had created, that is, participants who watched the video possibly evaluated their performance against what they saw in the video. Thus, to be able to complete the task with success one ought to replicate the video. Given that tasks in the video were completed in an optimal manner, attaining an equivalent level of success was not unchallenging. The results from the assessment of the tasks' ease of use seem to pertain to the same underlying issue. That is, older adults in the video condition seem to have been conditioned by the video, and because they were not able to complete the task with the same level of accuracy/dexterity as the person in the instructional video, they assumed the task as being more difficult than what it really was. An implication of this finding is that a video that appears to be complicated might lead older adults to assume that they are not very capable, and thus reject the application.

In order to assess older adults' acquired knowledge, participants were retested after a retention interval of approximately 12 days, a period during which participants did not have access to the application or smartphone. Despite some improvements in certain metrics, our results do not indicate consistent differences between sessions, which may suggest that the retention interval was enough to dissipate most of what older adults had learned in the first session. Only the results from Task 1, from participants in the control group, seem to show some retention between sessions. These participants were notably faster in the second session, which, given the ease of the task, may indicate that some learning occurred.

4.1   Gestures

With regard to the influence of learning condition in the type of gestures performed while interacting with the time picker, our results seem to suggest a relation between conditions and gesture performed: elders in both learning conditions were more likely to address the time picker with a swipe than participants in the control group. The swipe is arguably a less natural gesture than a tap, thus less likely to be inferred with ease. Even if brief, seniors in the learning conditions had a previous contact with the swipe, so they would only have to recall what they saw or did; whereas seniors in the control group would have to infer on their own how to manipulate the time picker. The result may be nevertheless cofounded to some extent with participants' previous experiences, since there was also a relation between the type of gesture performed and familiarity with smartphones, i.e. seniors who had used a smartphone before were more prone to swipe. Moreover, a closer analysis of participants in the control group who were able to swipe reveals that these seniors were the only ones in the control group who had experience with computers, and one even owned a touch device. These results support the idea that without prior knowledge, to infer a rather simple gesture such as swipe from the interface alone is not as natural as it may seem.

Although our results may suggest that both learning conditions attained some level of success in teaching older adults to swipe, it is not clear the extent to which seniors grasped the concept behind swiping – e.g. we cannot assert that seniors realized that a swipe is typically used to disclose hidden information. What we can at least hypothesize is that older adults in the learning conditions were able to develop an association between the swipe gesture and the action of changing the hour. For instance, one participant would start moving his hand over the screen, emulating the swipe, when asked to change the hour, even though he was on a screen that did not have any scrollable element; he just knew that in order to change the hour he had to do that gesture. While seniors were able to learn how to swipe with some level of success, further tests are needed in order to understand how well that concept was interiorized.

4.2   Limitations

A main limitation of this study lies on the sample, both in terms of size and in terms of older adults' representativeness. Thirty-three seniors distributed across three conditions took part in the study, which is a relatively small sample in particular when one considers the high variance in cognitive abilities and experience of participants.

The problem caused by the small sample is even more expressive in the tutorial condition, since we were only able to collect data from seven participants. Samples were also not entirely unbiased given that the study was divided in two phases and seniors in the second phase were assigned directly to that condition.

Older adults in this study also had a low educational background, and no experience, or almost no experience with computers and related technology. While older adults in this study may characterize a large portion of Portuguese seniors, they might not be representative of the overall senior population. By contrast with similar studies, the educational background of older adults in this study was considerably low. For instance, older adults in Mykityshyn's study [2] had on average 14 years of education, in contrast with approximately 7 years of seniors in this study. Given the small sample, an inhomogeneous group of seniors, and a not very representative sample, it is difficult to generalize the results with confidence.

5   Conclusion

In this paper we explored how effective two learning conditions – video and tutorial – were in teaching older adults to interact with a touch interface. We also looked at the long-term and short-term effects of the learning conditions for which we collected two data points. Despite noteworthy results in some metrics, we were not able to find significant differences between conditions, neither were we able to find consistent improvement across sessions. The problem may lie in the small and inhomogeneous sample; therefore further tests with better controlled samples may lead to more conclusive results. Further tests should also consider simpler and discrete tasks, in order to focus on the qualities of learning methods, and to not overload seniors' short-term memory.

Nevertheless, older adults in the study were able to learn. We found consistent improvements between trials within the same session, and older adults who had had previous contact with smartphones through usability testing achieved better results in their first session. The question is what the best strategies to instigate learning are, and for how long are older adults able to retain what they learn. Previous work showed that an interval of 24 hours does not produce a significant decline in performance [6]; whereas this present study and others [2] found a meaningful decline in performance after a longer period without access to the test material. Future work should also attempt to determine when a sudden decline in performance occurs in order to identify when the learning process has to be reinforced.

Acknowledgments. The work in this paper was supported by the ChefMyself project (aal-2012-5-120), co-funded by the Ambient Assisted Living Joint Programme and Fundação para a Ciência e a Tecnologia (FCT).

References

1. Rogers, W.A., Campbell, R.H., Pak, R.: A Systems Approach for Training Older Adults to Use Technology. In: Communication, Technology, and Aging: Opportunities and Challenges for the Future, pp. 187–208. Springer, New York (2001)
2. Mykityshyn, A.L., Fisk, A.D., Rogers, W.A.: Learning to Use a Home Medical Device: Mediating Age-Related Differences with Training. Human Factors 44(3), 354–364 (2002)
3. Mitzner, T.L., Fausset, C.B., Boron, J.B., Adams, A.E., Dijkstra, K., Lee, C.C., Rogers, W.A., Fisk, A.D.: Older Adults' Training Preferences for Learning to Use Technology. Human Factors and Ergonomics Society Annual (2008)
4. Leung, R., Haddad, C.T., Mcgrenere, J., Graf, P., Ingriany, V.: How Older Adults Learn to Use Mobile Devices: Survey and Field Investigations. TACCESS 4, Article 11 (2012)
5. Leung, R., Findlater, L., McGrenere, J., Graf, P., Yang, J.: Multi-Layered Interfaces to Improve Older Adults' Initial Learnability of Mobile Applications. TACCESS 3, Article 1 (2010)
6. Rogers, W.A., Fisk, A.F., Mead, S.E., Walker, N., Cabrera, E.F.: Training Older Adults to Use Automatic Teller Machines. Human Factors 38, 425–433 (1996)
7. Struve, D., Wandke, H.: Video Modeling for Training Older Adults to Use New Technologies. TACCESS 2, Article 4 (2009)
8. Sauro, J., Dumas, J.S.: Comparison of Three One-Question, Post-Task Usability Questionnaires. In: Proceedings of the SIGCHI Conference on Human Factors in Computing Systems, pp. 1599–1608. ACM, New York (2009)
9. Correia de Barros, A., Cevada, J., Bayés, À., Alcaine, S., Mestre, B.: User-Centred Design of a Mobile Self-Management Solution for Parkinson's Disease. In: 12th International Conference on Mobile and Ubiquitous Multimedia, Article 23, ACM, New York (2013)
10. Correia de Barros, A., Leitão, R.: Young Practitioners' Challenges, Experience and Strategies in Usability Testing with Older Adults. In: Encarnação, P., Azevedo, L., Gelderblom, G.J., Mathiassen, N. (eds.) Assistive Technology: From Research to Practice, AAATE 2013, pp. 787–792. IOS Press, Amsterdam (2013)
11. Rubin, J., Chisnell, A.L.: Handbook of Usability Testing: How to Plan, Design and Conduct Effective Tests. Wiley Publishing, Inc., Indianapolis (2008)
12. Fisk, A.D., Rogers, W.A., Charness, N., Czaja, S.J., Sharit, J.: Designing for Older Adults: Principles and Creative Human Factors Approaches. CRC Press, Boca Raton (2009)

Reassuring the Elderly Regarding the Use of Mobile Devices for Mobility

António Cunha[1], Paula Trigueiros[2], and Tiago Lemos[3]

[1] Universidade de Trás-os-Montes e Alto Douro, UTAD, Vila Real, Portugal
and
INESC TEC - INESC Technology and Science (formely INESC Porto)
acunha@utad.pt
[2] UNIDCOM/IADE – Unidade de Investigação em Design e Comunicação
and
FEUP - Faculdade de Engenharia da Universidade do Porto, Portugal
paula.trigueiros@gmail.com
[3] Universidade de Trás-os-Montes e Alto Douro, UTAD, Vila Real, Portugal
tcmlemos@gmail.com

Abstract. People facing threats of mobility loss have their self-confidence shaken and tend to reduce their physical activity. As is well-known, the decreased physical activity, particularly for the elderly, is one of the factors that contribute to accelerating the deterioration of their health with consequent loss of autonomy and quality of life. Today, GPS-based technologies available on mobile devices offer many solutions to help guide users around much of the world. However, there are several known factors that act as barriers to the use of these technologies, such as user unfamiliarity with these devices, the complexity of geographical information and the difficulty of typing the origin and destination locations. In this paper we propose a solution for mobile devices that seeks to promote user confidence in daily mobility, especially among the elderly. We present the main system functionalities and the interface design.

Keywords: Active aging, Mobile applications, daily mobility.

1 Introduction

It is an accepted fact that populations are aging in developed societies [1]. The decrease in mortality along with improvements in the quality of healthcare and better living and working conditions have led to greater longevity than in the past. A strategy which addresses population ageing should be organised in order to help create a cohesive and inclusive intergenerational society [2].

Information Communications Technology (ICT) is considered an important tool in helping to create this cohesive and inclusive society [3]. ICT can make key contributions to the independent living of the elderly, particularly in reducing expenses for health and care services, providing individual solutions and meeting individual needs, improving living standards and creating new business opportunities [4].

Usually the receptivity of the elderly to new technology is low, but in cases where its use entails obvious and relevant benefits to their lifestyle, they are very receptive [5].

C. Stephanidis and M. Antona (Eds.): UAHCI/HCII 2014, Part III, LNCS 8515, pp. 46–57, 2014.
© Springer International Publishing Switzerland 2014

Within ICT, the adoption of mobile devices (tablets and smartphones) has seen huge growth, given their features, such as communication ability, internet and phone, intuitive touch interaction, big and high resolution displays, light weight, high resolution cameras, sensors (GPS, compass, among others) and advanced computation ability. These features make them appropriate for assisting the elderly in their daily activities and afford a promising tool for improving their quality of life (QoL). Imaculada Plaza at [3] presents a comparison of seven quality of life components identified by older people and the expectations and needs of the aged in relation to mobile applications found in the literature:

Table 1. Comparison of quality of life components identified by older people and expectations and needs of the aged in relation to mobile applications found in the literature. Source: [3].

QoL component	Needs of older person
Family and other relationships/contact with others	Maintain social contact / communication device
Emotional well-being	Feeling safe and secure
Religion/spirituality	
Independence/ Mobility / Autonomy	Freedom of movement/ Memory and daily life activity aids/ Enjoyment/ Self-actualization
Social/ Leisure activities	Memory and daily life activity aids/ Enjoyment/ Self-actualization
Finances / standard of living	
Own health/health of other(s)	Healthier independent life

People facing threats of mobility loss, such as that related to the diagnosis of Parkinson's disease or the arrival of its first symptoms, have their self-confidence shaken and tend to reduce their physical activity (PA) in order to avoid hazardous situations. At such moments people start wondering: "... what if I become disoriented, how can I find my way back home?" or "... if I get lost, will my loved ones be able to find me?"

Physical activity is a well-known factor in healthy ageing and the lack of it has long been associated with chronic disease [6]. The decrease in PA in people, particularly the elderly, is one of the factors that contribute to an accelerating deterioration in their health, with consequent loss of autonomy and quality of life. Moderately frequent intense activity has significant cardiovascular and mental health benefits, and protects against osteoporosis, obesity and related disorders. Promoting physical activity in adults is a public health priority [7].

Today the technologies provided by personal mobile devices offer many solutions to help guide users, based on the Global Positioning System (GPS). These solutions can support and guide users over practically the whole planet, showing them the best route between two selected points.

However, there are several factors known to act as barriers to the use of these technologies, such as the fact that many people, and especially the elderly, are still not familiar with the use of these devices; geographical information as it is usually presented in these applications - maps and abstract schemas - is complex and often requires the introduction of names of origin and destination locations.

In this paper we propose an application for mobile devices that seeks to promote people's confidence in daily mobility. This solution focuses on that section of the population which is aged, gets about on foot or by public, lives alone, and may have one or more carers (among family, neighbours or professionals). We seek to help elderly people on the QoL of emotional well-being and fulfil their needs to feel safe and to enjoy healthier more independent lives.

In order to do so, we are designing and implementing an App prototype, on mobile devices named Compass&Magnifier (C&M). At this first stage, the requirements are based on brainstorming, on interviews with elder care professionals, on known eld-erly- related limitations and on other relevant work.

This paper is organized as follows: Section 2 refers to related work and Section 3 explains the methodology adopted for the development of our App. Section 4 depicts the main C&M system functionalities and the interface design. Finally, Section 5 summarises the paper and presents a synopsis of future work.

2   Related Work

Two main GPS technology-based strategies were identified for reassuring the aged in their everyday routines: to increase their sense of safety through easy/swift contact with their loved ones or carers; and to provide them with relevant information about their routine(s).

2.1   Increase Old People's Sense of Security through Easy and Rapid Contact with Their Loved Ones or Carers

There are several solutions based on GPS technology that aim to increase older adults' autonomy by increasing their sense of security when outdoors, and which also ease carers' concerns by reassuring them that they will be alerted if their loved ones be-come disorientated and need help.

Some of these solutions focus on senior citizens suffering from dementia, Alz-heimer's disease or other memory-related problems. They register and monitor the elderly's everyday routes, trigger alerts to carers if they are wandering off or lost, or notify carers if they are safe inside or around the home, or if they are making sched-uled visits to the doctor.

Within these solutions, the dedicated systems, such as special GPS bracelets, GPS necklaces (e.g. see [8]) or shoes (e.g. see [9]), are professional solutions and incur associated costs – usually users buy the device and sign up to a service on a paid monthly basis. However, these systems can cause stigmas to the users because they are specific to these problems. Such dedicated solutions are beyond the scope of this paper.

There are other solutions based on Apps that run in mobile devices. They overcome the stigma inconvenience because the mobile devices do not specifically concern themselves with these problems; they can even be considered fashionable.

Moreover the Apps are usually cheap and the mobile device Apps permit the user to benefit from many other forms of support. The smartphone prices are still high, but every day sees their prices falling and their power and sensors improving. If the user doesn't have one yet, probably he/she will obtain one soon.

There follows a description of a branch of Apps related to reassuring the elderly in their daily comings and goings.

The Apps focus on older adults and people in the initial stages of dementia, such as Alzheimer's patients, e.g AlzNav [10] and Tweri: The Alzheimer Locator [11] enables us to pre-define a safe geographical limitation zone and generate an alert to the user and to the carers, if the person passes beyond the defined limits.

These Apps also implement other functionalities, such as: SOS buttons, buttons that when pressed make a direct call to one predefined carer; and System failures, e.g. "out of battery", "loss of GPS signal" or "loss of GSM signal", which inform carers about user device status.

AlzNav App also generates a simplified walking navigator that is always able to point the user in the right direction in order to get back home. Other Apps promote the user's sense of security based on simplicity, e.g. One Touch SOS App [12]. The App implements SOS buttons that send the user a pre-defined contact address.

Since elderly people tend to have sight difficulties, Apps such as The Big Lancher [13] equip smartphone interfaces with large buttons and texts, thus enhancing user usability and consequently their sense of security. The Big Lancher also includes an SOS Button functionality.

The authors of Protege [14] developed an App for enhancing communications between the old adult and their carer. This App has a very good interface adapted for the elderly, and implements a substantial set of functionalities, of which we highlight: the SOS Button, which alerts in the event of a fall, or of no activity or a low battery; and carer inquiry messages, e.g. "how are you?" or "where are you?".

2.2   Providing the Elderly with Relevant Information about Their Routine

One way of reassuring a senior citizen is to inform him/her about his/her routine progress, e.g. "everything is ok!" or "you are late". Daily Commute [15] is an App that aims to make a prediction in relation to the user's daily travel and help him/her arrive on time. The App compiles user travel data over time to predict commute time each morning. Despite it not being an App specifically adapted for the elderly, the functionality enabling it to forecast "leave time" and "arrival time" can be very reassuring.

Real-time geographical information is another very important way of reassuring the aged. It can be re-assuring for an elderly person to be able to review a route in order to remember it or to see his/her progress in real time. Maps Apps, such as the widely known Google maps [16], are web-based services that provide detailed information about geographical regions and sites around the world. They usually provide visual road maps and satellite views. In some towns and cities, Google Maps offers "street views" comprising photographs taken from vehicles (3D views). This kind of App usually has too many functionalities or choices available at the same time, which may serve as a drawback to elderly users.

3   Methodology

As a methodology for design and development, we choose the user-centered design (UCD), since it tries to optimize the product around how the users can, want or need to use it. UCD was introduced by Norman and Darper [17], and became a recognized methodology among researchers in Human-Computer Interaction (HCI). It is characterized as a multi-stage problem solving process that requires designers to analyse and foresee how users are likely to use a product and test the validity of their assumptions with regard to user behaviour in real world tests with actual users.

There are several tools in the analysis of UCD, but those primarily used are *persona*, scenarios, and use cases. The persona is a fictional and life-like character that represents archetypal users [18-19]. It is described following field research, and since it is almost impossible to apply all user characteristics, there may often be several personas.

Scenarios is a fictional story about the "about the persona´s daily life" or a sequence of events with the *persona* as the main character. There can be best case scenarios, average case scenarios, or worst case scenarios, where, according to the main character's experience, either everything works out for the best, or he has an ordinary day in which nothing exciting or depressing occurs, or everything around him or her goes wrong. Scenarios can help us discuss potential designs with other designers and potential users [20].

The use case captures a contract between the stakeholders of a system and describes the system's behavior. It collects together different scenarios (different sequences of behaviour) [21].

3.1   Requirements

Following our research, we made an enquiry dedicated to people of 50 or more years old, concerning people's interest in using some devices in their everyday life, and into their frequency of use. This enquiry included questions regarding their self-evaluation, about their autonomy in terms of everyday tasks, and also about their comparative confidence and sense of wellbeing, in relation to others of the same age.

Up to the time of publication of this paper, we had 57 respondents, 39 of whom were aged between 50 and 60. For the upper ages we only had 18 responses. Nevertheless, these results showed that the few older people above the age of 60 use mobile devices only rarely, and those that do use them only use basic functionalities. The authors Ferreira et al [14] reported as a fact that they could not ask senior citizens what they expect from an Android mobile application / device due to their relative level of ignorance regarding the full possibilities of this technology.

So at this first stage, we decided to design a prototype, based on an initial set of requirements that could be considered to meet with better acceptance and greater success among the targeted persons. These requirements were based on brainstorming, interviews with eldercare professionals, research on elderly- related limitations and on similar mobile Apps.

We identified three main groups of requirements, which are listed and detailed below:

1. General aspects to consider: The App should focus on a few relevant tasks, closely related to daily routine, and use simple or well-known metaphors;
2. Considering the interface and layout design, it should provide selective user-friendly contents – directly connected to the task. The layout must be consistent throughout the menu's sequence and redundant on essential information or commands. It is also important to guarantee clear and familiar information, using cultural or acquired stereotypes in terms of tasks and colours, as well as to provide flexible interaction and error tolerant design, e.g. taking into consideration hand tremors and reduced sight. Finally, it is essential to assure feedback control (audible or tactile forms) and allow user preferences – such as volume control, type size, or voice commands.
3. The visual interface would benefit from the choice of an accessible typography, with large and clear font, presented in white or yellow, on a dark blue or black screen; and it is important to avoid overlapping the text with background patterns or images.

With "Dewsbury" [22], we agree that "One of the most complex and time-consuming elements of designing for people is actually the requirements process. In order for the final design to be accessible to and actually used by the Target group it is critical that this group is fully engaged in the design process".

The next step (beyond the scope of this paper) will be the evaluation of the prototype and a participatory redesigning with a group of older people, following UCD methodology.

3.2 Personas and Use Cases

Based on the uniqueness of our social and geographical territory (inland northern Portugal) and on our previous experience and research, we decided to focus on people living in a rural environment, in receipt of poor services and for the most part living a long way from main services and care providers.

Most of the elderly population targeted have poor literacy skills and have lived in that region almost the whole of their lives. They remained in their village while their younger relatives moved to the big cities.

Presented with these problems, we decided to evolve this interface, taking into account two different types of cases and problems, and two *persona*: Elderly people who remain in their own homes in a small village, facing problems of isolation and difficulties of covering distances; People that move to another area which is unknown to them – facing fears of uncertainty about their new environment.

To represent those two types, we created Maria (persona 1) and Leandro (persona 2). Their descriptions are as follows:

Persona 1: Mary, retired marketer.
Maria's goal: Maintain her routines and feel secure.

Maria is an 83-year-old widow who has always lived in her small rural village in northern Portugal. Despite not having had the opportunity to go to school, she learned to read, write and to do some maths.

Although retired, Mary continues to manage her small village shop (grocer's) and walks daily between home and work. During the walk she usually takes the opportunity to chat with her neighbours.

She raised three children, who live close to her. The youngest daughter lives with her two grandchildren several metres from her home and visits her daily, providing her with the necessary support. Her oldest son lives a little further away, but even so, Mary goes to have lunch with him every Saturday. Whenever the weather permits, she goes on foot. The middle child lives outside the village, so in this case Mary uses the phone to keep in touch.

Every weekend she attends mass, on Saturday or Sunday, depending on which day is the more convenient.

Usually she sleeps between 22:00 and 06:00, and for relaxation her favourite companion is the television.

As the years have gone by, she has had more difficulty in following her routines – she suffers from hypertension and varicose veins. She has been taking more and more breaks and having longer rests.

Mary cooks her own food and brings her groceries home daily. In the main she uses her gas stove and microwave oven. Despite having recently acquired a mobile phone and a washing machine, she finds it difficult to use them without assistance. She has never used a computer.

Use Case

— Maria's new smartphone has a C&M Application. Her son installed it in order that she could be confident in maintaining her daily mobility.
— Even when she feels tired on her way to the shop, she is confident that if she falls or lingers longer than usual, one of her children will be alerted and will probably contact her or will even come to help her.
— On the other hand, she can also find the nearest safe place, in case she decides to choose a different route. That is why she uses the C&M - she uses the magnifier icon on the main screen and selects her neighbour, based on house and face picture – she hates to dial and write names to contact! In dangerous situations she can always call for help using the main screen S.O.S shortcut.
— Once she is very near, she decides to ring and announce her arrival for a small chat… and rest!

Persona 2: Leandro Silva, ex-farmer.
Leandro's goal: Walk about in the city that he doesn't know, and feel safe there.

Leandro is 78 years old, and because his wife recently died, he was left alone and went to live with his son Joel in the city. He used to work as a farmer, having studied only up to the end of the 4th year of schooling.

This is the first time he has left his home town. Although Joel has enrolled him in the day care facility, he likes to walk around, to look at the magazines at the kiosk and to rest in a public garden in his locality. Once in a while there are some football games on the café's TV and he likes to go there and watch them. He would like to have a small pet – to keep him company during the day and to accompany him around the city. But Joel worries about his solitary wanderings tries to discourage him from doing so.

He performs his daily toilet on his own and manages to prepare tea or a simple meal – ever since Joel showed him how to use the main kitchenware.

In the evening he turns on the TV while waiting for the rest of the family to arrive home. Together they chat a little and eventually play some cards.

Use Case

— Every day, before going out, Leandro makes sure he doesn't forget his mobile phone. It has an app with a compass and a magnifier that reassure him about his way home...
— When he decides do walk around the corner he looks at the compass and con-firms that he is going in the right direction for the pharmacy – where he went two weeks ago to buy his medicine.
— He is sure about the way home, but in any case, he knows that if something hap-pened his son or the institution to which he usually goes in the afternoon would be contacted.

4   Compass and Magnifier

In order to define C&M App, we describe the functional system specification and interface design.

4.1   Functional System Specification

In Fig. 1 a C&M Unified Modelling Language (UML) Use Case is presented, in which we highlight the carer and elderly actors' functionalities.

Carer. The carer is the person responsible for setting up the application. Access to this part of the system requires authentication in order to avoid accidental or unau-thorized data changes. The management is composed of two different sets of func-tionalities.

On the one hand, the functionality "Manage System" allows the editing or valida-tion of the safety area, automatically estimated by the system based on historic users' routes and mobility variables such as time, locations, distances and user speed. These variables are automatically collected by the system, which produces a commutation profile in order to monitor users' behaviour during daily mobility. The Carer can ac-cess the commutation profile and validate or rectify it in order to properly adapt the system's monitoring to user needs. In addition, the system management includes the configuration of contacts that should receive the system's warnings in case of an ab-normal situation such as falls or long delays.

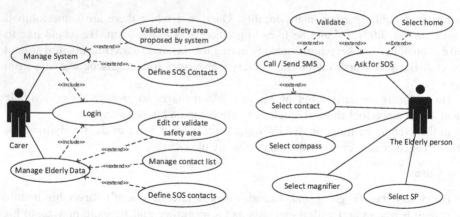

Fig. 1. C&M UML Use Case diagram

On the other hand, the functionality "Manage Elderly Data" concentrates the attention of the Carer on the elderly user. The definition of safety areas is one of its subtasks concerning the user's movement through exterior environments. If the user enters a zone outside the safe area, an SOS event is generated. The Carer can also manage the user contact list.

The Elderly Person. The elderly person is the central character in the system. On his/her needs everything hinges. He/she can select a safety point (SP) as destination from the available SP list on magnifier mode. Then he/she might follow the orientation provided by the compass mode, which indicates the path from the user location to the selected destination.

At any location, if the user selects the magnifier mode, the system sorts the SP according to distance in order to inform him/her about the current location and the nearest SPs. If the system detects that the user has strayed from the safety area, or that he/she has fallen or is not adhering to his/her scheduled or common routines, it will trigger an SOS event and suggest to the user an "Ask for SOS" action. If the user ignores the action and remains outside the safe zone, the system will send a message to the pre-selected contacts. Otherwise the user can cancel or confirm the action.

The "Ask for SOS" action can also be triggered by the user if he/she becomes frightened. In this case, the system automatically selects home as SP destination.

Finally, the user can contact any relatives on the contact list by voice or SMS.

4.2   Interface Design

The main design concepts of this App are the two common physical tools used daily to assist people in doing some tasks: the magnifier is used to help see and read information, and the compass is used to find the way.

The App aims to summarise and show most relevant information at a certain moment, in a single and permanent circle that doesn't change when the screen is being turned round, Fig. 2. The user does not need to search for the information as it is always in the same place.

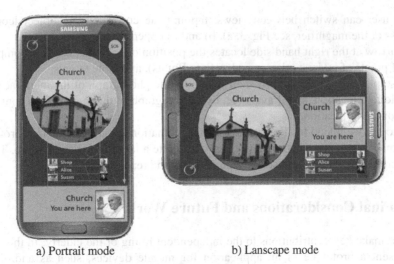

a) Portrait mode   b) Lanscape mode

Fig. 2. C&M layouts modes

The main screen can be presented as a magnifier view or as a compass view, Fig. 3.

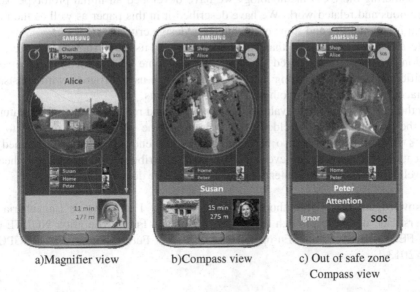

a)Magnifier view   b)Compass view   c) Out of safe zone
                                                   Compass view

Fig. 3. C&M views

When the user stops, the App screen shows the magnifier view, Fig. 3 a), which allows the user to select a certain target. When the user is moving, the App screen shows the compass view, Fig. 3 b), which gives directions to the selected target. If no target is selected, the user's home will be the system's default. For both views, the same circle occupies the centre of the screen. Alternatively appears the "handle" of the Magnifier or the "pointer" of the Compass.

The user can switch between views, tapping the corresponding object icon, the compass or the magnifier, see Fig. 3, a), b) and c) upper left icon.

An arrow at the right hand side locates the position of each menu that accompanies a list of points of interest (also named as Safe Points), available targets.

These places are identified by their name, by the photograph of the main façade of the building / location, and if available, by a photograph of the main person connected to that building/location.

Although we intend to allow some other combinations or styles, this first prototype of the interface is presented in dark blue, with quite a large font size in white. This is considered a good compromise between contrast and readability.

5   Final Considerations and Future Work

ICT can make key contributions to the independent living of the elderly. In this paper we present a prototype of an application for mobile devices, such as androids or smartphones, called Compass and Magnifier. It seeks to promote people's confidence in maintaining daily mobility, realizing the importance of those daily activities for active ageing.

Considering the UCD methodology we have developed an initial prototype based on previous and related work. We have described it in this paper as well as the main system functionalities and some of the interface design criteria.

We are aware of the fact that this work is still in its early stages. However, the solution we have encountered already satisfies some of the main requirements identified. It is based on strong metaphors and allows us to progress with consistent interfaces and menus, among other important statements.

In the next stage we will evaluate this prototype and redesign some of its features, with the participation of an elderly target group. Some requirements relating to the carer's point of view will also be developed. In the end we will have designed an application that helps to achieve our main goal: contributing to the elderly's health and wellbeing based on the potential of ICT and mobile devices.

Acknowledgements. The authors thank the FEUP – Faculdade de Engenharia da Universidade do Porto through the Project I-City for Future Mobility: NORTE-07-0124-FEDER-000064, and European Project FP7 - Future Cities: FP7-REGPOT-2012-2013-1.

References

1. Rowland, D.T.: Population Aging - The Transformation of Societies. Springer (2012)
2. Ministry of Labour and Social Affairs of the Czech Republic: Quality of Life in Old Age - National Programme of Preparation for Ageing for 2008 – 2012. MLSA, Prague (2008)
3. Plaza, I., Martín, L., Martin, S., Medrano, C.: Mobile applications in an aging society: Status and trends. J. Syst. Softw. 84, 1977–1988 (2011)

4. Gaßner, K., Conrad, M.: ICT enabled independent living for elderly. A status-quo analysis on products and the research landscape in the field of Ambient Assisted Living (AAL) in EU-27 (2010)
5. Burrows, A., Mitchell, V., Nicolle, C.A.: The over 50s and their motivations for using technology (2010)
6. Hallal, P.C., Andersen, L.B., Bull, F.C., Guthold, R., Haskell, W., Ekelund, U.: Global physical activity levels: surveillance progress, pitfalls, and prospects. The Lancet. 380, 247–257 (2012)
7. Commission of the European Communities: A white paper on a strategy for Europe on nutrition, overweight and obesity related health issues, http://eur-lex.europa.eu/LexUriServ/LexUriServ.do?uri=COM:2007:0279:FIN:EN:PDF
8. GPS Elderly Tracking System, http://www.tracking-system.com/for-consumers/gps-elderly-tracking-system.html
9. GPS Smart Shoe, GPS Shoes, GPS Devices, GTX Corp, GTXO, Track your loved ones. GPS Smart Shoe, Aetrex, http://www.gpsshoe.com/
10. AlzNav - Aplicações Android no Google Play, https://play.google.com/store/apps/details?id=pt.fraunhofer.navigator
11. Tweri: localizador Alzheimer - Aplicações Android no Google Play, https://play.google.com/store/apps/details?id=es.solusoft.tweri
12. One Touch SOS - Aplicações Android no Google Play, https://play.google.com/store/apps/details?id=com.ideophone.sos
13. BIG Launcher para Android, http://biglauncher.com/pt/
14. Ferreira, F., Dias, F., Braz, J., Santos, R., Nascimento, R., Ferreira, C., Martinho, R.: Protege: A Mobile Health Application for the Elder-caregiver Monitoring Paradigm. Procedia Technol. 9, 1361–1371 (2013)
15. Valley Rocket LLC: Daily Commute, https://itunes.apple.com/us/app/daily-commute/id499636507?mt=8
16. Maps - Aplicações Android no Google Play, https://play.google.com/store/apps/details?id=com.google.android.apps.maps
17. User centered system design: new perspectives on human-computer interaction. L. Erlbaum Associates, Hillsdale (1986)
18. Pruitt, J., Grudin, J.: Personas: Practice and Theory. In: Proceedings of the 2003 Conference on Designing for User Experiences, pp. 1–15. ACM, New York (2003)
19. Blomkvist, S.: Persona - an overview. In: Extract from the Paper The User as a Personality. Using Personas as a Tool for Design. Position Paper for the Course Workshop, Theoretical perspectives in Human-Computer Interaction, IPLab, KTH (September 3, 2002), http://tinyurl.com/y8kaojf
20. Human-computer interaction. Pearson/Prentice-Hall, Harlow, England (2004)
21. Cockburn, A.: Writing effective use cases. Addison-Wesley, Boston (2001)
22. Dewsbury, G., Sommerville, I., Bagnall, P., Rouncefield, M., Onditi, V.: Software Co-design with Older People. In: Clarkson, J., Langdon, P., Robinson, P. (eds.) Designing Accessible Technology, pp. 199–208. Springer, London (2006)

Towards Mobile Accessibility for Older People:
A User Centered Evaluation

José-Manuel Díaz-Bossini, Lourdes Moreno, and Paloma Martínez

Computer Science Department, Universidad Carlos III de Madrid,
Avda. Universidad 30, 28911 Leganés, Madrid, Spain
{josemanuel.diaz,lourdes.moreno,paloma.martinez}@uc3m.es

Abstract. As people age, they experience a decline in a wide variety of their abilities such as vision, hearing, mobility and so on. Mobile technologies could be used to improve their quality of life in a wide set of situations such as security, autonomy or personal communication. One of the main threats in the use of mobile devices by our elders is the accessibility barriers that exist on the devices and mobile applications. Unfortunately, addressing these issues is even harder in new devices like smartphones or tablets where there is not a proper set of guidelines focusing on this domain. Based on our own set of accessibility guidelines, an accessibility evaluation of two mobile applications with elderly involvement has been carried out in this work. The outcomes support the suitability of the set of accessibility guidelines proposed as a method to evaluate; on the other hand the data collected from the study with users provide interesting findings about the perception of the older users when they interacting with mobile applications.

Keywords: Accessibility, Older people, Android, Mobile Interfaces, evaluation.

1 Introduction

According to the European Commission [3] in early 2012, 17,8 % of the European population had 65 years old or over, and the 4,9 % had 80 years old or over. That is, almost a quarter of the European Population could be considered as older population. This number will grow up exponentially in the years to come.

Maybe older people don't use the mobile devices in the same way that other younger users but, in fact, what older users expect from mobile communications is not very different from what generic users expect; mainly, personal communication and services to improve their safety and quality of life [4].

Nevertheless, this trend will change in a few years from now, when the middle-age population becomes the new elderly population. We've all grown up using personal computers, mobile devices, and in general, any device that makes our lives easier.

In fact, now our elders use mobile devices to keep the contact with their families or use simple applications that help them in their daily basis. More and more, mobile devices and new technologies are used to improve the quality of life of older people by using for example Medical Assistance applications, smart houses, and so on.

C. Stephanidis and M. Antona (Eds.): UAHCI/HCII 2014, Part III, LNCS 8515, pp. 58–68, 2014.
© Springer International Publishing Switzerland 2014

Sadly, this improvement of the quality of life of our elders is not possible for everyone. In fact, there are a substantial number of people that is being excluded because they are affected with one, or more than one, disabilities.

Address accessibility issues are not a simple task but is even harder in the mobile context where the devices and technologies evolves faster than the accessibility problems are addressed.

In this paper, we proposed a checklist in order to improve the accessibility of mobile interfaces. This checklist mobile accessibility guidelines is an improved version of one developed previously. This checklist is being used to conduct expert evaluations. In order to demonstrate the suitability of this resource and conduct a more complete accessibility evaluation following a User Centered Design (UCD) approach [2], this paper includes the elderly users' participation in an evaluation of mobile Apps.

Section 2 shows the background and related work in this topic. Section 3 details the experimental design for the evaluation by older users of the Mobile applications. The analysis and the results of the study are discussed in Section 4. Finally, Section 5 exposes the conclusions and the future work of this research.

2   Background

As we said above, mobile devices and technologies are evolving so fast. This continuous evolution implies new challenges to be tackled. Accessibility issues have been, and will be, one of these challenges.

The Web Accessibility Initiative (WAI) from the World Wide Web Consortium (W3C) is working on adapt the Web Content Accessibility Guidelines (WCAG) and the User Agent Accessibility Guidelines in the mobile context [5].

Many authors have studied the accessibility and usability issues and propose many guidelines or a set of best practices that could be applied to the mobile context too [6], [7], [8].

Mobile operating system providers such as Google, Microsoft or Apple provide some guidance to develop accessible application for their operating systems [9], [10].

During years, mobile devices have not been designed with older people in mind and are often difficult for them to use and excluding them from the technologies. Several studies demonstrated that a mobile device or application, if carefully designed, can be used effectively by older people [11],[12].

Nowadays, we have better devices with better screens and powerful technologies that are most appropriated to be used by older people. Nevertheless, apps are not normally created with older users in mind.

Most of the studies developed to investigate mobile applications for older people share the same starting point: the important premise that "elderly people want to stay and live in their homes as independently and as long as possible" [13].

This is not a trivial issue, because older people are not a homogenous group of users, so design apps for older people is a hard task. In the literature, we can found several guidelines (mostly focused on web applications not in mobile apps) that try to address the design issues for older people [14] [15] [16].

3   Previous Work

The previous work [1] provided a set of guidelines to keep in mind in order to achieve accessibility in mobile interfaces for older people. This set is provided in a list of checkpoints or checklist. This checklist is the result of a review study of the literature, accessibility standards and best practices that are being performed in this knowledge area, by using of this check-list of accessibility aimed at elderly people, a survey of three mobile native Apps on Android platform was carried out by accessibility expert.

3.1   Checklist Mobile Accessibility Guidelines for Older People

A set of criteria collected from different sources and focused mainly on older people was provided.   This set of criteria has been improved, some of them has been erased; because some of them are good criteria to address accessibility issues, but they are not good enough to solve or to improve the accessibility for older people and they were replaced by another ones.

The different sources were accessibility standards and guidelines established by the W3C [5], from the literature [6], [7], [8] and finally from the accessibility best practices recommended by Apple and Google in their application developers guides [9], [10].

The result has been a checklist mobile accessibility for older people. This checklist is provided through barriers common to mobile device. The table 1 shows this checklist; a code and brief description of each checkpoint (barrier common) is described.

Table 1. Checklist proposed to address accessibility issues for older people

Code	Description of accessibility barrier
W3CP001	Information conveyed using color (for example, "required material is shown in red") with no redundancy.
W3CP002	Non-text objects (images, sound, video) without text alternative
W3CU001	Long words, long and complex sentences, jargon
W3CU002	Content spawning new windows without warning user.
W3CU003	Blinking, moving, scrolling or auto-updating content
WDG-TD	Unsuitable Target Design (larger targets, clear confirmation of target capture, etc.)
WDG-UG	Use of unsuitable Graphics or not accessible (Graphics should be relevant, images with alt tag, etc.)
WDG-BWF	Unsuitable design features for browser windows (Avoid scroll bars, only one open window)
WDG-CLD	Not accessible content and unsuitable layout Design (Language should be simple and clear, highlight important information, etc.)
WDG-UCD	Unsuitable design according to cognitive barriers (Provide ample time to read information, support recognition rather than recall)

Table 1. (*continued*)

Code	Description of accessibility barrier
WDG-UCB	Unsuitable Use of Color and Background (Colors should be used conservatively, background not in pure white or change rapidly in brightness between screens, insufficient contrast, etc.)
Android001	No provide redundant information for information only auditory (Make sure that audio prompts are always accompanied by another visual prompt or notification, to assist users who are deaf or hard of hearing)
Android 002	Forms difficult to understand. Interface controls have properly labels and these labels are understandable and descriptive
GB001	Opaque Objects. The page contains components (eg. a Flash object) that is totally opaque to screen readers
GB002	Too many links. A large number of links requires that users perform a lengthy and exerting activity when listening to all of them.

3.2   Accessibility Audit/Expert Evaluation

We performed the evaluation of three different apps [1]: Big Launcher [17], Fontrillo [18] and Mobile Accessibility for Android (MAA) [19]. These Apps have as aim to modify the default interface for another more accessible one.

An expert on mobile accessibility was carried out an evaluation. He tested each checkpoint of Table 1 for each App. The results of study indicated Big Launcher is the most accessible for older people of the three applications.

In order to conduct a more complete accessibility evaluation following a User Centered Design (UCD) approach with the elderly users' participation, a user tests are presented in this paper.

4   Experimental Design

We performed a study with the participation of older users. This study is composed of three different stages. First of all, older users had to perform some easy and day by day tasks with two applications. Second, we performed an interview to each user guided by a set of question that will be shown later on this paper. Finally, a user survey was carried out and the results are presented.

4.1   Object of Study

We focus this study on perform an accessibility evaluation of two different applications from the Google Play Store with real older users and taking into account the Checklist Mobile accessibility guidelines for older people (see Table 1).

The evaluation was performed with 8 participants (two men and six women) with ages between 65 and 82.

4.2   Sample APP's

The Apps of the sample modify the mobile interfaces to convert them in more accessible interfaces for people with disabilities or elderly people.

From three different apps (Big Launcher, Fontrillo and Mobile Accessibility) evaluated in previous work, we have removed the Mobile Accessibility for Android for this study, because although it is a really good accessible app, it is focused mainly on blind people and does not fit exactly with the study target.

The BigLauncher application was tested on its 2.3.4 version (latest version available). Since our latest analysis in the previous work BigLauncher doesn't evolve so much.

The evaluation of the Fontrillo Application has been made in its 1.1.2 version (latest version available). Since our latest analysis, in contrast to Big Launcher, Fontrillo has had a considerable number of changes. This version includes some new functionalities that increases the app value like an alphabetical ordered keyboard, screen to configure favorite apps, etc.

Figure 1 shows screenshots of the BigLauncher App on the left and Fontrillo App on the right.

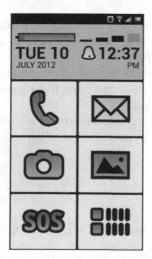 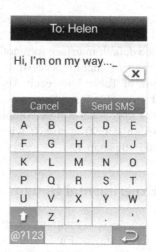

Fig. 1. Main screenshot of BigLauncher App (left) and text input main screenshot of Fontrillo App (right)

All these apps have good acceptance by users and they are highly scored in the Google Play Store. The score of Big Launcher App in the Google Play Store is 4,3 out of 5 stars and Fontrillo has 4,4 out of 5 stars.

4.3   Participants

In this study 8 users with ages between 65 and 82 years old have participated. The users had different cultural levels and different know-how in the use of Smartphones.

None of them have a severe disability but they have some visual, understanding or ability issues. The table 2 shows the characteristics of users.

Table 2. Users information

	U1	U2	U3	U4	U5	U6	U7	U8
Age	65	69	82	72	68	71	68	70
Device	LG optimus L5 II	Samsung Galaxy S	Galaxy S4	Huawei Ascend W2	Huawei Y300	Samsung Galaxy Ace	BQ Aquaris 5	Samsung Galaxy S
Disability	Glasses	N/A	Manual Dexterity, Glasses	Glasses	Glasses	Glasses	N/A	Glasses
Gender	Woman	Woman	Woman	Woman	Woman	Man	Man	Woman
Studies	Primary	Primary	Secondary	Primary	Primary	Primary	Primary	Primary
Smartphone used for	Calls, text	Calls, Texts	Calls	Calls, Text, Pictures	Calls, Text, Pictures	Calls	Calls, Text, Pictures	Calls
Problems using a Smartphone	Iconography, Small Fonts, Understand the apps	Understand the apps	Mobility. She uses a pointer device.	Iconography, Small Fonts	Iconography, Small Fonts	Iconography, Small Fonts	Understand the apps	Understand the apps and small fonts
Time using a smartphone	Over 2 years	Between 1-2 years	2 years	Less than 1 year	Between 2 and 3 years	Less than 1 yeas	Between 2- 3 years	Between 1-2 years

4.4 Procedure

We perform two different sessions with the participants. During the first one, perform a simple and brief explanation of our research. In the second session we teach them how to install the applications and demand them to perform some simple tasks with both applications. Finally, for each user we perform a structured interview with the use of a questionnaire based on the Checklist Mobile accessibility guidelines for older people (see Table 1).

We define a list of day-to-day tasks and a high-skilled task that the users should try to carry out with both applications. We didn't give them any support while they were carrying out these tasks.

The simple tasks included the following:

- Make a call
- Looking for a contact
- To add a contact

- Text a contact
- Review the calls list
- Take a picture
- Look for the picture you just take
- Search for whatsapp application and use it.

The high-skilled task consist on configure the emergency call number.

Each user has his/her own device and the accessibility tools, provided by the Android Operating System (TalkBack and the Explore by Touch) features were disabled (because they haven't got any severe visual disability).

4.5   Questionnaires

Once our users had performed the task commented on Section 4.4, we had an structured interview with each one. We conduct these interviews through a questionnaire (see Table 3) that has been designed based on the checklist (see Table 1). So besides that we carried out the evaluation of users, we have been able to validate the suitability of the proposed checklist comparing data resulting from the analysis of experts with users.

The questionnaire is composed by three different types of questions which allowed us to collect different data (qualitative and quantitative):

- Personal Questions: These questions allow us to collect data for statistical purposes (age, experience, etc.)
- Question based on each criteria of the checklist: These questions will be the core of our research and are based on the criteria established. Users must grade their answers between 1 to 5; where 1 mean totally disagree and 5 totally agree.
- Qualitative Questions: These questions are useful to obtain users opinion because answers are opened answers and users can explain their answers.

The complete collection of questions is shown on table 3.

Table 3. Questionnaire used in evaluation with elder users

Personal questions
Age
Mobile Device
Disability/Disabilities
Gender
Educational Level
Do you use your smartphone mainly for ...? (calls, internet, messages, ...)
Do you have any problem when you use your smartphone? (small fonts, understanding, ...)
How long have you been using a smartphone?

Table 3. (*continued*)

Questions based on the criteria (graded between 1 and 5)
The Application language is understandable   (W3CU001)
Popups makes me hard the use of the application (W3CU002)
Blink and scrolling makes hard to interact with the application (W3CU003)
Iconographies and links are larger enough to interact with them (WDG-TD)
Iconography is understandable (WDG-UG)
Popups or alert messages makes hard to use the application (WGG-BWF)
Application provides ample time to read the information important information appears highlighted (WDG-CLD)
Background colors and icons colors are appropriate   (WDG-UCD)
Interface buttons and controls have appropriate text captions (Android 001)
Audio prompts are always accompanied by another visual prompt (Android002)
There are so many links or buttons that make me hard to understand and to use the application (GB002)
Qualitative questions
Which application do you prefer?
What is the main strength of the application you choose?
What is the main weakness of the application you choose?
What is the main strength of the application **you didn't** choose?
What is the main weakness of the application **you didn't** choose?

4.6   Evaluation Method

Statistical and qualitative data have been produced by user answers.   These data have been used to provide the analysis and the discussion of the results. By the way, for each criterion, except for those related to the use of screen readers and high visual disabilities, we had a different question that could be graded from 1 to 5, the final result for each criterion/question will be the average between them.

In next section we provide the scores for each criterion and the analysis of the results.

5   Analysis and Results

Regarding to the user answers to questions based on the checklist. Table 4 shows the average and standard deviation between each answer. Both applications got similar scores. The standard deviations are small with a few exceptions; this data indicates that most of the users have close answers.

Most of the criteria have obtained high scores, with the exceptions of the answers concerning to the checkpoints W3CU002 and WDG-BWF. It is due to open new windows (Popups) without notice to users, multiple windows open or scrolls that hinder the use of interfaces in the two app. The answers concerning to the checkpoint GB002 get low scores, it is because users have the perception that the interfaces have too many links with the consequent effort involved access to many links for older people.

Table 4. Averages and the standard deviations of the user answers

Criteria	BigLauncher		Fontrillo	
	Average	St. dev.	Average	St. dev.
W3CU001	4,38	0,74	4,00	0,76
W3CU002	1,38	0,52	1,13	0,35
W3CU003	3,38	0,74	3,88	0,64
WDG-TD	4,25	0,71	4,50	0,53
WDG-UG	4,25	0,71	3,13	1,25
WDG-BWF	1,50	0,53	1,75	0,71
WDG-CLD	4,00	0,76	2,63	0,52
WDG-UCD	4,50	0,53	4,13	0,83
WDG-UCB	4,50	0,53	4,63	0,52
Android001	4,25	0,71	4,00	0,76
Android 002	4,63	0,52	4,38	0,52
GB002	2,50	0,53	2,38	0,74

The most valuated criteria were those that improve the interaction with the application like WDG-TD or WDG-UG for example; and those that improve the cognitive design like WDG-UCB or Android 002.

The results of the open questions indicate that the users remarked that BigLauncher app is so easy to use; they all committed the simple task and many of them even the high-level skilled task. Regarding Fontrillo app, most of them remarked that this application is more complete than BigLauncher but that it is a little harder to use and to understand. They all completed the easy tasks (but using a little bit of time that with BigLauncher). High-skilled task was only accomplished by two of them. Fontrillo has a minimum advantage over BigLauncher, but users prefer BigLauncher because, according to them, it was easier to use. In the other hand, users said that Fontrillo has more functionalities which they like as the alphabetical keyboard for text.

Users agree that both applications are accessible and useful for they needs but, as we said before, according to the qualitative answers most of them prefer BigLauncher because its interface is easier to use. This is because the BigLauncher interface is very visual, includes big icons with metaphors that users understand well. In this way, Fontrillo is not as visual. Also Fontrillo has transitions from left to right to move from one interface to another which users do not understand. Users understand better and are more comfortable with BigLauncher that includes only a main interface, and they do not need to navigate. Only two users (U5 y U7) chose Fontrillo and they were those that had been using smartphones since long time ago.

As a curiosity, the user (U5) said his favorite application was BigLauncher, however she changed his mind, and finally she decided that the best application was Fontrillo because it included a flashlight, and this functionality it is essential for her.

With regard to app versions evaluated in previous work, the new version of Fontrillo under study improves considerably the weaknesses that it had. New version accomplish with most of the criteria established. BigLauncher doesn't add new functionalities that could be useful for older people. Finally, in order to analyze the suitability of the checklist developed by the authors, the results of user reviews coincide with the evaluation carried out in previous work by the expert, this similarity of results indicates that the Checklist itself could be a valid tool to evaluate the accessibility of mobile applications for the elderly

6   Conclusions and Future Work

In this paper we continued with the research started in 2013 that tried to collect a set of accessibility criteria or best practices that could be applied to mobile interfaces for older users. We reviewed the set of criteria and improved it by adding new criteria and deleting those ones that don't fit well with our target audience.

In addition, and to test the suitability of our checklist, we performed an evaluation of two android applications, Big Launcher and Fontrillo, with eight users with ages between 65 and 82 years old. We designed a set of easy tasks that they had to perform and a set of questions that they had to answer after they have been using both applications.

According to the results, both applications get similar results, and users concluded that both applications would fit well for they needs; most of them, preferred Big Launcher because, according to their answers, is easy to use.

As main weaknesses, in this evaluation none of the users had any kind of severe disability, so criteria focused on address concrete accessibility issues such vision, hearing, and so on couldn't be correctly evaluated (they don't use any kind of accessibility tool such as Talkback).

We want to perform more studies over our checklist, next steps could be to make it extensible to iOS or Windows Phone applications and to extend this checklist to new features such as those that are task-oriented like call or info search or those that are context-dependent like videophone or desktop application.

Acknowledgements. This work was supported by the Regional Government of Madrid under the Research Network MA2VICMR [S2009/TIC-1542], by the Spanish Ministry of Education under the project MULTIMEDICA [TIN2010-20644-C03-01] and by the European Commission Seventh Framework Programme under the project TrendMiner (EU FP7-ICT 287863).

References

1. Díaz-Bossini, J.M., Moreno, L.: Accessibility to mobile interfaces for older people. In: 5th International Conference on Software Development and Technologies for Enhancing Accessibility and Fighting Info-exclusion (DSAI 2013), Vigo, Spain (November 2013)
2. Preece, J., Rogers, Y., Sharp, H.: Interaction design: Beyond human-computer interaction. John Wiley & Sons, New York (2002)
3. Andueza Robustillo, S., Corsini, V., Marcu, M., Vasileva, K., Estat, D.G., Marchetti, E., Empl, D.G.: EU Employment and Social Situation (February 2013)

4. Abascal, J., Civit, A.: Mobile communication for older people: new opportunities for autonomous life. In: Proceedings of EC/NSF Workshop on Universal Accessibility of Ubiquitous Computing: Providing for the Elderly, vol. 487 (2001)
5. Mobile Accessibility,
   `http://www.w3.org/WAI/mobile/Overview.html#covered`
6. Zaphiris, P., Ghiawadwala, M., Mughal, S.: Age-centered research-based web design guidelines. In: CHI 2005 Extended Abstracts on Human Factors in Computing Systems, New York, NY, USA, pp. 1897–1900 (2005)
7. Ownby, R.L.: Making the Internet a Friendlier Place for Older People. Generations 30(2), 58–60 (2006)
8. Barrier walkthrough - Giorgio Brajnik,
   `http://sole.dimi.uniud.it/~giorgio.brajnik/projects/bw/bw.html#nv_d7e55`
9. Accessibility | Android Developers,
   `http://developer.android.com/guide/topics/ui/accessibility/index.html`
10. Accessibility for Developers - Apple Developer,
    `https://developer.apple.com/accessibility/`
11. Goodman, J., Brewster, S., Gray, P.: Older people, mobile devices and navigation. In: HCI Older Popul., pp. 13–14 (2004)
12. Massimi, M., Baecker, R.M., Wu, M.: Using participatory activities with seniors to critique, build, and evaluate mobile phones. In: Proceedings of the 9th International ACM SIGACCESS Conference on Computers and Accessibility, pp. 155–162 (2007)
13. Plaza, I., Martín, L., Martin, S., Medrano, C.: Mobile applications in an aging society: Status and trends. J. Syst. Softw. 84(11), 1977–1988 (2011)
14. Zimmermann, G., Vanderheiden, G.: Accessible design and testing in the application development process: considerations for an integrated approach. Univers. Access Inf. Soc. 7(1-2), 117–128 (2008)
15. Sloan, D., Atkinson, M.T., Machin, C., Li, Y.: The potential of adaptive interfaces as an accessibility aid for older web users. In: Proceedings of the 2010 International Cross Disciplinary Conference on Web Accessibility (W4A), p. 35 (2010)
16. Hellman, R.: Universal design and mobile devices. In: Stephanidis, C. (ed.) HCI 2007. LNCS, vol. 4554, pp. 147–156. Springer, Heidelberg (2007)
17. BIG Launcher para Android, `http://biglauncher.com/`
18. Fontrillo: smartphones made simple!, `http://www.fontrillo.com/`
19. Android for the blind,
    `http://www.codefactory.es/en/products.asp?id=415`

Design of a Social Game for Older Users Using Touchscreen Devices and Observations from an Exploratory Study

Lilian Genaro Motti[1], Nadine Vigouroux[1], and Philippe Gorce[2]

[1] IRIT UMR 5505, Université de Toulouse 3 Paul Sabatier,
118 Route de Narbonne, 31062 Toulouse, France
`{lilian.genaro-motti,vigourou}@irit.fr`
[2] HandiBio EA 4322, Université du Sud Toulon Var,
Avenue de l'université, 83957 Toulon, France
`gorce@univ-tln.fr`

Abstract. Previous studies about tactile interaction by older adults show some important design considerations that should be applied in order to create more usable and accessible applications. The related results have been applied during the development of a serious game destined to support a social activity with older adults using touchscreen devices. An exploratory study investigates the use of touchscreen mobile devices by 17 older adults and 5 children. The results of an empirical observation allow a description of the participants' appreciation of touchscreen devices, a typology of common errors, the gesture strategies of tactile interaction and design proposals to support interaction.

Keywords: Serious game, interaction techniques, touchscreen, older adults, interaction error, participative user-centered method.

1 Introduction

Older adults' attitudes towards new technologies can interfere the way they perceive and interact with technologies. The subjective evaluation of handiness, control and ease of use of technologies can prevent from anxiety, misgivings and reluctance [1]. Touchscreen devices are perceived as ready-to-use and manipulate thanks to the mobility of the devices and direct interaction on the display screen [2]. Besides, the popularization of touchscreen mobile devices and their perceived usefulness are impacting their acceptance and older adults' motivations.

Digital games have entertainment and therapeutic values for older users [3]. They could be used to learn interaction techniques, prevent from technological exclusion and support social activities.

In order to evaluate the use of social and ludic activities to facilitate the discovering of touchscreen devices, we designed a serious game. The system "Puzzle Touch" is consisted of tactile puzzle games. The pieces of the puzzle representing parts of an image should be re-arranged by tactile interaction. The images used for the puzzle

C. Stephanidis and M. Antona (Eds.): UAHCI/HCII 2014, Part III, LNCS 8515, pp. 69–78, 2014.

games represented views of the city where the participants live in, extracted from old pictures, postcards, maps and engravings provided by the city hall archives.

Age-related changes on functional skills and little experience with technologies are pointed out as factors affecting usability issues of digital games [3]. Besides, older users special needs and difficulties have to be taken into account when designing or developing applications destined to their use. Several studies evaluated interaction techniques and interfaces for older adults and they provide important information to conceive more accessible and usable interactive systems.

This paper describes how the results of previous experiments were applied during the design of the social game "Puzzle Touch".

This game was installed on 7 handheld touchscreen devices with different screen sizes (3.5 to 10 inches) and allowing pen or finger interaction. 17 older adults (58 to 85 years old) participated of this exploratory study. 5 children (9 years old) were invited to join one group of participants in order to create inter-generational activity. The activity took place in a public place where the participants were used to take computer lessons.

The next section 2 presents some related work. Then, the conception phase presents how the related studies results have been included on the development of this system, on section 3. Our exploratory study is presented on section 4. Section 5 presents the results of this study, including participant's appreciation, a typology of common errors and an analysis of gesture strategies. Finally, section 6 presents a conclusion and some perspectives for future work.

2   Related Work

Several studies evaluated interaction techniques for older adults using touchscreen devices and provided guidelines and recommendations for conceiving more accessible and usable systems and applications [4–11]. Literature review about tactile interaction of older users shows that several parameters should be taken into account during the design phases of an application [12]. Some reviews focus on one specific situations of use, as recommendations for mobile phones [13] or the use of handheld computers [14].

Older adults are a heterogeneous populations due to the individual age related changes and the evolution of their characteristics [15, 16]. Several studies suggest participatory activities to conceive devices and systems, including future users during the development phases to get their point of view and feedback [14, 17]. However it is not easy to include older users on research studies [17]. One of the reasons is transport or displacement to the university or laboratory. Besides, controlled activities can be used for specific studies but they are sometimes very different than ecological and realistic situations of use. Some authors proposed group studies or working in pairs during the experiments in order to help users feel comfortable and observe the possibilities of partnership and support [18–20].

Older users could really benefit from some advantages of touchscreen and handheld portable devices. In addition to health care and medical assistance applications

[2, 21], games and ludic activities can be helpful to maintain social activities and networks [3, 22], providing cognitive stimulation and also initiating new users to technologies.

The next section describes how the results of previous studies about interaction techniques for older adults using touchscreen have been applied for conceiving a system destined to support a social activity with older users. Then, an exploratory study is conducted on a familiar place where participants were used to take computer lessons.

3   Conception of a System to Support a Social Activity with Older Users Using Touchscreen Mobile Devices

The objective of this system is to help older adults discovering touchscreen handheld devices and learning tactile interaction techniques. The serious game "Puzzle Touch" should also support a social activity, facilitating the acceptance and affecting user's attitudes towards new technologies. The observation of the interactions should provide information about the users' difficulties and strategies.

The system should be suitable to the different screen sizes of handheld devices. The chosen orientation mode is portrait so right handed and left handed users could use the same gestures. This configuration has also been successfully used in two previous studies [7, 22], by consequent targets will be initially placed at the bottom of the screen.

The system should support pen and finger interaction. This first version is single-touch: only one piece should be moved at the time.

Some studies about the gestures of interaction of older users indicate a preference for long gestures instead of taps [1, 8, 23, 24]. This system simulate drag and drop on the touch screen: the user touches to select a piece and slips his finger or pen through the screen to move the target (drag). When the user releases the touch, the target stops moving (drop).

Most studies about better target sizes concern only tap interaction. Tapping for selecting targets on vertical monitors (17 inches screen), authors recommend 16 mm targets width and 3 to 6 mm spacing for older users without motor impairment [4]. As the available handheld devices have smaller screen sizes, the system "Puzzle Touch" uses smaller targets sizes. One study concerning tap gestures on a small screen (4.3 inches) compares 5, 8 and 12 mm width targets for 9 targets placed on a 3x3 grid. Target spacing compared is 1 and 3 mm between targets. Authors describe better results when touch selection is followed by audio or audio tactile feedback and bigger target sizes [5]. Another study used 6 mm width targets on small screens size (3.7 inches) during digit input tasks. Results show better performances when the touch is followed by a magnifying visual feedback [9].

For this system, target sizes vary according to the number of puzzle pieces and the screen sizes. The system presents different numbers of targets: 9 large, 12 medium or 16 small pieces according to the game options. As the puzzle pieces are placed randomly in the bottom of the screen, it is not be possible to generate enough spacing between targets and targets can overlay. Our proposal is to add a visual feedback (the touched target is placed on the top of the others) and a thick black border (1 mm) replacing the space between targets (Fig. 1). Target sizes according to the number of puzzle pieces and the screen sizes are detailed on the Table 1.

Table 1. Target sizes according to the screen sizes of two different devices, Galaxy Note II (WXGA 1280x720 Super AMOLED) and Galaxy Note 10.1 (WXGA 1280x800 LCD)

Number of targets	Target sizes on 5 inch screen	Target sizes on 10 inch screen
9	25x16 mm	46x35 mm
12	19x19 mm	19x16 mm
16	35x35 mm	35x27 mm

The interactive system uses old images of the city (postcards, old pictures and engraving reproductions kindly provided by the city hall archive) as well as pictures of historical places. Puzzle games were generated from the selected images, cut on with 9, 12 or 16 rectangular pieces. Images had different colors (grayscale, soft colors or colored photography) and represented different subjects (landscapes, portraits, statues, objects, maps). A watermark is displayed on the background of the grid (30% opacity) (Fig. 2). The task consists of placing the targets on the grid (Fig. 3).

The system should be functional on different operational systems. HTML5, Javascript, JQuery and Php have been chosen as they support all the necessary interaction.

The Table 2 below synthetize the parameters that have been taken into account during the design phase.

Table 2. Characteristics and design choices for the system

Characteristics	Design choices
Task	Target selection, displacement and positioning on the grid
Gesture of interaction	Move (drag and drop)
Target size	Large, medium and small
Target color	Grayscale and color
Target number	9, 12 or 16
Target position	Bottom of the screen
Spacing between targets	Replaced by thick borders (1mm)
Feedback	Visual feedback

4   Exploratory Study

4.1   Methodology

The study was consisted of two sessions with two groups of users. It took place in a public place where the participants were used to take computer lessons. Each section last about 90 minutes:

- 30 minutes: 1) presentation and explanation about the main principles of the game, 2) exchange about the touchscreen devices and 3) interview about participant's previous experiences with puzzle, video games and use of information and communication technologies.
- 60 minutes: free playing, individually or in small groups (2 or 3). Participants were allowed to choose and try the different devices and input techniques. After each game, an electronic questionnaire asked user appreciation.

Data were collected through empirical observation and questionnaires. The interactive system recorded tactile interaction data on the touchscreen. The experimenter observed the activity, took notes and helped the participants to use the devices.

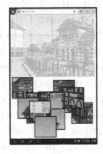

Fig. 1. One piece of the puzzle and the black border

Fig. 2. Screenshot of the puzzle game at the beginning. The targets are randomly placed at the bottom and the grid with a watermark is displayed at the top.

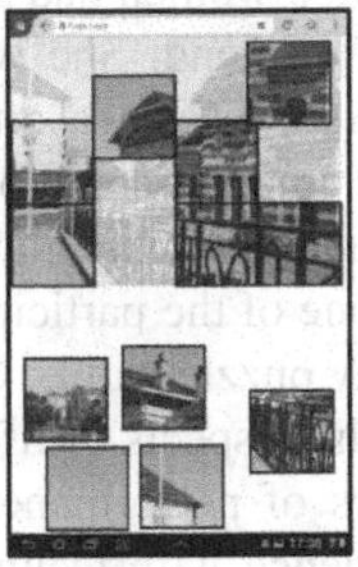

Fig. 3. Screenshot showing a state of the game

4.2 Apparatus

The system described on section 3 were installed in 7 handheld touchscreen devices with different screen sizes and allowing finger or pen interaction: 3 iPads with 9.7 inches screen, 1 Galaxy Note with a 10 inches, 1 Galaxy Note II with a 5 inches screen and a pen, 1 Samsung S3 with a 4.7 inches screen and 1 IPhone with a 3.5 screen.

Table 3. Characteristics according to the situation of use and user's choice

Characteristics	Used devices and situation of use
Situation of use	Inside a room, with tables and chairs, artificial lights and windows. Wi-Fi connection available. Monitors and instructors available to help if needed.
Device position	Handheld or fixed (over a table)
Screen sizes	3.5 to 10 inches, resolution 149 to 306 ppi
Screen orientation	Portrait mode (locked)
Input technique	Single-touch, with finger or pen

4.3   Subjects

The first group was composed of 6 older users, 2 men (58 and 76 years old) and 4 women (66, 67, 75 and 85 years old). The second group was composed of 11 older adults, 4 men (74 to 83 years old) and 7 women (70 to 87 years old) and 5 children, 2 girls and 3 boys (all 9 years old). Two women didn't want to tell their ages, but they had more than 65 years old and they were retired.

According to previous studies about older user's interaction with computers and touchscreen, the age-related changes on cognitive[9], motor [25] and visual skills [22] affect user's performances. The conditions of this study didn't allow measuring the user's skills. Nevertheless some effects related to manual dexterity have been observed and reported.

Three women had some difficulty to use the devices. One of them wore a splint on the right hand. She was right handed, she wasn't able to hold the devices but she could still uses her left hand or the right hand fingers to interact. One had arthritis and complained of some pain on the arms at the end of the section. One had arthrosis and deformation on the index finger. She used the middle finger to interact.

None of the participants were visually impaired uncorrected. All of them were able to play puzzle games with small 16 pieces, even on the 3.5 inches screen device.

Other aspects of life history and individual characteristics can also be used as predictors of performances such as education [20], health conditions [2] and previous experience with technologies [19, 26]. Most of the participants (12 of them) use a computer every day or almost every day. The children do not use a computer so often, but they have more frequent access to touchscreen devices. Only one older participant has a touchscreen tablet and uses it every day or almost every day.

All the participants have already played puzzle games, mostly with jigsaw shapes on cardboard. Only one older adult plays it regularly. Three older adults use to play electronic games almost every day (Facebook apps, online Flash games, computer games with conventional input techniques as mouse and keyboard).

5   Results

5.1   Participants Appreciation

The benefits of a social activity as shown by other studies about ludic activities and digital games seem to be confirmed [3, 22]. All the participants were pleased to learn how to use tactile devices with this entertainment activity. They said it was preferable to learn how to interact with an unknown technology during a ludic activity, without constraints or judgment. Playing games affected positively older users' attitudes towards technologies. They felt comfortable to ask the instructor or the more experienced users help when they had some difficulties during the activity. Working in pairs or in group help them learning to one from another, as practiced by some group studies [19, 20].

They were also able to discover solutions to common errors or difficulties together. For example, as the children had more experience with touchscreen devices, they were able to help the older users. Children helped the older ones to start interaction and also observed their main errors, providing solutions or correcting the gesture. Showing their interest on touchscreen devices, they encouraged older users to be more curious about it and try to discover new tips.

5.2   Common Errors during Touchscreen Interaction of Older Adults

Common errors have been observed and classified into four categories according to their causes: devices (Table 4), input techniques (Table 5) and interactive system (Table 6). This analyze must be completed through more broad studies.

Table 4. Common errors related to the device

Description	Proposals
Pushing physical buttons: turn off, volume controls. Small buttons are hard to find, to identify and to push.	Special case to hide physical buttons (i.e. inside a box with a flap, a slipping panel) New design and explicit buttons.
Touching soft buttons: back to home, back to another page, take screenshots. Soft buttons are hard to find and to identify.	Possibility of disabling soft buttons Define a constant location Better design for easier identification
Reflection on the screen	Protector film
Finger marks on the screen	Pen interaction, cleaning tissue
Problems to hand hold	Special case to prevent the device of slipping or falling down

Table 5. Common errors related to the input technique

Description	Proposals
Pen: Touches with the side of the pen, pen only works straight up	Pen could have touch points by the sides
Pen: Buttons change the interaction if pushed	Pen could have explicit buttons Pen buttons could be disabled by the user
Fingers: Single touch detection of another point of interaction	Identify accidental touches

Table 6. Common errors related to the interactive system

Description	Proposals
Pieces come back to the second touch position	Prioritize target interaction zone according to the context

Some errors or difficulties could be related to the user's skills or impairments. As the condition of this study did not allow measuring user's visual, cognitive or motor impairments, the table below only report some errors probably related to the individual manual dexterity (Table 7).

Table 7. Common errors probably related to the user's manual dexterity

Description	Proposals
Place the palm of the hand on the screen to control the movements of the fingers	Define interaction and non-interaction zones
Hiding the screen	Adapting target sizes
Unregistered touches (low capacitance, dry skin, fingers side or nails)	Pen interaction would be more convenient

5.3   Strategies for Touchscreen Interaction

Users adapt themselves according to the situation and device. Different strategies for interacting with the targets have been observed and analyzed. They are described on the table below (Table 8).

Table 8. Gestures and strategies of interaction on touchscreen by older users

Kind of gesture	Supported by the system	Proposals and support
Slipping the finger or the pen from the initial position to the final position: slowly	Yes	N.A.
Slipping the finger or the pen from the initial position to the final position: fast	No, the pieces arrive later	Optimize the system's performances
Small gestures pushing the piece	Yes	Smoothing the gestures Tutorial Online help to new users
Fast gestures, pushing the pieces as they would continue on the same direction	No, pieces stay where the finger released the screen	Similar to a swipe, test the direction and continue the trajectory of the targets

6   Conclusion and Planned Activities

Touchscreen devices and the system "Puzzle Touch" can be used to support game and inter-generational activities. This seems to facilitate the appropriation of new technologies.

The existing studies about tactile interaction of older adults are helpful but don't embrace all the different situations of use and the individual characteristics of this heterogeneous population. It is not possible to designers to determinate or to know in advance what kind of devices will be used neither the screen sizes nor position. Furthermore, all the characteristics of use have an effect on user's interaction. It is not possible either to preview user's abilities or impairment. So systems should be responsive and flexible [20].

The results of this exploratory study give important issues to design more accessible, usable and ergonomic interfaces. This observation method could be considered as a contribution for the participative user-centered method.

Following the results and the proposals of this study, a new version of our system "Puzzle Touch" can be released. The next version of this interactive system should support the use of different input techniques (pen, finger) but also or multi touch interaction. The detection of multi-touch should prevent accidental touches from interrupting the interaction, i.e. when the user touches outside the targets, it should not be considered to the game. Touching outside the gameplay area or pushing buttons should not interrupt the activity. A detailed analysis of older users' tactile gestures could provide more information to support their interaction.

Acknowledgements. PhD Scholarship Ciências sem fronteiras CNPQ Brazil (#237079/2012-7). We cordially thank the Espace multimédia de Meudon, its staff and the participants. We also thank the City of Meudon and the Meudon City Hall Archive for the images.

References

1. Umemuro, H.: Lowering elderly Japanese users? resistance towards computers by using touchscreen technology. Univers. Access Inf. Soc. 3, 276–288 (2004)
2. Piper, A.M., Campbell, R., Hollan, J.D.: Exploring the accessibility and appeal of surface computing for older adult health care support. In: Proc. 28th Int. Conf. Hum. Factors Comput. Syst., CHI 2010, vol. 907 (2010)
3. Ijsselsteijn, W., Nap, H.H., de Kort, Y., Poels, K.: Digital game design for elderly users. In: Proc. 2007 Conf. Futur. Play - Futur. Play 2007, Toronto, Canada, November 15-17, p. 17 (2007)
4. Jin, Z.X., Plocher, T., Kiff, L.: Touch screen user interfaces for older adults: Button size and spacing. In: Stephanidis, C. (ed.) HCI 2007. LNCS, vol. 4554, pp. 933–941. Springer, Heidelberg (2007)
5. Hwangbo, H., Yoon, S., Jin, B.: A study of pointing performance of elderly users on smartphones. Int. J. Hum. Comput. Interact. 29, 1–10 (2013)
6. Lepicard, G., Vigouroux, N.: Touch Screen User Interfaces for Older Subjects. In: Miesenberger, K., Klaus, J., Zagler, W., Karshmer, A. (eds.) ICCHP 2010, Part II. LNCS, vol. 6180, pp. 592–599. Springer, Heidelberg (2010)
7. Lepicard, G., Vigouroux, N.: Influence of age and interaction complexity on touch screen Color and position effects on user performance. In: 12th IEEE Ine-Health Netw. Appl. Serv (Healthcom), Int. Conf. e-Health Netw. Appl. Serv., pp. 246–253 (2010)

8. Hourcade, J., Berkel, T.: Tap or touch?: pen-based selection accuracy for the young and old. In: CHI 2006, pp. 881–886 (2006)

9. Tsai, W.-C., Lee, C.-F.: A study on the icon feedback types of small touch screen for the elderly. In: Stephanidis, C. (ed.) UAHCI 2009, Part II. LNCS, vol. 5615, pp. 422–431. Springer, Heidelberg (2009)

10. Chung, M.K., Kim, D., Na, S., Lee, D.: Usability evaluation of numeric entry tasks on keypad type and age. Int. J. Ind. Ergon. 40, 97–105 (2010)

11. Lee, J., Poliakoff, E., Spence, C.: The effect of multimodal feedback presented via a touch screen on the performance of older adults. In: Altinsoy, M.E., Jekosch, U., Brewster, S. (eds.) HAID 2009. LNCS, vol. 5763, pp. 128–135. Springer, Heidelberg (2009)

12. Genaro-Motti, L., Vigouroux, N., Gorce, P.: Touchscreen interaction of older adults: a literature review. In: AAATE 2013, Vilamoura, Portugal, September 19-22, vol. 33, pp. 837–843. IOS Press (2013)

13. Al-Razgan, M.S., Al-Khalifa, H.S., Al-Shahrani, M.D., Alajmi, H.H.: Touch-Based Mobile Phone Interface Guidelines and Design Recommendations for Elderly People: A Survey of the Literature, pp. 568–574 (2012)

14. Zhou, J., Rau, P.-L.P., Salvendy, G.: Use and Design of Handheld Computers for Older Adults: A Review and Appraisal. Int. J. Hum. Comput. Interact. 28, 799–826 (2012)

15. Sears, A., Hanson, V.L.: Representing users in accessibility research. ACM Trans. Access. Comput. 4, 1–6 (2012)

16. Hanson, V.: Age and web access: the next generation. In: Int. Cross-Disciplinary Conf. Web, vol. 44, pp. 7–15 (2009)

17. Dickinson, A., Arnott, J., Prior, S.: Methods for human – computer interaction research with older people. Behav. Inf. Technol. 26(4), 343–352 (2007)

18. Apted, T., Kay, J., Quigley, A.: Tabletop sharing of digital photographs for the elderly. In: CHI 2006, pp. 781–790. ACM (2006)

19. Harada, S., Sato, D., Takagi, H., Asakawa, C.: Characteristics of Elderly User Behavior on Mobile Multi-touch Devices. In: Kotzé, P., Marsden, G., Lindgaard, G., Wesson, J., Winckler, M. (eds.) INTERACT 2013, Part IV. LNCS, vol. 8120, pp. 323–341. Springer, Heidelberg (2013)

20. Gonçalves, V.P., Ueyama, J.: Um Estudo sobre o Design, a Implementação e a Avaliação de Interfaces Flexíveis para Idosos em Telefones Celulares. Simp. Bras. Fatores Humanos (2010)

21. Hollinworth, N., Hwang, F.: Investigating familiar interactions to help older adults learn computer applications more easily. In: BCS-HCI 2011 (2011)

22. Leonard, V.K., Jacko, J.A., Pizzimenti, J.J.: An exploratory investigation of handheld computer interaction for older adults with visual impairments. In: Proc. 7th Int. ACM SIGACCESS Conf. Comput. Access., ASSETS 2005, pp. 12–19 (2005)

23. Kobayashi, M., Hiyama, A., Miura, T., Asakawa, C., Hirose, M., Ifukube, T.: Elderly user evaluation of mobile touchscreen interactions. In: Campos, P., Graham, N., Jorge, J., Nunes, N., Palanque, P., Winckler, M. (eds.) INTERACT 2011, Part I. LNCS, vol. 6946, pp. 83–99. Springer, Heidelberg (2011)

24. Moffatt, K., McGrenere, J.: Slipping and drifting: using older users to uncover pen-based target acquisition difficulties. In: Proc. 9th Int. ACM ASSETS 2007, pp. 11–18 (2007)

25. Nicolau, H., Jorge, J.: Elderly text-entry performance on touchscreens. In: Proc. 14th Int. ACM SIGACCESS Conf. Comput. Access., ASSETS 2012, vol. 127 (2012)

26. Findlater, L., Froehlich, J.E., Fattal, K., Wobbrock, J.O., Dastyar, T.: Age-related differences in performance with touchscreens compared to traditional mouse input. In: CHI 2013, pp. 343–346. ACM (2013)

A Survey and Design Implementation of the Elder's Outgoing Preference: The Local Bus System

Jeichen Hsieh[1] and Chang-Chan Huang[2]

[1] Industrial Design Dept., Tunghai University, Taichung, Taiwan
jeichen@thu.edu.tw
[2] Landscape Dept., Tunghai University, Taichung, Taiwan
cchuang0516@thu.edu.tw

Abstract. In bus system, to provide appropriate services for passenger demand cannot be ignored. When the trend, low birth rate with senior citizens, is coming in our country, re-understanding bus passenger information needs and information behavior must be concerned in an being E-government. By information seeking (behavior) and participating observation the passengers, need and behavior are surveyed. After understanding the local bus system, the research suggests an information schema to solve the problem to fit the information meaning of the information seeking.

Keywords: Preference, Bus System, Information Seeking, Information Need.

1 Introduction

Since information delivery and immediately following nowadays as to existing bus system should have in response to change in the environment for new services and methods. Basically, the bus passenger demand and usage behavior are in consistency. The major behavior is nothing more than to go out wait a ride, on board, touch down destination, and get off the bus. If you consider the more intimate needs, of course, from the departure gate to reach the destination gate is the best. It is all the taxi service does. For the needs of today's senior citizens under physiology and mental from aging phenomena, how to help them on travelling is an E-government's responsibility. Application of scientific and technological strength of the Internet with some changes in the system would work in the environment and these demands could be fulfilled intimate on bus ride for the older.

2 Literature Review

2.1 Researches on Bus System

Previous studies [11][12][13][14][9][8]have revealed App, QR code, GPS and other Internet technology can be appropriately applied to the bus system, but really friendly

C. Stephanidis and M. Antona (Eds.): UAHCI/HCII 2014, Part III, LNCS 8515, pp. 79–87, 2014.

and caring, not a reasonable solution for the elderly on the user interface considerations. Remote areas where the bus does not match the cost-effectiveness has been developed in line with contemporary environmental consideration [6] [7].

2.2   Information Seeking

Bus information behavior covers the information needs, search, collect, organize, evaluate and use [10]. Kuhlthau believes that information needs are constantly revised, and will vary with changes in cognitive and constantly changing at all stages [3][4]. According to the extent Taylor described the needs as four [5]. Harter asks the essence of the original meaning [2]. Grover proposed eight stages that normal users seek mode [1].

3   Methodology

Participant observation is used to handle the problem and dig the information meaning, need, and behavior on the older area. Interview with a questionnaire also used to handle the psychological and physiological need of the older. Bus system is from the secondary data of the Government.

After the text edit has been completed, the paper is ready for the template. Duplicate the template file by using the Save As command, and use the naming convention prescribed by your conference for the name of your paper. In this newly created file, highlight all of the contents and import your prepared text file. You are now ready to style your paper; use the scroll down window on the left of the MS Word Formatting toolbar.

4   Implementation

By using human one resident and ten action assistant, a total of six months in Ishioka region interact with participants.   Particular focus is on the elderly community information needs and information behavior (Ishioka is a regional field of aging for the elderly). According to field situations understand the status of the local bus is not fulfilled completely. A case study in Longxing section of the area we found just two trips a day and it does not open on Saturday and Sunday. The main transport just provides students get on and off first. Time also caters for student-centered.

The residents are not taken into account at all. Most of the elderly in the ground based on agriculture, they always get up early to work and go home around 11:00 to rest, do not go outside ordinarily.

But organizing a major event in the field, uses the depth interview questionnaire to participants (62 samples), the information needs are most people are willing to participate in activities. In any public events, possible cause is that they have known each other. In the instruments that they come are walking, bicycles, electric cars, share a ride car or welfare organization and the initiative to provide public car carrier send dominated. Completely no public transport supports. Details and figures are as follow:

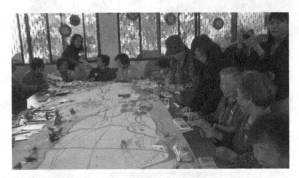

Fig. 1. Participants and activity 1: (Map Memory Puzzle)

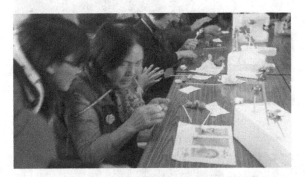

Fig. 2. Participants and activity 2: (Dough)

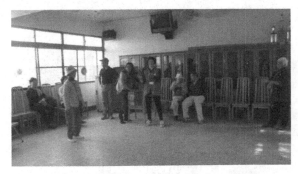

Fig. 3. Participants and activity 3: (Kara OK)

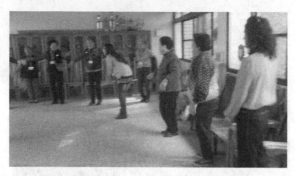

Fig. 4. Participants and activity 4: (Body movements)

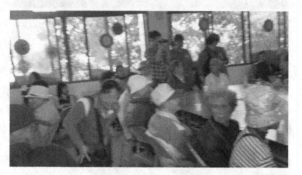

Fig. 5. Lunch together

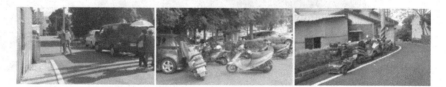

Fig. 6. Transportation used

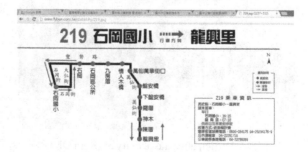

Fig. 7. Bus station name and stop sign

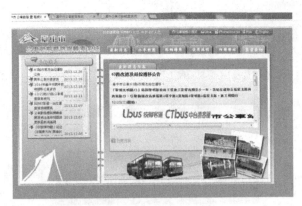

Fig. 8. Homepage of Bus Information System

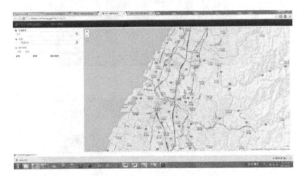

Fig. 9. Bus map and shift

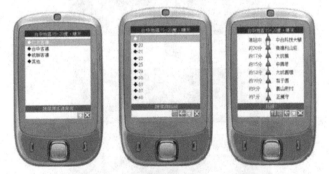

Fig. 10. Operating interface on phone

5   A Remodel Schema for Free Ride

A remodel schema is built based on three parts, the free and warranty car providers, E-center, and passengers in local area. The schema is as following by flowcharts:

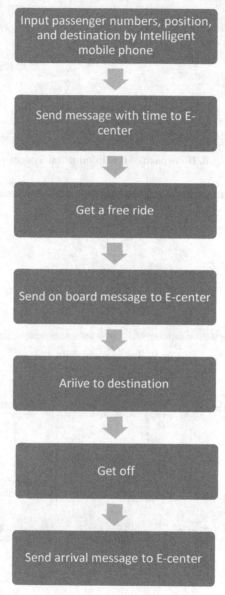

Fig. 11. Process of passenger side

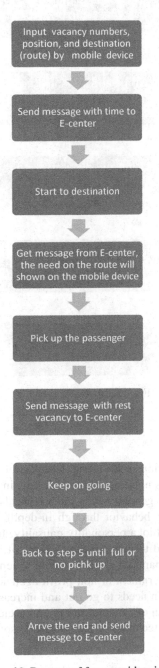

Fig. 12. Process of free provider side

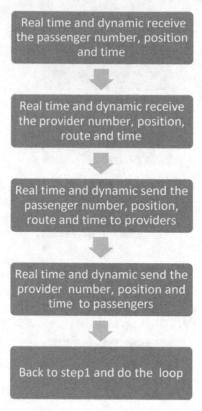

Fig. 13. Process of E-center

6   Conclusion

Because participant observation in the field (Ishioka) of height between the ground and the mountains, the bus is not cost effective results in relatively lower occupancy rates. An aging society with general needs push it needs to be re-considered. After studying information seeking behavior through in-depth interviews, learned that the elderly take a bus zone in Ishioka personality causality. In order to solve the elderly out by public instruments and to increase the chances of an elderly person to go out, we propose a ride by the dynamic real-time system schema, but it still rely on inter-mediate processing by E-government or non-profit agencies throughout the system. It is expected to solve the region needs to go out and increase the positive interpersonal interaction. But, the protection of personal safety and accident insurance needs further considerations. Engineering technology and network software are also need to be assessed.

Acknowledgment. The research is parts of   GREEnS project   supported by Tung-hai University. Thanks.

References

1. Grover, R.: A Proposed Model for Diagnosing Information Needs. School Library Media Quarterly 32(4), 95–100 (1993)
2. Harter, S.: Psychology Relevance and Information Science. JASIS 43(9), 602–615 (1992)
3. Kuhlthau, C.C.: Developing a Model of the Library Search Process: Cognitive and Affective Aspects. RQ 28(2), 232–242 (1988)
4. Kuhlthau, C.C.: A Principle of Uncertainty for Information Seeking. Journal of Documentation 49, 367–388 (1993)
5. Taylor, R.: Question-negotiation and Information Seeking in Libraries. College and Research Libraries 29, 178–194 (1968)
6. Lin, G.: Bus Estimated Arrival Time Study Under Unusual Circumstances Communications, Information Engineering of China University serving special class. Master Thesis (2011)
7. Qiu, R.: Green Energy Public Bicycle Design Research, National Taipei University of Education, Department of Art and Design. Master Thesis (2012)
8. Ye, Z.: Import Car Repair Business Operations of APP and QR Code Cum Inventory Management System Inventory - in NH's Case, Information Management, National Kaohsiung University of Applied Sciences Serving Special Class. Master Thesis (2011)
9. Yankee, F.: GPS Navigation and Positioning With Integrated PL, Department of Electrical Engineering, National Cheng Kung University. Master PhD Thesis (2001)
10. Yuji, C.: Taipei County Bus Ride Willingness by User Analysis and Research Programs to Improve the Road Network, National Chiao Tung University. Institute of Traffic and Transportation Engineering Thesis (1984)
11. Luo, Y.: By Travel Card Transaction Data to Explore the Origins and Destinations of Passengers Bus Routes, Tamkang University, Department of Transportation Management. Master Thesis (2004)
12. Huang, J.: Former Bus Line Dynamic Information System by User Behavior Research, Tamkang University, Transportation Management. Thesis (2003)
13. Chen, Q.: Intelligent Bus Stop Setting Research Standards, Central Police University, Institute of Traffic Management. Master's thesis (2000)
14. Yang, B.: Advanced Dynamic Bus Information System by User-effective Measure, Tamkang University, Transportation Management. Thesis (2000)

Understanding Independent Living Requirements:
A Study of Shanghai Seniors

Shan Huang[1] and Hua Dong[2,*]

[1] College of Architecture and Urban Planning, Tongji University, Shanghai, China
shan_huhu@aliyun.com
[2] College of Design and Innovation, Tongji University, Shanghai, China
donghua@tongji.edu.cn

Abstract. There are more and more empty-nested elderly in China, and they
need to maintain independent living with support from the family and the community. This paper discusses the meaning of independence in later life and the
crucial dimensions of independence. Interviews were conducted with 51 older
persons living in a community in Shanghai to understand the independent living
requirements from older people's perspective. Physical capabilities, typical
problems in daily living, and life styles were discussed, which offers insights
into how to improve independence in later life for older people living in
communities.

Keywords: Independence, older people, capability, activities of daily living.

1 Introduction

In China, families used to play an important role in caring for older people, as reflected by the Chinese traditional value of 'filial piety'. However, the 'One-child' policy
and the 'Reform and Opening-up' policy have resulted in more and more small-sized
families, which undermine the traditional family-based old age supporting pattern. A
qualitative study shows that the capacity of the family support for the elderly in urban
households in Suzhou (a city near Shanghai) has actually weakened, as is reflected in
financial support, daily life caring and emotional consultation [1].

Urbanization has resulted in more and more empty-nested elderly in China. The
studies on community care have reached growth peak since the publication of the
China's 12th Five-year Plan which emphasizes on giving priority to the development
of social service for the elderly.

Independence in later life is often understood as the ability to do everyday activities
without the reliance on others (physical independence). A supplementary understanding is not doing everything oneself but having control over one's life and choosing
how that life is led [2]. Independence is therefore related to people's decision making,
which includes thinking and communication capabilities (mental independence). Independence in later life is also related to social constructions [3] (social independence).

---

* Corresponding author.

C. Stephanidis and M. Antona (Eds.): UAHCI/HCII 2014, Part III, LNCS 8515, pp. 88–97, 2014.

Financial independence is critical as it affects an older person's ability to maintain and improve his/her physical as well as mental wellbeing (Figure 1). In Chinese urbanized area, an older person's economic support typically comes from pension and family support.

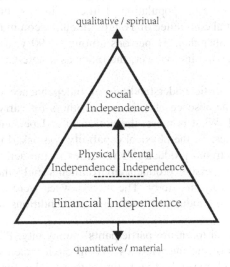

Fig. 1. The pyramid of independence dimensions

Physical independence depends to a great extent on one's physical/functional capability, likewise, mental independence relies on mental capability. That is, the more physical/mental abilities, the higher the independence. The mental status includes both the cognitive and emotional statuses. The cognitive ability is more obvious and greatly affects the physical ability, whereas emotional functionality such as depression is harder to recognize and diagnose. Inclusive design toolkit (available at: www.inclusivedesigntoolkit.com), an online toolkit presenting a model for the relationship between user capabilities and product experience, classifies user capabilities into 7 categories: vision, hearing, dexterity, reach & stretch, locomotion, thinking, communication [4]. The former five are related to physical capabilities, and the last two are concerned with mental abilities.

Social independence is located at the top of the pyramid. Secker et al. [5] proposes a two-dimensional model of independence, with one dimension reflecting the degree of reliance on others (physical/mental independence) and the other the subjective assessment of autonomy, desired level of choice and social usefulness (mental independence), which indicates that physical/mental independence could greatly reflect the degree of social independence.

Independence is not only a complex notion that includes multiple meaning, but also a mutable notion that should be thought as an unstable achievement [6]. Since the rate of capability decline in the disablement process is highly individual and people redefine the notion over time as their situation changes, it is necessary to go deep into individual levels to understand the real demands in the specific disablement pathway.

2   Methods

In order to find the independent living requirements from older people's own perspectives, in-depth interviews that last 1 to 1.5 hours were carried out. The older people living in communities were the population of interest in this study. With the help of the community residential committee of Tongji Xincun, a community near a University in Yangpu District, Shanghai, 51 persons among 60-90 years old were recruited. Two researchers (one as the interviewer, the other as a note-taker) were involved in every interview.

One of the individualistic understandings of independence is that the ability to function unaided and the absence of reliance on others for carrying out activities of daily living (ADL) [7]. What is more, the notion of independence differs to people with different capabilities. So the physical capability was asked firstly (especially the capability of using electronic products). Difficulties in the activities of daily living, and the link between a person, products/environments and other people were also taken into consideration in this study. The interviewees were asked to describe the conditions when they use products at home and the conditions when they go out for social activities.

Pseudonyms were used to ensure participants' anonymity. Pictures were taken to remind the researchers of the interviewees' living environments. All the interviews were audio-recorded and transcribed verbatim without delay for avoiding data missing, and all the data (interview notes and pictures) were put in a database for analysis.

3   Results

Based on self-report, the participants were divided into 4 levels of physical abilities in this study: very low, low, medium, and good. The summary of the participants' basic information is shown in Table 1.

Table 1. Characterization of participants

		Number of respondents
Couple / Individule	Couple	7(16%)
	Individule	37(84%)
Sex	Male	25(49%)
	Female	26(51%)
Age	61-70	8(16%)
	71-80	24(47%)
	81-90	19(37%)
Education	Illetracy or primary school	8(16%)
	Middle school or high school	15(29%)
	Junior college or above	28(55%)
Physical ability	0 (very low)	15(29%)
	1 (low)	6(12%)
	2 (medium)	21(41%)
	3 (good)	9(18%)

3.1   The Physical Capability

The participants' abilities of using everyday electronic products (e.g. mobile phones, cameras, computers, the automated teller machines – ATMs) were classified into four levels: very low (score 0), low (score1), medium (score 2), and good (score 3). The participants who scored 0 accounted for 51% (Table 2), which suggested a low level of use of electronic products in their daily life. The reasons could be summarized as:

- Some older people could not afford these products, or they regarded purchasing electronic products as an unnecessary expenditure.
- These products were too complicated for some older people to use.
- Some older people did not trust the virtual world, and they were more willing to accept tangible things, e.g. most of the participants took money out from the bank counter, rather than from the ATMs.

Table 2. Capability of using electronic products

Number of respondents	Capability of using electronic products
0 (very low)	26(51%)
1 (low)	6(12%)
2 (middle)	6(12%)
3 (good)	13(25%)

3.2   Typical Problems

The interviewees were asked to describe the conditions when they used products at home and the conditions when they went out for social activities. The qualitative data were classified according to user capability categories: dexterity, vision, hearing, mobility and memory.

Dexterity. Most products need manual handling, and older people's loss of dexterity (at various degrees) often makes physical manipulation out of control, which causes problems in daily activities. Almost all of the interviewees (19 out of 21) who got 0 or 1 in physical ability evaluation had difficulties in opening food packaging. It was difficult for them to tear apart packaging by hands without a pair of scissors, especially the small packs with zigzag openings. Figure 2 shows the powder sprinkled on the table when an interviewee aged 84 was making a cup of instant coffee.

Pulling a plug out of electronic sockets requires both fine pinch grip and reasonable pull force from one hand, and a push force from the other. It was a challenging task for the elderly, and most of them preferred a switch to a plug.

Some activities like using a key or a mobile phone require accuracy and dexterity simultaneously. Several participants felt it was hard to pinch a key and plug it into the keyhole. Using touchscreen phones also requires fine dexterity of the index finger. In this study, only two participants used touch phones, and both of them had difficulties in touching the correct point on the screen.

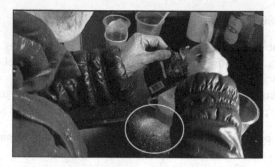

Fig. 2. Typical problem of opening food package

Typical problems in interaction with products caused by dexterity limit are listed as follows (Table 3):

Table 3. Typical problems caused by dexterity limit

Products	Dexterity functions	Typical problems
food package	pinch grip	cannot do this delicate task; have to do it with scissors or other tools;
plugs and sockets	pinch grip, pull force	need two hands working together;
mobile phone	push force	incorrect manipulations;
key	pinch grip, push force	hard to pinch a key and plug it into the keyhole.

Vision. Older people often wear a pair of reading glasses when reading texts. But some people, like Mrs. Zhao, preferred magnifying glass, because if she wore the reading glasses for a long time, the bridge of her nose would become uncomfortable (Fig. 3).

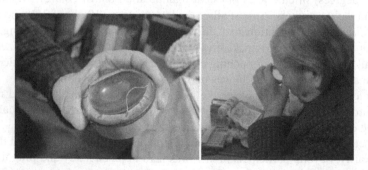

Fig. 3. Mrs. Zhao's magnifying glass

There were also many problems when older people interacted with digital devices and their instructions. For instance, many found following instructions difficult, and they need larger texts, higher contrast, and longer pauses between setting-up steps.

The study suggests that the visual functions of contrast sensitivity and usable visual field were more important to older people for outdoor activities. Many participants complained that conspicuous marks between stairs were lacking in public spaces, such as in the subway stations.

Hearing. Most of the participants complained about the product with sound prompt functions.

"I can't hear the sound of 'beep...beep...' when the washing machine finished work. I also often forget that I have had some clothes in the washing machine, which would be found a few days later. So I have to wash them again or just wait beside the washing machine when it is working." — Mrs. Zhang, 81 years old

Some participants usually ignored the alarm because of their declined hearing, which could be dangerous.

Mobility. Typical problems caused by mobility (the ability to move and walk) limit are as follows:

- The regular sofa is too soft and low, and it is hard for an older person to sit for a long time and stand up without help. Several participants had adapted their sofa /chair with cushions (Fig. 4).

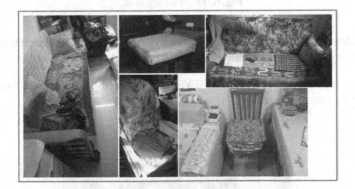

Fig. 4. The adapted sofa and chair

- Stairs with abrupt slopes or without armrests are very dangerous, and older people have to hold the armrests and move carefully step by step (Fig.5). They preferred the armrests made of wood to those of metal.

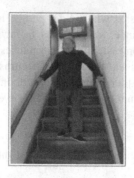

Fig. 5. The stair with wood armrest

- The bus footstep is often too high, so it is hard for an old person to get on the bus.
- Walking aids are often needed for those who cannot walk for a long distance (Fig. 6).

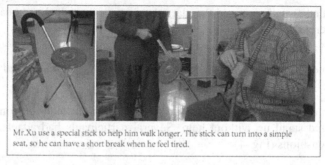

Mr.Xu use a special stick to help him walk longer. The stick can turn into a simple seat, so he can have a short break when he feel tired.

Fig. 6. The walking aids

Memory. Memory is a type of cognitive ability. According to the interview, the impact of memory loss on daily living is reflected in the following aspects:

- Many participants cannot remember TV channels, so they often write the channels down on a piece of paper (Fig. 7).

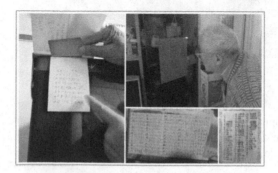

Fig. 7. The handwritten TV channels

- Commonly used small items, like remote controls and reading glasses, are often difficult to find when needed.
- Older people often forget to take medicines. Mrs. Qian had a pill box (Fig. 8), but it was useless for reminding her to take medicines on time.

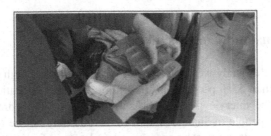

Fig. 8. Mrs. Qian's pill box

3.3   Life Styles

Two typical life styles were identified: following the traditional way, or accepting new things. Most of the participants preferred old things (e.g. traditional handcrafts, Beijing Opera and "Red song") that might evoke their memory of the youth.

"I like watching military TV programs and amateur singing contests, especially the 'Red song'. Once you are old, you are living on memory." — Mr. Huang, 75 years old

Many participants' hobbies in old age were related to their handcraft skills attained in younger age. For example, Mrs. Lou was a worker in a textile factory before retirement, and she was good at knitting. After retirement, she really enjoyed knitting jumpers and making shoes and shirts for her grandson.

It was observed that older people who had good physical capabilities, or had higher living standards, or had children living abroad, tended to accept the modern life style. They were interested in online shopping, playing computer games, learning English, and playing the piano. They wanted to catch up and make connections with the new world.

"I need to be up to date with news. It will be a little embarrassing if other people are talking about news that I don't know about. " — Mr. Lin, 78 years old

Social connection was also an important factor, especially for those who moved to Shanghai in later life. They often felt lonely for leaving away from their previous social circles:

"I don't like anything in Shanghai: the weather, the bank... I really want to go back to my original place and chat with my old friends." —Mrs. Lu, 84 years old

No matter what level of their living abilities, older people were reluctant to be dependent, and they desired to be connected with others. Mrs. Qian lost eyesight when she was young. But she managed to do a lot of things independently. The happiest moment for her was basking in the sun, meanwhile knitting jumpers and chatting with neighbors in the community garden, which made her feel like "a normal person". Mr. Xue lived alone, and he loved to go to the community garden to do exercise every morning. For him, it was not only for keeping fit, but also keeping connected with old friends and neighbors.

4   Discussions and Conclusions

The participants in this study were biased for their location and high education levels. There were more than 55% people who had junior college education or above. Although this made the interview easier, the sampling does not represent the general population of older people in Shanghai, and the results may not be generalizable. On the other hand, dependency can be seen as an indicator of importance for various needs. It means that the higher the dependency, the bigger the need. The people who are 71-85 years old accounted for 84% because of their higher level of dependency. So the study reflected well the old-old people's needs.

This community-based study helps capture many requirements for independent living, from older people's perspectives:

Physically, three quarters of the participants assessed their physical ability as 'very low', 'low' or 'medium'. Many of them had difficulties in interacting with everyday products because of their declined dexterity, vision, hearing, and mobility capabilities. More than half of the participants had very low level of interaction with electronic products.

Mentally, memory loss had caused many inconveniences in older people's daily life, from having difficulties in finding items to forgetting to take medicines on time.

Socially, when physical and mental abilities allow, older people enjoy socializing through community-based activities, such as exercises and chatting with friends.

Although literature suggests there is a link between physical independence, mental independence and social independence, this study did not investigate these relations in depth. Financial independence was not a focus of this study.

The findings have a lot of implications for design, which is further studied in follow-up research.

Acknowledgements. We thank all the people who participated in this research, and the help of the community residential committee of Tongji Xincun. Many postgraduate students at the College of Design and Innovation helped data collection, and our sincere thanks go to them.

References

1. Cheng Jianlan, A.: Research on the Elderly Supporting pattern in China: A Survey in Suzhou. Nanjin University, China (2012)
2. Brisenden, S.: Independent living and the medical model of disability. Disability, Handicap & Society 1(2), 173–178 (1986)

3. Plath, D.: Independence in old age: the route to social exclusion? British Journal of Social Work 38(7), 1353–1368 (2008)
4. Clarkson, P.J., Coleman, R., Hosking, I., Waller, S.: Inclusive design toolkit. University of Cambridge, Cambridge (2007)
5. Secker, J., Hill, R., Villeneau, L., Parkman, S.: Promoting independence: but promoting what and how? Ageing & Society 23(3), 375–391 (2003)
6. Schwanen, T., Banister, D., Bowling, A.: Independence and mobility in later life. Geoforum 43, 1313–1322 (2012)
7. Inclusive Design Toolkit, http://www.inclusivedesigntoolkit.com (accessed January 14, 2010)

Investigating the Effects of User Age on Readability

Kyung Hoon Hyun, Ji-Hyun Lee, and Hwon Ihm

Korea Advanced Institute of Science and Technology, Korea
{hellohoon,jihyun187,raccoon}@kaist.ac.kr

Abstract. This paper focuses on creating a guideline for style, line spacing, size, text box and age group combinations of Korean fonts for different electronic displays. Reading time and recall time were measured to analyze the readabilities among various typographical layouts. The importance of typographical elements were different among the age group: line height and font sizes are the most important element for 20s to skim through the documents; font style and line height for 30s; line height and font size for 50+. Although, 20s, 30s and 50s had similarities on recalling speed since the font size and the line heights were the two most important readability elements. Thus, it is clear that the typographical layouts need to be designed differently based on the target user of the design. The optimized font combination for readability was also generated.

Keywords: Font Readability, Conjoint Analysis, Korean Typography.

1 Introduction

Understanding the effects of the styles and the layout of the fonts on the readability of reading materials has been one of the primary subject of study for the wide range of disciplines such as interface design, typeface design, graphic design and other related fields. One reason for such phenomenon is the merits of effective space management. The management of screen real estate is critical for ensuring both aesthetics and high readability of the screen-based textual content [8]. However, the effectiveness of screen real estate management on readability can vary among the text of different display sizes and the age of target readers. According to Myung [7], the readability importance hierarchy comes in the following order: line-spacing (53%), font style (35%), followed by font size (12%). Furthermore, each product line of mobile phone differs in screen resolution, making large fonts unsuitable for mobile displays [4]. Therefore, the ideal combinations of font style and the layout should also change in accordance with the size of the display and the age group of the target users, since the layout must be transformed to accommodate the same amount of textual content on various screen sizes.

The readability of a text varies with the font style as well as the layout of the text. From the aspect of legibility, line-spacing, font face, and font size are the dominant factors [7]. Passage length and letter spacing also affect the legibility of the textual

C. Stephanidis and M. Antona (Eds.): UAHCI/HCII 2014, Part III, LNCS 8515, pp. 98–105, 2014.
© Springer International Publishing Switzerland 2014

material. Typically, a graphic design expert carefully constructs an ensemble of font style and layout, which consists of features such as line-spacing or letter-spacing that aim to increase the readability of the content, based on personal aesthetic preferences or subjective estimates on screen real estates. However, since the text layout and the font sizes are inevitably modified due to the various shapes and sizes of the display screens, it is important to understand the correlation among font style, screen size, and the age of the target users.

The objective of the paper is to create a guideline for combining style, line spacing, and size of Korean fonts for different age groups and for electronic displays that differ in orientation, a desktop monitor and a mobile phone, for example.. Analyzing the accuracy and the duration of reading activity of the readers among various font and layout combinations can help identify the optimal font and layout combinations for the different screen size among different age groups.

A conjoint analysis was conducted to measure the readability among different font styles, font size, line spacing, screen sizes, and age groups. A total of 54 combinations of fonts, line spacing, size, age group and screen size were evaluated. 3 font styles were analyzed for the evaluation – Gothic (san serif), Myeong-Jo (serif) and Pen (cursive) font styles from Nanum font family (Fig. 1). It is widely known that serif style typefaces provide better readabilities on printed material while san serif style displays better on screens [1]. However, this widely spread knowledge on serif and san-serif styled fonts may vary depending on the overall layout, the size of the font and screen sizes [2]. Three degrees of line spacing was used for this experiment (50%, 100%, and 150%). The age groups is form in 3 groups (20 ~ 29, 30 ~ 39 and 50 ~ 59).

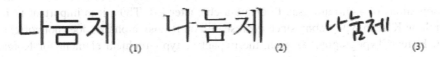

Fig. 1. Nanum font family: (1) Nanum Gothic; (2) Nanum Myeongjo; (3) Nanum Pen

According to Mo et al [6], the smallest Korean font size that are readable to the age group between 20 and 30 is 10.7 pt, and 16.6 pt for 40 and older. Therefore, we have evaluated 3 sizes: 10.7pt, 16.6pt, and 22.5pt.   Two representative instances of screen size was used: 1366x768 and 480x320 (most used PC screen and mobile phones resolution according to w3school's screen resolution statistics, and Android Market). Based on the possible combinations of the above features, the readability of each text in 4 categories was measured by the means of accuracy (counting error) and reading time (duration of reading the given text.

The results can be used in identifying optimal font size, font type and lay-out for presenting screen-based text on electronic display.

The readability of the font, font size and line height can be evaluated by measuring reading speed of the text [4, 7, 8]. Tullis et al [8] considered reading time and accuracy to compare the read-abilities among the four different font styles. The result showed that the reading time and the accuracy correlated to the font size, and the users preferred larger fonts. Arial, san serif font, and MS San Serif showed small differences in the degree of readability. This result contradicts to the field myth that the san serif displays better on screen than the serif fonts.

The performance of the readability is not only defined by the style of fonts and font size, but other typographical elements such line height, and the display size – bounding box [4, 7]. Huang et al [4] have investigated the impact of font size in various display resolution on text searching time. Different screen resolutions had varying optimal font sizes. For instance, 125 dpi with 3.8mm font size; 167 dpi with 2.6mm – 3.0mm; 200 dpi with 2.6mm; 250 dpi with 2.2-2.6 provides good readability for Chinese documents.   Line height is also found to be related to the readability of the writings along with other typographical elements such as font style, font size. Myung [7] have conducted researches on levels of importance of the typographical elements with Hangeul: Korean Fonts. The line-spacing has the relative importance of the 53%, font style has 35% and font size has 12%. Tullis et al [8] discovered that the font size actually is the most influential typo-graphical element in readability, but it contradicts what Myung [7] have measured. This may suggest that the typographical guidelines are not universally applicable for both Roman alphabet and Korean alphabet due to the structural dissimilarities. Roman alphabets are efficient due to its one-dimensional left to right alphanumeric letter composition [3]. However, Hangeul characters can be assembled in two-dimensional way similar to that of building blocks. The building blocks of the Korean letters are called Jamo, and at least two or three combinations of Jamo are used to create a character [5]. Thus, it is important to research on Korean typography since the research on Roman alphabet does not correlate with Korean Typography. As such, the impact of typographical element for Korean was investigated along with age group and text box sizes to pro-vide guidelines for using Korean typography.

2   Experiment

2.1   Test Subjects

15 test subjects were selected from the three age groups: 20 ~ 29; 30 ~ 39; 50 ~ 59. The experiment subjects were recruited from Korea Advanced Institute of Science and Technology, Daejeon, South Korea. The experiment texts were taken from the elementary school book's readings and exams. The character and objects' names were replaced with new names to reduce the opportunities for recognizing the readings. The experiment was conducted on a PC with a Dell Color monitor. The experiment materials were displayed on a self-developed program writ-ten on Python as shown in the Fig. 2.

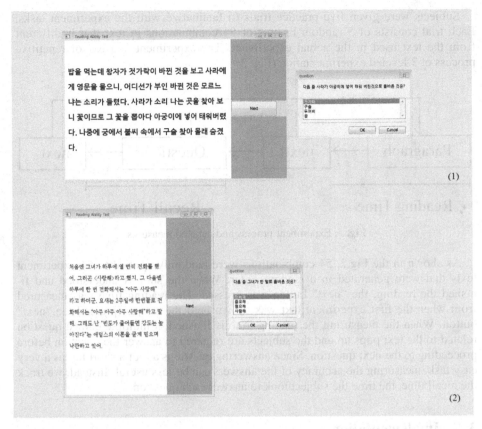

Fig. 2. User Interface for the readability evaluation is shown: (1) layout combination of Nanum Gothic, font size 16.6pt, line height 200%, 600x400; (2) layout combination of Nanum Myeongjo, 12.7pt, line height 200%, 320x480

2.2   Procedure

The experiment is to identify the optimized combinations of font style, font size, line height and text box for 3 different age groups. Nanum font family was used since it is the one of the most commonly used font family in Korea.   We have evaluated 3 sizes: 10.7pt, 16.6pt, and 22.5pt.   Three degrees of line spacing was used for this experiment (100%, 200%, and 300%). Two representative instances of screen size was used: 1366x768 and 480x320 (most used PC screen and mobile phones resolution according to w3school's screen resolution statistics, and Android Market).   Based on the 54 possible combinations of the above features, the readability of each text in 4 categories will be measured by the means of reading time (duration of reading the given text) and accuracy (duration of the recalling the answer).

Subjects were given five practice trials to familiarize with the experiment tasks. Each trial consists of 5 random layouts of 54 combinations in text that is different from the text used in the actual experiment. The experiment consists of repetitive process of 2-leveled experimentation (Fig. 3).

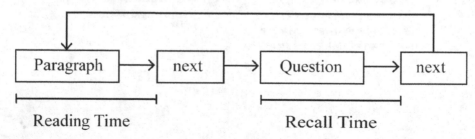

Fig. 3. Experiment process and targeted measures

As shown in the Fig.2, 54 combinations were randomly applied to 54-experiment texts that were generated in a random order. When the subject understood and finished the reading, the "next" button was pressed. The reading time was measured from when the first experiment text was shown until the subject pressed the "next" button. When the measuring the reading time is finished, a multiple choice question related to the text pops up and the subjects are required to answer the question before proceeding to the next question. Since answering questions about a short text is a very easy task, measuring the accuracy of the answers can be less useful. Instead, we track the recall time, the time the subject took to answer each question.

3   Implementation

3.1   Reading Speed

The total number of characters in experimentation paragraphs has the mean values of 100.53 and the median is 100. The reading speed of 54 typographical combinations are calculated with the formula from Myung [7]:

$$RS = \frac{\text{Number of total characters}}{\text{Search time}} \tag{1}$$

The search time in the above formula is equivalent to the reading time obtained from the experiment. A conjoint analysis is then conducted to using the calculated reading speed in order to identify significant typographic elements of readability. There were significant differences in the typographic elements influencing readability among the age groups (Fig. 4).   The significantly effective typographical elements for age group of 20 to 29 on readability are font size and line height (p-value < 0.039, r2 = 0.243). In contrast, font style is the most important typographical element for people in the age group of 30 to 39(p-value < 0.001, r2 = 0.427). The font style is the least important element to the age group of 50++ (p-value <0.02, r2 = 0.281).

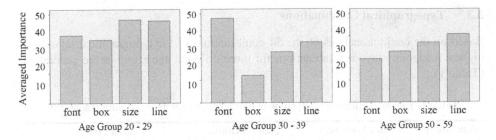

Fig. 4. Averaged importance of the typographical elements for reading speed of three age groups

3.2 Recall Speed

The recall speed is calculated using the response time of the subjects for answering the questions during each question session.

$$RcS = \frac{Number\ of\ total\ characters}{Response\ time} \tag{2}$$

The recall time was then applied to conjoint analysis to identify significant typographic elements on readability. As shown in the Fig. 5, here were significant differences on the typographic elements influencing readability among different age groups. The significantly effective typographical element for age group of 20 to 29 on readability is: line height, font size, font style and text box. The line height is most important to the age group of 20 – 29 (p-value < 0.005, r2 = 0.348)   when the age group of 30 to 39 (p-value < 0.006, r2 = 0.342)   and 50++ values the font size the most. Especially, the age group of 50++ is highly dependent on font size for their effective readability (p-value < 0.005, r2 = 0.452).

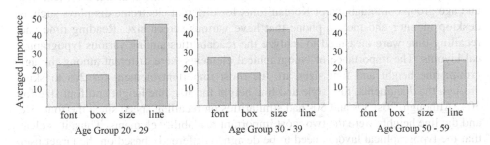

Fig. 5. Averaged importance of the typographical elements for recall speed of three age groups

The impact of the font size is different among reading speed and recall speed. It might be resulted from the skimming effect. The objective of reading is to skim through the paragraph as soon as possible to quickly overview the whole paragraph, therefore the larger font size may not always help.

3.3   Typographical Combinations

Based on the conjoin analysis on the 54 combinations of the typographical layouts, 3 highest readability layout combinations for three different age groups were generat-ed (Table 1).

Table 1. The most effective typographical combinations for the maximum readability

Age Group	Nanum Myeongjo	Nanum Gothic	Nanum Pen
20 – 29	Text box:480px Font size: 11pt* Line Height: 200%	Text box: 480px Font size: 17pt* Line Height: 300%	Text box: 600px Font size: 11pt* Line Height: 200%
30 – 39	Text box: 480px Font size: 23pt* Line Height: 200%	Text box: 600px Font size: 11pt* Line Height: 100%	Text box: 600px Font size: 17pt* Line Height: 100%
50 – 59	Text box: 600 Font size: 17pt* Line Height: 200%	Text box: 480 Font size: 17pt* Line Height: 300%	Text box: 480 Font size: 17pt* Line Height: 300%

* font sizes are rounded up for readability

Despite the importance of the font style, font size, text box and line height, the typo-graphical combination shows that different font requires different layouts to enhance the readability based on different age groups.

4   Conclusion

In this paper we attempted to create a guideline for style, line spacing, size, text box and age group combinations of Korean fonts for different electronic dis-plays such as desktop monitor and mobile phone that have various screen size. Reading time and recalling time were measured to analyze the readabilities among various typographi-cal layouts. The importance of typographical elements were different among the age group: line height and font sizes are the most important element for 20s to skim through the documents; font style and line height for 30s; line height and font size for 50+. Although, 20s, 30s and 50s had similarities on recalling speed since the font size and the line heights were the two most important readability elements. Thus, it is clear that the typographical layouts need to be designed differently based on the target user of the design. The optimized font combination for readability was also generated based on the experiment results which can be helpful reference for interface design-ers, typeface designers, and graphic designers to justify their designs, especially on responsive website designs. How other factors accompanied by age difference such as eyesight, memory, familiarity with electronic devices, and eye movement speed influ-ence the reading speed and recall time should be investigated in the future work.

References

1. Altaboli, A.: Investigating the effects of font styles on perceived visual aesthetics of website interface design. In: Kurosu, M. (ed.) HCII/HCI 2013, Part I. LNCS, vol. 8004, pp. 549–554. Springer, Heidelberg (2013)
2. Bernard, M.L., Chaparro, B.S., Mills, M.M., Halcomb, C.G.: Comparing the effects of text size and format on the readability of computer-displayed Times New Roman and Arial text. International Journal of Human-Computer Studies 59(6), 823–835 (2003)
3. Cai, D., Chi, C., You, M.: The legibility threshold of Chinese characters in three-type styles. International Journal of Industrial Ergonomics 27(1), 9–17 (2001)
4. Huang, D.L., Patrick Rau, P.L., Liu, Y.: Effects of font size, display resolution and task type on reading Chinese fonts from mobile devices. International Journal of Industrial Ergonomics 39(1), 81–89 (2008)
5. Jung, J.w., Lee, J.W.: Hangeul learning system. In: Pan, Z., Zhang, X., El Rhalibi, A., Woo, W., Li, Y. (eds.) Edutainment 2008. LNCS, vol. 5093, pp. 126–134. Springer, Heidelberg (2008)
6. Mo, S.-M., Kim, D.-M., Lim, C.-W., Park, T.-J., Lee, I.-S., Kong, Y.-G., Song, Y.-W., Jeong, M.-C.: Evaluations of Factors Affecting Legibility. Journal of the Ergonomics Society of Korea 28(4), 1–7 (2009)
7. Myung, R.: Conjoint analysis as a new methodology for Korean typography guideline in Web environment. International Journal of Industrial Ergonomics 32(5), 341–348 (2003)
8. Tullis, T.S., Boynton, J.L., Hersh, H.: Readability of fonts in the windows environment. In: Conference Companion on Human Factors in Computing Systems. ACM (1995)

Involving Senior Workers in Crowdsourced Proofreading

Toshinari Itoko[1], Shoma Arita[2], Masatomo Kobayashi[1], and Hironobu Takagi[1]

[1] IBM Research – Tokyo, 5-6-52 Toyosu, Koto, Tokyo 135-8511, Japan
{itoko,mstm,takagih}@jp.ibm.com
[2] The University of Tokyo, 7-3-1 Hongo, Bunkyo, Tokyo 113-8656, Japan
arita@cyber.t.u-tokyo.ac.jp

Abstract. Seniors have a wealth of knowledge and free time, so they are a promising workforce for crowdsourced tasks. Currently senior workers are hardly involved in real applications. We have started an experimental project that crowdsources proofreading micro-tasks to volunteer workers to efficiently produce accessible digital books. By design, the majority of the workers in this project are senior citizens. In this paper, we report the findings of our experiment in which we tested four working hypotheses about the behavioral characteristics of senior workers. We also discuss skill management to improve task performance and motivation encouragement for long-term involvement of senior workers.

Keywords: Senior Workforce, Elderly, Ageing, Micro-tasks, Crowdsourcing, Gamification, Accessibility.

1   Introduction

Crowdsourcing is recognized as a powerful tool for outsourcing manual tasks and is widely utilized in real applications. The tasks offered by typical crowdsourcing services are not demanding as regards the workers' physical locations or time, so they are highly suitable for a large number of non-fulltime workers. Seniors are an especially promising workforce for such tasks, especially in Japan where the population is aging rapidly [1]. However, there are no well-established methods for effectively involving senior workers in crowdsourced work. Our findings will help accelerate the development of methods to support crowdsourced applications with. In October 2013, in collaboration with the Japan Braille Library, we launched an experimental crowdsourcing project to convert printed books into an accessible digital text format, DAISY (Digital Accessible Information SYstem) [2], using the micro-tasking model proposed in [3]. As of January 2014, 178 participants including 83 seniors (age 60+) have registered and more than 1,200 hours of work has been completed. Since the crowdsourcing of proofreading is a well-known approach (e.g., [4][5][6]), our research focus was to develop methods to improve senior workers' long-term performance in crowdsourcing. These methods must be based on a deep understanding of their behaviors in practical applications. This paper is organized as follows. In Section 2, we introduce the implementation of our system and the experimental hypotheses.

C. Stephanidis and M. Antona (Eds.): UAHCI/HCII 2014, Part III, LNCS 8515, pp. 106–117, 2014.

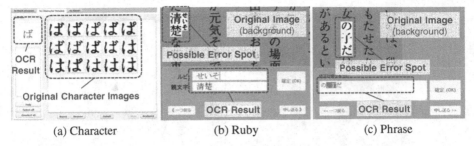

| (a) Character | (b) Ruby | (c) Phrase |

Fig. 1. Three types of crowdsourced proofreading interfaces

In Section 3, we report the results and notable findings. In Section 4, we discuss how to manage skills and motivate senior workers doing crowdsourced tasks.

2   Implementation and Hypotheses

Our experiment is designed to understand behavioral features of senior workers from two main perspectives: proofreading operations and mechanisms for encouraging motivation. Starting with the system design proposed in [3], we introduce additional implementation considerations and experimental hypotheses.

Total Involvement. We arranged the experimental website to improve the involvement of senior workers as shown later in this section. Given that senior citizens tend to have a desire to contribute to their society [7], seniors are expected to work more if the technical and motivational barriers are eliminated. Thus we start with this hypothesis:

(H1). Seniors will do more work than young workers.

2.1   Crowdsourced Proofreading Interfaces

Our system decomposes the proofreading process into three types of sub-tasks and provides a specialized view for each of them: Character, Ruby, and Phrase (Fig. 1). This is based on the observation that there are three kinds of typical OCR (Optical Character Recognition) errors in Japanese text: (a) repeated errors involving a specific character (i.e., a specific character tends to cause similar OCR errors throughout a book), (b) errors in ruby (a pair consisting of one or more Chinese-derived characters and a pronunciation gloss (displayed nearby in a smaller (ruby) font)), and (c) letter separation errors in phrases (as in English when "m" is read as "r" plus "n"). Since the Character view uses an interface from CONCERT [5], it has some English labels, which were not redesigned for the Japanese users. In comparison, the Ruby and Phrase views have relatively large buttons with Japanese labels. See [3] for details of the design of each view.

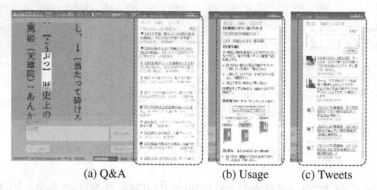

(a) Q&A   (b) Usage   (c) Tweets

Fig. 2. Screenshots of the sidebar of the proofreading interfaces

Differences in Competence. Several articles indicate that senior workers have more linguistic knowledge but weaker ICT skills and visual attention than younger workers [8][9]. We believe that Character requires more ICT skills and visual attention while Ruby and Phrase call for more linguistic knowledge, which leads to our second hypothesis:

(H2). Seniors will be relatively good at the Ruby and Phrase tasks while young workers are better at Character.

2.2   Mechanisms for Encouraging Motivation

With all three of our proofreading views, workers can start or leave the work whenever they want to. There are no quotas or scheduled hours. This makes participation easier, especially for people who have little time for volunteer work. However, this also means that they can always leave the project, and so we added additional mechanisms to encourage their long-term involvement. We used two approaches to achieve this goal: removing barriers to continuing participation and providing incentives for active participation. For barrier removal, our system has question-answer support, since a leading cause of quitting is when a worker cannot complete a difficult task. For incentive, a gamification mechanism provides workers with a variety of types of feedback in response to their contributions.

Question-Answer Support. Previous studies have indicated that senior citizens using ICT have stronger needs for support from other people compared to younger people [10][11][12], we carefully integrated a question-answer (Q&A) forum into the proofreading interfaces as illustrated in Fig. 2-a. The list of the latest questions, a link to the full list of questions, and a link to post a new question are always visible at the right side of the proofreading interfaces. This allows proofreaders to easily access the question-answer features whenever they need to during proofreading tasks. The Q&A forum can transfer knowledge about the language itself, the usage of the system, and the rules of proofreading, coming from the participants who know the answers to the participants who need to know. We anticipated that senior participants would post relatively more questions in the forum since they prefer guided support from other people and tend to dislike trial-and-error approaches [10]. In the sidebar, there are two other tabs. "Usage" shows brief instructions for the ongoing proofreading task with a link to the full instruction manual in PDF format (Fig. 2-b). Again, research shows senior citizens prefer to learn from manuals almost as much as they like support from other people, but they prefer to print documents rather than read them on screen. The "Tweets" tab offers a Twitter-like chat interface (Fig. 2-c) intended for frequent, informal communications among participants that could lead to a stronger sense of collaboration. Regarding the Q&A forum, we have a third hypothesis based on the previous research:

(H3). Seniors will ask more questions than the young workers.

Gamification. Rankings and badges are popular methods to motivate active participation in various types of online social systems. It is known that providing participants with feedback about their contributions can improve their motivation (e.g., [13]). Since crowdsourcing allows workers to freely start and leave their work whenever they want, motivation is needed for sustainable involvement. Thus we added gamification features to our system. They consist of (a) a ranking based on the number of completed tasks during the last 30 days, (b) badges based on completed tasks, (c) the accumulated numbers of completed tasks of each task type, (d) the worker's personal contribution to the last book the worker contributed to, as a percentage of all of the work done so far on that book, and (e) the number of books that the worker has contributed to relative to the total number of books in this project (Fig. 3). Note that (a) is a kind of competition between each worker and the other workers while (b) and (c) measure the worker's own efforts. The scores of (d) and (e) give a larger perspective on the worker's contribution. Since previous studies (e.g., [14]) showed that gamification mechanisms could benefit senior citizens as well as younger people, this leads to our fourth hypothesis:

(H4). Gamification features will more strongly encourage seniors than young workers.

2.3   Miscellaneous Design Considerations

Fig. 3 shows the portal page that the participants see after logging into the system. It consists of announcements to the participants at the top, large icons that link to the main features (e.g., proofreading or Q&A) in the middle, a gamification screen at the bottom, and links to download manuals and the chat interface on the right side. The portal page is designed not only for proofreaders but also for DAISY book users, i.e., people with print disabilities. The system provides them with forums to request new DAISY books, which can lead to new proofreading tasks. One of our goals is to keep this forum active, because a previous study reported that the lack of tasks can disrupt the momentum of participation in a micro-tasking system, and the lost

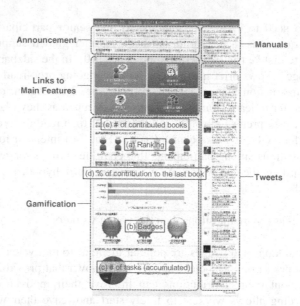

Announcement —

Links to
Main Features —

Manuals

(e) # of contributed books

(a) Ranking

(d) % of contribution to the last book

Tweets

Gamification —

(b) Badges

(c) # of tasks (accumulated)

Fig. 3. A screen shot of the portal page with the gamification display

participants may never return [15]. Finally, the system also provides a sandbox forum to allow participants to practice using the forum interface.

The website design for senior citizens involved many accessibility-related considerations. For example, their declining sensory and physical abilities require larger text and buttons [16]. Meanwhile, they often use inexpensive devices with small screens (e.g., XGA displays). Senior citizens may have difficulties in scrolling the pages, which imposes a design constraint that all of the needed information should be visible on one screen. Thus there is a trade-off between the sizes of the content and the screen. We used an iterative design process based on user feedback with experts deciding on the size of each component and their layout. Also, we iteratively improved the accessibility for the DAISY book users, who usually use a screen reader to access websites.

3   Experimental Results

In this section, we describe the results of our experiment in terms of the four hypotheses (H1–4) from Section 2. The experiment started on October 15, 2013. We analyze the data from this date to January 26, 2014 in this paper. In that period, 178 volunteers registered and 112 of them were "active workers", who did at least one task. They contributed more than 1,200 hours and proofread 136 books. The outcomes by types of tasks are summarized in Table 1.

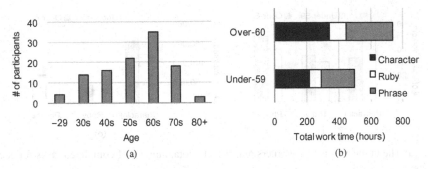

Fig. 4. (a) Age distribution of active workers and (b) Total work time (hours)

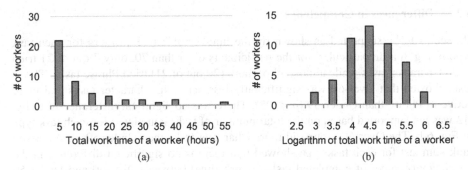

Fig. 5. Distribution of (a) the total work time (hours) and (b) the logarithm of (a)

Table 1. Proofreading Outcomes by Task Type

Task type	# completed	Total working time	# per hour
Character	279,390 tasks	553 hours	505 tasks
Ruby	77,930 tasks	180 hours	432 tasks
Phrase	137,070 tasks	500 hours	274 tasks

3.1   Total Involvement

The active workers had wide distribution of ages (Fig. 4-a). There were 56 active senior workers (Over-60) and 56 active younger workers (Under-59). The Over-60 group worked a total of 755 hours while the Under-59 group worked 514 hours (Fig. 4-b). The distribution of total work time for each active worker was not a normal distribution (Fig. 5-a). However, the logarithm of the total work time seemed to be normally distributed (Fig. 5-b), with statistical support from a Shapiro-Wilk normality test ($p > .05$). A Welch test showed that the logarithmic total work time for Over-60 was significantly longer than the Under-59 ($p < .05$). The average log values were 4.107 and 3.769 for Over-60 and Under-59, respectively.

(R1). H1 was supported. Over-60 worked significantly longer than Under-59.

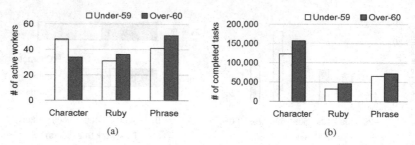

Fig. 6. (a) The number of active workers and (b) The total number of completed tasks for each task type

3.2   Differences in Competence

H2 seems to be supported as shown by the number of active workers for each task type in Fig. 6-a. In particular, for the participants older than 70, only 7 out of 21 tried to do Character tasks while almost all of them (20 out of 21) tried Phrase tasks. The χ^2 tests showed that Over-60 was significantly less active in Character tasks and more active in Phrase than Under-59 ($p < .05$). There was no significat difference in Ruby. H2 was not supported based on the total number of tasks completed for each task type in Fig. 6-b. The Over-60 group did more Character tasks than Under-59. A Wilcoxon rank sum test for each task type showed that there is no significant difference in the efficiency (number of completed tasks / work time) between Over-60 and Under-59 ($p > .05$).

(R2). H2 was partially supported. The Over-60 group was less likely to try Character tasks while they tried more Phrase tasks. However there was no significant difference in the efficiency metric between the Over-60 and Under-59 groups.

3.3   Question-Answer Support

During the experimental period, 60 questions were posted by proofreaders. The average numbers of questions for each active participant were 0.63 and 0.70 for Under-59 and Over-60, respectively. This result seems to confirm H3. However, the limited number of questions is too small to support a firm conclusion. Certain participants tend to post many questions, while 85% of the active participants did not post any. This result does not necessarily indicate that the Q&A forum is of no use for the majority of the participants. The data shows that 73% of the active participants accessed the Q&A forum and 59% read at least one Q&A thread. They may have gained knowledge from the Q&A forum even if they did not post any questions. In addition, several participants wrote question-like messages using the chat interface rather than the Q&A interface. This might indicate that if the system provides a quicker way to post questions, the participants would be encouraged to post more questions. Out of the total of 60 questions, 56 were answered by members of the library or development teams, only 1 was answered by other participants, but 3 received answers from both

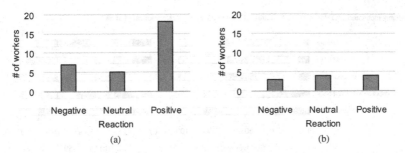

Fig. 7. Effects of the gamification display on the number of contributions for participants who (a) looked at the game metrics vs. (b) never looked at them

staff members and participants. All of the questions were answered within 24 hours. As regards the subjects of the questions, only 1 question asked for linguistic knowledge, while 33 asked for system usage information and 26 asked about proofreading rules.

(R3). H3 could be promising but our results were inconclusive. At least for the limited sample, seniors tended to ask more questions than younger participants.

3.4 Gamification

We added the gamification features to our system in the middle of the target period. Thus we can compare the results without and with the gamification. For analyses, we divided the participants into two groups: those who have looked at the gamification display and those who have never looked at it. We scored the game display as seen when a participant scrolled down the page and the mouse cursor moved over the game display. Fig. 7 shows the number of participants for whom the gamification features had positive, neutral, and negative effects, based on comparing the amount of contributions during each week before and after the introduction of gamification. For the group that looked at the game metrics, the numbers of participants with positive, neutral, and negative reactions were 18, 5, and 7, respectively. For the latter group that never looked at the game metrics, the numbers were 4, 4, and 3. This result seems to show some positive effects of the gamification display. We also compared the effects for senior and young participants and found no apparent effects related to age.

For further analyses, we conducted an online survey. We asked how each component of the gamification display motivated participants with a 5-point Likert scale from 1 (not motivated at all) to 5 (highly motivated). A total of 29 participants (22 senior and 7 young) responded to the survey. The results are summarized in Fig. 8. For the Over-60 group, the average values were 3.3, 3.0, 3.1, 3.6, and 3.6 for ranking, badges, the accumulated number of tasks, the percentage of contribution to the last book, and the number of contributed books, respectively. For the Under-59 group, the values were 3.3, 2.6, 2.6, 3.0, and 3.6. The majority of the respondents most preferred the display of the number of contributed books. In contrast, ranking, badges, and the accumulated number of tasks were least motivational according to self-reporting.

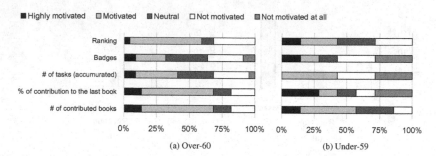

Fig. 8. Subjective evaluation of each gamification component

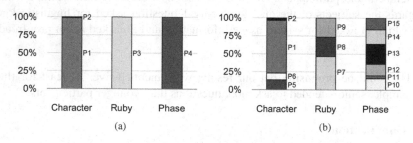

Fig. 9. (a) High-performers for a book vs. (b) long-tail workers accumulating work on a book. Each stacked rectangle represents the amount of the contribution of a worker to the book.

(R4). H4 could be promising but our results were inconclusive. At least for the limited sample, the participants who had looked at the gamification display tended to perform more tasks but no age-related effect was observed. At the same time, the subjective evaluation did indicate that the Over-60 group felt more encouraged than the Under-59.

4   Discussion

4.1   Effects of High-Performance Workers

As shown in Section 3.1, the senior participants tended to complete more work. However, we need to note that the total work performed by the workers was not normally distributed. A few high-performance workers contribute much more than others, and thus apparent tendencies in the total performance are dominated by their outcomes. For some books, almost all of the work was completed by one high-performance worker (Fig. 9-a). However, there are also some books that involved more than 10 workers completing a single book (Fig. 9-b). This observation indicates that the sustainability of micro-tasking community can involve both the contributions of high-performers and long-tail workers. More investigation of the differences among individuals will be needed. Note that the task performance depends not only on the

Table 2. Top X worker's performance by task type

TOP	Character			Ruby			Phrase		
	# tasks	Cumulative total	Age	# tasks	Cumulative total	Age	# tasks	Cumulative total	Age
1	85,269	30.5%	64	9,528	12.2%	49	24,948	18.2%	49
2	37,392	43.9%	57	6,305	20.3%	78	15,198	29.3%	76
3	35,407	56.6%	49	5,270	27.1%	76	10,769	37.1%	45
4	28,956	66.9%	45	5,227	33.8%	64	8,863	43.6%	64
5	27,919	76.9%	61	4,965	40.2%	42	7,525	49.1%	64
10%	6,836	87.6%	–	4,853	46.4%	–	4,426	63.1%	–
25%	957	96.3%	–	1,312	83.3%	–	1,236	86.4%	–
50%	133	99.4%	–	302	95.4%	–	292	97.0%	–

skills of each worker but also on the content and OCR quality of each book. It will be necessary to eliminate the effects of differences among books to assess the skills of individual workers. It is also notable that there were many seniors among the high-performers (Table 2). The involvement of active seniors will be a key to enhancing crowdsourcing applications.

4.2   Complementarity in Competencies

The results in Section 3.2 showed that the differences between senior and younger workers for each task type are observed in terms of trying to start work or not start while the differences are not clear in the performance metrics of the active workers. This may indicate that the dominating factors in the workers' decisions are changed before and after starting work. We had classified the proofreading sub-tasks based on the three competencies of linguistic knowledge, ICT skills, and visual attention. What are the unpredicted competencies? In the experiment, we noticed a fourth competency we called "task-specific knowledge", which may be the most important competency we recognized after starting work. In our context, this is knowledge about the editorial rules in proofreading. In fact, almost half of the questions posted in the Q&A forum asked about editorial rules. It is not hard to anticipate that few of the workers would have such knowledge in the beginning. The lack of task-specific knowledge about editing might mask significant efficiency differences between senior and younger workers, as discussed in Section 3.2.

4.3   Knowledge Transfer among Participants

The Q&A forum was essential for some of the participants, especially among the seniors. It provided them with crucial on-demand support while doing the work. The resulting answers in the Q&A threads also helped other participants with similar questions. In addition, we used the Q&A forum to iteratively update the downloadable instruction manuals. The communications in the forum allowed us to see what information the participants needed and helped us improve our system. However, the limited results during the experimental period were insufficient to evaluate the age-difference effect on need for Q&A, because there were too few questioners. Another problem for the future is to address the lack of mutual support in the Q&A system. During the experimental period, most of the questions were answered by administrators. One reason might be that most of the questions were related to the system usage or proofreading rules, both of which required expert knowledge that the participants had not yet acquired it. However, since the amount of work that can be done by administrators is limited, mutual support among participants is needed to improve the scalability and sustainability of the micro-tasking system. We are continuing our pilot study and we will examine whether the participants with longer experience are motivated to transfer their knowledge to novices.

4.4   Motivation Encouragement by Gamification

The results indicated that the gamification mechanism has certain positive effects in motivating participants. In addition, the questionnaire results showed that the seniors were more positive about the gamification than the younger participants. More specifically, seniors preferred the gamification components in a general way, while the younger participants favored specific metrics such as the number of contributed books and ranking. Among the gamification components, the visualizations of contributions were most preferred. In particular, the seniors did not like the visualizations of their own efforts or competition with other participants, whereas the younger participants tended to like the competitive aspects. This might be because our experiment involved volunteers who had intrinsic motivations to contribute to society by helping people with disabilities. Other types of tasks may call for other types of incentives. It is future work to examine what types of feedback are effective to encourage senior citizens to participate in other types of micro-tasks such as paid work not for social contribution as well as to assess age differences in the effects of gamification with a larger sample.

5   Conclusion

This paper described some of the characteristics of senior workers observed in a crowdsourcing system for proofreading tasks. The results showed that seniors tended to do more work than young workers. It was indicated that the Q&A and gamification mechanisms are particularly effective for senior workers. Also the potential of the multi-generational approach was shown. The involvement of both senior and younger workers allows gathering different competencies while micro-tasking allows decomposing a larger task into sub-tasks for each competency. Our future work will include individual skill management for performance improvements and individual motivation encouragement for long-term engagement. For skill management, preliminary findings were presented in [12]. For motivation encouragement, basic findings were discussed in this paper. Based on these insights, we will continue investigating elderly participation in crowdsourcing, including different types of tasks, such as paid work.

Acknowledgments. This research was partially supported by the Japan Science and Technology Agency (JST) under the Strategic Promotion of Innovative Research and Development Program. We thank Mr. Sawamura and other staff members of the Japan Braille Library for their support. We also thank all of the participants in our experiment.

References

1. Miura, T., Nakayama, M., Hiyama, A., Yatomi, N., Hirose, M.: Time-Mosaic Formation of Senior Workforces for Complex Irregular Work in Cooperative Farms. In: Stephanidis, C., Antona, M. (eds.) UAHCI 2013, Part II. LNCS, vol. 8010, pp. 162–170. Springer, Heidelberg (2013)
2. DAISY Consortium, http://www.daisy.org/
3. Kobayashi, M., Ishihara, T., Itoko, T., Takagi, H., Asakawa, C.: Age-based Task Specialization for Crowdsourced Proofreading. In: Stephanidis, C., Antona, M. (eds.) UAHCI 2013, Part II. LNCS, vol. 8010, pp. 104–112. Springer, Heidelberg (2013)
4. Bookshare, http://www.bookshare.org/
5. Neudecker, C., Tzadok, A.: User Collaboration for Improving Access to Historical Texts. Liber Quarterly 20(1), 119–128 (2010)
6. Chrons, O., Sundell, S.: Digitalkoot: Making Old Archives Accessible Using Crowdsourcing. In: Proc. HCOMP 2011 (2011)
7. Marmot, M., Banks, J., Blundell, R., Lessof, C., Nazroo, J. (eds.): Health, wealth and lifestyles of the older population in England: ELSA 2002. Institute for Fiscal Studies (2003)
8. Ouchi, Y., Akiyama, H. (eds.): Gerontology – Overview and Perspectives, 3rd edn. Univ. of Tokyo Press (2010) (in Japanese)
9. Staffing Mature Worker Survey, http://www.goldenworkers.org/images/publication/mature_workers_survey_2012_adecco.pdf
10. Leung, R., Tang, C., Haddad, S., McGrenere, J., Graf, P., Ingriany, V.: How Older Adults Learn to Use Mobile Devices: Survey and Field Investigations. ACM Trans. Access. Comput. 4(3), Article 11 (2012)
11. Czaja, S.J., Lee, C.C., Branham, J., Remis, P.: OASIS Connections: Results From an Evaluation Study. The Gerontologist 52(5), 712–721 (2012)
12. Kobayashi, M., Ishihara, T., Kosugi, A., Takagi, H., Asakawa, C.: Question-Answer Cards for an Inclusive Micro-Tasking Framework for the Elderly. In: Kotzé, P., Marsden, G., Lindgaard, G., Wesson, J., Winckler, M. (eds.) INTERACT 2013, Part III. LNCS, vol. 8119, pp. 590–607. Springer, Heidelberg (2013)
13. Farzan, R., DiMicco, J.M., Millen, D.R., Dugan, C., Geyer, W., Brownholtz, E.A.: Results from deploying a participation incentive mechanism within the enterprise. In: Proc. CHI 2008, pp. 563–572. ACM (2008)
14. McCallum, S.: Gamification and serious games for personalized health. Stud. Health Technol. Inform. 177, 85–96 (2012)
15. Takagi, H., Harada, S., Sato, D., Asakawa, C.: Lessons Learned from Crowd Accessibility Services. In: Winckler, M. (ed.) INTERACT 2013, Part I. LNCS, vol. 8117, pp. 587–604. Springer, Heidelberg (2013)
16. Web Content Accessibility Guidelines (WCAG) 2.0, http://www.w3.org/TR/WCAG20/

Leveraging Web Technologies
to Expose Multiple Contemporary Controller Input
in Smart TV Rich Internet Applications
Utilized in Elderly Assisted Living Environments

Evdokimos I. Konstantinidis, Panagiotis E. Antoniou, Antonis Billis,
Georgios Bamparopoulos, Costas Pappas, and Panagiotis D. Bamidis

Medical Physics Laboratory, Medical School, Faculty of Health Sciences
Aristotle University of Thessaloniki, Greece
evdokimosk@gmail.com

Abstract. This work describes a lightweight framework allowing internet applications to access controllers such as the Wii remote, Wii balance board and MS Kinect irrespective of proximity or configuration. This is achieved by utilizing predetermined schemas for encapsulating the controller information and transferring this data through standard internet communication technologies (RESTFUL services and Web Sockets) in platform independent, device naïve ways. These features of the framework provide Rich Internet Applications (RIAs) with ubiquitous access to sophisticated human computer interaction schemes for diverse uses. The proliferation of Smart TVs as central information hubs in elderly assisted living environments, along with the need for simple gesture control schemes for these demographics, provides one application of this framework. Thus, we demonstrate how this service can be incorporated for developing internet applications and how it can be utilized for providing intuitive interaction methods for RIAs deployed through Smart TVs in elderly assisted living environments.

Keywords: cross-device communication, smart home, elderly, ambient assisted living, ubiquitous communication technologies, exergaming serious gaming.

1 Introduction and Background

1.1 Introduction

It has become increasingly common for contemporary and novel input devices to find fertile ground with new tasks in the realm of Human Computer Interaction. Towards this end, depth imaging devices are considered as suitable candidates to substitute or complement traditional input methods for future applications and systems. With the introduction of Microsoft's Kinect depth imaging device and the release of powerful SDKs exploiting and enhancing its information (by providing both image and body skeleton information), users are enabled to control and interact with applications and

C. Stephanidis and M. Antona (Eds.): UAHCI/HCII 2014, Part III, LNCS 8515, pp. 118–128, 2014.
© Springer International Publishing Switzerland 2014

systems through natural postures/gestures, without touching a game controller. Recent literature promotes the usage of such devices as a trend for modern designs [1–5].However, one of the promising approaches on utilizing gaming input devices for new interactive designs, before the Kinect sensor was introduced in the market, had been based on Nintendo Wii remote control and Wii BalanceBoard. The former corresponds to the users' movements (accelerations) while the latter utilizes the body's center of mass. Both of the devices support wireless connectivity. Consequently, they can be utilized when there are movement restrictions due to limited space [6, 7].

Even more exotic sensors-as-controllers have been developed in order to facilitate specialized needs in human machine interface. Interface devices like Neurosky's Mindwave device utilize direct electroencephalography signals (EEG) to assess brain function [8, 9] and, with custom software, infer cognitive and emotional states and utilize them in a multitude of ways.

1.2   Background

Beyond mainstream gaming, unconventional controllers like Wiimote, Wii balance board and the Kinect found use in the field of ubiquitous computing [10]. The advent of integrated sensors/controllers like the Kinect has enabled this contextual utilization of user input [11]. Fusing unconventional controllers and streaming their input to the web provides interesting applications potential such as gestural user interfaces for increased productivity in the management of tiled display [6].Furthermore, in the field of cross device applications, the enabling of the user through the seamless integration of several diverse control devices, dictates implicitly the use of natural, unconventional and unobtrusive control schemes and control devices [12–14].

Focusing on enabling applications of cross-platform cross-device, ubiquitous computing the Smart Home is one of the most promising. Smart homes aim to augment people's lives through technologies that provide increased functionality, communication and awareness [15]. In that context Smart TVs are aiming to become the epicenters of interaction in smart homes. For one, due to the TV sets long lived existence there has been developed a strong familiarity with people of any demographic. For example, it has been suggested that there is a link between technology and area ownership of the home [16]. On the other hand, Smart TV sets have been successfully used for controlling aspects of the Smart Home [17].

While Smart Homes are an impressive quality of life enhancer for people of any age, they take a significance boost when seen within the scope of assisted living, and specifically in the area of elderly assisted living and quality of life improvement. In this field, contemporary controllers/sensors find significant use. For example, Kinect has been proven effective in monitoring the stance of a senior in order to anticipate and prevent balance loss [18], or the Wii suite of controllers (Wiimote, Wii board) has been used for enabling elderly people to increase their physical activity levels by engaging in games that utilize these controllers and drive the users to increased physical and psychological wellbeing [19]. In fact, research explored the utility of cognitive and physical training through computer games and provided significant conclusions, with results providing specific guidelines for topics as diverse as depression or interaction between generations [20, 21]. This kind of research has even coined a portmanteau term exergaming (exercise gaming) to describe computer software that facilitates mental and physical training in a computer gaming environment [20, 21].

1.3   Rationale

Incentivized by the presented context we developed a lightweight framework (Controller Application Communication framework – CAC framework) that allows internet applications ubiquitous access to controllers such as the Wii remote, Wii balance board MS Kinect and Neurosky Mindwave. This is achieved by using predetermined schemas for encapsulating controller information and transferring the data through standard internet communication technologies in a cross platform, and device independent way. In this work we briefly describe this framework and present the first technical assessment results from a developer base that implemented it in a small demo application. Additionally, we present a demo use case scenario of implementing this framework in an exergaming application of an elderly assisted living environment.

2   Materials and Methods

2.1   Description of the CAC Framework

The CAC framework [22] has the role of an intermediary, in order to allow the connection of a series of controllers to all applications that use the framework and require sensor input. The CAC framework functions as a number of loosely coupled services that

1. Encapsulate the raw information from the device, in a predetermined, structured albeit custom way
2. Format all requests for sensor/controller data from the applications, in a uniform, framework aware, data schema and
3. Utilize ubiquitous internet communication technologies (Websockets and RESTful web services) to make possible the transmission of requests and data from and to applications running on a multitude of platforms and devices, through a distributed server structure (Fig. 1).

The CAC framework exposes structures and functionalities specific for every supported input device. The appropriately formatted information is pushed from the devices to the service. A processing component of the framework acquires information from the device and passes it to the server. This component is either an application that uses the devices' libraries (e.g. Microsoft Kinect SDK) and drivers or, when technology allows, the exposed functionalities of the sensor/controller itself as it would become available by emerging ubiquitous computing technologies. This information (for example, the RGB stream of the Kinect or the weight of a person on the Wii Balance Board) is then either polled by the applications or pushed by the service to the applications. It must be noted that applications which consume the framework's communicated data can be either conventional computer applications or embedded software in custom hardware such as Smart phones, Smart TV sets, tablets, or robotic devices; in general, any piece of software, or hardware that can facilitate internet communication.

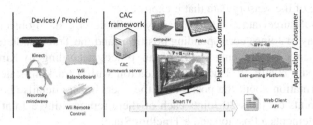

Fig. 1. Controller Application Communication (CAC) framework concept

Through the described provisions for custom but uniform across the framework encapsulation of controller data and application requests, as well as, with the use of the standard real time internet communication technologies, this framework facilitates device and platform independent communication between controller/sensor devices and relevant applications.

The next subsection presents the web client API that facilitates developers to incorporate the framework to web applications exploiting the usage of contemporary controllers.

2.2   CAC Framework's Web Client API

The CAC framework web client API (available information online at http://kedip16.med.auth.gr/cac-framework) brings contemporary input devices (e.g. Kinect, Wii, Mindwave) to modern web applications by utilizing the CAC framework in an easy to use way. The API isolates technological details (web sockets, restful calls) and gives the developers the capability to be more productive by allowing them to focus more on the exploitation of the controllers' information.

Table 1. Device object

Attributes	Description
DeviceID	The device hardware unique id
DeviceType	1:Skeleton
	2:Wiimote
	3:BalanceBoard
	4:Mindwave
	5:RgbColorImage
LastUpdateDateTime	The date and time of the last device capture
SessionID	The session ID the device belongs to.

The main data object delivered through the API is the Device Object which contains information regarding the device that streamed the data. Its attributes are depicted in Table 1. Depending on the device, the objects SkeletonSourceData, WiiSourceData, MindwaveSourceData and RGBVideoSourceData contain the transmitted information. The developer has access directly to those four structures. Each one of these structures apart from general attributes has its own information, coming from the nature of the sensory data that it captures.

The SkeletonSourceData contains an array of Skeletons. Each object of the array includes an array of Joints, corresponding positions and the TrackingState. The TrackingState represents the tracking status of an object according to Kinect (0: Not-Tracked, 1: PositionOnly, 2: Tracked). A skeleton with a tracking state of "position only" has information about the position of the user, but no details about the joints. The array of Joints contains 20 Joints each of them representing a Joint of the body. Each Joint implements a Position and a TrackingState.

The WiiSourceData contains AccelState (in case of wii remote controller) BalanceBoardState and ButtonState. The BalanceBoardState contains Weight in Kg, the CenterOfGravity (x and y axis) and the components of the weight at the 4 pressure sensors of the Balance Board (BottonLeft, BottomRight, TopLeft, TopRight). The ButtonState includes information of the buttons status being BalanceBoard or Wiimote.

The MindwaveSourceData contains the values of the processed EEG power spectrums (Alpha1, Alpha2, Beta1, Beta2, Delta, Gamma1, Gamma2, Theta), output of NeuroSky proprietary eSense meter for Attention, Meditation, and other future meters and signal quality analysis (can be used to detect poor contact and whether the device is off the head).

The RGBVideoSourceData contains the RGBVideo object which incorporates the width and height of the image and the base64String of the image data.

The consumption of the CAC framework through the API requires the developer to include the required javascript libraries, to define the unique session identifier [22] and to add the appropriate event listener to process the incoming packets. Table 2 implements the addEventListener for skeletonEvent, wiiEvent, while the MindwaveEvent and RGBVideoEvent can be used in the same way.

Table 2. CAC framework web client api example

```
document.addEventListener("skeletonEvent", function(e) {
    document.getElementById("y-position").value =
e.detail.SkeletonSourceData.Skeletons[0].Joints[0].Position.Y;
});

document.addEventListener("wiiEvent", function(e) {
    document.getElementById("weight").value =
e.detail.WiiSourceData.BalanceBoardState.WeightKg;
});
```

2.3   Evaluation of the Framework's Implementation API

In order to assess the technical feasibility and overall programming convenience of implementing this framework in realistic implementation scenarios, a user study was conducted. A demo web page was setup and a group of 17 programmers were asked to incorporate the framework client API into it. The participants had to include the required script files in order to read information from the devices and depict it through certain fields of the html page. The participants were provided with an API package of the framework in Javascript and its reference which contains descriptions of the API, its structures and short examples. The group of programmers needed to catch the data from a suite of controllers (MS Kinect, Wii Balance Board, Neurosky Mindwave) and populate the demo page with these data. The tasks that were to be implemented are summarized in Table 3. Fig. 2 demonstrates a developer's implementation with the demo page populated by the relevant data.

Table 3. Tasks to be implemented on the demo page by developers using the framework's javascript API

Task to be implemented	Relevant controller
Detect if User's hand is on the left or right of the User's center irrespective of height	MS Kinect
Display streaming RGB video	MS Kinect
Display the weight of the user	Wii Balance Board
Display the "Attention" [8] of the user (a measure of the User's attention level)	Neurosky Mindwave
Display the "Meditation" [8] of the user (a measure of the User's relaxation level)	Neurosky Mindwave

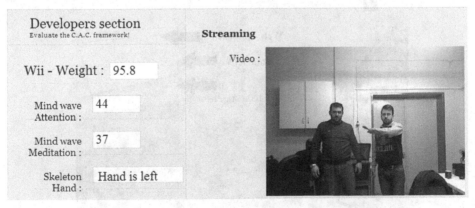

Fig. 2. The outcome web page after the completion of the task

After the implementation all developers were given a survey form to fill out in order to evaluate their experience with the API. Apart from a brief series of questions regarding programming experience and skills of this developer in different aspects of development, the survey explored the technical use specifications of the API (Ease of implementation, functionality, etc) and probed the developers for expressing their opinion regarding fields of application and some even more focused questions regarding the APIs potential as a facilitator of elderly assisted living control schemes. Apart from a couple of open ended probing questions all our questions contained responses rated on a five item Likert scale.

2.4   A Demo Use Case Scenario

Beyond the technical feasibility testing by the group of developers we have initiated, in the context of the USEFIL project [23], a demo use case in controlled lab environment in order to take away the look and feel of a real world application that would be empowered by the described framework. The aim of the USEFIL project is the creation of an unobtrusive elderly assisted living environment for both monitoring the elderly user's status and providing quality of life enhancers in the form of mental and physical exercise games. In that context the CAC framework was utilized for fusing the Wii and Kinect sensors in order to allow the elderly user to control and participate in several exergaming scenarios and for utilizing the Kinect as a monitoring sensor.

The demo use case that was tested thus far was a controlled experiment of an elderly user interacting with the exergaming suite repurposed into the USEFIL project through the Wii balance board and the MS Kinect sensor (Fig. 3). After the elderly user interacted with the demo platform a brief discussion took place where probing questions were asked regarding the user experience.

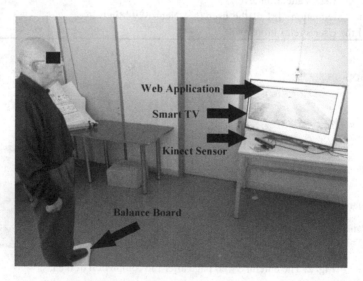

Fig. 3. Demo Use case of elderly exergaming scenario utilizing the CAC framework for fusing multiple controller data

3   Results

3.1   Developers' Survey

Most programmers who participated on this evaluation have reported good expertise regarding web technologies. On the other hand, they have on average little programming experience with sensing devices and programming apps for smart devices, such as SmartTVs and mobile devices. As it is presented in Fig. 4, none of the developers reported any difficulty in using the framework. The majority of the participants believe that the framework is functional and reliable, while most of them reported that they would adopt it within their applications. Furthermore, they believe that the CAC framework would provide added value to development on assisted living environments, while most of them think that the framework would enhance elderly accessibility to the web. The average time the developers spent to integrate the CAC framework was 13 minutes.

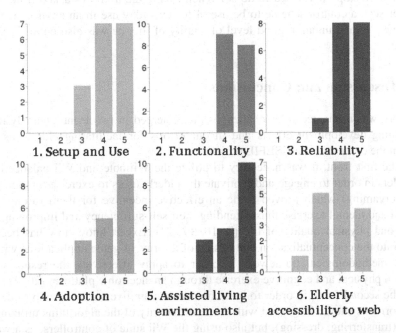

Fig. 4. Developers answers at the questions: 1. How would you rate the CAC framework regarding its setup and use?, 2. How would you rate the CAC framework regarding its functionality?, 3. How would you rate the CAC framework regarding its reliability?, 4. Would you adopt the framework within your applications?, 5. Do you believe that the CAC framework would provide added value to development on assisted living environments?, 6. Do you believe that the CAC framework would enhance elderly accessibility to the web? The x-axis represents Likert scale components (1-5), while the y-axis represents the count of programmers that specified the corresponding component.

When asked to spontaneously provide application fields for the CAC framework the participants of the survey mentioned exergames and physical training for elderly, but also went to more diverse fields such as map navigation, impaired people mouse substitute and monitoring applications.

3.2 Elder Users' Demo Use Case

When the elderly user was asked if the overall experience was a positive or a negative one he was enthusiastic that it was a positive one. When asked about the intuitiveness of the control interface the user mentioned that apart from a couple of glitches that led to the reset of the Wii balance board one time in order for it to work appropriately, the control scheme seemed to him very intuitive and non-intrusive. The user, however mentioned that the experience was a bit tiring, a fact that should be attributed at the battery of exergaming demo tests that he took. It should be noted that even though in the end he mentioned being tired, at the time of the experience, when asked if he would like to stop, he refused to do so. When finally the user was asked if he would consider such a control scheme to be useful for everyday use in an environment that would help him maintain a good level of quality of life, he was also enthusiastically positive.

4   Discussion and Conclusions

Our work was motivated from challenges that emerged in two fronts, namely in our exergaming development efforts and in our efforts for facilitating elderly assisted living in the context of the USEFIL project.

On the first front, it was necessary to utilize the Wiimote and Wii balance board controllers in order to engage and motivate the elderly users to exercise through gaming (exergaming) which proved to be an effective incentive for them to engage in physical and mental exercise thus extending their self-sufficiency and improving their mental and physical quality of life [7, 16, 17, 24]. Expert know-how has been invested into the conceptualization and design of a series of game applications within a specific methodological framework in order to apply effectively the results of research on physical and cognitive exercise through an electronic platform [20, 21].

On the second front, in order to infer an elder's cognitive state, a group of devices and algorithms should be fuzzed with the vast majority of the algorithms utilizing the Kinect (transferring, dressing), but also using the Wii suite of controllers, as a way of interaction with a smart TV set, which is the User Interface hub for the training applications, as well as a natural centerpoint for an assisted living environment [25].

From the results of the survey group it becomes clear that the described framework is an easy to use effective tool for fusing and streaming multiple controller/sensor input through the web. This can enhance further Rich Internet Applications (RIAs) with intuitive control schemes. While this provision is a nice interface enhancement in a general context, it takes a whole new importance in the area of elderly assisted living. It is noteworthy that even from this very controlled demo use case that was implemented with even a single elderly user the feedback was strongly positive.

While this work has largely fulfilled its purpose there is significant room for further work. With the advent of the emerging Internet of Things architectural paradigm [26], the switch from standard but ad hoc data formats to established namespaces becomes something far more than a novel improvement. Facilitating the transparent and ubiquitous interplay of devices and applications through frameworks and services like the one described here, becomes an important and viable avenue of research.

Acknowledgements. The work has been partially funded from the European Union's Seventh Framework Programme (FP7/2007-2013) under grant agreement no 288532. For more details, please see http://www.usefil.eu.

References

1. Son, J.P., Sowmya, A.: Single-handed driving system with kinect. In: Kurosu, M. (ed.) HCII/HCI 2013, Part II. LNCS, vol. 8005, pp. 631–639. Springer, Heidelberg (2013)
2. Le, H.-A., Mac, K.-N.C., Pham, T.-A., Nguyen, V.-T., Tran, M.-T.: Multimodal smart interactive presentation system. In: Kurosu, M. (ed.) HCII/HCI 2013, Part IV. LNCS, vol. 8007, pp. 67–76. Springer, Heidelberg (2013)
3. Chang, H.-T., Li, Y.-W., Chen, H.-T., Feng, S.-Y., Chien, T.-T.: A dynamic fitting room based on microsoft kinect and augmented reality technologies. In: Kurosu, M. (ed.) HCII/HCI 2013, Part IV. LNCS, vol. 8007, pp. 177–185. Springer, Heidelberg (2013)
4. Meneses Viveros, A., Hernández Rubio, E.: Kinect©, as interaction device with a tiled display. In: Kurosu, M. (ed.) HCII/HCI 2013, Part IV. LNCS, vol. 8007, pp. 301–311. Springer, Heidelberg (2013)
5. Mandiliotis, D., Toumpas, K., Kyprioti, K., Kaza, K., Barroso, J., Hadjileontiadis, L.J.: Symbiosis: An Innovative Human-Computer Interaction Environment for Alzheimer's Support. In: Stephanidis, C., Antona, M. (eds.) UAHCI 2013, Part II. LNCS, vol. 8010, pp. 123–132. Springer, Heidelberg (2013)
6. Lou, Y., Wu, W.: A Real-time Personalized Gesture Interaction System Using Wii Remote and Kinect for Tiled-Display Environment. In: 25th International Conference on Software Engineering and Knowledge Engineering, Boston, USA (2013)
7. Billis, A.S., Konstantinidis, E.I., Mouzakidis, C., Tsolaki, M.N., Pappas, C., Bamidis, P.D.: A game-like interface for training seniors' dynamic balance and coordination. In: XII Mediterranean Conference on Medical and Biological Engineering and Computing 2010, pp. 691–694. Springer (2010)
8. Neurosky Inc., Mindwave User Guide (2011),
   http://developer.neurosky.com/docs/lib/exe/
   fetch.php?media=mindwave_user_guide.pdf
9. Yasui, Y.: A brainwave signal measurement and data processing technique for daily life applications. J. Physiol. Anthropol. 28, 145–150 (2009)
10. Weiser, M.: The computer for the 21st century. ACM SIGMOBILE Mob. Comput. Commun. Rev. 3, 3–11 (1999)
11. Tan, C.S.S., Schoning, J., Luyten, K., Coninx, K.: Informing intelligent user interfaces by inferring affective states from body postures in ubiquitous computing environments. In: Proceedings of the 2013 International Conference on Intelligent user Interfaces, pp. 235–246. ACM, Santa Monica (2013)

12. Nebeling, M., Zimmerli, C., Husmann, M., Simmen, D., Norrie, M.C.: Information Concepts for Cross-device Applications. In: DUI 2013 3rd Work. Distrib. User Interfaces Model. Methods Tools. Conjunction with ACM EICS (2013)

13. Melchior, J., Vanderdonckt, J., Roy, P., Van: A model-based approach for distributed user interfaces. In: EICS 2011 Proceedings of the 3rd ACM SIGCHI Symposium on Engineering Interactive Computing Systems, pp. 11–20. ACM, Pisa (2011)

14. Paterno, F., Santoro, C., Paternò, F.: A logical framework for multi-device user interfaces. In: EICS 2012 Proceedings of the 4th ACM SIGCHI Symposium on Engineering Interactive Computing Systems, pp. 45–50. ACM, Copenhagen (2012)

15. Edwards, K.W., Grinter, R.E.: At home with ubiquitous computing: Seven challenges. In: Abowd, G.D., Brumitt, B., Shafer, S. (eds.) UbiComp 2001. LNCS, vol. 2201, pp. 256–272. Springer, Heidelberg (2001)

16. Hughes, J., Rodden, T.: Understanding Technology in Domestic Environments: lessons for cooperative buildings. In: Yuan, F., Konomi, S., Burkhardt, H.-J. (eds.) CoBuild 1998. LNCS, vol. 1370, pp. 248–261. Springer, Heidelberg (1998)

17. Cabrer, M., Redondo, R., Vilas, A., Pazos Arias, J., Duquw, J.: Controlling the smart home from TV. Consum. Electron. IEEE Trans. 52, 421–429 (2006)

18. Pisan, Y., Marin, J.J.G., Navarro, K.F.K.: Improving lives: using Microsoft Kinect to predict the loss of balance for elderly users under cognitive load. In: Proceedings of the 9th Australasian Conference on Interactive Entertainment Matters of Life and Death, IE 2013, pp. 1–4. ACM Press, New York (2013)

19. Jung, Y., Li, K.J., Janissa, N.S., Gladys, W.L.C., Lee, K.M.: Games for a better life: effects of playing Wii games on the well-being of seniors in a long-term care facility. In: Proceedings of the Sixth Australasian Conference on Interactive Entertainment, pp. 1–6. ACM, Sydney (2009)

20. Bogost, I.: Videogames and the future of education. Horiz 13, 119–128 (2005)

21. Görgü, L., Campbell, A., Dragone, M., O'Hare, G.: Exergaming: a future of mixing entertainment and exercise assisted by mixed reality agents. Comput. Entertain. - Theor. Pract. Comput. Appl. Entertain. 8 (2010)

22. Konstantinidis, E.I., Antoniou, P.E., Bamparopoulos, G., Bamidis, P.D.: A lightweight framework for transparent cross platform communication of controller data in ambient assisted living environments (2013)

23. Artikis, A., Bamidis, P.D., Billis, A., Bratsas, C., Frantzidis, C., Karkaletsis, V., Klados, M., Konstantinidis, E., Konstantopoulos, S., Kosmopoulos, D., Papadopoulos, H., Perantonis, S., Petridis, S., Spyropoulos, C.S.: Supporting tele-health and AI-based clinical decision making with sensor data fusion and semantic interpretation: The USEFIL case study. In: International Workshop on Artificial Intelligence and NetMedicine, p. 21 (2012)

24. Billis, A.S., Konstantinidis, E.I., Ladas, A.I., Tsolaki, M.N., Pappas, C., Bamidis, P.D.: Evaluating affective usability experiences of an exergaming platform for seniors. In: 2011 10th International Workshop on Biomedical Engineering, pp. 1–4. IEEE (2011)

25. Chen, W.: Gesture-based applications for elderly people. In: Kurosu, M. (ed.) HCII/HCI 2013, Part IV. LNCS, vol. 8007, pp. 186–195. Springer, Heidelberg (2013)

26. Atzori, L., Iera, A., Morabito, G.: The Internet of Things: A survey. Comput. Networks 54, 2787–2805 (2010)

Senior User's Color Cognition and Color Sensitivity Features in Visual Information on Web-Interface

Migyung Lee and Jinwan Park

Graduate School of Advanced Imaging Science, Multimedia & Film,
Chung-Ang University, Korea
miklee@naver.com, jinpark@cau.ac.kr

Abstract. At seeing from the viewpoint of HCI, the problems relevant to the use of smart devices like mobile phone, tablet PC are not limited to young people. Each user experiences smart devices with respectively different use abilities. When senior generations use smart devices, the color environment on a device's screen may take an important role in their usability. We conducted a survey targeting some senior generations with an application program for this experiment in various color environments on a tablet PC's screen. From the survey, we found that male and female senior generations preferred for larger text size and more distinctive brightness contrast between the text's color and the background color, and also preferred for opposite color combinations. Color arrangement commonly being preferred for by seniors was clear, dynamic high-chromatic color combinations, and unfavorable arrangements were dull, static low-chromatic color combinations. However, there were gender differences in 2nd and 3rd preferring color combinations. While female seniors preferred soft-feeling color combinations, but male seniors did hard-feeling color combinations. From this survey, we identified the existence of gender differences in the preferred color combinations as well as the senior people's general visual ability.

Keywords: Smart device, Aging Society, Senior Generation, Color Cognition, Color Combination.

1 Introduction

Recently from the HCI viewpoint, there are developing some studies for the efficient usability of smart devices targeting various user classes [1]. Of the web graphic user interface's factors, the visual information like texts, images, icons and menu are visual factors requiring a senior user's intuitive understanding, and they take important roles in information cognition [6, 13, 14]. It is know that for information to senior users having low visual-perceptual abilities, the most efficient way to deliver information should clearly use the color application to visual factors as well as should increase a text's explicitness and readability [10, 11, 12]. However, currently most interface designs are being developed around young generations, so it needed some researches

C. Stephanidis and M. Antona (Eds.): UAHCI/HCII 2014, Part III, LNCS 8515, pp. 129–137, 2014.
© Springer International Publishing Switzerland 2014

to experiment senior people's visual abilities [3]. So, this study set following hypotheses and conducted an experiment in a tablet PC environment.

H1: Senior generations will prefer for larger text sizes.

H2: Senior generations will prefer for more distinctive brightness contrast between the background color and the text's color.

H3: Senior generations will prefer for more distinctively contrasting color arrangements in graphic factors like menu and icons.

H4: Senior generations will prefer for harder-feeling, clearer color combinations rather than soft-feeling, dull color combinations.

2   Composition of Experiment Materials for Color Cognition

Through a previous survey, we selected 6 senior people, and then conducted the FGI(Focus Group Interview), and collected necessary color information for solving web-usability relevant problems. Experiment sample was based on Korea I.R.I's 'Hue & Tone 120 System', and was produced according to an American chromatologist, Faber Birren's arrangement principle. Figure 1 showed the 2-colors arrangement sample used in this experiment, and this sample was based on setting the suitable location on the color wheel. Through some color experts' verification process about 55 color arrangements in the 1st sample, the 55 colors were reduced into 26 arrangements consisting into the 2nd sample seen in right side.

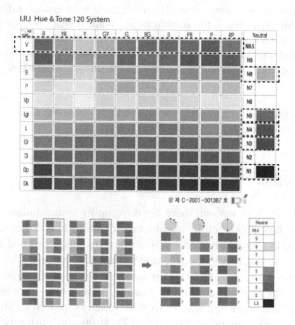

Fig. 1. Color Sample

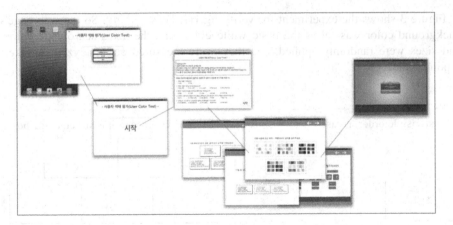

Fig. 2. System flow

Table 1. Application Development Brief

Application development information	
H/W	*Device: iPad 1 & 2 (not retina)*
S/W	*Tool: X Code,* Library*: UIKit*

3   Senior User Survey

We conducted a survey targeting 74 seniors (28 males and 46 females) ranging from early 50s to 70s in their ages. Specifically, 22 males and 44 females were 50s in their ages, and 6 males and 2 females were 60s in their ages. We provided only a brief explanation about the method and procedure to operate the application programs in a tablet PC. Average experiment time spent by these participants was within about 4 minutes.

3.1   Survey Methodology

In order to experiment senior generations' color cognition abilities, we proposed three questions. It was to investigate the background and text brightness and size preference measurement, preference of color combination for visual element, preference of the color combination. We conducted the SPSS 18.0 program for statistically analyzing the survey data, and conducted the cross analysis (cross-tab) in order to recognize respondents' characteristics by gender, and then used the chi-square ($\chi2$) value in order to identify both genders' characteristics difference.

For the arrangement evaluation and the preferred arrangements, each question item was transformed into each score and the t-text by gender was conducted in order to identify genders' differences.

Figure 3 shows the experiment for verifying H1, H2's validity. So the web page's background color was set as the basic white color, and the text's achromatic colors and sizes were randomly applied, and they were measured and analyzed in Likert 5-point scale.

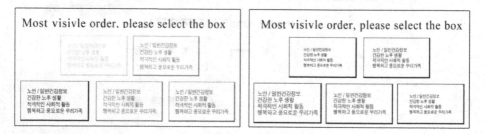

Fig. 3. Background and text color brightness & text size preference measurement

Figure 4 shows the experiment verifying H3's validity, so investigated if there were more preferred arrangement patterns in color combinations of graphic factors like menu and icons.

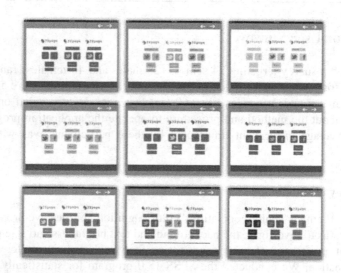

Fig. 4. Experiment of preference of the color combination for visual elements

Figure 5 shows the experiment verifying H4's validity, so investigated if there was any gender difference in senior generation's preference for arranged images. For this, experiment sample was made by based on Korea I.R.I's 'Color Image Scale'.

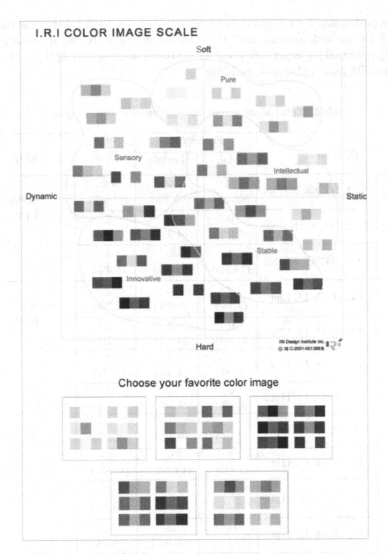

Fig. 5. Preference for Arranged color Images

3.2   Survey Result

First question is about the results of cross analysis (cross-tab) on the subjects' preference for the font brightness and the font size by gender. Statistical analysis is shown on Table 2.

For the font brightness, the response rate in order of 'N1.5, N3, N4, N5, N8' was absolutely higher in both genders, and the rates was 85.7% for male subjects and 95.7% for female subjects, respectively. As the result of chi-square (χ2) test, there was no significant difference between the both genders (χ2=3.988, p=.136). For the font size preference, the response rate in order of '17, 15, 14, 12, 11pt' was the highest as 57.1% for male subjects and 60.9% for female subjects, and the both genders generally preferred for larger font sizes. As the result of chi-square ($\chi2$) test, there was no gender difference ($\chi2$=6.144, p=.523).

Table 2. Statistical analysis of the experiment shown in Figure 3

Division		Participant		Total	$\chi2$ (p)
		Male	Female		
Text value	N1.5, N3, N4, N5, N8	24 (85.7%)	44 (95.7%)	68 (91.9%)	3.988 (.136)
	N1.5, N3, N5, N4, N8	0 (0.0%)	2 (4.3%)	2 (2.7%)	
	N1.5, N4, N3, N5, N8	4 (14.3%)	0 (0.0%)	4 (5.4%)	
Text size	14, 11, 17, 15, 12pt	2 (7.1%)	0 (0.0%)	2 (2.7%)	6.144 (.523)
	14, 12, 11, 15, 17pt	0 (0.0%)	2 (4.3%)	2 (2.7%)	
	14, 12, 15, 17, 11pt	0 (0.0%)	2 (4.3%)	2 (2.7%)	
	14, 15, 17, 12, 11pt	0 (0.0%)	2 (4.3%)	2 (2.7%)	
	15, 14, 17, 12, 11pt	2 (7.1%)	4 (8.7%)	6 (8.1%)	
	15, 17, 14, 12, 11pt	2 (7.1%)	6 (13.0%)	8 (10.8%)	
	17, 14, 15, 12, 11pt	6 (21.4%)	2 (4.3%)	8 (10.8%)	
	17, 15, 14, 12, 11pt	16 (57.1%)	28 (60.9%)	44 (59.5%)	
Total		28 (100.0%)	46 (100.0%)	74 (100.0%)	

Second question is about the more preferred arrangement patterns in color combinations method of graphic factors like menu and icons. Statistical analysis is shown on Table 3.

As the results evaluating whole arrangements, it was found that in most experiments, opposing color arrangements like the colors of red, yellow-red, yellow, and green-yellow generated the highest cognition rates.

Table 3. Statistical analysis of the experiment shown in Figure 4

Contrasting(C) Opposite(O) Similar color(S)	R	YR	Y	GY	PB	P	RP	Full
C – O - S	2 (2.7%)	24 (32.4%)	20 (27.0%)	12 (16.2%)	50 (67.6%)	50 (67.6%)	66 (89.2%)	224 (45.6%)
C – S - O	2 (2.7%)	0 (0.0%)	0 (0.0%)	2 (2.7%)	2 (2.7%)	2 (2.7%)	0 (0.0%)	8 (1.5%)
O - C - O	58 (78.4%)	48 (64.9%)	54 (73.0%)	60 (81.1%)	22 (29.7%)	20 (27.0%)	8 (10.8%)	270 (49.8%)
O – S - C	12 (16.2%)	2 (2.7%)	0 (0.0%)	0 (0.0%)	0 (0.0%)	2 (2.7%)	0 (0.0%)	16 (3.1%)
Full	74 (100.0%)	74 (100.0%)	74 (100.0%)	74 (100.0%)	74 (100.0%)	74 (100.0%)	74 (100.0%)	518 (100.0%)
χ2 (p):	114.993***(.000)							
***p<.001								

Finally, the third question was the experiment verifying H4's validity. Statistical analysis is shown on Table 4. Research hypothesis is senior generations will prefer for harder-feeling, clearer color combinations rather than soft-feeling, dull color combinations. As the results of this experiment, it was found that the response rate in order of '3-2-1-5-4' was 43.5% for female seniors, and the response rate in order of '3-2-4-5-1' was 42.9% for male seniors.

Table 4. Statistical analysis of the experiment shown in Figure 5

Division	Male	Female	Total	χ2 (p)
2-1-5-4-3	0(0.0%)	2(4.3%)	2(2.7%)	
2-3-5-4-1	0(0.0%)	2(4.3%)	2(2.7%)	
2-3-5-1-4	0(0.0%)	2(4.3%)	2(2.7%)	21.128*
2-3-4-5-1	4(14.3%)	8(17.4%)	12(16.2%)	(.012)
4-5-1-2-3	0(0.0%)	2(4.3%)	2(2.7%)	
3-2-5-1-4	4(14.3%)	0(0.0%)	4(5.4%)	
3-2-4-5-1	12(42.9%)	8(17.4%)	20(27.0%)	
3-2-1-5-4	0(0.0%)	20(43.5%)	20(27.0%)	
3-2-1-4-5	0(0.0%)	2(4.3%)	2(2.7%)	
3-4-2-5-1	8(28.6%)	0(0.0%)	8(10.8%)	
Total	28(100.0%)	46(100.0%)	74(100.0%)	

4   Discussion and Conclusions

We surveyed 74 senior people to investigate senior generation's color cognition and color sensibility. This study's hypotheses verification and its conclusion are as follows.

H1: Senior generations will prefer for larger text sizes. Seeing the Table 2 Experiment about the brightness difference between the background color and the text color, and the text size, it was found that senior generations preferred for more distinctive brightness contrast and also larger font sizes. As the results of chi-square ($\chi 2$) test, there was no significant difference between the both genders.

As the results of Table 2, it was identified that senior generations preferred for more distinctive brightness contrast between the background color and the text color.

H2: Senior generations will prefer for more distinctive brightness contrast between the background color and the text's color. As the results of Table 2, it was identified that senior generations preferred for more distinctive brightness contrast between the background color and the text color.

H3: Senior generations will prefer for more distinctively contrasting color arrangements in graphic factors like menu and icons.

As the results evaluating whole arrangements, it was found that senior generations preferred for 'the opposing color arrangements' the most and they preferred for clear contrasts.

H4: Senior generations will prefer for harder-feeling, clearer color combinations rather than soft-feeling, dull color combinations. This hypothesis was exactly coincided in the term of both genders' most favorite color combinations. It was found that senior generation's most favorite color arrangements were clear, dynamic high-chromatic color combinations, and their unfavorable arrangements were dull, static low-chromatic color combinations. However, there were gender differences in 2nd and 3rd preferring color combinations. While female seniors preferred soft-feeling color combinations, but male seniors did hard-feeling color combinations.

The results of this study identified that color cognition was similarly appeared according to a man's age, that is, a generation's visual ability, and clear color contrasts were needed so that seniors could conveniently cognize colors. Besides, it was found that the arrangement preference had some subjective, sensitive characteristics, so it showed some differences in both genders. We hope that the results of this study will actively be utilized at setting color plans while designing a web interface.

References

1. Norman, D.A.: The Design of Everyday Things. Basic Books, New York (2002)
2. Overbeeke, C.J., Djajadiningrat, J.P., Hummels, C.C.M., Wensveen, S.A.G.: Beauty in usability: forget about ease of use! In: Green, W.S., Jordan, P.W. (eds.) Pleasure with Products: Beyond Usability, pp. 9–18. Taylor & Francis (2002)
3. Gero, J., Bonnardel, N. (eds.): Studying Designers. University of Sydney, Sydney (2005)

4. Norman, D.A.: Emotional Design: Why We Love (or Hate) Everyday Things. Basic Books, New York (2005)
5. Norman, D.A.: Introduction to this special section on beauty, goodness, and usability. Human- Computer Interaction 19(4), 311–318 (2004)
6. Valdez, P., Mehrabian, A.: Effects of color on emotion. Journal of Experimental Psychology: General 123, 394–409 (1994)
7. Buckalew, I.W., Bell, A.: Effects of colors on mood in the drawings of young children. Perceptual and Motor Skills 61, 689–690 (1985)
8. Elliot, A.J., Maier, M.A., Moller, A.C., Friedman, R.: Color and psychological functioning: the effect of red on performance in achievement contexts. Journal of Experimental Psychology: General 136, 154–168 (2007)
9. Soldat, A.S., Sinclair, R.C., Mark, M.M.: Color as an environmental processing cue: external affective cues can directly affect processing strategy without affecting mood. Social Cognition 15, 55–71 (1997)
10. Nielsen, J.: Designing Web Usability: The Practice of Simplicity. New Riders Publishing, Indianapolis (2000)
11. Elliot, A.J., Maier, M.A.: Colo rand psychological functioning. Current Directions in Psychological Science 16(5), 250–254 (2007)
12. Valdez, P., Mehrabian, A.: Effects of color one motions. Journal of Experimental Psychology 123(4), 394–409 (1994)
13. Kwallek, N., Lewis, C.M., Robbins, A.S.: Effects of office interior color on workers' mood and productivity. Perceptual and Motor Skills 66, 123–128 (1988)
14. Walters, J., Apter, M.J., Svebak, S.: Color preference,arousal, and the theory of psychological reversals. Motivation and Emotion 6(3), 193–215 (1982)

The Analysis and Research
of the Smart Phone's User Interface Based
on Chinese Elderly's Cognitive Character

Delai Men, Dong Wang, and Xiaoping Hu[*]

School of Design, South China University of Technology
Guangzhou Higher Education Mega Centre, Panyu District, Guangzhou, P.R. China, 510006
huxp@scut.edu.cn

Abstract. With the rapid development of modern information era, smart phones have become an irreversible trend to replace the tradition ones. With the trend of aging population in China, we can't underestimate the rapidly growing population of the Chinese elderly people and increasingly demanding for smart phone. The UI, which is short for user interface, is referred to the collection of interactive methods between phone users and interior phones system. And the research on UI is becoming more and more important in the research of smart phone. By doing the survey which combined the elderly's cognition with the smart phones' UI design, the thesis is aimed at acquiring the methods of UI design for elderly people so that the smart phones can conform to them better. In this way, the smart phones' functions can be totally applied to them and elderly people's vision enjoyment can be improved.

Keywords: Elderly people, User interface, Smart phone, Design method, Elderly's cognition.

1 Introduction and Background

1.1 The Trend of Aging Population

There is growing aging phenomenon with the rise of aging population throughout the world. According to the World Health Organization [1], all across Asia, the number of people who is age of 65 and above is expected to increase dramatically over the next 50 years. For this region, the population of this age group will increase by 314 percent—from 207 million in 2000 to 857 million in 2050. What should we do in face of the aging century? These issues are also being confronted in the West where population aging is more advanced. But the process of population aging is much more rapidly in Asia than Western countries, and it will occur in some Asian countries in the earlier development of their economies.

---

[*] Corresponding author.

C. Stephanidis and M. Antona (Eds.): UAHCI/HCII 2014, Part III, LNCS 8515, pp. 138–146, 2014.

For about two decades of speculation and anticipation, aging population has finally arrived with a demographic and social reality in China. Two and a half decades ago, when we started to pay attention to the aging population in early days, China's population aged 60 and above was only 7.6 percent, and those aged 65 and above constituted only 4.9 percent of the total population [2]. In 2005, more than 140 million people in China are 60 years or older, a population size that exceeds the total population of Japan, and approximately the same as the total population of Bangladesh or Russia [3]. What is more, as aging population continues, we can't underestimate it.

1.2   The Trend of Smart Phones in China

Based on the latest data published by the global technology research and consulting company Gartner, the whole smart phone sales of 2013 is 968 million which had a increase of 42.3 percent by the last year. And it's the first time that smart phone have exceed the unsmart phones that the smart phone has the 53.6% sales in the whole sale volume of mobile phone. China has the distinct contribution on the smart phone selling with the fast increasing rate by 86.3% in 2013. Because the Chinese elderly has the low utilization on smart phone, it will have an enormous potential market.

1.3   The Specialties of the Elderly People When Using Smart Phone

Due to their aging, many elderly people suffer from the declination of cognitive, motor and physical abilities. Many of them experience difficulties using certain features when interacting with their mobile phones, especially technology of shifting from keypad to touch-screen mobile user interfaces.

2   Methods

2.1   Determining the Target People of the Study

The research is only focus on the permanent residents in China who's age is between 60 and 90 years old. And it's available whether they have smart or not. The sample contains 50 elderly people which come from different provinces in the north China, east China and south China. Because of the low density of elderly people and the distance barriers, the elderly people in the west China is out of the survey.

2.2   Card Testing

This study was to determine the operating acceptability, the cognitive preferences and the consumer demands of the smart phones' UI for people older than 60 years; some testing card were prepared for this propose. Then the final testing card was formed after some necessary modification.

The testing cards contain five parts. The first part is the general information of the audience and the second part is the detailed content of their mobile phone. The third part is about their operation acceptability of the smart phones' UI and the forth part is aimed at analyzing the cognitive preference of the UI with different color, structure or visual effect, etc. The fifth part of the testing is to get the core consuming factors of the elderly when choosing the smart phone.

2.3   Data Analysis

The data was collected and the SPSS software was used to analyze the frequency distribution.

3   Literature Review and Related Research Work

3.1   The Lack of Survey of Elderly People

The design process of smart phone interface runs through four basic interactive design processes: identifying the Target User Group, defying 3D UI Context, building interface Prototype, and evaluating [4]. But there are no talent companies concentrated on the Chinese elderly people in China and all the best-selling smart phones and the UI are created for the young people who have the enormous consuming power. So the research on the Chinese elderly people is very little.

Therefore, we can no more underestimate the rapidly growing population of the Chinese elderly people and their growing need of smart phone.

3.2   The Importance of Smart Phone's UI for the Chinese Elderly

As one of the most important elements of smart phone functions, UI determines the comfort level when people use the smart phone and the enjoyment when they watch it. It can not only improve the phone operability but also ease users' memory pressure. Some elders especially the new generation have become the users of smart phone, accounting for their special cognition, there exists quite differences from the general individuals as for the elders' using customs and cognitive styles. Although the global aging problem has become more and more remarkable, the research on elderly people's smart phone is still in the initial stages. Besides, few people pay attention to the research of their smart phones' UI.

3.3   The Aim of This Paper

The aim of this paper is to get the acceptability and the preference of different smart phone's UI for the Chinese elderly people through the investigation by using the card testing and questionnaire. Then we'll analyze the demographic, the elderly people's information of their mobile phone, the cognitive preference of the elderly people and their demands after the investigation. In the end of this paper, we can conclude the main principles when designing the smart phone's UI for the Chinese elderly people.

3.4   Related Work

The Japanese Company Fujitsu have created one famous smart phone "Raku Raku", which is made for the elderly. The Raku Raku – which means "comfortable" or "easy" in Japanese – comes with large app icons and text, and can even slow down a caller's voice so that they can be understood better [5].Though it's design for the elderly, its interface is very colorful and it uses the Android 4.0 Ice Cream Sandwich system which is very young. And it eventually gets the Considerable income.

Apple Inc supposed their products just like iPhone and iPad were designed for the consumer aged from "one to 100". It just across the youth demographic and are age friendly products. IPhone has the easy interface which is very harmony and its visual effect is very enjoyable. But in China not every elderly people can afford the iPhone and it does not suits every elderly people as the icons are too complex to them.

Most smart phones on the market, however, use Google's Android OS. Because Android is to some extent open source, however, individual phone handsets have different versions of the interface. The interface is very multiple and garish and it's not easy to handle it. Windows Phone has taken great strides, and although the interface is flashy and full of bright colors, it is the simplest mobile operating system to users [6].

The Samsung Company was going to make one smart phone targeted towards the elderly and the disabled. The functions are very useful for the elderly people, but the specific of the UI is rarely mentioned.

4   Results

4.1   Demographic

The demographic of the survey contained two value of number: number of persons/percentage in this paper.

The sexual distinction, the age level, the education background and the income of per month of the 55 elderly people who have been investigated was shown in Table 1.

Table 1. The information of the elderly

	Categories	F	%
Sex	Male	24	43.6%
	Female	31	56.4%
The age level	60-70	37	67.3%
	70-80	18	32.7%
The Education Background	Primary School	17	30.9%
	High School	32	58.2%
	Undergraduate	6	10.9%
The income/month	Below 1000 RMB	1	1.8%
	1000 RMB-2000 RMB	37	67.3%
	2000 RMB-3000 RMB	15	27.3%
	3000 RMB-5000 RMB	2	3.6%

4.2   The Information of Their Mobile Phone

The information of their mobile phone was determined by the questionnaire and the results are showed in the Table 2. It mainly subscribes the section of their phones' price and the purchase channel.

Table 2. The information of their using mobile phone

	Categories	F	%
Brand	Apple	5	9.1%
	Samsung	22	40%
	Nokia	19	34.5%
	Other	9	16.4%
Mobile Phones' Price	0-500 RMB	19	34.5%
	500 RMB-1000 RMB	17	30.9%
	1000 RMB-2000 RMB	6	10.9%
	2000 RMB-3000 RMB	5	9.1%
	Above 3000 RMB	8	14.5%
The Approach to Get the Mobile Phone	Bought by themself	12	21.8%
	Bought by their children	43	78.2%

4.3   The Elderly's Cognitive Preference

The elderly's cognitive preference of their mobile phone was got by the Card Testing and the results are shown in the Table 3. It contained the preference of composition, style and color, and different kinds of smart phones have been tested of its color.

Table 3. The elderly's Cognitive Preference

	Categories	F	%
Screen Lock	Pass word	9	16.4%
	Four directions slide	15	27.3%
	Long press the middle key	7	12.7%
	Just slide switch	24	43.6%
Composition	Horizontal composition	5	9.1%
	Vertical composition	31	56.4%
	It does not matter	19	34.5%
Interface Composition of Main Page	ISO	20	36.4%
	Android	9	16.4%
	Windows 8	17	30.9%
	Other	9	16.4%
Interface of Messaging	ISO	23	41.8%
	Android	8	14.5%
	Windows 8	17	30.9%
	Other	7	12.7%

Table 3. (*continued*)

Interface of Dialing	ISO	8	14.5%
	Android	16	29.1%
	Windows 8	29	52.7%
	Other	3	5.5%
Interface of Social Software	Facebook	41	74.5%
	WeChat	2	3.6%
	QQ	9	16.4%
	Sina Microblog	3	5.5%
The Tonality of Main Page	Light coffee	17	30.9%
	Green	4	7.3%
	Orange	15	27.3%
	Ocean blue	3	5.5%
	Purple	5	9.1%
	Yellow	1	1.8%
	Red	4	7.3%
	Brown	6	10.9%

4.4   The Elderly's Demands and Needs

The elderly's demands and needs of their mobile phone was got by the questionnaire and the results are shown in the Table 4.

Table 4. The elderly's demands

	Categories	F	%
The Influence by UI	Obvious	34	61.8%
	Un-obvious	21	38.2%
Change the UI Frequently	Yes	13	23.6%
	No	42	76.4%
The Ideal UI's Style in the Future	Scientific	2	3.6%
	Brief & Simple	49	89.1%
	Interesting	4	7.3%
	Fashion	0	0%
The Central of Smart Phone's UI	Harmony	18	32.7%
	High deficiency execution	21	38.2%
	Conform to your visual habits	12	21.8%
	Visual enjoyment	4	7.3%

5   Discussion

5.1   Demographic

Through the results of the demographic, we can find that the female is more than male, it's mainly because the lifespan of Chinese female is longer than Chinese male.

The education background results can tell us that the Chinese elderly people have the low degree of education for only 10.9% people are undergraduate. Most of their income is between 1000 RMB/month to 3000 RMB/month, and the income between 1000 RMB-2000 RMB owns 67.3% of all the subjects. So it determines the consuming power is enough to buy smart phones and it's a large market based on the huge population of elderly in China.

5.2   The Information of Their Mobile Phone

Through the brand using data, we can find that the Samsung has the maximum users with 40% and Nokia still have the 34.5% of users though Nokia has the little brand share in the whole market of China. The updating speed of elderly's mobile phone update speed is much slower than the youth and the middle-aged people. 34.5% of the mobile phone is 0-500 RMB and 30.9% of the mobile phone is 500-1000 RMB. So their mobile phones' price is a little low relatively but it does not mean there is no market prospect on the elderly for there's still 24.5% people whose mobile phone is above 1000 RMB. Considering the approach of getting the mobile phone, we can conclude that the main purpose they get the mobile phone is for their children. So the update rate of their mobile phone is sometimes depending on the youth and the middle-aged people and the elderly people is passive on the choosing of their smart phones.

5.3   The Elderly's Cognitive Preference

The "just slide switch" get the 43.6% and the "pass word" only get 16.4% indicated that the elderly didn't like to make the screen lock too complex to enter the main page. The 56.4% elderly choose the vertical composition and 34.5% elderly has no sense of this difference. The main page of ISO 7 gets the maximum number of 36.4% and then followed the interface of windows 8 with the number of 30.9%. At the interface of messaging, ISO 7 also gets the maximum number 41.8%. And Windows 8 with the 30.9% of the elderly is followed. We can get that the ISO 7's and Windows 8's optical design is very useful for the special group. At the interface of dialing, 52.7% elderly people choose the Windows 8 and this number is much higher than other ones. The Windows 8's dialing interface is very simply which only has the number, some simply boxes and the number field. We can indicated that the elderly need simply operation more than visual effect when they meet the mobile phone's functional interface they use frequently.

We put four kinds of social software in the Card Testing which the style and composition is very different from the other ones. The interesting thing is that the Facebook's interface get the maximum number 74.5% in spite they have never used this software for it's not feasible in mainland China. The reason why they choose Facebook is that they thought the Facebook's main interface structure is still the same as their mobile phone's and it's very direct and clearly, but the other ones is not the same and they should take more time to learn from it. We can indicated that they have used to the interface structure of they used before and their thoughts have been fixed and they don't want to change it. The tonality of the main page is tested by the smart phone with one main hue. Most of the elderly people like the light coffee and orange. It shows that the Chinese elderly people who like the bright and brisk color will be fond of orange and they like the gentle color will like the color light coffee.

5.4   The Elderly's Demands

Through the data of the survey, we can find that above one half of the elderly care about the mobile phones' UI. Only 23.6% elderly people want to change the UI frequently and on the contrary 76.4% elderly does not. So the elderly need one stable UI so that he can drive well. Of 89.1% elderly people's ideal UI are brief & simply ones, it indicated that they want their mobile phone more simply than present. And 38.2% elderly people think the central of smart phone's UI is high efficiency execution and 32.7% think harmony is the central. Only 7.3% elderly people think the visual enjoyment is the central of the smart phone's UI. So we can conclude that the Chinese elderly have no sense of the enjoying play of the smart phone and they are very practical.

6   Conclusions

After the analysis of the results and the discussion, we can find the elderly people's characteristics when using their mobile phone and the principles when design the UI for them. Though the research, we can conclude that:

1)   The education background results can tell us that the Chinese elderly people have the low degree of education, so the interface should use simply words and compositions.
2)   Although the Chinese elderly's mobile phone is mainly below 1000 RMB, there is still enormous potential market based on the population of China elderly.
3)   The interface designed for the elderly should keep connect with the previous mobile phone which is mainly used by the elderly people, and it's better to use the same UI structure so they can operate the smart phones smoothly.
4)   The smart phones' screen lock should not be too complex and it's not good to set the pass word as the screen lock.
5)   The interface of smart phone can be more brief and simple in the future.
6)   The UI design for Chinese elderly people should remain stable.

Acknowledgment. The project supported by Guangdong Natural Science Foundation under the Grant No.: S2012010008234, and Institution of Higher Education Internal Foundation for Humanities and Social Science Research Project under the Grant No.: x2sjN8130350.

References

1. World Health Organization: Active Aging: A Policy Framework (2002),
   http://www.who.int/aging/publications/active/en/index.html
2. Banister, J.: Implications of the Aging of China's Population. In: Poston, D., Yaukey, D. (eds.) The Population of Modern China, pp. 463–490. Plenum Press, New York (1992)
3. Feng, W., Mason, A.: Population aging in China: Challenges, opportunities, and institutions. In: Transition and Challenge: China's Population at the Beginning of the 21st Century, pp. 177–196 (2007)
4. Preece, J.: Yvonne Rogers and Helen Sharp. Interaction design beyond human-computer interaction, pp. 119–120. John Wiley & Sons, Inc. (2002)
5. Smart-phones struggle to connect with the elderly,
   http://www.cnbc.com/id/101045757/
6. Smart-phone for the elderly: buying advice, http://www.pcadvisor.co.uk/buying-advice/mobile-phone/3371979/smartphone-for-elderly-buying-advice/

Ergonomic Principles to Improve the Use of Cognitive Stimulation Systems for the Elderly: A Comparative Study of Two Software Tools

Gabriel Michel, Eric Brangier, and Mélissa Brun

Lorraine University, PErSEUs, UFR SHA, Île du Saulcy, 57006 Metz, France
{Gabriel.Michel,Eric.Brangier}@univ-lorraine.fr,
myla-melissa@hotmail.fr

Abstract. The aim of our communication is to present results of an evaluation of two cognitive stimulation software tools ("ProfessionalTool" and "StudyTool") and to give recommendations to improve their usability. The evaluation was conducted using a test user on a group of 32 seniors (average age 78.19 years) and a group of 15 people (mean age 30.47 years). The "ProfessionalTool" software includes thirty exercises targeting different cognitive skills. The second software – "StudyTool"- has been designed by our team applying user-centered design. The performances of these interfaces were measured using a questionnaire of satisfaction and a heuristic inspection observation grid, based on ergonomic criteria. The scores obtained by each group and each method of data collection were calculated and compared. An important result is that the number of problems encountered by users in the cognitive stimulation tasks is M=10.09 with ProfessionalTool; i.e. a senior user remained stuck for ten minutes on a settings screen. The results of the questionnaire also indicate problems concerning visual ergonomics guidelines, workload, control and error handling, uniformity and consistency, significance and compatibility. This experience highlights the importance of ergonomics in cognitive stimulation software. Their adaptation to a specific public need is often insufficient, especially as the users have troubles with memory and attention. Our study enables us to make a positive contribution of ergonomic human- computer interaction to cognitive stimulation. Beyond the actual effect of cognitive stimulation that is no longer in doubt, the challenge is to support the use and empower the user. This is only possible through tailored interactions.

Keywords: Ergonomics, User Experience, Gamification, Persuasive Technology, Emotional Design, Motivation.

1 Introduction

Population aging is above all a social and demographic problem. In Europe, the percentage of people aged over 65 years old rose from 7,5% to 12,5% between 1950 and 2000, according to forecasts this percentage could be as high as 30% by 2050 [6].

C. Stephanidis and M. Antona (Eds.): UAHCI/HCII 2014, Part III, LNCS 8515, pp. 147–154, 2014.
© Springer International Publishing Switzerland 2014

In France for example, INSEE (the french statistical agency) estimates that the over 65's will represent 20,1% of the population by 2020 (13 million) and more than 26% by 2050 (over 18 million). A third of the population will be over 60 years old by 2050, compared to one in 5 people in 2000. The proportion of over 60's in the total population will be higher than the under 20's. In other industrialized countries like Japan, Italy, and Germany the phenomenon of population aging is even more critical [1]. Even in China it has been forecast that 23% of the population will be over 65 by 2050. According to the World Health Organization there will be 2 billion people aged 60 and over by 2050.

As well as the expected labor shortage in the countries hit, this population aging phenomenon will be accompanied by health problems, such as dementia, cognitive impairment, depression, inability to adapt, lack of self efficacy and social isolation, making this population dependent and vulnerable [2]. It will therefore be very valuable to develop efficient mechanisms aiming to reinforce and improve the life functions of the elderly, both for individuals and societies and their efforts to cope with what appears to be a demographic revolution [2].

All existing research shows that being active enables seniors to keep a positive image of themselves, to expand their horizons and to conserve a well being which defies the stereotypes associated with their age.

Among these activities, cognitive stimulation can be the answer to maintaining this well-being by means of regular brain training. These tools, combined with ergonomic knowledge, and specific criterion for this population can provide access to intellectual stimulation using technology which until now has been out of their reach [3].

We will start with a brief overview of cognitive stimulation, then go back to the domain of technology and seniors before presenting our tests and discussing the results.

2   Cognitive Stimulation and Aging: A Rapidly Expanding Domain

The current aging of the population has lead to an increase in research programs aiming to find solutions to cognitive impairment and neurodegenerative diseases. For most people cognitive stimulation is still considered as the non drug related management of Alzheimer's disease. But today cognitive stimulation isn't just stimulating cognitive functions such as memory, attention and problem solving through classical exercises. It is a comprehensive educational approach which is cognitive but also psychological and social. It is in fact a concept which is currently expanding in many different directions. The populations targeted are not only elderly people who are ill, but all categories of the population, professionals who use it, applying it to different domains.

The idea is to solicit functions which are less frequently used as people get older. The positive effects of cognitive stimulation in the repetition of the tasks involved are observed. Performance scores vary considerably before and after the training, and closely depend on the basic intellectual level of the participants [4] For people with various types of mental retardation, we will refer to cognitive remediation which we observed, enabled a certain amount of progress [5]. Its approach is focused on the reconstruction of the person's inherent abilities, encouraging meta-cognitive processes rather than gaining new knowledge [6].

Previously cognitive stimulation only concerned patients suffering from dementia, but gradually concerned elderly people and people with mental disabilities. Nowadays we hear more and more about the development of CS systems for all categories of the population.

Coming back to seniors, apart from CS, we are already aware of the advantages of using the internet [7]: social interaction, learning, searching for subjects of personal interest, being able to keep up with the latest news, online banking, developing online social networking, online shopping, keeping in contact with friends and family. After the web which is increasingly becoming a part of seniors' lives, CS systems are foreseen as being among the services which will see their use by this population grow rapidly. This will happen as soon as they become more accessible financially and in terms of usability.

3   Seniors and Technology

Even today Technology is not accessible to everybody and presents an obstacle for a considerable number of seniors. The complexity of certain interactions, the large amount of information on the same page, the speed this information is presented at, all these features make it difficult for them to search, and even more so for people with mental disabilities [8]. Most of the time, just by simplifying the interface would be enough to noticeably increase user performance. An assessment made of several websites show that usability for seniors was only 2,8% for text spacing, 5,8% for guidance and navigation, 9,5% for audio and video animations, 25% for hypertext links, and 38% for the efficacy of the Site Map etc. Even if the tasks were performed successfully, user efficiency , satisfaction and preference levels are not fulfilled [6].

Very few interfaces are adapted to elderly people, even in the domains where universality is essential, for example, the electronic vote [9]. Even if there is a large amount of knowledge which enables seniors to access technology today [10], especially specific ergonomic guidelines, they are not often taken into consideration by the designers. This is the case for cognitive stimulation software programs too.

We initially carried out an ergonomic inspection of several cognitive stimulation software programs. This assessment of the consistency with the guidelines for seniors showed that all the software programs contained errors, proving that the ergonomic guidelines had not been taken into account at the conception phase.

4   Ergonomic Evaluation

4.1   Method

The evaluation was carried out using a user test, a satisfaction questionnaire and an observation grid. The questionnaire consisted of a data sheet and a satisfaction evaluation, based on Bastien and Scapin criteria [11]. It included 6 categories and

18 items presented in the form of a 5 point Likert scale. The observation grid accounted for the occurrence of difficulties, participants' remarks, timing of sessions and the number of game requests expressed by our participants.

4.2   Presentation of the Interfaces

Two cognitive stimulation exercises were tested. The first one was the « Displaced characters » from the ProfessionalTool software program (a well known software in the field of cognitive stimulation softwares), which aims to boost mental functions, particularly those of seniors. This program appears to be the most popular one used in France, the one most often mentioned in articles about cognitive stimulation and the most common one on the internet. ProfessionalTool consists of thirty exercises targeting different cognitive skills. We chose one of the most typical which is a memory training exercise (see Fig.1).

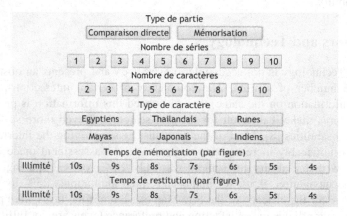

Fig. 1. ProfessionalTool settings screen

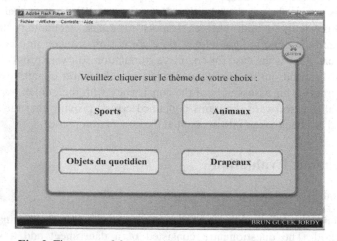

Fig. 2. First page of the parameters of the StudyTool Software

This exercise of ProfessionalTool is a memory training exercise using slightly abstract figurative characters (hieroglyphics etc.). After memorizing these characters, they are displayed again but have to be recognized among other different pictures.

The second exercise of image memorization was designed for this study applying user centered design (see Fig.2). Initially, several adjustments were made to the memory training software program following well known ergonomic guidelines. To be able to guarantee the exercise usability both in substance and in form, we pretested a group of seniors. This approach enabled the final version of the exercise to be designed.

4.3   User Tests

In our user centered research we set about to test interaction as thoroughly as possible. We allowed for discussion time with the participants before each session to enable them to feel confident and able to ask any relevant questions, making sure that they could handle the tools, especially the mouse, particularly the participants with little practice.

The test period began with filling in the data sheet , followed by the test user and ending with the satisfaction questionnaire. This procedure was repeated for each software being studied.

Population Details. Our sample was made up of a total of n = 47 participants. For the group of seniors the number of participants were n = 32 the average age was 78,19 yrs old with 87,5% women and 12,5% men. As for the younger control group n= 15 with an average age of 30,47 years old, 73,3% of whom were women and 26,7% men. 9,4% of the seniors had already used technology compared to 93,3% for the control group. The volunteers were either met in their homes or at a retirement home, which had displayed notices informing the residents of the study. The seniors were divided into 2 groups: A and B, group A began by testing ProfessionalTool, group B began with the StudyTool software. The groups formed were of the similar age and had the same level of computer skills.

Results. Only part of this study will be presented here. It deals with observation of the problems encountered. We compared the number of problems encountered, their frequency per minute, and finally the game time calculated per session (see Table1).

Regarding the number of problems encountered the feedback was very enlightening. For the senior group , the average number of problems is 8,63 lower for our version (M= 1,47 ED= 1,46) than for ProfessionalTool's (M= 10,09 ED= 4,30). The same tendency was found for the control group with a noticeably lower average for our version (M= ,60 ED= ,74) than for ProfessionalTool 's (M= 8,93 ED= 4,99). This result can be applied generally to the control group (p= ,000 < ,05) as well as to the senior group (p= ,000 < ,05).

Table 1. Results of the assessment of problems of use (Senior group)

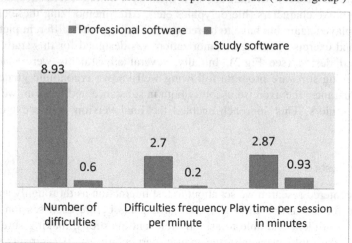

For the senior group the average frequency of the occurrence of problems is (M= ,00 ED= ,000) for our version. It is significantly lower (p= ,000 < ,05) than ProfessionalTool's (M= 1,50 ED=,55). For the control group the average is also lower for our version (M= ,20 ED= 1,63) than for ProfessionalTool' (M= 2,70 ED= 1,63). This result can be applied generally (p= ,000 < ,05).

Significantly, for interaction time (p= ,000 < ,05), the session times for our senior group, are clearly lower for our version (M= 1,49 ED= ,65) compared to ProfessionalTool's (M= 6,16 ED= 6,15). The situation is similar for the control group with a lower average time for our version (M= ,93 ED= ,17) than for ProfessionalTool 's (M= 2,87 ED= 1,36). This tendency can also be applied generally (p= ,000 < ,05).

This tendency also appears for the control group with a much lower average for our version (M= ,60 ED= ,74) than for ProfessionalTool's (M= 8,93 ED= 4,99).

The results of the satisfaction questionnaire also indicate problems concerning visual ergonomics guidelines, workload, control and error handling, uniformity and consistency, significance and compatibility. Taken as a whole the results of the evaluation eventually showed that ProfessionalTool has a low level of usability in terms of efficiency and the occurrence of user errors.

5   Discussion

This experience highlights the importance of certain ergonomic aspects of cognitive stimulation software. Their adaptation to a public with specific needs is often insufficient. This experience also underlines the necessity of the support of ergonomic recommendations (feed-back, usage intention, persuasion techniques engaging interaction, reinforcement...) and more generally, using an ergonomic approach to improve interface quality therefore enhancing use and acceptance of these tools. We must point out that these ergonomic improvements do not only benefit the population targeted, but also significantly benefit the control population; this is a typical result in research which is destined, in theory, to populations with specific needs.

6   Conclusion

Our study demonstrates the almost total lack of ergonomic considerations at the concept phase of the SC systems and to prove the positive effect of their inclusion. Beyond the actual effect of cognitive stimulation that is no longer in doubt, the challenge is to support the use and empower the user. This is only possible through tailored interactions..

According to [12, 13, 14, 15] these results give weight to the importance of the concept of "Perception of Gamification". This experience shows clearly that the lack of gamification implies a lower usage. Cognitive stimulation systems have to introduce persuasive technologies and graphic design to explain the interface's appearance and users commitment. To a certain degree, gamification will amplify the use of software. It would thus appear as a decisive factor for the design of a successful human-technology relationship beyond classic theories of technology adoption and use.

However, it relies on motivators dealing with nonfunctional needs; the usefulness of a system is not covered despite its importance, notably on work context. It thus questions the contribution of Gamification to casual systems, especially considering the kind of motivation triggered. We state that Gamification is about creating an interactive universe that would be simple, beautiful, appealing and engaging. It implies a will to mislead the user by modifying the core meaning of use: the conflicting relationship between elderly and cognitive stimulation.

Some Gamification upholders are currently talking about he concept of significant Gamification [14, 15, 16], calling for user-centered game elements selection. It would be interesting to apply gamification criteria in order identify design rules that could be generalized in cognitive stimulation software.

Going beyond the scope of this research, we are currently working on a set of specific guidelines (intended for the designers of these systems) in which we incorporate knowledge from persuasion technology to enable enhanced acceptance and efficiency of these systems.

References

1. Study University of Louvain, http://www.uclouvain.be/cps/ucl/doc/.../ML_article_chastel_veillissement.doc
2. World Health organization. Active aging: A policy framework. CITY: World Health Organization, (2002), http://whqlibdoc.who.int/hq/2002/WHO_NMH_NPH_02.8.pdf (September 1, 2011) (retrieved)
3. Lemaire, P.: La personne âgée, psychologie du vieillissement. De Boeck, Bruxelles (2005)
4. Auffray, C., Juhel, J.: Effets généraux et différentiels d'un programme d'entraînement cognitif multimodal chez la personne âgée. L'année Psychologique 101(1), 65–89 (2001)

5. Büchel, F., Paour, J.L.: Déficience intellectuelle: déficit et rémédiation cognitive. Enfance 57(3), 227–240 (2005)
6. Hart, T.A.: Evaluation of websites for older adults: how 'senior-friendly' are they? Usability News 6(1) (February 2004), http://www.surl.org/usabilitynews/61/older_adults.asp (accessed)
7. Kolodinsky, J., Cranwell, M., Rowe, E.: Bridging the generation gap across the digital divide: Teens teaching internet skills. Journal of Extension 40(3) (June 2002), http://www.joe.org/joe/2002june/rb.html
8. Lewis, C.: HCI and cognitive disabilities. Interactions 13(3), 14–15 (2006)
9. Michel, G., Klein, M.: Utilisabilité et discrimination: étude préliminaire des machines à voter françaises. In: Actes de la Conférence IHM 2008. ACM Digital Library, Metz (2008)
10. http://www.w3.org/WAI/
11. Bastien, J.M.C., Scapin, D.L.: A validation of ergonomic criteria for the evaluation of user interfaces. SIGCHI Bulletin 23, 54–55 (1991)
12. Marache-Francisco, C., Brangier, E.: Gamification experience: UXD with gamification background. In: Blashki, K., Isaias, P. (eds.) Emerging Research and Trends in Interactivity and the Human-Computer Interface, pp. 205–223. IGI-Global (2013)
13. Marache-Francisco, C., Brangier, E.: Perception of Gamification: between Graphical Design and Persuasive Design. In: Marcus, A. (ed.) DUXU 2013, Part II. LNCS, vol. 8013, pp. 558–567. Springer, Heidelberg (2013)
14. Marache-Francisco, C., Brangier, E.: Redefining Gamification. In: Blashi, K. (ed.) Proceedings of IADIS International Conference Interfaces and Human Computer Interaction 2012, pp. 227–231 (2012)
15. Marache-Francisco, C., Brangier, E.: Process For Gamification: From The Decision Of Gamification To Its Practical Implementation. In: The Sixth International Conference on Advances in Human oriented and Personalized Mechanisms, Technologies, and Services, CENTRIC 2013, Venice, Italy, October 27-November 1 (2013) ISSN: 2308-3492; ISBN: 978-1-61208-306-3
16. Duplàa, E., Kaufman, D., Sauvé, L., Renaud, L., Signalova, T., Emmanuel, T.: Méthode de spécifications de jeux sérieux adaptés aux ainés. Actes de l'atelier « Serious games, jeux épistémologique numériques ». In: EIAH 2013, pp. 14–18 (2013), http://eductice.ens-lyon.fr/EducTice/ressources/journees-scientifiques/atelierSG-EIAH2013/ActesatelierSG-EIAH2013

Assessing the Elderly's Emotional Responses while Interact with Movies Enriched with Additional Multimedia Content

Kamila Rios da Hora Rodrigues, Cesar A.C. Teixeira,
and Vânia Paula de Almeida Neris

Department of Computer Science, Federal University of São Carlos/UFSCar, Brazil
{kamila_rodrigues,cesar,vania}@dc.ufscar.br

Abstract. The elderly population is faced with barriers when using new Information and Communication Technologies (ICT). These barriers include their low ability to read, as well as fears or lack of involvement with the media content. With the interactivity provided by the interactive Digital TV (iDTV), it is possible to attract greater interest among this audience. This paper provides data from a case study conducted to analyze the emotional responses of the elderly when interacting with a movie enriched with additional multimedia content. This content was added in excerpts with narrative structures that can trigger feelings of doubt or dissatisfaction and require reasoning or prior knowledge of the subject. The results suggest that the elderly prefer to watch TV more passively and without the intervention of other media. Considering the results a set of good practices and strategies was formulated for the design and of TV programs for this audience.

Keywords: Interactive Digital TV, Narrative Structures, Additional Multimedia Content, Emotional Responses, Elderly and Interaction Design.

1 Introduction

Television plays several roles in the lives of the elderly. It is probably their main source of information and entertainment. Some researchers believe the use of media and leisure have come to be almost indistinguishable in the daily lives of elderly people [1]. They have also suggested that television replaces lost social contacts for elderly viewers and helps them maintain an ongoing sense of participation in society and overcome feelings such as alienation and loneliness [1], [2], [3], [4]. However, this sense of participation and satisfaction provided by TV may be reduced if the viewer experiences physical and cognitive difficulties, which are typical of elderly people, such as the loss of hearing, vision or understanding of what is broadcasted [2], [5].

In the guide for the development of interactive TV services for elderly viewers, Carmichael [2] states that, to find an appropriate solution for the elderly, it is necessary to know this public and the difficulties experienced on account of their age. Important issues should be taken into account when designing interactive television services for these viewers.

In the context of interactive TV media, it is possible to offer additional content, with the purpose of displaying extra media information. This solution may provide the

C. Stephanidis and M. Antona (Eds.): UAHCI/HCII 2014, Part III, LNCS 8515, pp. 155–166, 2014.
© Springer International Publishing Switzerland 2014

viewer with a more valuable experience at the end of the TV session [6]. With regard to the elderly audience, interactive TV should provide them with an opportunity to extend the use of TV so that it includes similar activities to the Internet. The elderly can look for information, customize their viewing habits, carry out activities related to e-commerce (shopping, using banking services etc.) and interact with other viewers, by playing an increasingly active role [5].

In this study, additional multimedia content refers to extra information added to TV media in excerpts containing complex narrative structures with the aim of offering something more to the viewer, how to clarify, inform, criticize or make suggestions [6].

In a previous study, which appeared in HCII 2013 [5], we showed that additional content solution can assist the elderly viewer to be more closely engaged with iDTV. It can also help them to appreciate TV programs, especially by involving viewers in the media plot and making the TV experience more interactive and playful. The case study allowed evaluating the behavior of the elderly viewer after interactions with additional content previously added to a TV program. We investigated which additional media formats are more appropriate for the studied group. This previous study also included the formalization of some lessons learned and recommended good practices for the design of additional content for the elderly viewer [5].

This paper provides data from another observational case study conducted to analyze the emotional responses of elderly viewers - during and after the interaction - at this time to a movie that was enhanced with additional multimedia content. This content was added in excerpts including narrative structures that may induce feelings of doubt or dissatisfaction and require reasoning or prior knowledge about the subject. The results allowed a new set of good practices and strategies for the design and enhancement of TV programs for this audience.

The case study was conducted for eight months with elderly people from a Brazilian Reference Center for Social Assistance (CRAS in its Portuguese acronym). During this that period, the elderly group interacted with different devices such as tablets, smartphones, and printers. In two of these meetings, they were involved in activities with an interactive Digital TV. In this study eight elderly people were invited to watch a fourteen- minute long fiction movie. The emotional response of the audience was measured by means of the approach adopted by Xavier [7] and took account of three different methods and techniques.

This paper is structured as follows: Section 2 describes the main narrative structures used in film production and examines the inclusion of additional multimedia content in TV programs. Section 3 analyzes the observational case study conducted with the elderly audience. Section 4 discusses the results. Section 5 discusses some of the lessons that have been learned and investigates the question of good practices for the design of interactive additional content for elderly viewers. Section 6 summarizes the conclusions.

2   Narrative Structures and Additional Multimedia Content

For many people, including the elderly, the difficulties in monitoring a single medium often appear while the program is being shown and may be related to the content displayed. These situations occur because cinematographic art is formed of a complex system of languages that are always difficult for the viewer to understand [8]. New technologies are also engendered in the media systems and configure another phase of this art. These changes require the viewer to have new cognitive skills to ensure a successful outcome from the narratives [8]. The way that someone receives and interprets a given message, in a given context, depends on issues related to the way this message was sent and his/her earlier experiences [8], [9].

The filmic narrative consists of a sequence of events. During this sequence, the characters move in a given space. The script of the narrative is based on action and this involves characters, time, space and conflict [8], [9]. The narrative structures that can be found in movies include metalinguistic resources that may require greater cognitive skills and lead to situations that appear confusing to the viewer. These structures mean that there is complex narrative thread. The most commonly used technical devices in filmic narratives are: a) a change of temporal plane (flashback or flash forward), b) intermittent cursor (e.g. music to create suspense in scenes of tension, filming techniques to highlight something) c) metalinguistic resources and hypermedia (direct citations, self-referencing, external references that require prior knowledge by the viewer to understand), d) linear and non-linear characters (the role played by the character is explained slowly and causes changes in the direction of the plot), e) metalanguage (using other languages to merge different kinds of information. These overlapping languages may derive from other media such as paintings, photographs and comic strips, for instance) [8]. These resources make the narratives and outcomes of these media more complex. Several cognitive competences are needed by the viewers to ensure a good outcome obtained from the entertainment products. These include intellectual skills; such as reasoning and logic, sensory skills; such as attention and perception, and social and creative skills [9]. We believe that, in some situations, the use of narrative structures may trigger feelings of doubt or dissatisfaction. The viewers may get lost at various times during the movie if they are not attentive or lack any related prior knowledge. In view of this, these authors propose the use of additional information to support the television viewers' experience at times when there are incidents in the narrative structures that prevent the movie from having a successful outcome. Studies on additional multimedia content point towards the need for ´static solutions´. Some authors combine interactive Digital TV with hypervideo. The additional information is combined with the objects shown in the scenes and hyperlinks are embedded in the video being transmitted. The viewer can access the additional information by selecting a point on an area of the image displayed [10].

Although it is a useful solution, it fails to take account of the need to support the different viewers' profiles and their specific features. It also overlooks some of the difficulties and the fact that, for example, when the elderly public uses new technologies, it often rejects them.

Carmichael [2] argues that when offering products or interactive television services, the provider will have more chances to attract this audience if the service is combined with a menu (choice of options). Obrist et al. [4], however, warn that it is necessary to address the usability factors that are offered on screens as a set menu, because the elderly often encounter difficulties in using these interactive TV resources.

In light of these difficulties, designers and HCI professionals have the task of analyzing which features must be developed. This analysis must be carried out in partnership with the final users so as to meet their requirements for interaction with the additional content available. There is also a need to determine how best to display and interact with the features so that they are not rejected and the interactive experience can provide pleasurable and satisfying moments.

In the context of this research, thought should be given to the question of a suitable design for the display of content, which must be flexible and allow additional multimedia content to be provided for different viewers' profiles, including the elderly. In the light of this scenario, this paper presents results from an observational case study conducted with eight elderly viewers. The practice allowed an evaluation to be conducted of the emotional responses of a particular sample of elderly people and some good practices and strategies were formulated for the design of additional content for this audience.

3   Observational Case Study

The case study conducted with elderly people evaluated some aspects of the way this audience interacts with movies and with the additional content offered in some excerpts from this media. The main purpose was to analyze the emotional responses of the elderly when they interact with movies which are created with the aim of making use of narrative structures that induce feelings such as doubt, confusion, tension, or dissatisfaction. Alternatively they may require from the viewer some type of reasoning and/or previous knowledge of the subject being addressed.

It is believed that interaction with these excerpts and narratives can influence and define the effects of the viewer´s emotional experience. If this impact is negative, it might make the viewer more hesitant about using TV and its new available resources.

The case study was conducted at a Reference Center for Social Assistance (CRAS) run by the City Hall of São Carlos-SP-Brazil. This center is frequented by an elderly group of people aged between 60 and 85, with an average monthly income of around $ 300.00, a low level of literacy and little experience in the use of technology. The elderly take part in physical, recreational and cultural activities. The aim of the partnership established between the researchers involved in this work, the City Hall and CRAS, as well as participating and collaborating with the existing physical, recreational and cultural activities, was to disseminate information about how the new ICT can be accessed and used, while taking account of the range of abilities and competences of the elderly population, as well as their manner of interacting with these technologies. As a result, the research and extension work conducted at CRAS provided for this public the access to devices such as smartphones, tablets and high-end TV sets with touch sensitivity.

The environment planned for the case study simulated a living room with a couch, a television set and remote control. The elderly group was invited to participate in an activity that consisted of watching a fiction movie that lasted for fourteen minutes. The eight elderly volunteers were divided into pairs in a way that took account of similarity in profiles, such as age group, level of schooling, physical mobility abilities and skills /experience in using a TV set. Two of the pairs formed a part of a "control group" and watched the film with no additional multimedia content, while the other pairs formed a part of the "treatment group" and watched the same media enhanced with additional content on occasions when the narrative structure was thought to be complex. The additional content included media in text, audio or image formats.

3.1   Planning

Objectives of the Case Study: To analyze the degree of satisfaction of the elderly viewer when watching movies and observe whether this increases with programs that are enhanced with additional multimedia content in parts where the narrative structure is complex.

Hypothesis: It is believed that the elderly audience will obtain more satisfaction if they watch TV programs that are enhanced with explanatory additional content, which is made available on occasions when there might be doubts about the meaning. Alternatively, there might be additional content that can display relevant information.

Method and Prepared Questionnaires and Forms: A group of viewers was subjected to observation during a TV session to evaluate the emotional experience of the elderly viewers when they watch a movie with additional multimedia content. After the session, the group answered an evaluation questionnaire and took part in discussions to clarify significant points of the research. Some forms and questionnaires were prepared which included the following: a) a participant observation form, b) a SAM pictographic questionnaire (Self-Assessment Manikin) [11], c) a Brazilian protocol for research with Human Beings and, d) Authorization for Capture of Name, Image and Sound. The observation form supported the researchers in the analysis of the interactions and emotional reactions (gestures and facial expressions) and reported useful information about the viewers during the session.

Media: The media employed in the study was approximately fourteen minutes long and its genre was fiction. The choice of the media took into consideration information that had been collected from a profile questionnaire which had been given to this group of elderly people at the beginning of the project. The researchers sought for media that would arouse the interest of the audience, with a length of time that was compatible with the period they spent doing CRAS activities. It comprised excerpts of narrative structures that might cause doubt, misunderstanding or dissatisfaction, or excerpts that required some previous knowledge from the viewer. The elderly from the treatment group watched the movie which had been enhanced by three additional content. The first was included in textual format and contextualized a flashback scene. The second was in the format of text followed by an image and was incorportated in a scene with an external reference that required the viewer to have previous knowledge. The third was also included in a scene with an external reference; it was in audio format and supplied useful information for clarifying the context. The additional content were shown in parts of the movie when there was no speaking so as to avoid the loss of the main audio content. The added information was shown at the same time as the movie, and did not allow the video to be stopped so that the additional multimedia material could be enjoyed.

Interactivity Icon: In the ten seconds that showed the additional content before, an icon that indicated its presence was displayed in the upper right-hand corner of the

TV screen where it remained for five seconds. The screen on which the media was shown was 21.5 inches in size and the action icon for the additional content was a static interface feature occupying approximately 3% of the screen.

Figure 1 (a) illustrates one of the additional contents that has been included with image and text formats, Figure 1 (b) illustrates the screen showing the interactivity icon and, Figure 1 (c) shows the elderly viewers participating in the TV session.

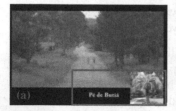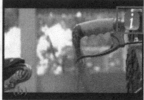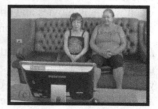

Fig. 1. a) Additional content added to the Textual and Image formats; b) Interactivity icon displayed in the displayed media; c) Elderly viewers participating in the TV session

3.2   Interaction with the Movie

In this stage, the pairs were invited to watch the movie, one at a time. At the beginning of the session, the viewers were informed of how the session was going to be conducted and that they were free to leave it at any time.

The elderly could interact with each other during the session. At the same time, the researchers analyzed the viewers in accordance with the ´Brazilian protocol for research with Human Beings´, and filled out the observation form that involved describing the gestures and expressions that arose during the session. The images of the viewers' faces and bodies were captured during the session for subsequent evaluation.

In the second period, at the end of the movie session, each viewer filled out the SAM form and took part in a discussion in which they were questioned about the experience they had undergone in the session. The discussion was conducted with the aim of obtaining, (in the most spontaneous manner possible), information about the feelings experienced during the movie. The discussion was also designed to obtain information that could allow an evaluation to be carried out of on the displayed interface solution (for the "treatment group" – movie with additional content).

3.3   Methodology for Assessing the Collected Data

The hybrid approach adopted by Xavier [7] was employed to evaluate the data collected during the TV session. The approach is used for the evaluation of the emotions of users when they interact with information systems. On the basis of the experiments, the authors found that, when used in an isolated manner, approaches for emotional evaluation may yield imprecise results. To overcome this problem, Xavier combined methods and assessment tools that exist in the literature. The approach takes into account different stakeholders such as users and experts, in addition to using data collected at different times of the evaluation, and involving interaction before, during and after the interaction.

The Xavier's approach is based on the semantic model for emotions proposed by Scherer [12]. The model is composed of a structure in a circular format that categorizes distinct emotions through the staggering of four main hemispheres: Valence, Arousal, Goal Conduciveness and Coping Potential. When an evaluation is conducted with users, this model takes account of the observation of components such as physiological responses, subjective feelings, cognitive appraisal, behavioral tendencies and motor expression. Xavier [7] determines a set of methods and tools for each component, which can be used to collect information.

Only three of these components were evaluated in this case study, which are: subjective feelings, motor expression and cognitive appraisal. These components were chosen because they are the most closely related to satisfaction, which is the focal point of our research. Among the assessment tools listed by Xavier [7], we have adopted: the SAM [11] questionnaire to evaluate subjective feelings; Discourse Analysis of Collective Subject (ADSC in Portuguese) [13] for cognitive appraisal and, analysis of Emotion Heuristics [14] to evaluate motor expression.

SAM [11] is an evaluation method that uses pictograms and addresses issues relating to the affective quality of a computing system. With SAM, it is possible to evaluate three dimensions of a person when using a computer system: Pleasure, Arousal and Dominance. The SAM questionnaire used in this study evaluated two affective dimensions: pleasure and arousal, which are categorized in this research as ´satisfaction´ and ´motivation´, respectively.

The ADSC method allows a qualitative analysis to be conducted of the user's discourse and is evaluated on the basis of the number of occurrences of keywords in the user's speech during the interaction. After establishing the keywords, these are evaluated for similarity of meaning [13]. In this study, the discourse analysis was used to evaluate the filming, the data collected from observation and the semi-structured interviews.

A set of twenty-three emotion heuristics was used to analyze the motor expression and these represent the viewer's behavioral patterns when interacting with TV programs or movies. These heuristics are called TV Emotion Heuristics (TVEH) [14] and allow a comprehensive assessment of the emotional response of the viewers. Some of the TV Emotion Heuristics are as follows: Restless feet and/or legs, Physical Adjustments, Shaking one´s head, Moving one´s hands, Crying, Breathing deeply, Sleeping/dozing off/yawning, Watching everything in a scene or paying attention, Brow Raising, Gazing away, Smiling, Hand Touching the face. The heuristics observation was carried out based on a video with the capture the user's interactions. The heuristics can be classified as Positive, Negative or Neutral. However, if the evaluator does not feel the urge to make a characterization, or has doubts that the occurrence of that heuristic cannot be directly related to the media on display, he/she should use the 'Nothing Can Be Concluded'. Therefore, the user experience and the feelings associated with this experience should be defined based on an interaction scenario and interventions arising from them.

The video, that lasts approximately 50 minutes and contains images collected in the case study with the elderly from CRAS, underwent a heuristic evaluation of five evaluators, following the Molich and Nielsen [15] recommendations for heuristic evaluation. One of them was considered to be inexperienced, three had little experience and one of them was an expert in the method. The classification of the experience took into account the number of times that the evaluators applied the heuristic evaluation of emotions. Thus, the following classification was considered: above 5 applications: expert evaluator; 2-5 applications: evaluator with little experience; 0-1: inexperienced evaluator.

The application of the hybrid proposal proposed by Xavier [7] allows the specialist to infer if an information system is capable of eliciting a positive, neutral or negative emotional response in the users. The approach is divided into three stages: 1) Selecting Measures, 2) Generalization of Results and, 3) Incidence Octants.

In the *Selecting Measures* stage, the designer has to identify what measures will be used to evaluate the user's experience. In this case study, as mentioned earlier, the components evaluated were subjective feelings, motor expression and cognitive appraisals.

Table 1 illustrates the hybrid proposal in Stage 1 and for each of the three components used, describes which were the assessment methods adopted, the moment that this evaluation was carried out and who was responsible for the final decision when the evaluation of each component was conducted.

Table 1. Instantiation of the Selecting Measures stage

Emotion Component	Method and Domain Evaluated	Moment	Responsible Evaluator
Subjective Feeling	SAM –> *Satisfaction Domain*	Post-interaction	User
	SAM –> *Motivation Domain*	Post-interaction	User
Motor Expression	Emotion Heuristic + Observation –> *Satisfaction Domain*	Post-interaction and During the interaction	Specialist Group
Cognitive Appraisal	Interview (ADSC) + Observation –> *Motivation Domain*	Post-interaction and During the interaction	Specialist

In the *Generalization of Results* stage, each of the measures collected has its result evaluated individually and, for each measure employed, the designer must generalize the collected results in positive, neutral or negative terms. In the sequence, it is necessary to relate each result to the respective hemisphere (four octants) and consider the positive and negative side of each domain. According to Xavier [7], neutral results are not related in the octants of the semantic emotional space [12].

To carry out the *Incidence Octants*, the specialist must increment the octants of the semantic model on the basis of the results of the evaluated measures. The results obtained from the application of Stages 1 and 2 are described in the next section.

4   Results

The results obtained from each method and emotion component, that take account of the control groups (CG) and treatment group (TG), are summarized in Table 2. In this stage each elderly person had his/her experience evaluated as positive (+), negative (-) or neutral (0).

In Stage 2, the results computed for each method are generalized. In Stage 3, the octants incidence is evaluated. The designer must relate each positive or negative result to the respective hemisphere which is considered to be a positive or negative domain evaluated by the measure. In this instantiation, only two domains were evaluated: Satisfaction and Motivation.

Table 2. Evaluation of the elderly people´s (E) emotional experience

Emotion Component	Method	Evaluation (Positive +, Negative -, Neutral 0)
Subjective Feeling	TG: SAM - Satisfaction	E1= + E2 = + / E5 = + E6 = +
	CG: SAM - Satisfaction	E3 = + E4 = + / E7 = + E8 = +
	TG: SAM - Motivation	E1 = + E2 = + / E5 = + E6 = +
	CG: SAM - Motivation	E3 = + E4 = + / E7 = - E8 = +
Motor Expression	TG: Emotion Heuristic	E1 = - E2 = - / E5 = 0 E6 = -
	CG: Emotion Heuristic	E3 = + E4 = + / E7 = 0 E8 = +
Cognitive Appraisal	TG: Observation + Interview	E1 = + E2 = + / E5 = - E6 = -
	CG: Observation + Interview	E3 = + E4 = + / E7 = 0 E8 = +

When carrying out the incidence process in the octants, the specialist must compute how often a given octant was determined by the results of the measures adopted. The hemispheres related to the domains of Motivation and Satisfaction are north/south, east/west, respectively.

Taken as a basis the results shown in Table 2, Figure 2 illustrates the application of Stages 2 and 3 of the hybrid approach for each viewer, and also takes account of the partial and total evaluation of the groups for each domain evaluated. In accordance with the hybrid approach, the neutral results are not related to the octants of the emotional semantic space. Figure 2 (a) illustrates the results for the treatment group and (b) refers to the control group. The elderly people represented by number 1, for example, had positive results when viewed in the motivation domain evaluated by SAM, interview (ADSC) and observation (Table 1). The two measures are generalized in the respective hemispheres. This procedure is carried out for all the elderly and for all results of the applied methods. After the partial results have been obtained, these measures are added and represented in another hemisphere (Final Evaluation).

By means of the octants incidence process is possible to verify that the end result of the emotional responses for the control group (CG) coincides with the responses for the treatment group (TG). In both groups the emotional responses were concentrated in octant 7/8 (as illustrated in Figure2).

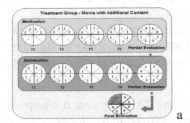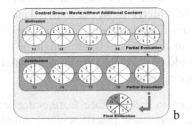

Fig. 2. Octants Incidence: a) for TG group and, b) for CG group

According to the hybrid approach and Scherer's semantic space [12], emotions concentrated in this octant suggest a positive experience. For the satisfaction domain, it can be understood that the viewers felt satisfied and had a pleasurable experience. In the case of the motivation domain, the indications are that they were interested and enthusiastic. This evidence can be confirmed in statements from viewers: "I found it very cool and funny", "Very interesting". However, with regard to the hypothesis that the elderly public might feel more satisfied when watching movies enhanced with additional content, the results point to the rejection of this hypothesis. These results corroborate those of previous research studies [5] and suggest that this profile of elderly viewer prefers to watch TV more passively, without the need for any kind of interaction, effort or intervention from other media on the main media. Given this information, it is necessary to reevaluate the purpose of offering interactive and additional content to this audience, because it is possible that this audience just wants to obtain the information and has no interest or inclination to interact with it.

5   Lessons Learned and Good Practices for the Design

The case study provided us evidence that elderly viewers constitute an audience with particular needs, which are not only physical but also 'affect-cognitive'. If they want the TV content to be more interesting for this audience, especially for the elderly with profiles similar to those studies here, the producers of this 'content' must think of new strategies and the possibility of offering more flexible content and interface solutions.

As regards the physical and emotional characteristics of the elderly in the interaction with additional content, there are a number of strategies that arise from our studies with this audience (and are also based on the literature) which include the following:

- Providing familiar interface element which do not require memorization and which might be more intuitive;
- Providing flexible and adaptive interfaces to define the profile of elderly viewers and their preferences. The likelihood of the elderly wanting to interact with the content might be higher if the provision of content took account of the pre-defined profile;
- Helping them to understand the new paradigm and the new possibilities it opens up by offering a playful and attractive design;
- Offering only what is needed at that time and also, if possible, respecting the preferences indicated. A great deal of information and opportunities for interaction may leave the elderly viewer bewildered and lost;
- Additional content, which is very important as a form of information, as a public utility or is related to health, might be provided in a compulsory mode. This strategy should be used for situations in which it is very necessary to ensure that the information reaches the elderly.

With regard to the interface features for interactive TV programs, it was possible to formulate some good practices which could be employed in the design of the interaction with additional content for the elderly viewer. These good practices supplement those that were initially proposed as a result of the first meeting with the elderly group [5], as well as supporting the practices described by Carmichael [2]. They also take into consideration some factors that arose from the study carried out by Obrist et al, [4]. These good practices are as follows:

- The interactivity icon should be attractive, preferably animated, larger than 3% of the display screen and available at the top left-hand corner of the screen (respecting the natural reading orientation for Western viewers);
- The way of displaying the additional textual content, for these viewers, must be different from that proposed by the Brazilian regulatory agencies [16]. It is suggested that the content with subtitles is displayed on the upper part of the screen because the visual exploration of the underside part of the screen only happens on a second occasion [4];
- The elderly may not associate the interactivity icon (interface element) on the TV screen with the same color button on the remote control. We should seek to overcome this problem to that does not require memorization or association with colors. One alternative is to define a single button on the remote control that can activate the interactions;
- In the design of the interface, (apart from considering a study about size and the disposition of text fonts), account should also be taken of a study about colors and contrast. A white font on a yellow background is not advisable. White fonts on a black background are preferable for a configuration format that allows more effective reading [16].

The profile of the elderly that has been studied here reveals that they adopt a more passive posture while watching TV. This characteristic may result from different influences ranging from low literacy and little experience with technology to characteristics related to ´affect-cognitive´ issues. The implementation of these practices is expected to reduce the effects on this audience resulting from their rejection of the more interactive contents, and allow them to enjoy the interactivity services provided, as well as enabling them to appreciate TV programs such as movies and give them live positive experiences.

6   Conclusion

The data collected from the study provide evidence that there is a demand for interface features that are more flexible and better suited to the needs of the elderly. These features also make it necessary to take account of the physical and emotional characteristics of the elderly viewer when designing interactive interfaces. The study also revealed that the elderly viewers from the studied sample seem not to mind the presence of complex narrative structures in the media. As they adopted a more passive posture during the session, many of these structures are not identified, understood or absorbed in the context of movies. The same occurs when there is additional content included. The results of the data collected from the application of the hybrid approach suggest that there is no difference in the emotional responses between the ´control´ and ´treatment´ groups that were produced by either the presence of narrative structures or the additional content supporting them. However, these results only take account of the profile of one particular viewer. Elderly people with a higher degree of literacy and who are users of new ICTs may show a more active posture and interact in a different manner with interactive TV content. Nevertheless, these assumptions require further study before they can be corroborated. We believe in immersing elderly viewers in new forms of communication. Moreover, there is a widespread belief that it is possible to digitally include these people by making them undergo experiences provided by the new ICTs, by making use of services without leaving home and enjoying pleasurable moments in the company of good TV programs.

Acknowledgements. We would like to thank CAPES for its financial support. We are also grateful to the physical educator João Carlos, the Sao Carlos City Hall and the coordination staff of CRAS.

References

1. Neugarten, B.: The meanings of age. University of Chicago Press, Chicago (1996)
2. Carmichael, A.: Style Guide for the Design of Interactive Television Services for Elderly Viewers. In: Independent Television Commission (ITC), England (1999)
3. Fouts, G.T.: Television Use by the Elderly. Canadian Psychology 30(3), 568–577 (1989)
4. Obrist, M., Bernhaupt, R., Tscheligi, M.: Interactive Television for the Home: Na ethnographic study on user's requirements and experiences. International Journal of Human-Computer Interaction 24(2), 174–196 (2008)
5. Rodrigues, K., de Almeida Neris, V.P., Teixeira, C.A.C.: Interaction of the elderly viewer with additional multimedia content to support the appreciation of television programs. In: Kurosu, M. (ed.) HCII/HCI 2013, Part III. LNCS, vol. 8006, pp. 227–236. Springer, Heidelberg (2013)
6. Rodrigues, K.R.H., Melo, E.L., Nakagawa, P.I., Teixeira, C.A.C.: Interaction with Additional Content to Support the Understanding of Television Programs. In: Proceedings of the IX Brazilian Symposium on Human Factors in Computing Systems, IHC 2010, Belo Horizonte -MG, Brazil, vol. 1, pp. 91–100 (2010) (in Portuguese)
7. Xavier, R.A.C.: A hybrid approach for evaluating the users' emotional experience. Master Thesis. PPG-CC, UFSCar, São Carlos, SP, Brazil (2013) (in Portuguese)
8. Barthes, R., et al.: Structural Analysis of the Narrative: Semiotic Researches, 4th edn., Vozes (1976) (in Portuguese)
9. Eisenstein, S.M.: The Film Sense. In: Leyda, J. (ed.), Harcourt Brace Jovanovich, Inc. (1975)
10. Leon, A., Gradvohl, S., Iano, Y.: Combining Interactive TV and Hypervideo. IEEE Latin America Transactions 5(8) (December 2007) (in Portuguese)
11. Bradley, M.M., Lang, P.J.: Measuring emotion: The Self-Assessment Manikin and the semantic differential. Journal of Behavior Therapy an Experimental Psychiatry 25(1), 49–59 (1994)
12. Scherer, K.R.: On the Nature and Function of Emotion: A Component Process Approach. In: Approaches to Emotion, pp. 293–317. Erlbaum, Hillsdale (1984)
13. Gondim, S.M.G., Fischer, T.: The discourse, the Discourse Analysis and the Methodology of the Collective Subject Discourse in Intercultural Management. Journal of Interdisciplinary Centre for Social Development and Management CIAGS 2(1), 9–26 (2009)
14. Rodrigues, K.R.H., Teixeira, C.A.C., Neris, V.P.A.: Heuristics for assessing emotional response of viewers during the interaction with TV programs. In: Proceedings of the 16th International Conference on Human-Computer Interaction 2014, Springer, Heidelberg (to appear, 2014)
15. Nielsen, J., Molich, R.: Heuristic evaluation of user interfaces. In: CHI9, Seattle, WA, April 1-5, pp. 249–256 (1990)
16. ABNT Brazilian Association of Technical Standards. NBR 15290: Accessibility in communication on television - Accessibility in TV Captions (2005), http://portal.mj.gov.br/corde/arquivos/ABNT/NBR15290.pdf (accessed on January 2014)

Improving Text-Entry Experience for Older Adults on Tablets

Élvio Rodrigues, Micael Carreira, and Daniel Gonçalves

INESC-ID, Rua Alves Redol, 9, 1000-029 Lisboa, Portugal
{elvio.rodrigues,micaelcarreira}@ist.utl.pt,
daniel.goncalves@vimmi.inesc.pt

Abstract. Touchscreen interfaces are increasingly more popular. However, they lack haptic feedback, making it harder to perform certain tasks. This is the case of text-entry, where users have to constantly select one of many small targets. This problem particularly affects older users, whose deteriorating physical and cognitive conditions, combined with the unfamiliarity with technology, can discourage them from using touch devices. In this study, we analyze the performance and behavior of 20 older adults when inputting text on a tablet. We tested a baseline QWERTY keyboard, as well as 2 variants that use text prediction in order to aid seniors typing. From our results, we derive a set of design implications that aim to improve the performance and usability of virtual touch keyboards, specifically for the older users.

Keywords: Older adults, Text-Entry, Tablet, Pre-Attentive Interfaces.

1 Introduction

In our daily life, we find ourselves surrounded by multi-touch technology, which gained popularity in the past few years through mobile devices such as tablets and smartphones. This enables new opportunities and forms of social interaction, instant information access, constant availability and higher control of the surrounding environment. Since touch screens allow users to directly interact and manipulate the information displayed on the screen by touching it, they are considered to be one of the most natural interaction technologies [7].

This is an opportunity for user groups that, until now, have shown some resistance in adopting technology. The fact that this technology interface relies more on software than hardware makes it highly flexible, and thus easy to adapt to users' needs. This offers the opportunity to design more accessible systems [4]. However, it has the disadvantage of lacking the haptic feedback of physical buttons, making it harder to accurately select targets. This characteristic hampers certain tasks, such as text-entry, where the user has to constantly select one of many small targets. Moreover, since text-entry is a task transversal to many applications, it particularly affects users that have difficulties in aiming and performing movements that require precision.

C. Stephanidis and M. Antona (Eds.): UAHCI/HCII 2014, Part III, LNCS 8515, pp. 167–178, 2014.
© Springer International Publishing Switzerland 2014

That is the case of older adults, whose deteriorating physical and cognitive conditions combined with the unfamiliarity with technology, deprives them from the innumerous opportunities created by touch devices. Furthermore, the lack of experience with the QWERTY layout can discourage them from using this technology. Although there is a large body of work that tries to understand the touch behavior and improve the typing experience on touchscreens, studies that target older adults are few. Since the requirements for senior users are different due to the declining of their motor and cognitive abilities, the solutions found for young adults may not be suited for seniors.

Therefore, we performed a study to better understand how we can improve the typing speed and/or reduce the error rate of older adults on tablets. Also, we take into account that older people may have little or no experience with the QWERTY layout, and thus developed 2 QWERTY keyboard variants that aim to aid older adults typing. We performed a user study with 20 senior participants. Then, we systematically analyzed the performance of each variant, thoroughly discussing the touch patterns found and the errors committed by the older adults.

Our main contribution is a thorough understanding of text-entry performance on tablets by senior users. We found that visual changes on the keyboard decrease the typing speed, without improving error rate; older adults systematically hit targets to the bottom and to the side of the hand used to type; single touch and a threshold between key taps can be used to reduce accidental insertions; and when a vertical slide occurs between rows, 96.4% of the times users want the character in the above row.

2   Related Work

Generally, older users easily adapt to touch technology. Loureiro et al. [10] analyzed different aspects of 8 touch based tabletop interfaces for the seniors. In all surveyed works, they concluded that touch yields a natural, direct and intuitive way of interaction with a device, allowing easier human-computer interaction for older people.

Stone [15] argue that, considering older people degraded physical capabilities, this kind of interfaces should have multiple sizes for fonts, buttons and icons. To solve the problem of text-entry, authors propose a gesture that allows switching from the traditional QWERTY keyboard (26 buttons), to a 12 button mobile phone interface (0-9*# layout), or even a binary interface. However, no implementation or experimental evaluation was performed.

Other researches have focused on optimal target size, spacing and positioning to improve the usability of touch interfaces for older users [9]. Indeed, Hwangbo et al. found that the target size is an important factor in pointing performance [8]. They recommend square targets with a side of at least 12mm. They also found that when target size reaches this level, the spacing between targets looses importance. However, these studies neglect the particular case of text-entry, which can be considered one of the most difficult tasks to perform on touch devices, due to the large number of targets and small key size and spacing.

Nicolau et al. [13] focused on the particular problem of text-entry. They performed a user study with 15 seniors, measuring the speed and accuracy of participants while performing text-entry tasks, both on a smartphone and a tablet. They also analyze users hand tremor profile and its relationship to typing behavior. Authors derive a set of guidelines for accessible virtual keyboards for seniors. However, the user study was performed using only the QWERTY keyboard, no alternatives were tested.

Although the body of work regarding older adults is relatively small, there is a extensive body of work focusing on average adults. Henze et al. [6] argue that shifting touch events can improve the typing error rate. Authors found that touch events are systematically skewed towards the lower-right corner of keys. Findlater et al. [4] opted for an adaptive keyboard. He evaluated two personalized keyboard interfaces specifically for ten-finger typing, both of which adapt their underlying key-press classification models. One of the keyboards also visually adapts the location of keys. Results have shown that only the non-visual keyboard improved typing speed and error rate.

As noted by Cheng et al. [3], people use different hand postures to type on tablets depending on how they were holding these devices. The authors developed iGrasp, a keyboard that automatically adapts its layout and position based on how the device is held. Another way to reduce the error rate of soft keyboard usage is through language models. Several approaches to highlight keys have been studied which involve making the rendered keys larger or smaller, depending on their likelihood [1]. The authors reported that users were faster and more accurate with this variant than with the regular QWERTY keyboard. Gunawardana et al. [5] developed a method that expands or contracts the keys' underlying area, keeping the visual feedback intact, based on a language model. A simulation suggests that it reduces the error rate.

As we have seen, previous studies are mainly focused on finding solutions for able-bodied adults. Although some studies have already analyzed the touch patterns and the optimal target size and spacing for senior users, none have presented and tested different alternatives to improve the typing experience for older people.

3   Developed QWERTY Variants

Due to the lack of haptic feedback, text-entry remains slower and more error-prone on touch devices than on traditional computer keyboards. Since one of our goals is to aid new users to input text, without hindering older users who are already experienced with QWERTY keyboards, we developed alternative keyboards based on the QWERTY keyboard layout. After developing the regular QWERTY keyboard to serve as a baseline, we developed 2 variants, which are described in the following subsections. These were the variants that achieved the best results in our previous study [14]. These variants use letter or word prediction to anticipate what the user is going to write. Detailed information about the text prediction algorithm is not the focus of this paper and has been previously published in [14]. The keyboards were implemented as a Windows Modern UI application for Windows 8.

Color Variant. The Color variant uses the developed letter prediction algorithm to highlight the next most likely letters for the current word (Figure 1a). We expect this variant to perform better than the regular QWERTY keyboard, especially if the user is not acquainted with the QWERTY layout, which might be the case of older adults. By highlighting the most likely letters, senior users may find the desired letter quicker. We also expect that users make fewer errors by noticing they are about to press a key that is not highlighted, or by acknowledging they missed or omitted a key press.

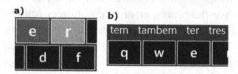

Fig. 1. (a) Color variant; (b) Predicted words variant

We decided to highlight 4 keys, since a previous study [1] concluded that it was the optimum number between 1, 2 and 4 keys. The highlighted key changes its color from black to gray to avoid the cultural connotations associated with particular colors (e.g.: the green and red colors may have positive and negative connotations, respectively). We also increase the size of the key's label. The highlight is continuous: the more probable the letter, the brighter the color and bigger the label on the key.

Predict Words Variant. This variant is an alternative already used in some touch devices. While the user is typing, a list of the most likely words is shown in a horizontal ribbon above the keyboard (Figure 1b). If the word the user wants to write is on the suggested list, he can save some key touches by tapping it so the full word, along with a space character, will be inserted. While this solution is fairly popular among younger users, it may be inadequate for older users. Since there is a cognitive effort required to process the list of suggested words, it might be harder for this group of users to divide their attention between the actual typing and the scanning of the suggestions' list. We opted to suggest 4 words to achieve a balance between the success rate of the prediction and the cognitive effort required to process the suggestions list.

4   User Study

In this user study we evaluate the typing performance of older adults using the developed variants in comparison with the traditional QWERTY keyboard.

Participants. Twenty participants, 15 females and 5 males, took part in the user study. Their age ranged from 61 to 92 years old, but the most prevalent age group was from 71 to 90 years old (75% of participants). Two participants used only the left hand to type, 5 used both hands, and the rest used only their right hand to type.

No participant had severe visual impairments. We also assessed users' capabilities regarding task-specific tremor, by asking them to draw an Archimedes spiral with each hand without leaning the hand or arm on the table [2]. None of the participants presented accentuated hand tremor. No participant had used a touchscreen device before. Although 17 participants had used the QWERTY keyboard whether in type-writers and/or personal computers (17 participants), most of them (12) reported to have little or no experience with QWERTY keyboards.

Procedure. The user study had two main phases: training and evaluation. At the beginning of the first phase, we explained how to use the virtual keyboard. Users were asked to type on the developed traditional QWERTY keyboard and the 2 variants. Participants were free to type in the position they found more comfortable. During the training phase, participants were allowed to type 2 sentences per keyboard variant.

In both phases, the task consisted in copying a sentence that was displayed at the top of the screen. After typing the sentence, the user could proceed to the next sentence by pressing a button. Copy typing was used to reduce the opportunity for spelling and language errors. Both required and transcribed sentences were always visible. The sentences were chosen randomly from a set of 88 sentences, such that no sentence was written twice per participant. Each sentence had five words with an average size of 4.48 characters and a minimum correlation with the language of 0.97. These sentences were extracted from a Portuguese language corpus of another study [12]. In order to avoid different correction strategies by the users, the delete key was removed. Participants were instructed to continue typing if an error occurred.

On the evaluation phase, participants were instructed to type the sentences as quickly and accurately as possible. Each user was asked to type 5 sentences for each variant, being the first one still trial (it did not account for the results). The order of tested variants was random to avoid bias associated with experience. In the end, users were asked to answer a survey with some demographic data, as well as satisfaction regarding each variant. The whole process took approximately 1 hour per participant.

Apparatus. A Samsung ATIV Smart Pc Pro 11.6" was used in the study. Each key has 20mm of width and 15mm of height. Visually, there is a space of 2mm between keys, horizontally and vertically. However, our implementation does not allow pressing between keys: each touch is always assigned to a key. This makes the keyboard more responsive, thus avoiding the frustration of performing a touch that does not produce a character. All participants' actions were logged through our evaluation application, so posterior analysis could be performed.

5   Results

By analyzing the log data produced by our application, we are able to draw conclusions on input speed and accuracy for each keyboard variant. We also focus on types of errors and their main causes. We performed Shapiro-Wilkinson tests of the observed values for Words Per Minute (WPM), Minimum String Distance (MSD) and types of errors to access if dependent variables were normally distributed. If they were, we applied parametric statistical tests, such as repeated measures ANOVA, t-test, and Pearson correlations. If measures were not normally distributed, we used nonparametric tests: Friedman, Wilcoxon, and Spearman correlations. Bonferroni corrections were used for post-hoc tests.

Input Speed. To assess typing speed, we used the WPM [11] text input measure calculated as:

(transcribed text - 1) x (60 seconds / time in seconds) / 5 characters per word

Figure 2a illustrates WPM by variant (without outliers). As expected, we found a correlation between input rate, QWERTY experience and number of hands used to type. A repeated measures ANOVA revealed significant differences between keyboard variants on text-entry speed ($F_{(2,30)}=3.84$, $p<0.033$). Bonferroni post-hoc tests showed significant differences between QWERTY and Color variant, meaning that users type significantly slower with the latter. This result contradicted our hypothesis that inexperienced users, who are not acquainted with the QWERTY layout, would benefit from the Color variant. We believe that the main reason for the lower input rate in the Color variant is that the highlighting of the keys was distracting. However, no user reported this. We also noted that, in some cases, despite the correct letter was the only one highlighted by the Color variant, some participants took a long time to find that letter on the keyboard. This means that some seniors were not paying enough attention to the highlighted keys, excluding them from the benefits of the suggestion.

Regarding the Predict Words variant there was no significant difference when compared with the QWERTY keyboard. However, only 7 of the 20 participants accepted at least one suggested word from the list during evaluation; the remaining 13 participants used the Predict Words variant as a normal QWERTY keyboard. Still, we did not find a correlation between text-entry speed on Predict Words variant and interaction methodology, i.e., if the participant accepted suggested words or typed as a normal QWERTY keyboard.

Quality of Transcribed Sentences. To measure the quality of typed sentences we used the MSD error rate, calculated as:

MSD(required text, transcribed text) / Max(required text, transcribed text) x 100

Figure 2b illustrates the MSD error rate by variant. A repeated measures ANOVA did not reveal significant differences between keyboard variants ($F_{(2,32)}=1.044$, $p=0.364$). Opposed to the results obtained on input speed, no correlation was found between quality of transcribed sentences and previous experience with QWERTY keyboards and number of hands used.

We expected both *Color* and *Predict Words* variants to outperform the QWERTY keyboard regarding MSD. Although we are not sure why the *Color* variant did not outperform the QWERTY keyboard, several situations occurred that are important to report. For instance, one participant ended up typing a word similar to the expected one because the *Color* variant suggested it, and he tapped the suggested letters without thinking too much. This is an issue related with the prediction algorithm.

Since the system does not always suggest the right letter, the user still has to pay attention to the suggested letters. Sometimes it seemed that participants were afraid of tapping a certain key if the system was not suggesting it, especially after tapping a sequence of keys correctly suggested. The performance of the *Color* variant was also affected by the fact that older users made many errors. This means that the *Color* variant cannot make good suggestions, because once there is an error in the current word, the system is not able to correctly predict the sequence of letters intended by the user.

The *Predict Words* variant also had a MSD similar to QWERTY, mainly because most participants (13) did not accept any suggestion. From the remaining 7, only 3 accepted a high number of suggested words (between 9 and 11 suggestions). From these, 2 participants had worst results in the *Predict Words* variant when compared with QWERTY. This happened because sometimes, when accepting a suggested word (located at the top of the keyboard), users tapped below the intended area, selecting a key from the top row of the keyboard instead. Another common error is to tap the space bar after accepting a suggested word. This counts as an insertion error because after accepting the suggested word a space is automatically inserted. Therefore, the use of the *Predict Words* backfired because participants ended up making mistakes they would not make in other situations.

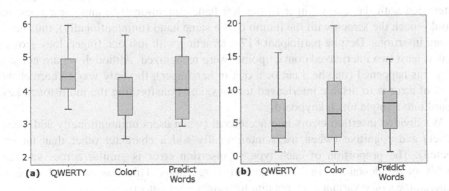

Fig. 2. (a) Participants' WPM by variant; (b) Participants' MSD by variant

Typing Errors. We classified the types of input errors using MacKenzie's et al. categorization [11] (substitutions – incorrect characters, insertions – added characters, and omissions – omitted characters). In some cases, we assign a more specific categorization to errors, but when we do, we explain the differentiation.

In Figure 3, we can verify that insertion errors are the most common type of error committed by senior participants. This type of error is unevenly distributed through all the participants: participants #2 and #17 are responsible for 62% of all insertion errors. Omissions were the second most common error type, followed by substitutions. The *Predict Words* variant was not analyzed thoroughly regarding typing errors, because most of the participants used it as a QWERTY keyboard.

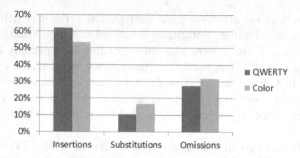

Fig. 3. Contribution of each type of error for the total amount of errors

Insertion Errors. We found that most of insertions (more than 60% of all insertions) occurred due to multiple interleaved points of contact, i.e., the second point of contact occurs before the first one is released. Since this insertion error exists because the keyboard is multi-touch, it is relevant to assess if this kind of error is mostly committed by participants who used both hands to interact with the keyboard. However, no correlation was found between number of hands used and multiple points of contact insertions.

We found that this type of accidental insertion was committed mostly by participants #2 and #17, which interacted with just one hand. We noted that participant #2 interacted with the index finger of her left hand (intentionally), and sometimes she would touch the screen with the thumb of the same hand (unintentionally), thus generating insertions. Despite participant #17 interacting with just one finger, logs showed that at least two interleaved contact points were recognized. Although we are not sure why this happened (maybe a cut or a dirt in her finger), the only way to correct this kind of error is to disable interleaved touches, i.e., transforming the multi-touch keyboard into a single touch keyboard.

We divided insertion errors into accidental (when users unintentionally add a character) and cognitive (when users intentionally add a character other than the expected). The proportion of each type of insertion error is similar across variants: 81.6% of accidental vs. 18.4% of cognitive insertions. This was expected since, in general, the *Color* variant does not aim to correct insertion errors.

Substitution Errors. We considered two types of substitution errors: neighbor (instead of touching the intended key, users touch an adjacent key) and cognitive (when users touch a different key from the expected) substitution errors. After analyzing the touch data, we found that touch points are skewed to the bottom and slightly to the right for users that interacted with their right hand. Other studies have also reported this result [13, 6]. We also found that the horizontal direction of the shift was related to the hand being used to type. For users that used their left hand, we could not verify the pattern across all keyboard, but it could be that our data might not be enough (only 2 participants used the left hand). Regarding participants that used both hands, we verified that the left side of the keyboard has its touch points skewed towards the bottom-left, while the right side of the keyboard has its touch points skewed towards the bottom-right. These results were true for both QWERTY and Color variant, which means that highlighting keys does not influence aiming. We verified that shifts have a bigger vertical deviation (Mean=13px; SD=11.5px) when comparing to the horizontal deviation (Mean=4.5px; SD=14.7px), for all typing methods. We also found that the vertical shift increases gradually, from the top to the bottom row (average vertical deviations: row1=11px; row2=14px; row3=18px; row4=20px).

In the QWERTY keyboard, users committed 29 neighbor substitution errors and 9 cognitive substitution errors. However, users significantly committed more cognitive substitution errors on Color variant (Z=-1.845, p=.065); they committed 30 neighbor and 30 cognitive substitution errors. We verified that in 65.5% of cognitive substitutions the user inserted a character that was highlighted by the Color variant. And, in the remaining 34.5%, the expected key was highlighted, but it did not prevent the user from inserting an erroneous character which was not highlighted. We also noted that in 20.7% of the cognitive substitution errors both expected and inserted keys were highlighted. Despite acknowledging this result, we could not find a justification for it.

Omission Errors. We subdivided omissions into 3 sub-categories: failed (the user presses an empty space instead of the intended key – only applicable to the keys in the edges), slide (the press action was in a different key when compared to the release action) and cognitive (user forgets to insert an expected character). Omission errors had approximately the same proportion across variants, being the cognitive most frequent (52%), followed by slide (27%) and failed (21%) omissions. We also found that forgetting to enter a blank space between words was a common issue among older people (44.8% of the total cognitive omissions), most likely due to a lack of practice in typing on computers. Since the Color variant highlights the next most probable keys, it would be expected that, if correct, the suggestion could minimize omissions. Still, cognitive omissions were as frequent as on the QWERTY keyboard. When further analyzing this type of error, we found that in 65% of cognitive omissions the expected key was highlighted. However, the next key taped by users (which was an error), was highlighted only in 22% of the cases. This means the Color variant was often helping the participant, but still they pressed an erroneous key that was not highlighted 78% of the time.

The slide omissions differ from the previous, because the user presents the intention to type a character, but fails in the execution. It occurs when the user presses and lifts his finger on different keys and therefore no output is generated. We classified slide omissions in three subcategories: (1) correct land-on, characterized by the finger landing on the intended key, and then sliding to another key; (2) correct lift-off, characterized by the finger landing on a neighbor key, and then sliding to the intended key; (3) and accidental slide, on which the user has no intention to tap either of the keys. The first type accounted for 36.4% of the slide omission errors, the second 57.6% and the third 6%. We found that all the errors classified as correct land-on, ended always in a key below the intended one; that is, the slide was always performed from the top to the bottom. Contrary to this, 89.5% of the errors classified as correct lift-off, ended in a key above the pressed one. On the remaining cases the slide was performed from the right to the left. This means that when a user performs a slide starting at a key in a given row, and lifts his finger on a key in the row above, we are

100% sure that the user intended to tap the key in the row above. When the slide is downwards, in 85.7% of the times, the user also wants the key in the row above (the key were he landed his finger). In the remaining 14.3% times, we do not know what the intentions of the user were, since the slide was accidental. This pattern was also verified for the Color variant. We hypothesize that this occurs because when the user slides down, it is because he is already moving his hand to the rest position, bellow the tablet. When the movement is upwards, it is a corrective movement, because the user adjusted the touch position in a contrary motion to the resting position. This pattern, to our knowledge, has not been reported by any other study, presenting an opportunity for improvement of virtual keyboards.

User Satisfaction. At the end of the user study participants were debriefed and asked about their preferred keyboard. We also collected comments during and after the test about their opinion regarding the several keyboard variants. When asked about their satisfaction (5-point Likert scale) regarding each variant, participants gave a higher rate to the QWERTY keyboard (Mean=3.8; Median=4), closely followed by the Color variant (Mean=3.75; Median=4) and finally by the Predict Words variant (Mean=3.1; Median=3). Still, 6 participants rated the Color variant with the highest score (5), while only 1 participant rated each of the remaining keyboards with the highest score. Statistically significant differences were only found between Predict Words and the other variants; participants were not as satisfied when using Predict Words.

Some users also reported that the tablet was too sensitive, referring to the fact that it is easy to make typing mistakes by lightly touching the device. A participant reported that it was faster to type with the *Color* variant, referring to a specific case when the system was able to always suggest the right letter. Some participants told us that the *Color* variant was really helpful but, in order to take full advantage of it, paying attention was necessary. When participants were asked about why they did not use the suggestions presented in the *Predict Words* variant, most participants said it was a feature too complex and they would need more practice in order to correctly use it.

6   Design Implications

From our results, we derive the following design implications.

- **Keep visual changes to a minimum.** As verified in the user study, visual changes that aim to focus the user attention on the most probable keys have a negative impact in text-input speed. Also, the *Color* variant had twice the cognitive substitution errors, when compared with the traditional QWERTY. Therefore, visual changes should only occur to give feedback about the pressed and released key.
- **Shift the touch points to the top and to the opposite side of the hand the user is using to type.** Our results confirmed that users who used only their right hand to interact with the virtual keyboard had a tendency to touch on the bottom-right of targets. This means that users will benefit from a top-left shift of their touch points to compensate the tendency. Conversely, users who only used their left hand

benefit with a top-right shift of their touch points. Users who interact with both hands will benefit from a top-left shift on touch points performed on the right side of the keyboard, and a top-right shift of the touch points performed on the left side of the keyboard. If it is not possible to detect the user's hand posture, an upward vertical shift of touch points will also benefit users.

- **When a vertical slide occurs between two keys of subsequent rows, produce the character in the row above.** When users perform a vertical slide from one row to a subsequent row (up or down), 96.4% of the times the user intends to select the key from the row above. In the remaining 3.6% times, we do not know exactly the intentions of the user were, since the slide was an accidental touch.
- **Choose single touch over multi-touch.** Older users have different necessities and capabilities. Regarding a generic keyboard that should fit all types of older users, single touch is the best choice. The quality of the sentences of the 2 most problematic participants in our user study increased drastically, while it only slightly prejudiced some other participants and had no effect at all on most participants.
- **Omit touch interactions that are below a certain threshold.** Sometimes, the older users would quickly and accidentally insert two characters instead of one. This occurs due to poor coordination and hand tremor. These insertions are characterized by a reduced time interval between the release of the first key and the press of the second key. Therefore, to enhance older adults' error rate, we can omit interactions that occurred below a certain time threshold.

7   Conclusion

Given the increasing use of touch mobile devices and, in particular, tablets, this study is timely and pertinent. The use of tablets by older citizens brings into sharp focus the need to bridge the gap between our aging population and advances in information technology. This is particularly important for tasks that are difficult to perform on touch devices, such as text-entry.

In this study, we investigated the text-entry performance of 20 older adults on a touch-based device. Our user study featured 3 virtual keyboards: traditional QWERTY, Color and Predict Words variants. We found that users typed faster with the traditional QWERTY keyboard. Regarding the quality of transcribed sentences, no significant differences were found across variants. We also found that older adults have difficulties using Predict Words variant mainly because it was too complex and they needed more training to use it. Lastly, we identify some design implications that should improve typing accuracy and encourage researchers to create more effective solutions for older adults. Future research should apply the design implications described here and investigate their effect on text-entry performance.

Acknowledgements. This work was supported by the Portuguese Foundation for Science and Technology (FCT): individual grant SFRH/BD/72735/2010; project PAELife AAL/0014/2009; and project PEst-OE/EEI/LA0021/2013.

References

1. Al Faraj, K., Mojahid, M., Vigouroux, N.: BigKey: A virtual keyboard for mobile devices. In: Jacko, J.A. (ed.) HCI International 2009, Part III. LNCS, vol. 5612, pp. 3–10. Springer, Heidelberg (2009)
2. Bain, P., Mally, J., Gresty, M., Findley, L.: Assessing the impact of essential tremor on upper limb function. Journal of Neurology 241, 1 (1993)
3. Cheng, L.-P., Liang, H.-S., Wu, C.-Y., Chen, M.Y.: igrasp: grasp-based adaptive keyboard for mobile devices. In: Proc. of the SIGCHI Conference on Human Factors in Computing Systems, CHI 2013. ACM (2013)
4. Findlater, L., Wobbrock, J.: Personalized input: improving ten-finger touchscreen typing through automatic adaptation. In: Proc. of the SIGCHI Conference on Human Factors in Computing Systems, CHI 2012, pp. 815–824. ACM (2012)
5. Gunawardana, A., Paek, T., Meek, C.: Usability guided key-target resizing for soft keyboards. In: Proc. 15th International Conference on Intelligent User Interfaces (2010)
6. Henze, N., Rukzio, E., Boll, S.: Observational and experimental investigation of typing behaviour using virtual keyboards for mobile devices. In: Proc. of the SIGCHI Conference on Human Factors in Computing Systems, CHI 2012. ACM (2012)
7. Holzinger, A.: Finger instead of mouse: Touch screens as a means of enhancing universal access. In: Carbonell, N., Stephanidis, C. (eds.) UI4ALL 2002. LNCS, vol. 2615, pp. 387–397. Springer, Heidelberg (2003)
8. Hwangbo, H., Yoon, S., Jin, B., Han, Y., Ji, Y.: A study of pointing performance of elderly users on smartphones. International Journal of Human-Computer Interaction (2013)
9. Jin, Z.X., Plocher, T., Kiff, L.: Touch screen user interfaces for older adults: Button size and spacing. In: Stephanidis, C. (ed.) HCI 2007. LNCS, vol. 4554, pp. 933–941. Springer, Heidelberg (2007)
10. Loureiro, B., Rodrigues, R.: Multi-touch as a natural user interface for elders: A survey. In: 2011 6th Iberian Conference on Information Systems and Technologies, CISTI (2011)
11. MacKenzie, I.S., Soukoreff, R.W.: Text entry for mobile computing: Models and methods, theory and practice. Human Computer Interaction 17, 2–3 (2002)
12. Nicolau, H.: Disabled 'R' All: Bridging the Gap between Health- and Situationally-Induced Impairments and Disabilities. PhD thesis, Instituto Superior Técnico (2013)
13. Nicolau, H., Jorge, J.: Elderly text-entry performance on touchscreens. In: Proc. 14th International ACM SIGACCESS Conference on Computers and Accessibility (2012)
14. Rodrigues, É., Carreira, M., Gonçalves, D.: Improving text entry performance on tablet devices. In: Interação (2013)
15. Stone, R.: Mobile touch interfaces for the elderly. In: Proc. of ICT (2008)
16. Yin, Y., Ouyang, T.Y., Partridge, K., Zhai, S.: Making touchscreen keyboards adaptive to keys, hand postures, and individuals: a hierarchical spatial backoff model approach. In: Proc. SIGCHI Conference on Human Factors in Computing Systems, CHI 2013 (2013)

AgeCI:
HCI and Age Diversity

Samuel Silva[1], Daniela Braga[2], and António Teixeira[1,3]

[1] Institute of Electronics and Telematics Engineering, University of Aveiro, Portugal
[2] VoiceBox, USA
[3] Dep. of Electronics, Telecommunications and Informatics Engineering,
University of Aveiro, Portugal

Abstract. We present an overview of recent works in which age is an important driving factor for Human-Computer Interaction design and development. These serve as starting grounds to discuss current practices and highlight challenges that might serve as beacons for future research in the field.

Keywords: age diversity, overview.

1 Introduction

Age related approaches to HCI, with some notable exceptions, are nowadays strongly focused on the elderly [20] boosted by applications in areas such as ambient assisted living [40] and, although to a lesser degree, on children. Nevertheless, age related characteristics of different age groups [48,39] make it important that users are not just divided in two (elderly and remaining users) or three (children, adults and elderly) categories. Even when the physical and cognitive characteristics of users seem equivalent, intrinsic differences in motivation and social needs as observed, for example, between teenagers and adults [49], might pose challenges regarding which methodologies to use to include them in the design process, elicit opinions or collect data.

The challenges posed to HCI by age diversity have led researchers to follow different methodologies to support design and development and assess user performance using different modalities, devices and user interfaces. We consider that the community might profit from an integrated view regarding how age associated characteristics/differences are addressed, not necessarily coinciding with an universal design approach. This should highlight and contribute to a first level of organization of the plethora of design and development methods that can be used by researchers in order to improve their work for specific age groups.

This paper is intended to present a general overview of the literature covering age-related issues and methodologies in HCI by focusing on the most recent surveys, studies, trends and challenges (mostly published after 2010) on the subject.

C. Stephanidis and M. Antona (Eds.): UAHCI/HCII 2014, Part III, LNCS 8515, pp. 179–190, 2014.

While selecting the surveyed literature we wanted to cover works regarding different age groups in four main categories: input/output modalities, target devices,applications and contributions to guidelines and methodologies. This provides us the grounds to highlight aspects that we consider might profit from further attention and discussion by the HCI community.

This article is organized as follows: Section 2 presents a brief overview (given the range and complexity of such matters [48]) of human characteristics affected by age, the motivating factors for differenced/adaptable approaches in HCI design and development; Section 3 presents a survey on recent literature regarding HCI works for which age is a driving factor covering aspects concerning different input/output modalities, the target devices, applications (and their graphical user interface) and main contributions on the form of reviews, guidelines and methodologies (and frameworks); Section 4 discusses some of the challenges depicted by the surveyed literature and some desirable routes for future work in the field; finally, section 5 presents some conclusions.

2   Age Related Characteristics

Literature is prolific in describing ageing effects and these can be felt at different levels in the individual. It is nevertheless important to consider intrinsic characteristics of particular age groups that might affect performance, for example due to early levels of motor skills development.

Researchers should consider physical, motor and perceptual limitations and cognitive changes, but must also contemplate socio-cultural aspects regarding other factors such as social integration (e.g., the need to fit a certain social group), cultural backgrounds and how different resulting mental models are used to organize information, influencing performance [39,57].

Physical and sensorial — Children might exhibit limitations due to their height, arms length and finger and hand size [47]. Furthermore, their motor skills might still not be mature enough resulting, for example, in visual-motor dis-coordination [25], reduced precision and inability to perform fine movements [48,5]. Although evolution occurs continuously, studies show that, important improvements in these aspects occur between six and eight years of age [25] and they refine and get more consistent by the age of 12 [2].

Physical performance is progressively affected by ageing resulting in reduced fine motor skills [11], strength and speed, sometimes leading to tremors. It is important to note that even if these aspects are not very pronounced, the effects of long term immobility might also pose problems, such as articulation and muscle pain, precluding certain interaction gestures/positions (e.g., long time standing or with arms in a fixed/rigid position). With age, a decreasing sensibility is also observed in hands and fingers. Physical limitations, although not expected to directly affect interaction, might pose problems. For example, if a user has trouble walking and uses a walking aid (cane or frame), the hands will have to deal with it and are less available for interaction.

With age, vision is affected in many different ways and naturally occurring changes often include reduced visual acuity, with decreased focus on near objects, different colour perception, increased sensibility to glare and decreased brightness perception [30,57]. These may also be aggravated by diseases such as diabetes.

Hearing loss is also observed with a particular emphasis on low volume sounds and higher frequencies [52].

Cognitive — Such as happens with the motor skills, the cognitive skills of young children are also under development [48,31] and vary much with age. One important characteristic is that children have short attention spans [10,47], i.e., the amount of time they manage to focus on a particular task is small. Attention is also much more easily given to aspects that stand out, even if they are not relevant to the current task [48] (e.g., coloured animated clown on screen instead of the instructions to reach the next stage). Furthermore, small children might have limited or no spelling skills.

Teenagers also present some important cognitive differences when compared with children and adults. These differences affect judgement, decision-making and risk-taking [49]. Teenagers are more willing to take risks and have a strong desire for autonomy and to develop an individual identity [16,41]. Furthermore, they seek association with peers and are highly susceptible to their influence (e.g., brands, technologies, clothes).

With advancing age, changes are felt affecting memory, information processing and intelligence. Working memory is used as a working space for storing information which needs to be readily available or used to perform decisions and comprehend written and spoken language [57]. Its decline therefore results in a slowdown in learning new (large amounts of) information, but also in a reduced capability to process complex information. This, added to increasing times to access long term memory elements, significantly affects the time required to perform tasks.

Changes to intelligence can be explained recurring to the concepts of fluid and crystallized intelligence [48,6]. Fluid intelligence refers to the ability to reason abstractly and to adapt to new situations despite of acquired knowledge. On the other hand, crystallized intelligence deals with the ability to use skills, knowledge and experience accumulated through the years. While both types of intelligence increase during childhood and early adulthood, between the ages of 30 and 40, fluid intelligence starts to decline while crystallized intelligence continuously increases and only starts declining much later in life [6]. By reviewing the literature regarding web navigation, Hanson [20] points out that crystallized intelligence is a particular advantage for older adults towards younger adults when faced with complex ill-defined tasks that require some thought and benefit from acquired experience.

Is is also important to understand that people can sometimes present several limitations. Even if taken individually they are of minor gravity, they might interact with each other resulting in a performance degradation that is far superior than that expected for the individual disabilities. [18,20].

It is important to note that all these age related effects are subject to individual variability precluding treating each of the age groups as a homogeneous group [32,43] and further stressing the importance of using proper methodologies that help design HCI for age diversity.

3   HCI for Age Diversity

To provide an overview of the various aspects involved we briefly analyse how research in the field can yield insight on the age-related aspects influencing user performance concerning different input/output modalities, devices and applications and how these results have contributed to propose guidelines and methodologies that might support further (systematic) developments. Notable previous surveys regarding specific age groups are those by Wagner et al. [54], for the elderly, and Read et al. [42] for children).

3.1   Interaction Modalities

The many existing modalities are not equally adequate or adopted by the users of different ages. Several recent studies investigated preferences and user performance.

Weiss et al. [56] remark that studies on modality preference are often restricted to younger users. In their study, they addressed the effects of age on modality preference (speech, touch and 3D gestures), but no evidence of such effects was found.

The most common interaction modality for desktop computers is the mouse. Mouse pointing performance has been assessed for particular age groups (e.g. children [25]) or comparing among age groups (e.g. young adults, adults and elderly [21]). In summary, main findings show evidence that speed and accuracy improve with age, for small children and that adults tend to perform better than young adults and the elderly. The latter, although performing slower than the remaining age groups did not commit more errors.

Interfaces using touch have been increasingly used, as a result of the technological advances in the field. Herztum et al. [21] and Findlater et al. [15] show that touch screens are easily used by the elderly and their use reduced the performance gap between young and older adults when compared to performances on traditional desktops (a survey on multi-touch for elders can be found in [29]). Jochems et al. [24], present a comparative study for three input devices (mouse, touch screen and eye-gaze control) and conclude that, irrespective of age group, touch screens attain the best performance (shorter execution time), most notably for elderly. Culen et al. [13] briefly describe a set of experiments also using touch with elderly, in different application scenarios, and analyse some of the challenges faced in using such technology regarding, e.g., how motor disabilities affecting movement accuracy might affect usage. Hwangbo et al. [23] report that older adult performance in pointing tasks can be improved by adding audiotactile feedback. Rodrigues et al. [45] assessed how different QWERTY keyboard variants, on touch screens, influenced young and old adults performance.

Regarding interaction with touch screens and focusing on gestures, Aziz et al. [5] assessed which gestures (e.g., tap, drag-and-drop, pinch, spin) children from two to twelve years old were able to use and found some evidence that children bellow age four had difficulty in performing some of the gestures. In a study by Arif et al. [4], older adults seemed to favour pen gestures (faster; better accuracy) instead of touch and no such effect was observed on children. Furthermore, according to Stoessel [50], gestures result in improved performance and satisfaction for the elderly who mostly favour single-finger gestures.

Anthony et al. [2] assess the performance of children and adults while using a touch screen and identify performance differences between the two age groups along with several technical challenges to use this modality. For example, gesture recognition modules have a poorer performance for children gestures and it is advisable that age-specific recognizers are trained. Furthermore, the gestures should be tailored in order to make conceptual sense to the child.

Jochems et al. [24] present a study where eye-gaze is combined with different methods for input validation (keyboard space key, foot pedal and speech) with an advantage for the keyboard key, mostly due to user familiarity with the keyboard vs the foot pedal and to time coordination problems between the moment an object is fixated and the speech input is performed.

Speech interfaces have also been subject to user performance assessment, in particular considering the elderly. Aman et al. [1] provide some insights about well known issues regarding automatic speech recognition problems with the elderly [53] and how to cope with them. Portet et al. [38] assess acceptability of voice interfaces in a smart home context. Although with a particular focus on the elderly, the authors perform a user study involving different age groups and conclude for overall acceptance provided the system does not drive users to a lazy lifestyle. Considering children and speech interfaces, an example, involving conversational agents, can be found in Prez-Marin [35].

Sometimes, when choosing the input/output modalities it is relevant to not only consider the specific motor and cognitive characteristics and limitations of the target age group (and context) but also how these will impact on other aspects, such as skills development in children. The work by Antle et al. [3] is a good entry point to these concerns. The author conducts a study in which children use three different ways of interacting with a spatial puzzle task (physical, graphical and tangible interfaces). For example, the mouse and graphical user interface, although serving the intended purpose, favoured a trial and error approach which might limit skills development for which the tangible interface was more suited.

3.2 Target Devices

As interaction modalities are not of universal use in all situations - be it devices or even concrete applications - they are, in most occasions, tightly related with the device used. Nevertheless, researchers have also assessed user performance considering devices (mobile phones, tablets, interactive TVs, desktop computers, etc.) as a whole, in different application scenarios. Boosted by the recent technological developments and current research trends, mobile devices are the most assessed platform.

Leung et al. [27] have performed a study in order to understand how the elderly learn to use mobile devices. By conducting the study for three groups (young adults, adults and older adults) they were able to identify which aspects were specific of older adults. For example, older adults significantly used less trial and error and preferred to learn alone. Therefore, better support should be provided for trying out tasks. A thorough review regarding handheld computers and their use by older adults can be found in Zhou et al. [59].

In a study by Zhou et al.[60], they conclude that the use of mobile phones is guided by age-dependent user requirementsand that older users had more difficulties than younger users to use multi-tap and touch and hold features.

Perrinet et al. [36], while studying different methods to input text using virtual keyboards in digital television applications, have detected significant differences in writing speed and error rates among age groups (not including children) even considering just expert users.

3.3 Applications

Regarding the evaluation of overall user performance and satisfaction using complete applications (i.e., with no specific focus on the platform or particular modalities, but on the graphical user interface), it is also important to approach users according to their characteristics and age related approaches have been proposed.

Website usability, considering the age factor, has been addressed by several authors. Punchoojit et al. [39] observed that age influenced the performance of users on different culturally oriented sites. Bergstrom et al. [46] used eye tracking while assessing the usability of websites, comparing young and older adults. They observed that older adults looked to the centre of the screen more frequently, looked to the peripheral left less frequently and took longer to look to the top periphery. Martens et al. [31] cover the design challenges and children's performance in using digital resources (review in Wirtz et al. [57]).

Game development and other applications, mostly for educational purposes, have also been addressed [51,33,34] advocating for participatory design and proposing methodologies to elicit contributions from children at different levels of the design and development cycle.

Studies have also focused on how individual elements in the graphical user interface can be modified to improve understandability to certain age groups (e.g., mobile device icons [26]) or performance in pointing and selection (e.g., target expansion [22]) and on how particular input modalities affect the way graphical user interfaces should be designed (e.g., touch [2]). Brajnik et al. [8] conclude that the inclusion of specialists (on-screen tutors) and tool tips does not have the same positive impact in older adults as in young adults probably due to the potential benefits of such design choices being out-weighted by the increasing complexity of the user interface felt by older adults.

3.4   Methodologies, Guidelines and Heuristics

Regarding children, the works by Read and colleagues have covered several aspects of child computer interaction and a recent review of the field can be found in [42].

Guha et al. [19] review the literature on Cooperative Inquiry and propose how this method can be used to support design with (and to) children by analysing a set of wrong assumptions concerning the work with children as design partners. Since children, nowadays, differ considerably from those of ten years ago given they are more independent and information active, the methods used must, therefore, consider such differences. The authors also emphasize, including examples taken from their experience, that adults working as proxies for children simply do not work as expected and methods have been proposed to tackle age-related issues (e.g., children's short attention spans [34,9]) or harder situations involving children with special needs (e.g., [17]).

Developing games involving children has been addressed, for example, by Tan et al. [51] and Moser et al. [33] by proposing methodologies that guide children's involvement along all the design and development cycle. Rounding et al., [47] discussed evaluation of user interfaces by children. Brown et al. [10] identify challenges of conducting usability studies, designed for adults with young children and found that issues like the smaller attention span of small children and the influence of the research setting (academic usability lab) need to be seriously considered in these cases.

Poole et al. [37,41] look into interface design for teenagers and provide a general description of notable cognitive/emotional and physical changes, assess the different challenges in research involving this age group and propose a set of best practices. Fitton et al. [16] point out that teenagers require a different approach than children or adults and that they might provide valuable insights regarding aspects for which younger children are too young and adults lack the technical skills. They gather a set of research questions concerning, for example, the methods used to engage teenagers in participatory design or which contexts (school, home, research lab) might be more appropriate to work with them.

Barros et al. [7] evaluate a mobile user interface for the elderly. Multiple evaluation stages are performed and a wide set of recommendations for inclusive design and design for older adults. In a similar approach, Ferreira et al [14] present a methodology using elderly centered design to support the development of a mobile application. Zhou et al. [59] and Liu et al. [28] present a literature review regarding the use of handheld computers by the elderly and provide a set of recommendations regarding input/output, menus, main required functions and applications.

Lynch et al. [30] discuss the importance of accounting for differences regarding elderly performance on websites and propose weighted heuristics to assess the usability of websites for this age group. Instead of putting all the heuristics at the same level the authors, based on input by older adults, proposed different weights for each, according to their importance, and managed to predict, based on the heuristics, differences in elderly performance for three websites.

4   Discussion

Considering the reviewed literature we identify several aspects deserving further attention from the HCI community and concerning age-related factors.

With the rapid technological advances, previous evaluation studies need to be reviewed — One very important aspect, as stressed by Hwangbo et al. [23], is that previous studies covering human performance for different input devices should be constantly reviewed since recent advances in technology might have considerable impact [6]. For example, extrapolating evaluation results gathered for mobile phones to smartphones is not straightforward as user requirements and expectations shift [60];

Lack of simultaneous assessment of performance for multiple age groups limits generalization of outcomes and comparison with other studies — Researchers often consider only specific age groups (e.g., children or adults) when assessing their performance using particular modalities or devices. This, although providing data for a particular scenario, only allows indirect comparisons between age groups. In fact, in most cases, even if the main purpose is to address the needs of a specific age-group, it is important to include additional groups in order to provide insight into which are the unique needs of the target group [27]. In an interesting article by Martens [31], the author points out that even the diversity among different age-stages, for children, should motivate duplication of previous studies to cover these intrinsic differences. Therefore, evaluation studies that assess performance for a wide range of ages would allow a greater insight into age differences and provide additional value to HCI;

Designing for adults and then adapting to another age-group can hinder more adequate solutions — One important aspect to consider is that it is still common that children and old adults are only involved in the design process at the time of the first prototypes. This, although valuable, works to modify an existing technology/approach, usually developed by adults, to cope with age related limitations instead of considering the broader context and a possible different approach to the problem from the start [58,40];

Ageing does not always translates to cognitive disadvantage — Contrary to what is common belief in HCI, Ball et al. [6] show evidence that older adults have some advantage in familiar tasks which depend on crystallized intelligence, i.e., skills learned over a lifetime and are outperformed by young adults when presented with unfamiliar tasks which profit from fluid intelligence (ability to deal with unknown situations). If these aspects are well understood, tasks can be designed to profit from them as previously highlighted.

Systematic multidisciplinary approach to understanding age-related characteristics and their impact is important — A systematic assessment of the physical and emotional characteristics of different age groups along with the challenges they pose to the individual and to HCI, and a collection of experimental results and best practices derived from the literature (in the line of what is proposed by Revelle [44], for children, and by Poole et al [37], for adolescents) might provide an important contribution to the HCI community.

Systems Used by Diverse Ages Should Aim for Coping with Diversity — Most works in the literature aim for approaches focused in particular age groups, rarely considering age diversity. It would be interesting to see works that gather efforts to develop devices, interaction patterns and user interfaces that can cope well with age diversity and the related challenge of intergenerational co-design (e.g., [58]). The effort of providing adaptive user interfaces is already performed, to some extent, in multimodal scenarios, to cope with different user limitations [] and might also be considered for age diversity.

Age estimation, e.g. [12], to the best of our knowledge, has not been used in the context of HCI design and might make it possible that, based on different user models, the interface could be age customized.

Research and evaluation methods must be adequate to the subjects ages and environment — The methodologies followed, for example, to elicit information from users, including them in the design process, should consider their physical and cognitive characteristics and account for the environments in which the systems will be used [42]. It is also important not to look into age groups with a set of preconceived ideas, but to actually test if these ideas have real impact considering the target users and context [20,55].

5 Conclusions

As mentioned, this paper does not aim to be a thorough survey of age-related aspects in HCI design, development and evaluation. Its purpose is to gather recent literature that spans what researchers are currently doing regarding age diversity. From the surveyed literature it is clear that several challenges still need to be tackled by the community or might provide clues for new research lines. Overall, age-related issues are being addressed for some age groups, but some of the research still relies on a preconceived idea of their characteristics, on adapting existing designs instead of building new ones, including users since design, and lacks methodologies that allow comparison among studies.

This article is just the first stage of what we consider should be a systematic approach to HCI for Age Diversity and many improvements to the presented work are possible (some of them not considered here due to a lack of space). For example, the surveyed works should gradually cover older publications and be organized according to a taxonomy that allows looking into the literature through different angles (age groups, devices, etc.).

Acknowledgements. Research partially funded by IEETA Research Unit funding FCOMP-01-0124-FEDER-022682 (FCT-PEst-C/EEI/UI0127/2011) and project Cloud Thinking (funded by the QREN Mais Centro program, ref. CENTRO-07-ST24-FEDER-002031).

References

1. Aman, F., Vacher, M., Rossato, S., Portet, F.: Speech recognition of aged voice in the aal context: Detection of distress sentences. In: 2013 7th Conference on Speech Technology and Human - Computer Dialogue (SpeD), pp. 1–8 (October 2013)

2. Anthony, L., Brown, Q., Tate, B., Nias, J., Brewer, R., Irwin, G.: Designing smarter touch-based interfaces for educational contexts. Personal and Ubiquitous Computing, 1–13 (2013)
3. Antle, A.N.: Exploring how children use their hands to think: an embodied interactional analysis. Behaviour & Information Technology 32(9), 938–954 (2013)
4. Arif, A.S., Sylla, C.: A comparative evaluation of touch and pen gestures for adult and child users. In: Proc.12th Int. Conf. on Interaction Design and Children, pp. 392–395. ACM, New York (2013)
5. Aziz, N.: Children's interaction with tablet applications: Gestures and interface design. Int. J. of Computer and Information Technology 2(3), 447–450 (2013)
6. Ball, R., Hourcade, J.P.: Rethinking reading for age from paper and computers. Int. J. of HCI 27(11), 1066–1082 (2011)
7. Barros, A.C., Ao, R.L., Ribeiro, J.: Design and evaluation of a mobile user interface for older adults: Navigation, interaction and visual design recommendations. In: Proc. DSAI (2013)
8. Brajnik, G., Giachin, C.: Using sketches and storyboards to assess impact of age difference in user experience. Int. J. of Human-Computer Studies (2013) (in press)
9. Brewer, R., Anthony, L., Brown, Q., Irwin, G., Nias, J., Tate, B.: Using gamification to motivate children to complete empirical studies in lab environments. In: Proc.12th Int. Conf. on Interaction Design and Children, pp. 388–391 (2013)
10. Brown, Q., Anthony, L., Brewer, R., Irwin, G., Tate, J.N.B.: Challenge of replicating empirical studies with children in hci. In: Proc. RepliCHI 2013 (2013)
11. Cheong, Y., Shehab, R.L., Ling, C.: Effects of age and psychomotor ability on kinematics of mouse-mediated aiming movement. Ergonomics 56(6), 1006–1020 (2013), pMID: 23586659
12. Choobeh, A.: An averaging technique for improving human age estimation algorithms. In: Proc. Communication Systems and Network Technologies (CSNT), pp. 868–870 (2013)
13. Culén, A., Bratteteig, T.: Touch-screens and elderly users: A perfect match? In: Proc. ACHI, pp. 460–465 (2013)
14. Ferreira, F., Almeida, N., Rosa, A.F., Oliveira, A., Pereira, J.C., Silva, S., Teixeira, A.J.S.: Elderly centered design for interaction — the case of the s4s medication assistant. In: Proc. DSAI (2013)
15. Findlater, L., Froehlich, J.E., Fattal, K., Wobbrock, J.O., Dastyar, T.: Age-related differences in performance with touchscreens compared to traditional mouse input. In: Proc. SIGCHI Conf. Human Factors in Comp. Systems, pp. 343–346 (2013)
16. Fitton, D., Read, J.C.C., Horton, M.: The challenge of working with teens as participants in interaction design. In: Proc. CHI 2013 EA Human Factors in Computing Systems, pp. 205–210. ACM, New York (2013)
17. Frauenberger, C., Good, J., Alcorn, A., Pain, H.: Conversing through and about technologies: Design critique as an opportunity to engage children with autism and broaden research(er) perspectives. Int. J. of CCI 1(2), 38–49 (2013)
18. Gregor, P., Newell, A.F., Zajicek, M.: Designing for dynamic diversity: Interfaces for older people. In: Proc. Fifth Int. ACM Conference on Assistive Technologies, pp. 151–156. ACM, New York (2002)
19. Guha, M.L., Druin, A., Fails, J.A.: Cooperative inquiry revisited: Reflections of the past and guidelines for the future of intergenerational co-design. Int. J. of CCI 1(1), 14–23 (2013)
20. Hanson, V.: Technology skill and age: what will be the same 20 years from now? Universal Access in the Information Society 10(4), 443–452 (2011)

21. Hertzum, M., Hornbaek, K.: How age affects pointing with mouse and touchpad: A comparison of young, adult, and elderly users. Int. J. of HCI 26(7), 703–734 (2010)
22. Hwang, F., Hollinworth, N., Williams, N.: Effects of target expansion on selection performance in older computer users. ACM Trans. Access. 5(1), 1:1–1:26 (2013)
23. Hwangbo, H., Yoon, S.H., Jin, B.S., Han, Y.S., Ji, Y.G.: A study of pointing performance of elderly users on smartphones. Int. J. of HCI 29(9), 604–618 (2013)
24. Jochems, N., Vetter, S., Schlick, C.: A comparative study of information input devices for aging computer users. Behaviour & Information Technology 32(9), 902–919 (2013)
25. Lane, A.E., Ziviani, J.M.: Factors influencing skilled use of the computer mouse by school-aged children. Computers & Education 55(3), 1112–1122 (2010)
26. Leung, R., McGrenere, J., Graf, P.: Age-related differences in the initial usability of mobile device icons. Behaviour & Information Technology 30(5), 629–642 (2011)
27. Leung, R., Tang, C., Haddad, S., Mcgrenere, J., Graf, P., Ingriany, V.: How older adults learn to use mobile devices: Survey and field investigations. ACM Trans. Access. 4(3), 11:1–11:33 (2012)
28. Liu, S., Joines, S.: Developing a framework of guiding interface design for older adults 56, 1967–1971 (2012)
29. Loureiro, B., Rodrigues, R.: Multi-touch as a natural user interface for elders: A survey. In: Proc. 6th Ib. Conf. on Inf. Sys. and Tech. (CISTI), pp. 1–6 (2011)
30. Lynch, K.R., Schwerha, D.J., Johanson, G.A.: Development of a weighted heuristic for website evaluation for older adults. Int. J. of HCI 29(6), 404–418 (2013)
31. Martens, M.: Issues of access and usability in designing digital resources for children. Library & Information Science Research 34(3), 159–168 (2012)
32. Meiselwitz, G., Wentz, B., Lazar, J.: Universal usability: Past, present and future. Foundations and Trends in Human-Computer Interaction 3(4), 213–333 (2010)
33. Moser, C.: Child-centered game development (ccgd): developing games with children at school. Personal and Ubiquitous Computing 17(8), 1647–1661 (2013)
34. Nicol, E., Hornecker, E.: Using children's drawings to elicit feedback on interactive museum prototypes. In: Proc.11th Int. Conf. on Interaction Design and Children, pp. 276–279. ACM, New York (2012)
35. Pérez-Marín, D., Pascual-Nieto, I.: An exploratory study on how children interact with pedagogic conversational agents. Behaviour & Information Technology 32(9), 955–964 (2013)
36. Perrinet, J., Pañeda, X.G., Cabrero, S., Melendi, D., García, R., García, V.: Evaluation of virtual keyboards for interactive digital television applications. Int. J. of HCI 27(8), 703–728 (2011)
37. Poole, E.S., Peyton, T.: Interaction design research with adolescents: methodological challenges and best practices. In: Proc.12th Int. Conf. on Interaction Design and Children, pp. 211–217. ACM, New York (2013)
38. Portet, F., Vacher, M., Golanski, C., Roux, C., Meillon, B.: Design and evaluation of a smart home voice interface for the elderly: Acceptability and objection aspects. Personal Ubiquitous Comput. 17(1), 127–144 (2013)
39. Punchoojit, L., Chintakovid, T.: Influence of age group differences on website cultural usability. In: Proc. 9th Int. Conf. ICT and Knowledge Eng., pp. 5–12 (2012)
40. Queirós, A., Cerqueira, M., Martins, A.I., Silva, A.G., Alvarelhão, J., Teixeira, A.J.S., Rocha, N.: Icf inspired personas to improve development for usability and accessibility in ambient assisted living. In: Proc. DSAI 2013 (2013)
41. Read, J.C.C., Horton, M., Iversen, O., Fitton, D., Little, L.: Methods of working with teenagers in interaction design. In: Proc. CHI 2013 EA Human Factors in Computing Systems, pp. 3243–3246. ACM, New York (2013)

42. Read, J., Markopoulos, P.: Child-computer interaction. Int. J. of CCI 1(1), 2–6 (2013)
43. Renaud, K., Blignaut, R., Venter, I.: Designing mobile phone interfaces for age diversity in south africa: "one-world"versus diverse "islands". In: Kotzé, P., Marsden, G., Lindgaard, G., Wesson, J., Winckler, M. (eds.) INTERACT 2013, Part III. LNCS, vol. 8119, pp. 1–17. Springer, Heidelberg (2013)
44. Revelle, G.: Applying developmental theory and research to the creation of educational games. New Directions for Child and Adolescent Development 2013(139), 31–40 (2013)
45. Élvio Rodrigues, Carreira, M., Gonçalves, D.: Developing a multimodal inferface for the elderly. In: Proc. DSAI (2013)
46. Romano Bergstrom, J.C., Olmsted-Hawala, E.L., Jans, M.E.: Age-related differences in eye tracking and usability performance: Website usability for older adults. Int. J. of HCI 29(8), 541–548 (2013)
47. Rounding, K., Tee, K., Wu, X., Guo, C., Tse, E.: Evaluating interfaces with children. Personal and Ubiquitous Computing 17(8), 1663–1666 (2013)
48. Santrock, J.W.: Life-Span Development. Mc-Graw Hill (2011)
49. Steinberg, L.: Cognitive and affective development in adolescence. Trends in Cognitive Sciences 9(2), 69–74 (2005)
50. Stoessel, C.: Gestural Interfaces for the Elderly Users: Help or Hindrance? Ph.D. thesis, Technischen Universität Berlin (2012)
51. Tan, J.L., Goh, D.H.L., Ang, R.P., Huan, V.S.: Child-centered interaction in the design of a game for social skills intervention. Comput. Entertain. 9(1), 2:1–2:17 (2011)
52. Teixeira, A.J.S., Pereira, C., e Silva, M.O., Alvarelhão, J., Silva, A., Cerqueira, M., Martins, A.I., Pacheco, O., Almeida, N., Oliveira, C., Costa, R., Neves, A.J.R., Queirós, A., Rocha, N.: New Telerehabilitation Services for the Elderly. In: Handbook of Research on ICTs for Healthcare and Social Services: Developments and Applications, pp. 109–132. IGI Global (2012)
53. Vipperla, R., Renals, S., Frankel, J.: Ageing voices: the effect of changes in voice parameters on asr performance. EURASIP J. Audio Speech Music Process. 2010, 1–10 (2010)
54. Wagner, N., Hassanein, K., Head, M.: Computer use by older adults: A multidisciplinary review. Computers in Human Behavior 26(5), 870–882 (2010)
55. Wandke, H., Sengpiel, M., Sönksen, M.: Myths about older people's use of information and communication technology. Gerontology 58, 564–570 (2012)
56. Weiss, B., Möller, S., Schulz, M.: Modality preferences of different user groups. In: Proc. ACHI, pp. 354–359 (2012)
57. Wirtz, S., Jakobs, E.M., M., Z.: Age-specific usability issues of software interfaces. In: Proc. 17th World Concress on Ergonomics (2009)
58. Xie, B., Druin, A., Fails, J., Massey, S., Golub, E., Franckel, S., Schneider, K.: Connecting generations: developing co-design methods for older adults and children. Behaviour & Information Technology 31(4), 413–423 (2012)
59. Zhou, J., Rau, P.L.P., Salvendy, G.: Use and design of handheld computers for older adults: A review and appraisal. Int. J. of HCI 28(12), 799–826 (2012)
60. Zhou, J., Rau, P.L., Salvendy, G.: Age-related difference in the use of mobile phones. Universal Access in the Information Society, 1–13 (2013)

Personalized Hand Pose and Gesture Recognition System for the Elderly

Mahsa Teimourikia, Hassan Saidinejad, Sara Comai, and Fabio Salice

Department of Electronics, Information and Bioengineering
Politecnico di Milano
via Ponzio 34/5, 22100, Milan, Italy

Abstract. Elderly population is growing all over the globe. Novel human-computer interaction systems and techniques are required to fill the gap between elderly reduced physical and cognitive capabilities and the smooth usage of technological artefacts densely populating our environments. Gesture-based interfaces are potentially more natural, intuitive, and direct. In this paper, we propose a personalized hand pose and gesture recognition system (called HANDY) supporting personalized gestures and we report the results of two experiments with both younger and older participants. Our results show that by sufficiently training our system we can get similar accuracies for both younger and older users. This means that our gesture recognition system can accommodate the limitations of an ageing-hand even in presence of hand issues like arthritis or hand tremor.

Keywords: gestural interaction, gesture recognition system, elderly.

1 Introduction

According to demographic studies, elderly population is growing all over the globe. This demographic shift is a by-product of lower fertility and better health conditions leading to lower mortality among older persons. The number of older persons aged 60 or over is projected to be 2 billion in 2050, three times the number in 2000, comprising 22 percent of the world population [1]. It is believed that population ageing will have significant socio-economic consequences for which a preparation is needed [2]. The WHO Active Ageing framework [3] considers health, safety, independence, mobility, and participation as the five higher level needs of the older persons for a higher quality of life. The important role ICT can play in this context is widely recognized [4]. For instance, AAL (Ambient Assisted Living) is a joint European project focused on the usage of ICT to help older persons in ageing well and is supported by the biggest EU Research and Innovation program, Horizon 2020.

For the realization of the inclusive society of future in which age and capability related discriminations are lifted and the older persons have the same opportunities as others, "Design for All" plays a central role. It concerns the design of products, services, and applications with accessible and adaptable interfaces for

C. Stephanidis and M. Antona (Eds.): UAHCI/HCII 2014, Part III, LNCS 8515, pp. 191–202, 2014.
© Springer International Publishing Switzerland 2014

special users like the elderly [4]. As far as the interfaces are concerned, novel human-computer interaction systems and techniques are required to fill the gap between elderly reduced physical and cognitive capabilities and the smooth usage of technological artefacts increasingly populating their environment.

Gesture-based interfaces have been around for several years and are considered to be potentially more natural, creative, and intuitive [5]. Gesticulations could be done with different body parts. [6] states that the hand is the most effective part of the body for communication through gestures. [7] supports this idea by analysing the gesturing literature and finding that hand-based gestures are at the top. [8] lists a set of requirements for effective hand-gesture interfaces which indicate two major research challenges: one concerns technical issues on the machine side to guarantee responsiveness, recognition accuracy, gesture spotting, etc; the other concerns interaction design issues on the human side like the gesture vocabulary size, learnability, comfort, etc.

Gesture-based interaction design is even more challenging for elderly people mainly due to their reduced physical and cognitive capabilities. Effects of ageing on sensory modalities, perception, cognition, and movement control are described in [9]. One of the challenges of hand gesture-based interfaces for the elderly lies in confronting the impacts of ageing on the hand. Research and studies in geriatrics suggest that for elderly people, both men and women, degenerative changes in musculoskeletal, vascular, and nervous systems lead to hand function degradation in terms of handgrip and finger-pinch strength, maintaining pinch force and posture, and dexterity of manual movements [10]. Other challenges include hand tremor which concerns involuntary shaking of the hand, and joint pains due to arthritis. These restrictions in hand functionality could impede an effective interaction with the interface. However, despite these age-related issues, studies like [11], comparing younger and older participants, suggest that age is not an exclusion factor for gestural interaction. We think that personalization could make gestural interaction more accessible and adaptable to some age-related issues, especially for an ageing hand.

In this work, we propose a vision-based hand gesture recognition system leveraging intuitive and natural poses and gestures of the hand that can be personalized. This system (called HANDY) is flexible enough to be trained (with a small number of trainings) for a variety of hand poses and gestures that meet the user's specific needs. In order to evaluate the system, we conducted two experiments: the first one on younger adults and the second one on older adults. We measured recognition accuracy of the system in both cases and qualitatively evaluated the difficulty of hand pose creation and gesture performance. Our results show that by sufficiently training our system we can get similar accuracies for both younger and older users. This means that our gesture recognition system can accommodate the limitations of an ageing-hand even in presence of hand issues like arthritis or hand tremor.

The following parts of the paper are structured as follows. In Sect. 2 we briefly review the work which has been done in the areas of gesture recognition systems, gesture interaction design, and gesture interaction and its applications for the elderly. Section 3 introduces the different parts of our gesture recognition system (HANDY). Section 4 is devoted to the description of our two experiments on younger and older adults. The results of the evaluation are discussed in Sect. 5. Finally, in Sect. 6, we present our conclusions and our future research path.

2   Background and Related Work

2.1   Hand Gesture Recognition Systems

Gesture recognition methods fall into two broad categories: wearable-based and vision-based [12]. Data glove is an example of a wearable sensor (e.g., [13]) which can provide accurate measurements of hand pose and movements. However, wearable sensors are commonly costly and intrusive. Vision-based techniques can be divided into two broad approaches [14]: model-based approaches that take advantage of a 3D or 2D model of the hand and appearance-based approaches which are used to extract the features of the visual data for gesture recognition. Model-based approaches usually suffer from high complexity in implementation and cannot be used in live applications. Appearance-based approaches use RGB or depth data or both as input. Our framework falls into this category. In our system, we will take advantage of the body tracking information extractable from Kinect SDK, so that depth thresholding (to locate and segment the hand) can be done regardless of the position of the hand.

Zhu and Pun [15] use Kinect depth data for extracting the trajectory data sequence of the hand movements, but, do not consider hand postures. In a similar way, [16] and [17] introduce a gesture recognition approach that considers the motion and shape information of the hand using depth data. However, the hand shape is considered to remain the same during the gesturing and pose estimation is done once at the beginning of the gesture. In another study by Chen et al. [18] HMM continuous gesture recognition is proposed considering the spatial and temporal features of the gestures. Yet, a small number of poses is recognized in this approach and the posture of the hand does not change while performing the gesture. HMM has been adopted also in the work by Starner et al. [19] for American Sign Language (ASL) recognition. To recognize the sign language they have ignored the detailed shape and pose of the hand and have only considered, coarse hand pose, orientation, and the trajectory of the gesture through time, and used such information as input for the recognition system. In a more recent work, Molina et al. [20] proposed an approach for static pose estimation and dynamic gesture recognition. They successfully recognized the gestures that include the change in the hand postures. They obtained an accuracy of 90% for recognition of combination of static hand postures and dynamic gestures.

Differently from these approaches, we consider hand poses and gestures composed of their combinations: hand poses are modeled by their skeleton, and time series analysis algorithms and HMM techniques are used to recognize sequences of hand poses. Using these techniques also personalized gestures can be defined and more flexibility can be added in case of gesture evolution.

2.2   Gestural Interaction for the Elderly

In general, gestural interaction was recognized as an important form of communication already in early studies (e.g., [21]). There has been a lot of research studying 3D spatial hand gestures. For instance, [22] studies freehand pose-based gestural interaction for novice users. [23] conducts a user study to understand users' preferences to manipulate digital content on a distant screen. Gestures represent an important aspect towards Natural User Interfaces. However, according to [24] even if gestures represent a useful addition in the interaction, many gestures are neither natural nor easy to learn or remember. Also [25] believes that the currently available systems are not natural, since they require to learn predefined artificial gestures, typically depending on the device or the application. This makes specific users like elderly reluctant to approach such applications.

As for the elderly, the very first question to face with is whether gestural interaction is even suitable for them taking into account their age-related sensory, motor, and cognitive impairments. In [11], authors describe the results of their devised experiment in which they compare the performance of younger and older participants in terms of accuracy and speed for a set of 42 one finger touch gestures. Their findings show a significant impact of the age only on the speed and not on the accuracy of the performance. And thus, they conclude that there is not anything intrinsic to gestural interaction which prevents the elderly from using it. They mention some motor problems from the literature which could be potential barriers for gestural interaction for older users: reduced wrist flextion and extension, less efficient perceptual feedback system, not having enough force for quick movements, having more submovements, and problems in performing continuous movements and movement coordination.

There are different application domains that could benefit from gestural interfaces. Gesture-based interfaces in smart homes for elderly with mobility impairment is one of the applications. Authors of [26] present an implemented gesture-based interface for elderly people for communication with an assistive robot in the context of a smart house. Defining six word signs (defined based on baby signs), using a monitor-mounted webcam, colored gloves, and Hidden Markov Models for gesture recognition, they claim to reach a recognition accuracy of 94.33%. Exergame is another potential application of gestural interaction for elderly that mainly focuses on physical well-being and rehabilitation. In [27], authors have developed two mobile games for the elderly using 3D gestural interaction for rehabiliation purposes. They concluded that gesture recognizer performance in terms of spotting quick gestures and ignoring unintended ones plays an important role in usability measures. Moreover, they consider familiarity and naturalness as two factors important in engaging older users in mobile gestural games. In another study [28], authors present the results and findings of two studies concerning gesture set design for a full-body motion-based game for institutionalized elderly people. They argue that user specific abilities are usually ignored by game designers. So, considering physical limitations, intuitiveness of the gestures, and learning easiness, they suggest a gesture set comprised of

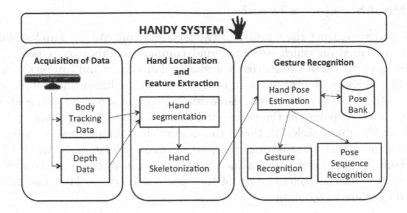

Fig. 1. The HANDY Gesture Recognition System

four static and four dynamic gestures. Discussing the results, they conclude that adaptability of the interaction is essential because of the heterogeneous participant abilities, either physical or cognitive. Finally, gestural interaction could be used in multimodal interfaces, especially those involving speech and gesture. In [29], authors describe a user study concerning speech and gesture interaction. The study takes place in an ambient assisted living lab with an intelligent wheelchair for assisted mobility and smart furniture for device control.

Our work is independent from the applications: it focusses on the possibility of personalizing the gestures taking into account also the characteristics of the hands of the elderly.

3   The Handy System

Figure 1 depicts the architecture of the HANDY system for hand gesture recognition. The description of the different parts of the architecture follows. A more detailed explanation of our gesture recognition system is presented in [30].

3.1   Hand Localization and Segmentation

This part of the system is responsible for locating the position of the hand and tracking it through time. RGB and depth information are extracted from Kinect sensors to locate and track the hand. NiTE skeletal tracking is used which gives the position of the wrist and the center of the hand. This information is used to perform hand segmentation with depth thresholding. Depth thresholding is an easy and quick way for real-time hand segmentation and it can be greatly beneficial for separating the hand from the background to exclude the effects of cluttered or dynamic backgrounds.

3.2 Hand Skeleton as Feature

In this part we extract the features of the located hand. We use hand skeletons as features based on which we define and compare different hand poses. The skeleton is a graph that summarizes the shape of an object and can be employed as an efficient shape descriptor for object recognition and image analysis. In order to obtain the skeleton of the hand, the Voronoi Diagram algorithm [31] is applied on the boundary points of the segmented hand, followed by a pruning process to extract the main skeleton. Using this approach, defining new postures can be as easy as saving a snapshot of the posture into the system. In the HANDY framework, the user can perform the custom poses in front of the Kinect and the system saves the skeleton data of the specified poses for later use in hand pose and gesture recognition.

3.3 Hand Pose Estimation

Extracted features of the hand are analyzed in this part to estimate the hand pose. Hand pose estimation refers to the recognition of a single posture of the hand. Hand poses are defined based on their corresponding skeletons. In the proposed approach, each user is initially required to make a pose bank consisting of a series of reference hand poses which are used later for pose estimation based on a similarity measure. Dynamic Time Warping [32], an algorithm for comparing time series, is used for the similarity estimation of two skeletons. Skeleton points are ordered as DTW applies on mono-dimensional time series. Moreover, for a fair comparison, the skeletons are normalized to be transition and scale insensitive.

3.4 Gesture Recognition

The aim of this part of the system is to analyze the sequence of the hand pose features to recognize the performed gesture. The HANDY system is able to recognize generic (dynamic) gestures. Each gesture is represented by a sequence of hand poses defined in our hand pose bank. A gesture gets sampled during its performance and each sample frame is analysed and the hand pose is extracted and mapped to the closest hand pose in the pose bank using our pose estimation method. Due to the stochastic nature of gesture performance by the users, we adopted Hidden Markov Models (HMMs) to represent each gesture. It is worth noting that misrecognition of an intermediate hand pose and assignment of the closest hand pose from the bank is tolerated by the gesture recognition mechanism thanks to HMMs. Using HMMs for gesture recognition, training is needed before the system be able to recognize the gestures. In practice, the recognition system encodes a user gesture into a sequence of hand poses and calculates the probability that the sequence belongs to one of the trained gestures. The trained gesture which obtains the highest probability is chosen as the performed gesture.

4   Methodology

We conducted two studies to evaluate our gesture recognition system regarding its effectiveness for older users. The rest of this section is dedicated to the explanation of these two studies.

4.1   Experiment 1: Younger Participants

Seven younger subjects without any hand problems participated in the first study (average age=29, SD=6.3). The study took place in our lab environment. At the beginning a brief explanation of the system was given along with the necessary instructions on its use. The participants were guided to record 21 static hand poses in order to build up the hand pose bank and then train the system with a set of five more generic gestures. The participants were asked to perform 20 trainings for each gesture followed by 30 test gestures in order to evaluate the recognition accuracy. Gestures had a fixed length of 1 second, and were sampled 10 times during their performance. Figure 2 depicts a generic hand pose bank created by a participant. Five generic gestures are illustrated in Fig. 3. The hand poses in the pose bank and the gestures were designed by the authors. Gestures contain key point poses in their performance which belong to the hand pose bank. In [30], we have explained in detail the technical aspects concerning the number and choice of hand poses in the pose bank as well as for the gestures. Finally, participants were asked to comment on the difficulty of hand pose shaping and gesture performance.

The recognition accuracy of the system was evaluated under two scenarios: 1) the system is trained and used by a single participant; 2) the system is trained by other participants and then used by another participant, so the training data of the whole set of participants is used for the gesture recognition.

4.2   Experiment 2: Older Participants

In the second study, 10 elderly people volunteered to participate (7 females, average age=68.5, SD=4.45). In the first part, they were asked to carry on a lighter version of the same test which had been done on younger subjects in order to evaluate how age affects the recognition accuracy of the system. Among

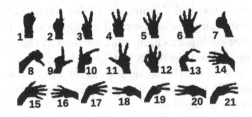

Fig. 2. Hand pose bank consisting of 21 static hand poses

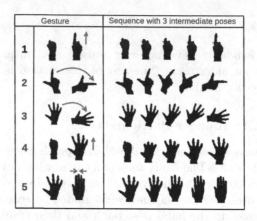

Fig. 3. Five gestures younger participants were asked to perform

the older participants we had one case of arthritis, one case of hand deformity, and one case of hand tremor. Like in the previous experiment, after explaining the purpose and potential applications of such gestural interaction system and providing the participants with required instructions on how to shape hand poses and how to perform gestures, they were asked to register 21 hand poses to create the pose bank, and then perform a set of 3 gestures instead of five with lower training sets. This was done to lessen the physical burden. In some cases, particularly hand deformity and arthritis, the final hand pose bank contained a reduced number of reference hand poses (minimum = 13). The recognition accuracy of the system was evaluated just for the scenario where the system is used by single person. In case of hand tremor, the participant was asked to keep the pose for a certain amount of time (1 second in our tests) and more than 1 sample was taken from the hand pose (10 in our case). From these 10 samples, the most repeated hand pose was considered as the estimated hand pose. Using Hidden Markov Models was another alternative to tackle hand tremor: sampling the hand poses in 1 second and considering the hand pose as a gesture.

5   Results and Discussion

5.1   Experiment 1: Younger Participants

As mentioned before, a total of 7 younger adults participated and completed the test. No significant change was observed in the results. Table 1 summarises the obtained results for each participant and for each of the gestures (previously depicted in Fig. 3) in the first scenario in which the system is trained and used by a single user as well as for the second scenario where the system is trained by other participants and used by a new participants. Participants P6 and P7 were asked to use their left hands.

For the second scenario (S2) only the training sets of the 5 participants that used their right hand were considered. In average, slightly less accurate results were obtained in scenario 2 (S2:96%) with respect to scenario 1 (S1:97%). This suggests that with external training data for some universal gestures, initial training is not needed. Participants were asked to rank the gestures based on their difficulty. Gestures involving difficult hand manoeuvres like wrist rotation (gestures 2 and 3, see Fig. 3) were commented to be the most difficult ones.

Table 1. Recognition Accuracy (%) for Experiment 1 - Younger Participants

	Gesture1		Gesture2		Gesture3		Gesture4		Gesture5	
	S1	S2	S1	S2	S1	S2	S1	S2	S1	S2
P1	100	100	90	90	100	100	96.6	100	100	93.3
P2	100	100	100	100	100	100	100	96.6	100	100
P3	100	100	100	100	96.7	100	96.6	86.6	100	96.6
P4	90	100	100	96.6	100	93.3	100	80	100	90
P5	83.3	96.6	100	93.3	100	93.3	76.6	100	96.6	100
P6	86.6	-	80	-	100	-	100	-	100	-
P7	96.6	-	100	-	100	-	96.6	-	93.3	-

5.2   Experiment 2: Older Participants

For the second study on older participants, 10 older persons volunteered to participate but only 6 of them completed the test (for reasons which will be mentioned). One of the participants was left-handed and thus performed the gestures with his/her left hand. Each test was done in one session. Most of the tests were done in an institute for elderly education (run by elderly themselves) and a few of them in our lab environment. Each test started with a general friendly talk describing the system and its potential applications setting a smooth start for the rest of the test. At the beginning, elderly participants were asked to specify their preferred interaction modality with technological artefacts and what applications they could think of using hand gestures. Five (out of 10) chose voice as their preferred interaction modality. They argued that this modality is easier to use and more natural. Three participants preferred traditional (keyboard, mouse) interaction modality. Having already learned how to use it, satisfaction of current small needs, and its tangibility and physical interaction were among the mentioned reasons. Finally, one participant chose touch interaction and one participant the gestural interaction. It is worth mentioning though that only this last participant was aware of potential applications of gestures having known TV sets controllable by hand gestures. When asked if they come up with any ideas for an application using hand gestures, most of them had a difficult time fantasizing one. A participant suggested it as a way to facilitate difficult manipulative tasks (like a door handle requiring much force to be turned). Another one mentioned mobility problems of the elderly and usage of gestures to issue commands from a fixed position.

In the next stage, we asked the participant to register the hand poses to create the pose bank. Required instructions were given orally; they needed to wave to draw the attention of the hand tracking mechanism and then keep the hand stable for a couple of seconds. Some participants (including the participant suffering from arthritis) mentioned that some hand poses were uncomfortable (specifically poses 4,20,21,15,17,19, see Fig. 2). The participants with hand deformity (suffering from Dupuytrens contractur) could perform only poses involving the first three fingers: if it would be possible to choose the input modality, he definitely prefers voice communication. He was not forced to go on with the test.

Afterwards, older participants were asked to complete a reduced version of the same gesture performance test done by younger participants. The number of gestures was reduced to 3 (gestures 1,2, and 5, see Fig. 3). Furthermore, rather than 50 training and test performances for each gesture, they were asked to do only 25 performances for training and test. The fatigue caused by the complete test had become evident in a mini pilot test. However, even with a lower number of required performances, three participants left the experiment at this point. We think this happened not only because of fatigue due to gesture performance but also because of lack of motivation. So, a more cheerful training phase through a game and/or having several test sessions could be beneficial. For the participant with hand tremor, the part of the system handling tremor was activated.

An average gesture recognition accuracy of 80% was achieved (compared to 90% range for younger participants). The main factor responsible for the lower recognition accuracy is less training numbers for elderly participants. Indeed, if we decrease the training number for younger participants, accuracy drops into the 80% range (similar to elderly results). Online training (training when the system is in use) could compensate for the lower numbers of training at the beginning. It is important to note that although hand problems like arthritis might lead to less accurate hand pose estimations but using HMMs diminishes these less accurate estimates at gesture performance level.

6   Conclusions and Future Work

In this work we proposed a vision-based hand gesture recognition system which is able to estimate user hand poses based on a personalized hand pose bank. Moreover our system is able to recognize generic hand gestures represented as stochastic sequences of hand poses modeled by HMMs. Furthermore, we conducted two experiments to investigate the potential benefits of our system for elderly people.

Our results show that our system is flexible enough to accommodate some of the physical limitations elderly people suffer from, mainly limitations related to an ageing hand, like hand tremor and arthritis. This was achievable in our system mainly thanks to personalizable hand poses and hand gestures. Thus, we think personalizability is an important ingredient of an effective gestural interaction system especially for users with specific needs.

There is still a lot to do to fill the gap between the technical requirements and human factors requirements for an effective, natural and inclusive gestural interaction system especially for specific users like the elderly. A gesture recognition system with high potentiality for personalization (flexible gesture definition with no or minimal decrease of accuracy) could be a suitable solution. The strength of personalization lies in the fact that it is a natural (and sometimes unconscious) way to adjust the gestural interaction to one's physical -and even cognitive- capabilities. This requires further investigation and is what we plan to examine in the future: evaluating the potential benefits of personalization on gestural interaction for specific target users like the elderly.

Acknowledgements. We would like to kindly thank Marina Peduzzi and Guido Tosatto for helping us organizing meetings and sessions with our elderly participants. We also deeply thank Auser Università Popolare Como for its collaboration with us.

References

1. UN: Department of economic and social affairs (desa) world population ageing 2009. DESA, United Nations, New York (2009)
2. UN: Review and appraisal of the progress made in achieving the goals and objectives of the programme of action of the international conference on population and development, 1999 report. United Nations publication, Sales No. E.99.XIII.16 (1999)
3. Kalache, A., Gatti, A.: Active ageing: a policy framework. Advances in gerontology= Uspekhi gerontologii/Rossiiskaia akademiia nauk. Gerontologicheskoe Obshchestvo 11, 7–18 (2002)
4. Malanowski, N., Ozcivelek, R., Cabrera, M.: Active ageing and independent living services: the role of information and communication technology. European Communitiy (2008)
5. Rautaray, S.S., Agrawal, A.: Vision based hand gesture recognition for human computer interaction: a survey. Artificial Intelligence Review, 1–54 (2012)
6. Erol, A., Bebis, G., Nicolescu, M., Boyle, R.D., Twombly, X.: Vision-based hand pose estimation: A review. Computer Vision and Image Understanding 108(1), 52–73 (2007)
7. Karam, M.: PhD Thesis: A framework for research and design of gesture-based human-computer interactions. PhD thesis, University of Southampton (2006)
8. Wachs, J.P., Kölsch, M., Stern, H., Edan, Y.: Vision-based hand-gesture applications. Communications of the ACM 54(2), 60–71 (2011)
9. Fisk, A.D., Rogers, W.A., Charness, N., Czaja, S.J., Sharit, J.: Designing for older adults: Principles and creative human factors approaches. CRC press (2012)
10. Ranganathan, V.K., Siemionow, V., Sahgal, V., Yue, G.H.: Effects of aging on hand function. Journal of the American Geriatrics Society 49(11), 1478–1484 (2001)
11. Stößel, C., Wandke, H., Blessing, L.: Gestural interfaces for elderly users: help or hindrance? In: Kopp, S., Wachsmuth, I. (eds.) GW 2009. LNCS, vol. 5934, pp. 269–280. Springer, Heidelberg (2010)
12. Murthy, G., Jadon, R.: A review of vision based hand gestures recognition. International Journal of Information Technology and Knowledge Management 2(2), 405–410 (2009)
13. Camastra, F., De Felice, D.: LVQ-based hand gesture recognition using a data glove. In: Apolloni, B., Bassis, S., Esposito, A., Morabito, F.C. (eds.) Neural Nets and Surroundings. Smart Innovation, Systems and Technologies, vol. 19, pp. 159–168. Springer, Heidelberg (2013)

14. Garg, P., Aggarwal, N., Sofat, S.: Vision based hand gesture recognition. World Academy of Science, Engineering and Technology 49(1), 972–977 (2009)
15. Zhu, H.M., Pun, C.M.: Real-time hand gesture recognition from depth image sequences. In: 9th Int. Conf. Computer Graphics, Imaging and Visualization (2012)
16. Liu, X., Fujimura, K.: Hand gesture recognition using depth data. In: Proceedings of the Sixth IEEE International Conference on Automatic Face and Gesture Recognition, pp. 529–534. IEEE (2004)
17. Binh, N.D., Shuichi, E., Ejima, T.: Real-time hand tracking and gesture recognition system. In: Proc. GVIP, pp. 19–21 (2005)
18. Chen, F.S., Fu, C.M., Huang, C.L.: Hand gesture recognition using a real-time tracking method and hidden markov models. Image and Vision Computing 21(8), 745–758 (2003)
19. Starner, T., Weaver, J., Pentland, A.: Real-time american sign language recognition using desk and wearable computer based video. IEEE Trans. on Pattern Analysis and Machine Intelligence 20(12), 1371–1375 (1998)
20. Molina, J., et al.: Real-time user independent hand gesture recognition from time-of-flight camera video using static and dynamic models. Machine Vision and Applications 24(1), 187–204 (2013)
21. Baudel, T., Beaudouin-Lafon, M.: Charade: Remote control of objects using free-hand gestures. Commun. ACM 36(7), 28–35 (1993)
22. Freeman, D., Vennelakanti, R., Madhvanath, S.: Freehand pose-based gestural interaction: Studies and implications for interface design. In: IHCI, pp. 1–6 (2012)
23. Lee, S.S., Chae, J., Kim, H., Lim, Y.K., Lee, K.P.: Towards more natural digital content manipulation via user freehand gestural interaction in a living room. In: Proc. UbiComp 2013, pp. 617–626 (2013)
24. Norman, D.A.: Natural user interfaces are not natural. Interactions 17(3), 6–10 (2010)
25. Malizia, A., Bellucci, A.: The artificiality of natural user interfaces. Commun. ACM 55(3), 36–38 (2012)
26. Lee, T.-Y., Kim, H.-H., Park, K.-H.: Gesture-based interface using baby signs for the elderly and people with mobility impairment in a smart house environment. In: Lee, Y., Bien, Z.Z., Mokhtari, M., Kim, J.T., Park, M., Kim, J., Lee, H., Khalil, I. (eds.) ICOST 2010. LNCS, vol. 6159, pp. 234–237. Springer, Heidelberg (2010)
27. Sunwoo, J., Yuen, W., Lutteroth, C., Wünsche, B.: Mobile games for elderly healthcare. In: Proceedings of the 11th International Conference of the NZ Chapter of the ACM Special Interest Group on Human-Computer Interaction, pp. 73–76. ACM (2010)
28. Gerling, K., Livingston, I., Nacke, L., Mandryk, R.: Full-body motion-based game interaction for older adults. In: Proceedings of the 2012 ACM Annual Conference on Human Factors in Computing Systems, pp. 1873–1882. ACM (2012)
29. Anastasiou, D., Jian, C., Zhekova, D.: Speech and gesture interaction in an ambient assisted living lab. In: Proceedings of the 1st Workshop on Speech and Multimodal Interaction in Assistive Environments, pp. 18–27. Association for Computational Linguistics (2012)
30. Teimourikia, M., Saidinejad, H., Comai, S.: Handy: A configurable gesture recognition system. In: 7th Int. Conf. on ACHI (2014) (accepted for publication)
31. Aurenhammer, F.: Voronoi diagrams: A survey of a fundamental geometric data structure. ACM Computing Surveys (CSUR) 23(3), 345–405 (1991)
32. Berndt, D.J., Clifford, J.: Using dynamic time warping to find patterns in time series. In: KDD Workshop, Seattle, WA, vol. 10, pp. 359–370 (1994)

Easy Handheld Training: Interactive Self-learning App for Elderly Smartphone Novices

Yosuke Toyota[1], Daisuke Sato[2], Tsuneo Kato[1], and Hironobu Takagi[2]

[1] KDDI R&D Laboratories, Inc., 2-1-15 Ohara, Fujimino, Saitama, 356-8502 Japan
{yo-toyota,tkato}@kddilabs.jp
[2] IBM Research - Tokyo, 5-6-52 Toyosu, Koto-ku, Tokyo, 135-8511 Japan
{dsato,takagih}@jp.ibm.com

Abstract. Smartphones have great potential for elderly people to enrich their lives. Elderly people, however, hesitate to use smartphones compared to younger people due to several factors such as anxieties about the difficulties of unfamiliar devices and the lack of daily assistance. Moreover, a conventional research reported that elderly IT novices struggled with basic operations in the first stage. Hence, we tried to find the common issues faced by the elderly with no previous smartphone experience and then created an interactive self-learning application (app) of the basic smartphone operations. Our demonstration app was designed to give "hands-on" experience by using integrated real videos. Results of usability testing showed that the subjects easily learned by themselves how to operate the smartphones without background information. The subjective evaluation results showed that the app engaged the interest of the subjects and also gave them confidence about acquiring operational skills by themselves.

Keywords: Interactive self-learning app, real videos, elderly people, user interfaces, smartphones.

1   Introduction

Smartphones such as Android phones and iPhone have great potential for elderly people by helping them to maintain their independence and enrich their quality of life (QoL) [1]. Smartphones improve their lives by not only providing the means of daily communication, but also giving strong support to health care, providing an intelligent navigation service, giving access to knowledge resources, and connecting them to valuable online services. However, it is difficult for many elderly people who are information technology (IT) novices to use IT devices like feature phones, smartphones and PCs. We use the term "feature phone" as the mobile phone, typically having a phone number pad, other than the smartphone here after. The elderly people have barriers that prevent them from trying smartphones out as reported by other studies. Some of these barriers are the fear of failure and anxieties about the difficulty of learning the various functions [1], [2]. Weilenmann et al. [3] described another barrier

C. Stephanidis and M. Antona (Eds.): UAHCI/HCII 2014, Part III, LNCS 8515, pp. 203–214, 2014.
© Springer International Publishing Switzerland 2014

facing elderly IT novices in the case of texting using feature phones. They reported that elderly feature phone novices have problems related to mundane and seemingly simple skills such as pressing the keys. This finding is not different from what we found in our observational survey in the case of the basic smartphone operations. We know from interviews with experienced lecturers of smartphone classes for elderly people and the participants in their classes that elderly people with no previous smartphone experience struggle with basic operations such as tapping a touchscreen, even though they have experience of using feature phones and PCs. All of these barriers make them hesitate to use IT devices. While young people often have helpful friends or coworkers who support their daily use and web searches for more information, many of the elderly people do not have such supporters and resources [1], [4], [5]. Therefore, we need new elderly friendly ways to overcome these barriers.

In this paper, a video-based interactive self-learning app is proposed for use by elderly IT novices. We want to offer a way of self-learning smartphone operations with apps that run on the smartphones. Another objective is to find a new learning method and a way to increase enthusiasm for learning how to use smartphones. To address these objectives, we conducted an observational survey and interviews. Based on the findings from these survey and interviews, a prototype app was designed. The app was used for user testing with the elderly. We also evaluated the comprehensibility of the instructions delivered by our video-training app. Our research design is shown in Figure 1.

This paper first reviews related work. The detailed design began based on user observations, and its effectiveness was verified by a pilot study and a primary study. Finally, the results of our research are discussed leading to our conclusions and future works.

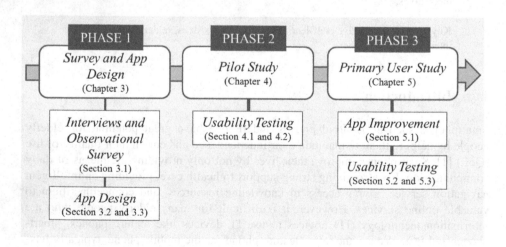

Fig. 1. Research Design

2   Related Work

Many studies have tried to assist IT novices, including elderly people, in making use of IT devices such as PCs, feature phones and smartphones. For the purpose of assistance, two strategies have been studied. Customizable user interfaces (UIs) have been proposed in order to provide user-friendly UIs for IT devices [6], [7], [8]. Olwal et al. [6] provided a customizable UI on feature phones and smartphones. Automatic personalization of the UI for PCs was also proposed (e.g. [7], [8]). Although such customizable UIs are able to simplify complex interfaces, the IT novices need a way of learning the basic operation of such devices.

Another strategy is a learning method for IT devices. Several investigations have focused on self-learning methods. They allow people to learn how to use the devices regardless of having helpful friends or coworkers who support their daily use. However, it is required easy-to-understand explanations and instructions for IT novices (e.g., avoiding technical jargon and complicated explanations). Hence, graphical tutorials using images and videos were studied for elderly IT novices [1], [9], [10]. Digmayer et al. [9] evaluated a video tutorial of a specific web site for troubleshooting. They reported that graphical tutorials were more effective than textual tutorials for the elderly. The same result was reported by Spannagel et al. [11]. However, their software did not offer "how-to" information. Struve et al. [10] evaluated effectiveness of a training method using video. Their research focused on a ticket vending machine. They reported that training methods for other software and system were their future work even though their findings were useful for future studies.   Leung et al. [1] developed a prototype named "Help Kiosk". Their prototype was able to support elderly people with interactive software on a PC to enable them to learn how to do tasks on smartphones. They tested two tasks, "adding a contact" and "setting an alarm", by using it. It is difficult for elderly IT novices to use their prototype because the knowledge about the basic operations of PCs and smartphones are required. It is not able to support with learning of basic operations that are tough tasks for them [3].

3   First Prototype of Interactive Self-learning App for Elderly Smartphone Novices

3.1   Survey on Behavior of Elderly People in Smartphone Classes

In order to find a better way of providing learning support to elderly smartphone novices, we conducted interviews and observed smartphone classes for elderly smartphone novices. This approach was based on two hypotheses: 1) Experienced lecturers' methods are available for app design. 2) We are able to obtain information about elderly people's barriers related to the first step in learning basic smartphone operations by observing participants practicing these operations in classes. First, we interviewed experienced lecturers of smartphone classes. Second, we made observations during their lectures and conducted interviews with class participants. The purpose of the latter approach is to confirm details of the issues revealed by the interviews with the lecturers and get new information useful in a consideration of learning methods for our app. The results of these interviews and observations were utilized in the design of our app.

The following two issues, (a) and (b), came to light as a result of the interviews with the lecturers. These were confirmed in the observational survey of their classes and interviews with class participants. Moreover, the issue, (c), and three other findings, (d), (e) and (f), were revealed as a result of the class observation:

- Issues revealed by our interviews and observation:

  (a) Elderly smartphone novices often press the screen too strongly or for too long. As a result, touch sensors in the screen misrecognize their action as a long tap.
  (b) Elderly people with no previous smartphone experience are confused by the sudden screen blackout caused by the auto sleep function. They mistakenly believe that the blackout indicates the phone battery is flat or a device fault has occurred.
  (c) Elderly people with no previous smartphone experiences cannot figure out what to do when they see the lock screen before they learn what it is and how to unlock it. They do not know what action to take when they see an icon with an arrow or a padlock.

- Findings from our observation:

  (d) It is not difficult for elderly people to master basic operations and how to use basic applications if lecturers coach them carefully. The most important factors are mimicking lecturers' examples about gestures and receiving prompt feedback from lecturers on operational errors made when using smartphones.
  (e) Elderly smartphone novices enjoy practicing the common touch screen gestures on smartphones such as dragging, flicking, and pinching in/out. They seem to feel that they are in control of their smartphones when learning and doing such gestures are seen as a first step.
  (f) Playing game apps with simple rules entertains elderly people. Multimedia feedback entertains them and is a clear guide to right or wrong action. They enjoyed playing with the apps used in the classes even during breaks.

3.2   Features of Our First Prototype

To address the common issues faced by participants in the smartphone classes listed in the previous section, we selected two sets of tasks for practice using our app. The first is a set which includes tapping, how to resume from sleep mode and unlocking the lock screen. These tasks were selected to address the issues (a), (b), and (c) shown in the previous section. The other is a set of basic map operations. We selected these actions because map apps are some of the most popular smartphone app and required the commonly used touch panel gestures of dragging, flicking, and pinching in/out related to the finding (e) shown in the previous section. Hence, elderly people are able to learn not only how to use a major smartphone app but also how to use typical gestures according to the situation such as confirming details of particular locations and checking the route to their destination over a large area.

After the tasks for our app were selected, we designed the first prototype app for elderly smartphone novices based on the findings (d) and (f) described in the previous section and the guidelines from other studies (guidelines for designing training programs [12], and multimedia instructional programs for elderly people [13], [14]). Our app was designed to have the following features:

- Features related to the guidelines:

- Our app presents "how-to" information in a procedural step-by-step format.
- Images and colored shapes are used for graphical tutorials. Colored shapes, such as circles and ellipses, show the points where fingers need to be placed or the end points of the operations of dragging and pinching. Arrows denote the directions of the path from start points to end points of the operations. Animations and real videos were used to explain how to operate the smartphone.
- The shapes described above are deformed dynamically depending on user operation in order to provide feedback. This feedback indicates whether or not the operations were executed correctly. The app changes color to show completion of the operation.
- Each step of the operation is explained in considerable detail without using technical terms so that people with no previous smartphone experience are able to understand the video tutorials naturally and easily. In addition, we chose appropriate font sizes and colors taking the characteristics of elderly people into consideration [12].

- Features related to the findings in the survey:

- Opportunities for "hands-on" experience are provided immediately after instructions are given on the app. These steps were devised to achieve the same effect as mimicking the lecturers' gestures in the actual smartphone classes.
- In accordance with the guidelines, our app provides real-time feedback. The app plays sound effects that indicate whether the user operations are correct or not. We selected game-like sound effects for feedback. When users perform an incorrect operation, messages pop up on the app explaining the correct operation. Users are made aware of their mistakes and get information on correct operation instantly.

The guidelines [12] indicate that graphics are sometimes better than actual pictures (e.g., photograph and real video) as they provide better cues and less clutter. It depends on the elderly knowledge and learning experiences of the individual person. Hence, we used both graphics and real video to ascertain which was the more effective in a range of scenarios.

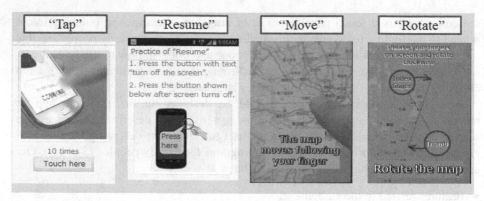

Fig. 2. Screen shots of instructions of our app ("Tap", "Resume", "Move", and "Rotate")

3.3   Implementation of Our First Prototype

Six tasks for training basic smartphone operations or map operations were implemented as follows. (Four screen shots related to the implemented function are shown in Figure 2.):

— *Tap: How to do a short tap on the screen.* A video tutorial (auto replay) and a button with the text "Press here for a short time" are displayed on the screen. If the button was pressed too long, the app displays the pop-up text, "Press it for a slightly shorter time".
— *Resume: How to turn the screen on from sleep mode.* Explanatory text and a static image are used to explain the operation for waking up the phone from sleep mode. In addition, a software button for sleep is placed under the instructions.
— *Unlock: How to unlock the lock screen.* A slider button is located below a video tutorial (auto replay) on the screen.
— *Move: How to move the map.* Two colored circles show start and end points of dragging on the map. An arrow and text shows the direction of dragging and descriptions of how to operate, respectively.
— Zoom in/out: How to scale the map by pinching with two fingers.
— *Rotate: How to rotate the map clockwise/anticlockwise.* Two colored circles show the start points of pinching or dragging using two fingers. Arrows and text were used in the same way as in the other map tutorial.

4   Pilot Study

4.1   Experimental Design

Our first prototype was implemented on a Samsung Galaxy S III with a 4.8-inch 1280x720 HD screen. We conducted one-on-one usability testing in a laboratory setting as shown in Figure 3. Ten elderly people aged 61-76 years (mean 67.6, SD 4.63) with no previous smartphone experience were recruited. They were retired workers from an IT company. They were all paid for participating in the experiment. The experiment duration was around 2 hours for each subject, including interviews using a paper-and-pencil questionnaire and a semi-structured interview. A camera recorded all operations on the smartphone. We conducted questionnaires using a 5-point Likert scale to ascertain subjects' impressions of smartphones and the usability of our prototype. The experiment began with an explanation on the purpose of our study and how the experiment would be conducted. The subjects answered the questions about their sensory perception and cognition related to the results of the experiment. In addition they answered questions on their use of feature phones if they had one. We conducted a semi-structured interview before they used our prototype app. They performed the app tasks without receiving any explanation on smartphones or our app. Tasks were given to them in order of increasing difficulty (e.g., tasks using dragging and flicking were given after the tasks that required tapping, tasks using two-finger gestures were given after tasks using one-finger gestures). The subjects performed all the tasks by themselves without our support. They answered the questionnaire about the difficulty of tasks in two parts. The first part was after finishing basic operational tasks on the smartphones, and the second part related to tasks involving the operation of our map app. Moreover, we received their subjective feedback about our app and smartphones through their answers to a questionnaire administered after they had finished all tasks.

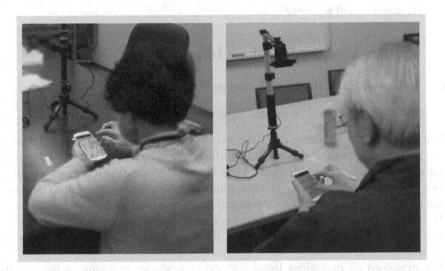

Fig. 3. The one-on-one usability testing in a laboratory setting

4.2   Experimental Results

The tutorial on tapping was subjectively evaluated as easy by all subjects with a median rating of 1.5 on a scale from 1 (very easy) to 5 (very difficult). Half of the subjects commented that the practice sessions for tapping were very boring. On the other hand, instructions about how to resume and how to rotate the map were hard to understand. The median scores were 4.0 (disagree) on a 5-point scale to the question, "The explanations are comprehensible." We found that 6 out of 10 started training before completion the video tutorials, which were displayed on the same screen with a button or a slider.

The major findings from the pilot study were as follows:

(a) It was difficult for the subjects to give their attention to both the video and the button or the slider at the same time. We displayed the video tutorial and buttons on the same screen; the subjects who gave attention to the button did not notice the video. A few subjects said "Was a video played on the same screen?". They knew that something was on the screen with the button; however, they did not recognize it as the video due to lack of attention.

(b) Real videos were better than graphics for these subjects. It was difficult for them to understand instructions, especially operations that required several steps, using a graphic and text; on the other hand, they commented "I am able to easily understand the real video which shows a demonstrator doing basic operations on the smartphone and using the map app. I preferred using the same smartphone as the one shown in the video for learning." and "It was difficult for me to learn operations with several steps when the instructions were provided via graphics and text only".

5   Primary User Study with an Improved App

5.1   Improvement on the First Prototype

We improved our app based on the results of the pilot study:

— We displayed the button or the slider below the video player after completion of the first playback of the video tutorial to focus the subjects' attention on the video tutorial. In addition, we added verbal and visual information that draws their attention to the video. Verbal explanations about the operation were added to the video data. This also compensates for the situation where visual information in the video is overlooked. We highlighted the button or the slider using colored frame borders and pop-up messages to shift attention from the video tutorial to the button or slider.
— We explained all operations using real video as shown in Figure 4 because the subjects commented that real video was easy to comprehend.
— The procedures for "Resume" include a few important parts. These parts were explained step-by-step in the video. To avoid overlooking these parts, we emphasized important scenes in the video using freeze-frame shots with colored shapes and text.
— We added training on long taps in order to make elderly people understand the difference between short taps and long taps in terms of the time duration their finger should be placed on the screen.

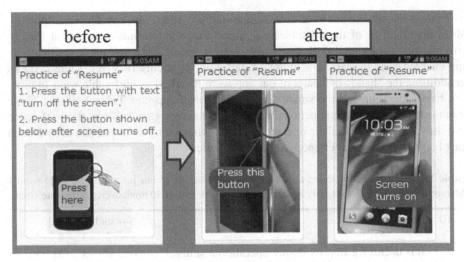

Fig. 4. Screen shots of our video tutorials about "resume" before and after improvement

5.2   Study Setup

We conducted usability testing with 40 subjects belonging to four different groups of elderly people (8 were alumni of an IT company, 22 were from human resource centers for elderly people, and the others were recruited by an online research firm). All subjects had no previous smartphone experience. Fifteen out of 40 had no experience using smartphones and feature phones. Twenty-three men and 17 women were 60-81 years (mean 70.6, SD 5.14). Other conditions were the same as those of the pilot study. The experimental procedure of the primary user study was same as that of the pilot study.

5.3   Experimental Results with Usability Improvement

As a result of improving the resume tutorial, the median score for the comprehensibility question, "The explanations are comprehensible", improved from 4.0 to 2.0 (p < 0.01) on a scale from 1 (strongly agree) to 5 (strongly disagree). The statistical differences in the questionnaire scores between the two studies were evaluated by the Mann-Whitney's U-test. In the "Resume" tutorial, the median score for the comprehensibility question improved from 4.0 to 2.0 (p < 0.01). According to the comparison between the scores for the question, "Further explanations are necessary", in the two studies, adding multimedia feedbacks (e.g., the speech instruction and colored shapes) helped the elderly to understand the operation of smartphones without overloading them with confusing information. The score improved from 2.0 to 4.0 (p < 0.01) on a scale from 1 (strongly agree) to 5 (strongly disagree). The median scores for difficulty about the tap practice in the two studies did not change significantly from 1.5 to 2.0 (1: very easy, 2: easy), although we added the practice of long taps and explanations about the differences between a short tap and a long tap.

Table 1 shows the answers to the questionnaire about our app and smartphones. More than 82.5 % of the 40 subjects reported that our tutorials were useful for improving their operational skills (see Table 1, ID 1 and 2). They felt that a self-learning app enabled them to learn how to use a smartphone by themselves (see Table 1, ID 2). In addition, the "hands-on" parts of our app were regarded as preferable ways to practice basic operations on the smartphone and the map app (see Table 1, ID 3). These results showed that our instructional video tutorials were gave subjects the confidence that they could improve their operational skills when using smartphones even though they had no previous experience with mobile devices.

Table 1. The number of selected answers about impressions of our tutorials on a scale from 1 (Strongly disagree) to 5 (Strongly agree). Several people out of 40 unanswered some questions.

ID	Questions	5-point Likert scale				
		1	2	3	4	5
1	It is useful for improving my operational skills	0	0	3	21	12
2	I had a feeling that I could make better use of a smartphone by doing more training on my own.	0	0	2	23	11
3	The "hands-on" parts of the app were useful for me.	0	0	0	22	13
4	It was delightful for me to try new things.	0	1	2	24	9
5	It would encourage me to buy a smartphone	0	3	5	19	8
6	I would like to use a smartphone more.	0	1	8	17	10
7	I had a feeling that I was able to take advantage of a smartphone.	0	5	8	19	4

Thirty-three out of 40 answered that they found trying new things to be enjoyable (see Table 1, ID 4). In this case, they learned what smartphones are and how to use them (basic operations and usage of the map app). Several subjects commented that "I feel like learning more about smartphones.", "I would like to go to a mobile phone shop to ask about smartphones." and "I feel like buying a smartphone before I go back home today". The effects on their interest in smartphones and buying motivation can be seen from the answers to our questionnaire (see Table 1, ID 5 and 6). Our tutorials reduced their fear of smartphones and anxieties about the learning difficulties for the various functions. The subjects who answered "neither agree nor disagree" or "disagree" to question ID 5 did not have an interests and/or needs. The subjects using feature phones do not like a lot of extra functions and prefer to keep it simple with function that allow them to make phone calls, and send mail and take photos. The subjects who did not use feature phones were interested in mobile phones. The subjects who answered "neither agree nor disagree" or "disagree" to question ID 6 worried about difficulties in relation to specific smartphone operations. These subjects made comments about them in the free description parts of our questionnaire such as "I could not get used to the operational feelings of the smartphone/touch screen.", "The operation of rotating the map was too difficult for me.", and "I failed to perform operations using two fingers". The subjects who answered "neither agree nor disagree" or "disagree" to question ID 7 made similar comments as in the case of question

ID 6. It is important for elderly people with no previous smartphone experience to learn how to operate smartphones using tasks that are not too difficult for them. In our studies, we gave the subjects tasks in order of increasing difficulty. However several subjects felt that some tasks were too difficult for them due to the variations in subjects' knowledge and experience about IT devices. This issue was solved by adding a method that allowed the degree of success for each task to be rechecked and retried where necessary. Moreover, a way to manage the level of difficulty of tasks and the pace of learning depending on their personal skills is useful.

6   Conclusions and Future Work

In this paper we have presented our interactive self-learning app for elderly smartphone novices. Our app was designed based on the findings of a survey on smartphone classes for elderly people and two experiments (pilot study with 10 people and primary study with 40 people). In the experiments, the elderly people with no previous smartphone experience were able to learn how to perform several basic smartphone operations and how to use a typical map app. A multimedia instructional program using real video comprising an instruction part and a "hands-on" practice part were shown to be effective for learning "how-to" information. We verified that our app not only raised the interest of the subjects in smartphones but also gave them the confidence that they acquire the needed skills to use smartphones. In the future, we will evaluate our app in field trials including elderly people with different IT backgrounds and interests.

References

1. Leung, R., Tang, C., Haddad, S., Mcgrenere, J., Graf, P., Ingriany, V.: How Older Adults Learn to Use Mobile Devices: Survey and Field Investigations. ACM Transactions on Accessible Computing (TACCESS) 4(3(11), 1–33 (2012)
2. Zajicek, M.: Interface Design for Older Adults. In: Proceedings of the 2001 EC/NSF Workshop on Universal Accessibility of Ubiquitous Computing: Providing for the Elderly (WUAUC 2001), pp. 60–65 (2001)
3. Weilenmann, A.: Learning to Text: An Interaction Analytic Study of How Seniors Learn to Enter Text on Mobile Phones. In: Proceedings of the SIGCHI Conference on Human Factors in Computing Systems (CHI 2010), New York, pp. 1135–1144 (2010)
4. Poole, E.S., Chetty, M., Morgan, T., Grinter, R.E., Edwards, W.K.: Computer Help at Home: Methods and Motivations for Informal Technical Support. In: Proceedings of the SIGCHI Conference on Human Factors in Computing Systems (CHI 2009), New York, pp. 739–748 (2009)
5. Kiesler, S., Zdaniuk, B., Lundmark, V., Kraut, R.: Troubles with the Internet: The Dynamics of Help at Home. Human-Computer Interaction 15(4), 323–351 (2000)
6. Olwal, A., Lachanas, D., Zacharouli, E.: OldGen: Mobile Phone Personalization for Older Adults. In: Proceedings of the SIGCHI Conference on Human Factors in Computing Systems (CHI 2011), pp. 3393–3396. ACM Press, New York (2011)

7. Liu, J., Wong, C.K., Hui, K.K.: An Adaptive User Interface Based on Personalized Learning. IEEE Intelligent Systems Archive 18(2), 52–57 (2003)
8. Weld, D.S., Anderson, C., Domingos, P., Etzioni, O., Gajos, K., Lau, T., Wolfman, S.: Automatically Personalizing User Interfaces. In: Proceedings of the 18th International Joint Conference on Artificial Intelligence (IJCAI 2003), California, pp. 1613–1619 (2003)
9. Digmayer, C., Jakobs, E.-M.: Help Features in Community-Based Open Innovation Contests. Multimodal video tutorials for the elderly. In: Proceedings of the 30th ACM International Conference on Design of Communication (SIGDOC 2012), pp. 79–88. ACM Press, New York (2012)
10. Struve, D., Wandke, H.: Video Modeling for Training Older Adults to Use New Technologies. ACM Transactions on Accessible Computing (TACCESS) 2(1(4), 1–24 (2009)
11. Spannagel, C., Girwidz, R., Löthe, H., Zendler, A., Schroeder, U.: Animated Demonstrations and Training Wheels Interfaces in a Complex Learning Environment. Interacting with Computers 20(1), 97–111 (2008)
12. Fisk, A.D., Rogers, A.R., Charness, N., Czaja, S.J., Sharit, J.: Designing for Older Adults - Principles and Creative Human Factors Approaches. CRC Press, Boca Raton (2004)
13. Mayer, R.E., Moreno, R.: Nine ways to reduce cognitive load in multimedia learning. Educational Psychologist 38(1), 43–52 (2003)
14. Moreno, R.: Learning in high-tech and multimedia environments. Current Directions in Psychological Science 15(2), 63–67 (2006)

Health and Rehabilitation Applications

On Clinical, Philosophical, Ethical and Behavioural Concepts for Personalised *Insilico* Medicine Supporting "Co-production of Health"

Niels Boye

Klinisk Informatik, Aarhus, Denmark
niels.boye@kliniskinformatik.dk

Abstract. Telemedical technology is constructed with the purpose of *compensating distance* in delivery of healthcare provisions within institutional frameworks utilizing supply-side-driven service models and ICT to "organise the delivery of healthcare". The aim of this paper is to outline "a framework of understanding" (clinical, philosophical, and ethical concepts) that uses technology to deliver personalised *insilico* medicine for use in daily demand-driven "Coproduction of Health" - and hence, *take advantage of distance* from healthcare resources and make health management of a chronic medical condition inclusive and pervasive in society; however, still founded in evidence-based medicine including use of computer-supported behavioural science models to "organise the consumption of health". Personalised *insilico* supported "Coproduction of Health" encompasses the five levers of change compiled by the high level eHealth2020 task force of the EU - #1: My data, my decisions, #2: Liberate the data, #3: Connect up everything, #4: Revolutionise health, and #5: Include everyone. The framework uses the WHO definition of health and the concept of "health capital" and introduces the "Digital Health Continuum" from 100% citizen to 100% patient and the associated ranges of "professional healthcare delivery" and "co-produced health management"- thus fusing and augmenting current supply-side driven service models with an ICT-supported and demand-side driven service model. *Insilico* personalised medicine implemented through the Coproduction of Health service-model is to be seen as a paradigmatic example of mobilizing - for the individual - all available health resources within social hubs empowered by design of innovative and collaborative frameworks to align otherwise conflicting, silo-shaped, and scattered interests.

Keywords: health, wellbeing, evidence-based medicine, telemedicine, prevention, non-communicable chronic diseases, NCDs, information and communication technology.

1 Introduction

Information and Communication Technology (ICT) for use in telemedicine has been designed to compensate for distance of a patient to institutional based healthcare.

C. Stephanidis and M. Antona (Eds.): UAHCI/HCII 2014, Part III, LNCS 8515, pp. 217–227, 2014.
© Springer International Publishing Switzerland 2014

The innovations gained in this context have been of incremental type and introduction and first implementations of such telemedical services have stimulated only minor secondary changes in organisation and business models within the healthcare sector. Seen in a societal perspective, it has been difficult to obtain reasonable cost-benefit ratios in large scale demonstrators of telemedical services when evaluated using gained Quality of Life indicators [1].

"Co-production of health" (CpH) is a coherent, compatible, complementary, augmenting, and demand-driven service-model in relation to conventional healthcare service models, where ICT is used to take advantage of distance from institutional healthcare for an active citizen with a health problem by creation of cross-sectional and -organisational ecosystems – which including also healthcare based resources. In CpH ICT is used to communicate, implement, and render operative evidence-based-medicine in societal settings and in the daily context of the individual citizen. The Co-production of Health service-model can only be real in an advanced, ubiquitous ICT-infrastructure able to recruit and exploit conventional and unconventional resources for health management.

Establishment of "integrated care" in Europe has been easier said than done probably due to the tradition in how healthcare is organised. CpH can however offer a platform for:

- Using knowledge as a tool of coordinating cross-organisational formal and informal care meaning "evidence-based, personalised, *coordinated* care and *insilico* medicine" - the European way of "integrated care".
- Support an extended corporate-social-responsibility of e.g. the food and beverage sector, meaning that commodities in the future will be sold with digital information transmitted in a format that allows for further electronic processing in relation to context and health of an individual person.
- Make knowledge on health and prevention of non-communicable chronic diseases pervasive in society.
- Support business-models based on knowledge-share principles.

This paper will not deal with the above macro-organisational issues of CpH, but describes an amalgamated, descriptive ontology for Co-production of Health with the aim of contributing to the overall framework of future design and implementation of ICT for Health and Wellbeing.

2   Materials and Methods

2.1   Creating a Framework for Understanding Health in the Context of CpH

The starting point of this work was taken in World Health Organisations definition of health from 1948, which has been unchanged since: "*Health is a state of complete physical, mental and social well-being and not merely the absence of disease or infirmity*" [2]. This definition can be criticized for not being operative and for the use of the word "*complete*" in relation to three non-independent criteria: "*physical, mental and social wellbeing*". However, if instead perceived as a vision or a theoretical goal for efforts in relation to gaining personal "health capital"[3], the definition becomes rather operative. The term "health capital" was introduced in 1972 by Michael Grossman, who aimed at constructing an economic model for the commodity "good health" and the related stock of "health capital" using a "shadow price" principle that depends on many other variables besides the price of medical care. This was the introduction of welfare economics that later was continued by among others by the Nobel Prize laureate Amatya Sen [4]. Both Grossman and Sen view citizens as both consumers and producers of health and verify theoretically that the commodity "good health" has conceptual distinctions from other goods, which should be taken into account when building service models, value creation models and the associated business models.

2.2   Advancement in the Framework of Understanding:

The FP-7 Support action project PREVE (FP7-ICT-2009.5.1- #248197) was a series of workshops on: "Directions for ICT Research in Disease Prevention" with selected experts receiving pre-workshop materials prepared by the project consortium[1]. The project-results are summarized and published in a Whitepaper [5] and serves as a part of the advancements in the framework of understanding of health reported in this paper. The behavioural aspects are based on a mutual US-EU funded workshop: "International Workshop on "New Computationally-Enabled Theoretical Models to Support Health Behavior Change and Maintenance" October 16-17, 2012 in Brussels, Belgium" [6].

3   Results

Figure 1 depicts on the horizontal axis the conceptual development in ICT in the last decades, where the technology has matured from being expert-operated, corporate-centred, discrete systems to now a day's also include individual user-centred, layman-controlled, pervasive ICT-infostructures. On the vertical axis is depicted the conceptual development in medicine from the patient as a "passive patient object" receiving care to being proactive in gaining health capital. The combined development in the two domains - health and ICT - enables the new models and concepts reported in this paper.

---

[1] Consortium and core-persons in PREVE: VTT Finland – Niilo Saranummi (coordinator); San Raphaelle Hospital, Milan, Italy - Alberto Sana; UPV, Valencia, Spain – Vicente Trevor, M Teresa Meneu Barreira, Aarhus University - Niels Boye.

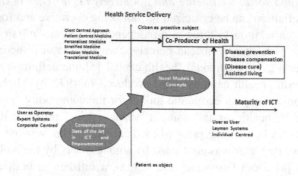

Fig. 1. Disruptive innovation towards Co-production of Health is enabled by multi-axial incremental innovations

The supply side service-model of conventional healthcare has a number of components. Figure 2 depicts these supply-side model-components in relation to an arbitrary "Digital Health Continuum (DHC)" from 100% citizen to 100% patient. The provisions are divided in a professional range and in a co-production range.

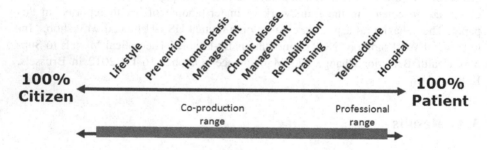

Fig. 2. The Digital Health Continuum fuses supply-side service models (Lifestyle -> Hospital) into two demand-side service models: Co-production of Health and Healthcare professional range

The PREVE project surveyed the biomedical literature in relation to clinical impact of self-care in relation to the eight most significant and lifestyle modulated.

Non-communicable Chronic Diseases (NCDs). During the discussions in the expert-groups a descriptive matrix from The Danish Council for Prevention was modified and compiled into the so-called Danish Matrix Reloaded depicted on figure 3:

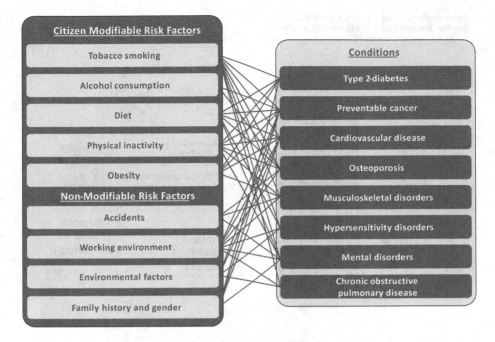

Fig. 3. The Danish Matrix Reloaded (see text for details)

Our original figure is interactive and the "evidence connections" of impact of specific self-care can be shown from single risk factors (citizen view) or from single health conditions (healthcare view); furthermore they can be combined in multiple risk factors (lifestyle view) or multiple conditions (comorbidity view). "Family history and gender" is a placeholder for genetic information.

"Personal medicine" is a vision originating in the idea of "tailor-made" drugs for the single individual. Due to regulatory and safety perspectives, it will be a vision that is difficult to accomplish for a foreseeable future. Other expressions which implies that "one size *does not* fit all" in medicine are "stratified medicine" and "precision medicine". Medical evidence is not directly based on information on individual health-trajectories, but on knowledge gained by scientific methods as depicted in figure 4 (in the left side of the figure). These statistical-based clinical and epidemiological methods imply a grouping of the participants in the trial. This grouping is defined by inclusion and exclusion criteria for participation in a trial. The highest grade of medical evidence is achieved, if a number of well-conducted trials with similar grouping by meta-analysis show matching results. In the professional conducted clinical process personalisation in relation to the single patient is done utilizing the statistically derived evidence-base containing a "non-existing average patient" with a relevant condition. The evidence is broad into action for the individual patient in the context of the single individual (right side of the figure 4) and hence tailored to that individuals' particular health problems.

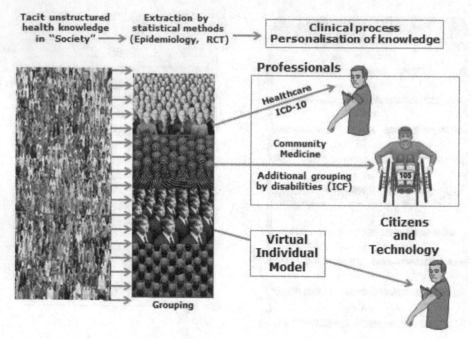

Fig. 4. The process of building health knowledge for evidence based medicine (left part of figure) and the process of personalizing this evidence in the clinical process (right side of figure) by healthcare professionals and by technology (virtual individual model), citizens (and professionals) in co-production of health

In co-production of health a similar mechanism is to be built using computational power and a Virtual Individual Model (VIM) that can personalise and contextualize the knowledge.

Figure 5 displays the societal boundary conditions of the Virtual Individual Model - that functions as an *insilico* digital avatar of the single individual. Choice architecture describes the way in which decisions may (and can) be influenced by how the choices are presented in order to influence the outcome [7]. Hence, the Virtual Individual Model provides personal preferences parameterization of an advanced "recommendation engine" where computational power will survey data on options, choice- possibilities and -architectures and fuse these with data from advanced sensors and furthermore, relate the information thus created to health knowledge in real time. The model with the *insilico* digital avatar in the centre is an example of "emphatic ICT-systems" that assist in bridging the gap between behavioural science theories and practical living with a chronic non-communicable disease [8].

The ethics governing our healthcare in Europe are directs descendants of the abstract principles in the Hippocratic oath with three main components: autonomy, justice and beneficence ("do good") - or at least non-malfeasance ("do no harm") - in relation to the patient [9]. These abstract ethical principles are also in force in

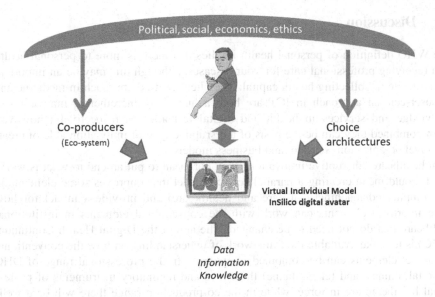

Fig. 5. Co-production of health is using technology to make health management demand-driven, pervasive, and inclusive in society by supporting cross-sectional ecosystems able to recruit unconventional resources and provide personalized recommendations in context

co-production of health but the implementation is slightly different from contemporary healthcare as discussed below.

Table 1 gives a comparison of some characteristics of the two complementary methods for building health capital.

Table 1. High Level Characteristics of Healthcare and Coproduction of Health

Health care	Coproduction of health
Patient	Citizen
Provisions	"Good health commodities"
Reactive to disease	Proactive in relation to health
Empowerment	Responsibility and Response-ability
Closed data repositories	Open data, "big data-technologies"
Document oriented	Model driven
Classifications	System biology framework
Sector	Eco-system
Regulated marked	Open, mature marked
Institutional ethics	Universal ethics

4   Discussion

The WHO definition of personal health implies that there is more to personal health than receiving professional care for your diseases, although this may be an important pre-requisite in collecting health capital. The client-centred approach in medicine and the user-centred approach in ICT are both achieved by incremental innovation in knowledge and services in health and digital technologies respectively; however, when combined they can be the basis of a disruptive type of innovation able of creating novel organisation- service- and business models.

In healthcare "disruptive innovation" may not mean to put an end to what is working. It could mean creating a parallel service-model that improves some elements in the complicated machinery of care and health(care) and provide a model for how these improved elements can work with the conventional elements in institutional healthcare that do not need to be changed. The aim of the Digital Health Continuum (DHC) is to make available the framework of understanding on how the conventional and novel elements can be combined in synergy. In the professional range of DHC (hospital, clinics, and telemedicine) the ethics and regulatory instruments of professional healthcare are in force, while in the co-production range there will be a well-defined mixed responsibility and response ability between professional and lay-men resources operated on a common knowledge base.

The high-level eHealth2020 taskforce of the EU has compiled five levers for change of healthcare using Information and Communication Technology (ICT) [10]: #1 My data, my decisions, #2: Liberate the data, #3: Connect up everything, #4: Revolutionise health, and #5: Include everyone. Co-production of health is a containment of these levers and has abilities to "package" them into a coherent method or a service-model compatible with the current service-models of healthcare e.g. lifestyle management augmenting primary, secondary, and tertiary prevention of non-communicable chronic diseases. Since healthcare has a daily and very efficient, well-organised production to look after, the lever "#4 Revolutionise health" should not be perceived as making profound changes current healthcare operation, but the knowledge and data contained in healthcare should be liberated and communicated in an agreed electronic format with the aim of "organising the individuals consumption of health" with the use of behavioural science models.

The Danish Matrix Reloaded should in the context of this paper be seen qualitatively. Based on already existing medical evidence there are self-care opportunities that can be personalised according to condition, disease state of condition, and identifiable risk factors. Hence, a personal "mix" of self-, informal-, and professional-care including the use of an individualised mix of pharmaceuticals and doses are within reach as a full functioning substitute for "personalised medicine". Personalised-, stratified-, or precision-medicine requires that current and future health-knowledge can be meticulous and detailed activated. This will on the other hand demand a finer granulation in computing methods and in grouping of data in more dimensions than usual in clinical medicine. These additional dimensions must include biomarker mark-up and other molecular medicine annotations [11]. A biomarker is anything that can be used (and measured) as an indicator of a disease, a disease state, or a physiological state.

In the early stages of a chronic disease the trajectory and outcome is very suscepti- ble to life-style management - performed in synergy with conventional treatment - since the disease process is not gone to near completion and to a clinical overt state with irreversible lesions, where only supportive therapy is possible. The advances in molecular medicine enabling the utilisation of biomarkers for early diagnosis and interception of chronic diseases will therefore prompt for alternative trajectory types to conventional institutional healthcare using ICT for pervasive knowledge handling in eco-systems, and taking advantage of distance to healthcare institutions. A positive psychology focus mainly on health and obtaining the "the good life" despite an NCD could be a side-effect of CpH.

In the industrial society "knowledge was power". Nowadays knowledge is in princi- ple a shared resource, but often in bits and pieces and without the proper (individual) context and some of these pieces are furthermore of inferior quality. The "power" in the knowledge-society lies in the ability to fuse, filter, relate, and operationalise knowledge, whether it is derived from the internet or from scientific information ob- tained by scientific methods based on grouping and statistics, which can be considered distant to "personalised medicine". The Virtual Individual Model will have the purpose of combining, filtering, and relating information, and hence upgrade information to individual knowledge that can be operationalised with an impact on personal health in the WHO definitions scope; hence tailoring of the general knowledge to specific knowledge in context of the individual. The division of the Digital Health Continuum in complementary professional- and co-production range is important in relation to this. Citizen in need for healthcare should not be deprived from professional attention by a technological solution; the professional health resources will however create more impact, if in-context, personalised knowledge in "professional grade" is at hand for the citizen wishing a good and healthy life despite a chronic disease.

A prerequisite for the development of emphatic systems for personal health is an algorithmic, model-driven approach to data handling. Taking the GPS-navigation system based software and hardware as an example on a model-driven "micro- decision support system". You have the analogue problem of getting from A to B. This is converted to a digital representation of the problem and the possible solution is calculated on the basis of digital description of the appropriate geography (options and choice architectures) and the digital result is converted to an analogue display (e.g. a map). There are challenges in this. The two conversions of analogue informa- tion to data and back after the calculation must be with high validity as also the digital representation of options and choice architectures. Since a Virtual Individual Model for Health will receive much more heterogeneous input data compared to what is coming out of a GPS-satellite also the data-foundations quality, quantity, and com- patibility are major challenges.

Since care was part of the Church's business-model centuries ago "care has been something that we give to each other in Europe" - in principle a societal task, that has been "tendered out" by to some extent different methods in the European countries. Complicated organisational and financial systems are built to ensure high professional standards, equal access to healthcare, an effective isolation of the patients from the true costs of healthcare, and a cost-effective operation of each link in the chain of a healthcare process. The abstract ethical principles originating in the Hippocratic Oath are in the healthcare systems given a tangible implementation dependent of social, cultural, technical and societal conditions. The present healthcare systems are designed to respond to acute diseases and embodies concepts of autonomy, informed consent, privacy, equal access etc. which reflect these particular systems, practices, and institutions. Autonomy is typically conceived of as *a right* to reject a treatment recommended by professionals, or in general as a right to free choice. Justice is understood as any citizens' *right* to equal access to services available within the health care system. In implementing of the five levers of the EU eHealth2020 taskforce one must be careful not to confuse the abstract principles with how these principles are currently implemented in healthcare, since such confusion may lead to cyclical argumentations. ICT can contribute to an expansion in the principles of autonomy and justice and in line with history make care coproduced in society in an open, deregulated - but mature and transparent - marked. Autonomy in CpH would be a right to manage your health and get the data that is needed for this (EU taskforce eHealth2020 lever 1). Justice would in CpH be different from the current implementation in distribution-ethics of standardised healthcare provisions and will also include the complementary right to personalised *insilico* medicine with own responsibility and response-ability. Persons who take advantage of this additional right are not violating the equal access principle in the healthcare sector for professional produced provisions, on the contrary - co-production is expected to free resources and create overall additional impact.

In essence CpH will for healthcare institutions and installations mean "core-business as usual", but complemented and augmented by "an outreach" to society employing evidence-based knowledge as the coordinating mechanism in health eco-systems. *Insilico* personalised medicine implemented in the Coproduction of Health service-model is seen as a paradigmatic example of mobilizing for the individual all available health resources in social hubs with design of innovative and collaborative frameworks to align otherwise conflicting, silo-shaped, and scattered interests.

Finally, on the societal level is lifestyle because of welfare is on the brink of threating the same welfare both in the Western and in the third world according to both OECD and WHO (see inset). Addressing

> **Diseases that break the bank**
> *"The worldwide increase of non-communicable diseases is a slow-motion disaster, ... These are the diseases that break the bank. Left unchecked, these diseases have the capacity to devour the benefits of economic gain. ... A recent World Economic Forum and Harvard University study estimates that, over the next 20 years, non-communicable diseases will cost the global economy more than US$ 30 trillion, representing 48 percent of global GDP in 2010. ... non-communicable diseases deliver a two-punch blow to development. They cause billions of dollars in losses of national income, and they push millions of people below the poverty line, each and every year."* (MARGARET CHAN, Director-General, WHO, addressing the UN General Assembly 2011)

prevention and retardation of impacts on lifestyle related disorders on all levels in society by employing an online, distributed problem-solving production model should therefore have high priority.

References

1. Henderson, C., Knapp, M., Fernández, J.-L., et al.: Cost effectiveness of telehealth for patients with long term conditions (Whole Systems Demonstrator telehealth questionnaire study): nested economic evaluation in a pragmatic, cluster randomised controlled trial. BMJ 346, 1035 (2013), doi:10.1136/bmj.f1035 (published March 22, 2013)
2. Preamble to the Constitution of the World Health Organization as adopted by the International Health Conference, New York, June 19-22 (1946), Signed on 22 July 1946 by the representatives of 61 States (Official Records of the World Health Organization, no. (2), p. 100) and entered into force on 7 April 1948
3. Grossman, M.: On the Concepts of Health Capital and the Demand for Health. Journal of Political Economy 80(2) (March-April 1972)
4. Sen, A.: Development as Freedom. Oxford University Press (1999) ISBN-13: 978-0-19-289330-7
5. http://preve-eu.org
6. http://www.behaviorchange.be
7. Johnson, E.J., Shu, S.B., Dellaert, B.G.C., Fox, C., Goldstein, D.G., Haeubl, G., Larrick, R.P., Payne, J.W., Schkade, D., Wansink, B., Weber, E.U.: Beyond nudges: Tools of a choice architecture. Marketing Letters 23, 487–504 (2013)
8. Nilsen, W.J., Pavel, M.: Moving Behavioral Theories into the 21st Century. IEEE Pulse, 25–28 (September/October 2013)
9. Beauchamp, T., Childress, J.: Principles of Biomedical Ethics, 6th edn. Oxford University Press (2009)
10. http://epractice.eu/en/library/5362646
11. Bousquet, J., Anto, J.M., Sterk, P.J., et al.: Systems medicine and integrated care to combat chronic non-communicable diseases. Genome Med. 3(7), 43 (2011)

Training and Learning in e-Health Using the Gamification Approach: The Trainer Interaction

Pierpaolo Di Bitonto, Nicola Corriero, Enrica Pesare,
Veronica Rossano, and Teresa Roselli

Department of Computer Science, University of Bari via Orabona, 4 – 70125 Bari - Italy
{veronica.rossano,teresa.roselli,enrica.pesare}@uniba.it,
{nicolacorriero,pierpaolodibitonto}@gmail.com

Abstract. One of the basic conditions to learn is motivation. Thus it is essential for learning environments to motivate the students to proceed into the learning process. Several researches propose the inclusion of new technological trends, such as the Gamification, to engage the users. In this paper the solution adopted in UBICARE system, where the Gamification approach has been used for training and learning purposes, is presented. The Gamification was used in the simulation of clinical cases aimed to both empower the patients to adopt healthy life-style and train the medical and paramedical staff about diagnostic procedures, therapeutic interventions and follow-up of patients. In particular, the paper presents the trainer interaction that is useful in order to keep the system up to date over time and to allow the definition of clinical cases tailored on the basis of users' needs.

Keywords: e-health, gamification, game based learning, learning by doing.

1   Introduction

The effectiveness of the learning by doing and the game based learning approaches has been largely documented in the literature [9, 15, 16, 17, 18]. In the latest years, the Gamification approach has revealed the value of game-based mechanics to create meaningful learning experiences in non-gaming contexts. "Gamification" is an informal umbrella term for the use of video game elements in non-gaming systems to improve user experience and user engagement. In other words, the Gamification can be defined as the use of game mechanics, dynamics, and frameworks to promote desired behaviours into domains like marketing, politics, health and fitness [1].

The mechanisms and dynamics of the game increase user's engagement and stimulate their active participation enhancing the learning outcomes. This is one of the crucial issues in e-learning: the learning experience will be more effective the more the participants will be involved and active in it and not merely passive users of a content.

In this perspective, the Gamification in learning processes can be a solution to achieve excellent training goals. Moreover, the use of gamification approach in e-learning environments addressed to e-health domain is not new. The entertainment

C. Stephanidis and M. Antona (Eds.): UAHCI/HCII 2014, Part III, LNCS 8515, pp. 228–237, 2014.

and fun that the game adds to the learning process is essential to engage the patients in learning how to manage and preserve their health status. This is particularly successful when the users are young, but it has been proved that also adults can be attracted to the games [10, 11, 12, 13, 14]. In *Pain Squad* [6], for example, the gamification approach is used to keep kids and teens with cancer engaged and motivated to complete their pain surveys twice a day. In *Septris* [7], instead, it is used to provide a practical approach to train medical and paramedical staff to manage daily activities of the patient, the therapy and the critical events.

In order to understand the role of gamification in education it is necessary to study in depth how the elements of the game can support the three dimensions of learning: cognitive, emotional and social [2, 8].

In the *cognitive area* the gamification can provide challenges perfectly tailored to the player's skills, in fact, the difficulty of the challenges increases as the skills of the player. Moreover, to propose specific problems and to encourage the students to set attainable sub goals for themselves that are proximal and specific are features that motivate the players. Those properties represent the basis of the game experiences and the gamification approach that are particularly useful to support students during the learning process.

In the *emotional area* the game involves a wide range of user's emotions: curiosity, frustration, and joy. The game often provides positive emotional experiences, and in case of negative ones, it encourages the players to use and transform them. One of the standard examples of negative emotional experience in a game is the defeat. Usually, the game implies repeated failures and often the only way to learn how to play is to repeat the game several times, each time the player learns something. In order to maintain a positive relationship between the player and his/her failures, the game provides rapid feedbacks to encourage the player to try until s/he succeeds. In traditional learning, instead, the feedbacks are not immediate and the students have few opportunities to try the exercises and when they can, the risks are high since the failures are monitored. The result of this process is anxiety and desire to escape. On the contrary, the gamification approach creates a learning environment in which any attempt is rewarded, in fact, when a failure occurs the player can correct her/his mistakes over and over again. Thus, the defeat becomes a necessary part of the learning process and students can see the failure as an opportunity, rather than being overwhelmed or become helpless and fearful.

In the *social area* the game experience allows players to experience new identities and roles, asking them to take decisions according to different points of view. For example, in most of video games players can take on roles that are imaginary, but sometimes they involve the players in real situations and environments. Moreover, the gamification allows to publish and share the achievements, which otherwise might remain invisible. In traditional learning, teacher traditionally provides the recognition, but in the gamified environments players can reward each other encouraging them to participate to the class/community.

On the basis of those premises it is possible to assert that a well-designed learning system that uses gamification approach can help students to assume meaningful and productive roles for learning [2].

For these reasons in the UBICARE (UBIquitous knowledge-oriented HealthCARE) project, aimed at creating a social network to share clinical data and knowledge in order to favour the de-hospitalization of patients suffering from peritoneal dialysis and chronic heart failure, the Gamification approach has been used to both empower the patients to adopt healthy life-style and train the medical and paramedical staff about diagnostic procedures, therapeutic interventions and follow-up of patients [3, 4]. In particular, the paper describes the UbiGame component that support the acquisition of skills related to the treatment protocols and diagnostic procedure. The main innovation introduced in the UbiGame component of the UBICARE project with respect to the available solutions in the literature, is the trainer profile, which allows users to create new games according to specific users' learning needs. The paper describes the trainer interaction, which allows new simulations to be built in order to keep the system up to date.

The paper is organized as follows: the next section describes the whole UBICARE system, section 3 describes the Simulation of clinical cases component, section 4 supplies an example of the trainer interaction and finally, some conclusions and future works are proposed.

2   The UBICARE System

In order to meet the final aim of the project, to allow the communication and information sharing between different figures involved in the patient management, the UBICARE system has been developed according to the social network paradigm. In particular, the missions of the system are to empower patients and caregiver in the disease management and to support and train medical and paramedical staff on specific procedures and guidelines. From a technological point of view, the offered services have been implemented using hybrid architecture, based both on plug-in and SOA (Service Oriented Architecture), to ensure the scalability of the whole system, as detailed in [4].

The *Health Care Network* (1) (Fig. 1) is the core of the system: it is a social network based on the open source framework ELGG (www.elgg.org). The use of an open source framework has allowed the developers to focus on design and development of the services to be offered by the system to better meet the functional requirements of the application scenarios.

The *Data Acquisition* plug-in (2) allows the collection of basic data useful for patient's management and monitoring. It uses both automatic acquisition, using medical devices, and manual acquisition of parameters monitored daily by the patient/doctor/paramedic. The *Patient Monitoring* plug-in (3) allows doctors and caregivers to be continuously informed about the health conditions of the patient. In particular, on the basis of the data collected using the Data Acquisition plug-in could be sent both automatic alerts, to regularly remind of controls and to point out critical events, and manual alerts, to aware the patients of some events that can be critical for their health. The *Knowledge Management Service* plug-in (4) is the e-learning component devoted to the e-learning activities and allows the sharing of educational

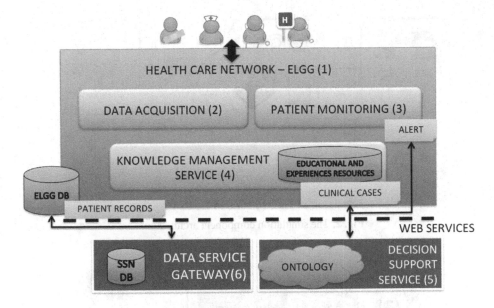

Fig. 1. The UBICARE system architecture [3]

resources among the community of users. In particular, the services available are the suggestion of personalized learning resources, simulations of clinical cases to train learners to deal with the main problems of their diseases, and the management of experience to share information about both official guidelines and medical protocols.

The *Decision Support Service* (5) is a web service that aims at supporting the medical and paramedical staff in managing the patient. In particular, it is able to suggest alternative therapies, to send automatic alerts based on patient monitoring, and to select interesting case studies to be used in learning and training processes. The *Data Service Gateway* (6) is a service infrastructure that allows the integration and interoperability of data in the whole system. The component ensures the extensibility of the system, the decoupling between distributed components, the transparency of the communication model, and the integration of the system with all different management systems of existing patient records (SSN DB in the figure).

3   The Simulations of Clinical Cases: UbiGame Component

The simulation component, named UbiGame, is part of the *Knowledge Management Service*. Starting from real medical records it builds a realistic problem, in order to allow specific skills about treatment protocols and diagnostic procedure to be acquired. In order to improve usability and maintainability of the component, the user interface and the decisional engine were split. A web service was built to retrieve all useful information for the simulation experience and to provide real patient data to help users to learn best practices in real case studies.

From the user perspective, the game consists of a web environment where a clinical case is defined according to a detailed patient clinical record, his/her actual

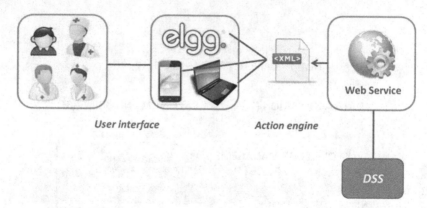

Fig. 2. The simulation component architecture

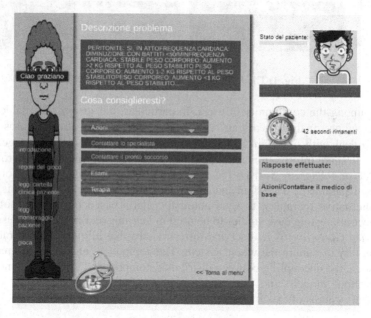

Fig. 3. The simulation game

monitoring parameters and the user profile and learning needs. The simulation of clinical cases is mainly addressed to general practitioners and paramedical staff, which have to be empowered to take care of patients according to standard protocols and to manage any critical state of health of the patient [5].

The simulated patient asks to the expert (the player) what to do in order to improve her/his health status. The possible alternatives proposed to the player are: therapies, actions and examinations. The player has to respond to the patient within 90 seconds to prevent the patient from getting worse. The time is visualized by means of a counter and an avatar indicates the worsening of the patient by images (Fig. 3). The player's answer could be completely wrong, correct or partially correct. In the first two cases, the game ends, while in the latter case a bonus of 5 seconds is given to allow the player to provide the correct answer.

When the simulation ends, a summary supplies detailed information about the game just ended. In particular, a detailed feedback is supplied for and against each possible answer.

UbiGame offers different scenarios to the different players according to the specific knowledge and skills that they should acquire. In particular, in the system have been defined the: caregivers, patients, nurse, general and specialist physicians. The professional figures involved in the patient's management are organized in a pyramidal hierarchy.

Patient and caregiver profile is the lower profile within UbiGame. The game goal for caregivers is to point out only real problems and train them to call a doctor or a medical institute only when necessary. Nurse is a medium profile: s/he is able to identify simple problems, to check therapy and to support patients and caregivers by suggesting who can solve particular problems but they can not take decisions about therapy, and they have to redirect patients to general or specialist practitioner. General practitioner, instead, is asked to solve simple/medium problems according to their skills, such as change therapy or recognize critical events by suggesting the appropriate actions. In this way, the patient will refer to the specialist only if necessary. The specialist physician indeed handles problems with a high level of difficulty. His goal in UbiGame is to test the system and to suggest possible specialist advice.

The main problems in the gamification approach applied to learning contexts are the addiction to the system and the scalability of the didactic contents. In this view, it is important to involve the player in the game updating process. The main aim of the updating process is to extend the player experience, over the time, before s/he, as naturally happens, get bored and finds the game repetitive and monotonous.

To avoid the mentioned problem of addiction, a trainer, among the different users of the game, has been defined. The trainer can create new simulation sessions and modify an existing one. The updating actions can be required because players can send feedbacks about the quality of the simulation game and in order to suggest improvements.

4   The Trainer Interaction

As said before, the goal of the Trainer within UbiGame is to create and to manage the simulations of clinical cases. The Trainer profile is not necessary a specialist. As previously mentioned the profiles are organized in a pyramidal hierarchy, thus the trainer of each level can create a simulation game for the levels below him. For example, a nurse can create a game for patient, caregiver and other nurses. The main idea is to provide different kind of games with different difficulty levels and on the basis of the actual users' learning needs (Fig. 4).

When a trainer starts the game interaction, the system selects a real patient profile within a specific trainer specialization context: cardiology or nephrology. For each specialization a set of real patient records are stored in the UBICARE database.

Trainer has to complete selected user profile by choosing some real monitoring data (Fig. 4). From the menu, the trainer can select one or more items to better fit the user's learning needs and to represent the patient.

The selected data will be used during the game simulation and represent the reasons that led the patient to seek an expert opinion. After the selection of the clinical profile, the trainer selects the action that would be suggested to the patient. The actions are divided into three categories: Examinations, Therapies and Generic Actions. A set of predefined actions is listed in the database, but if necessary the trainer can insert new actions that will be available in the next interactions.

In this way, according to his own experience, a trainer can customize general best practice to meet specific clinical cases. Moreover, in order to keep the simulations up to date, each specialist in the community can suggest changes to any game in UbiGame, to provide a different point of view of a particular clinical case. The Trainer, creator of the simulation, can accept the suggestions or not.

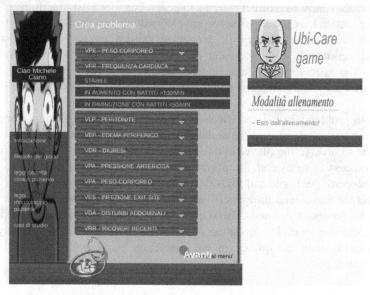

Fig. 4. Creation of new simulation – selection of monitoring data

4.1   The External Action Engine: The Web Service

The whole system is constantly interfaced with the remote web service, which is responsible for all data provided to the players. Rules, medical records, monitoring data and possible answers are all generated in real time from the web service to every request. Moreover, the web service stores all the games played by each player and its related statistics.

The webserver provides two kinds of simulations. The first one is automatically generated by the DSS that is used within the UBICARE system to implement the decision support service. Through a series of background calls to the DSS web

service, the UbiGame generates a set of simulations of real clinical cases using clinical profiles and actions coherent with the knowledge base of the DSS.
The second kind of simulation is generated starting from clinical profiles manually introduced by trainer. Using a simple interface (Fig. 5), in fact, the trainer can add and manage the monitoring data, their values and the possible problems related to them. Like in the previous case, the action engine of UbiGame will use those data in order to build a set of simulations on the basis of the data inserted by the trainer.

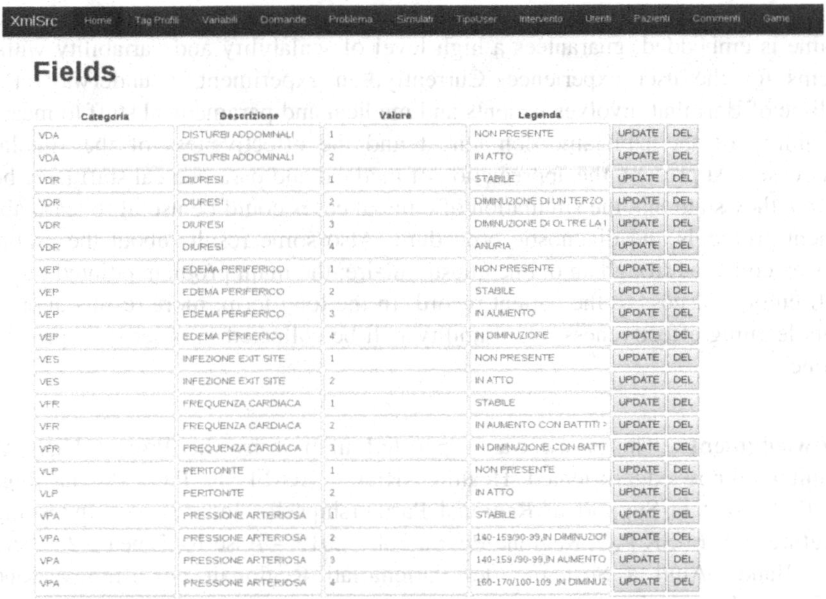

Categoria	Descrizione	Valore	Legenda		
VDA	DISTURBI ADDOMINALI	1	NON PRESENTE	UPDATE	DEL
VDA	DISTURBI ADDOMINALI	2	IN ATTO	UPDATE	DEL
VDR	DIURESI	1	STABILE	UPDATE	DEL
VDR	DIURESI	2	DIMINUZIONE DI UN TERZO	UPDATE	DEL
VDR	DIURESI	3	DIMINUZIONE DI OLTRE LA I	UPDATE	DEL
VDR	DIURESI	4	ANURIA	UPDATE	DEL
VEP	EDEMA PERIFERICO	1	NON PRESENTE	UPDATE	DEL
VEP	EDEMA PERIFERICO	2	STABILE	UPDATE	DEL
VEP	EDEMA PERIFERICO	3	IN AUMENTO	UPDATE	DEL
VEP	EDEMA PERIFERICO	4	IN DIMINUZIONE	UPDATE	DEL
VES	INFEZIONE EXIT SITE	1	NON PRESENTE	UPDATE	DEL
VES	INFEZIONE EXIT SITE	2	IN ATTO	UPDATE	DEL
VFR	FREQUENZA CARDIACA	1	STABILE	UPDATE	DEL
VFR	FREQUENZA CARDIACA	2	IN AUMENTO CON BATTITI >	UPDATE	DEL
VFR	FREQUENZA CARDIACA	3	IN DIMINUZIONE CON BATTI	UPDATE	DEL
VLP	PERITONITE	1	NON PRESENTE	UPDATE	DEL
VLP	PERITONITE	2	IN ATTO	UPDATE	DEL
VPA	PRESSIONE ARTERIOSA	1	STABILE	UPDATE	DEL
VPA	PRESSIONE ARTERIOSA	2	140-159/90-99,IN DIMINUZIO	UPDATE	DEL
VPA	PRESSIONE ARTERIOSA	3	140-159 /90-99,IN AUMENTO	UPDATE	DEL
VPA	PRESSIONE ARTERIOSA	4	160-170/100-109 ,IN DIMINUZ	UPDATE	DEL

Fig. 5. UbiGame Web Server: A subset of health problems of the patient

When a user asks for a simulation of a clinical case in the system, both the sets defined as previously described are used to select the one that best fits the user's learning needs.

5 Conclusions

The gamification approach can improve motivation and keep user engaged in order to make the learning process more effective. This is particularly useful in those contexts in which the learning is a necessity and, thus, often not pleasant. In the e-health field, for example, there are situations in which both patients and caregivers are forced to acquire knowledge and skills to improve their life-style. Moreover, the gamification approach could be helpful also to professional figures for acquiring new skills. These premises have led to the adoption of the gamification approach to design and build the simulation of clinical cases component, embedded in the Knowledge Management

Service of the UBICARE system. In order to make realistic the interaction with the learning environment, real patient records are used to build the simulated clinical cases. In addition, in order to keep the system up to date over time and to allow the definition of clinical cases tailored on the basis of the users' needs, a trainer profile has been added among the players. The trainer is a special profile that can easily add new simulations based on her/his own experience and update her/his game according to the feedbacks of the community. This is one of the strengths of UbiGame component, since allow the contents (the simulations) to be continuously renewed both automatically using the knowledge base of the DSS and manually using the trainers' expertise. Moreover, the use of an external web service, in which the logic of the game is embedded, guarantees a high level of scalability and variability without problems for the user experience. Currently, an experiment is underway at the Polyclinic of Bari that involves patients and medical and paramedical staff to measure the usability of the UbiGame component and the effectiveness of the simulated clinical cases. At present, the appreciation of medical and paramedical staff have been collected, they state that the simulation of clinical cases could be useful to learn about treatment protocols and diagnostic procedure. Also some results about the usability have been collected trough an online questionnaire; the main problem pointed out was the difficulty of access to the patient record. In the long term, more results about the patients learning effectiveness and usability will be collected in order to improve the component.

Acknowledgments. This work was supported in part by the Project UBICARE (UBIquitous knowledge-oriented HealthCARE) - EU-FESR P.O. Puglia Region 2007-2013 Grant in Support of Regional Partnerships for Innovation - Investing in your future (UE-FESR P.O. Regione Puglia 2007-2013 – Asse I – Linea 1.2 - Azione 1.2.4 - Bando Aiuti a Sostegno dei Partenariati Regionali per l'Innovazione - Investiamo nel vostro futuro).

References

1. Zichermann, G., Cunningham, C.: Gamification by Design: Implementing Game Mechanics in Web and Mobile Apps. O'Reilly Media, Sebastopol (2011)
2. Lee, J.J., Hammer, J.: Gamification in Education: What, How, Why Bother? Academic Exchange Quarterly 15(2) (2011)
3. Di Bitonto, P., Di Tria, F., Roselli, T., Rossano, V., Berni, F.: Distance Education and Social Learning in e-Health. International Journal of Information and Education Technology 4(1), 71–75 (2014)
4. Berni, F., Corriero, N., Pesare, E., Rossano, V., Roselli, T.: A Knowledge Management Service for e-health. In: ICERI 2013 Proceedings, pp. 488–493 (2013) ISBN: 978-84-616-3847-5
5. Corriero, N., Di Bitonto, P., Roselli, T., Rossano, V., Pesare, E.: Simulations of clinical cases for learning in e-health. International Journal of Information and Education Technology, International Conference on Information and Education Technology (ICIET) (January 2-3, 2014)

6. Pain Squad app, http://www.campaignpage.ca/sickkidsapp/files/MediaRelease_Cundari_PainSquadApp.pdf

7. Stanford University – Septris Game, http://cme.stanford.edu/septris/game/SepsisTetris.html

8. Illeris, K.: The three dimensions of learning: Contemporary learning theory in the tension field between the cognitive, the emotional and the social. Krieger, Malabar (2003)

9. Papastergiou, M.: Digital Game-Based Learning in high school Computer Science education: Impact on educational effectiveness and student motivation. Computers & Education 52(1), 1–12 (2009)

10. Jun Kiat Ong, M.: Gamification and its effect on employee engagement and performance in a perceptual diagnosis task, Master dissertation, Master of Science in Applied Psychology, University of Canterbury

11. Kato, P.M., Cole, S.W., et al.: A Video Game Improves Behavioral outcomes in Adolescents and Young Adults With Cancer: A Randomized Trial. Pediatrics 122(2), 305–317 (2008)

12. Piccinno, E., Vendemiale, M., Tummolo, A., Ortolani, F., Frezza, E., Torelli, C., Di Bitonto, P., Rossano, V., Roselli, T.: New technologies for promoting hypoglycaemia self-management in type 1 diabetic children. In: 9th Joint Meeting of Paediatric Endocrinology, Milan, September 19-22 (2013)

13. Di Bitonto, P., Roselli, T., Rossano, V., Frezza, E., Piccinno, E.: An educational game to learn type 1 diabetes management. In: The 18th International Conference on Distributed Multimedia Systems, Miami Beach, USA, August 9-11, pp. 139–143. KSI Press, Skokie (2012) ISBN: 1-891706-32-2

14. Lieberman, D.A.: Interactive video games for health promotion: Effects on knowledge, self-efficacy, social support, and health. In: Street Jr., R.L., Gold, W.R., Manning, T.R. (eds.) Health Promotion and Interactive Technology: Theoretical Applications and Future Directions, pp. 103–120. Lawrence Erlbaum Associates Publishers, Mahwah (1997)

15. Prensky, M.: Digital Game-Based Learning. McGraw-Hill, New York (2001)

16. Lepper, M.R., Malone, T.W.: Intrinsic motivation and instructional effectiveness in computer-based education. In: Snow, R.E., Farr, M.J. (eds.) Aptitude, Learning, and Instruction: vol. 3. Conative and Affective Process Analyses, pp. 255–286. Lawrence Erlbaum, Hillsdale (1987)

17. Rieber, L.P.: Seriously considering play: Designing interactive learning environments based on the blending of microworlds, simulations, and games. Educational Technology Research & Development 44(2), 43–58 (1996)

18. Rosas, R., Nussbaum, M., Cumsille, P., Marianov, V., Correa, M., et al.: Beyond Nintendo: design and assessment of educational video games for first and second grade students. Computers & Education 40(2003), 71–94 (2003)

Challenges When Engaging Diabetic Patients and Their Clinicians in Using E-Health Technologies to Improve Clinical Outcomes

Brian Edward Dixon[1,2,3], Abdulrahman Mohammed Jabour[1],
Erin O'Kelly Phillips[4], and David G. Marrero[4,5]

[1] Department of BioHealth Informatics, School of Informatics and Computing,
Indiana University, Indianapolis, IN, USA
{bedixon,ajabour}@iupui.edu
[2] Center for Biomedical Informatics, Regenstrief Institute, Indianapolis, IN, USA
[3] Center for Health Information and Communications, Department of Veterans Affairs,
Veterans Health Administration, Health Services Research and Development Service,
Indianapolis, IN, USA
[4] Diabetes Translational Research Center, School of Medicine, Indiana University,
Indianapolis, IN, USA
{ekokelly,dgmarrer}@iu.edu
[5] Department of Endocrinology, School of Medicine, Indiana University,
Indianapolis, IN, USA

Abstract. Diabetes mellitus (DM) is a chronic disease affecting more than 285 people worldwide and the fourth leading cause of death. Increasing evidence suggests that many DM patients have poor adherence with prescribed medication therapies, impacting clinical outcomes. Patients' barriers to medication adherence and the extent to which barriers contribute to poor outcomes, however, are not routinely assessed. We designed a dashboard for an electronic health record system to integrate DM disease and medication data, including patient-reported barriers to adherence. The dashboard was pilot tested at multiple ambulatory clinics to examine whether integrated electronic tools can support patient-centered decision-making processes involving complex medication regimens for DM and other chronic diseases. During pilot testing, we encountered several challenges when engaging patients and clinicians in using the dashboard as well as a portal used to gather self-reported psychosocial information directly from patients. In this paper we explore those challenges and suggest methods for better supporting the adoption and use of e-health technologies to improve care delivery processes as well as health outcomes for populations like diabetic patients.

Keywords: Medication Adherence, Type 2 Diabetes Mellitus; Computerized Medical Records Systems, Personal Health Records, Physician-Patient Relations, Drug Monitoring, Patient-Centered Care.

C. Stephanidis and M. Antona (Eds.): UAHCI/HCII 2014, Part III, LNCS 8515, pp. 238–247, 2014.
© Springer International Publishing Switzerland 2014

1 Introduction

Diabetes mellitus (DM) is a chronic disease affecting more than 285 people worldwide and the fourth leading cause of death. Globally the prevalence of DM continues to rise at nearly epidemic rates, driven by urbanization, growing increases in obesity, and aging of populations [1]. Findings from several studies investigating the quality of DM care reveal a discrepancy between system-level disease management strategies and outcomes [2-6]. In essence, even though there are improved treatment strategies, expected outcomes are not occurring at a commensurate level. Therefore greater emphases on patient-level factors that may explain DM intervention outcomes are being explored.

One such factor is adherence to complex medication regimens. Increasing evidence suggests that patients with diabetes often have poor adherence with prescribed medication therapies [7, 8]. However, the reasons why patients do not take their medications as prescribed are poorly understood [9]. Previous studies on adherence have relied on patient self-report data on medication use, or they have used more "objective" measures such as gaps in prescription coverage or technologies to determine if patients are taking their medications. An example is electronic MEMS caps, which document when a pill bottle is opened [10-12]. All of these approaches have limitations which include accuracy; reporting and response bias; or limited effect size [13].

Despite existing evidence and efforts, patient-reported barriers to medication adherence and the extent to which those barriers contribute to poor DM outcomes are not currently assessed routinely in clinical practice [14]. Indeed, few have assessed the role of barriers perceived by patients to medications use and how perceived barriers may be addressed by intervention.

To address medication adherence issues facing individuals with complex medication regimens, we developed a clinical information system to electronically integrate the capture and presentation of information regarding DM patients' disease management, medication adherence, and perceived barriers to adherence [15]. The system combines objective data regarding medication possession ratios with laboratory and point-of-care testing data as well as patient-entered data on perceived barriers to adherence. By routinely capturing patient-reported barriers and integrating such information at the point-of-care with other electronic health data, we seek to better inform DM therapy decision-making processes.

In this paper, we describe the system and our experience pilot testing the system in three primary care clinics. During the pilot testing, we encountered several challenges when engaging patients and clinicians in using both the dashboard as well as a portal designed to gather patient-reported barriers to medication adherence. Here we discuss those challenges and suggest methods for better supporting the adoption and use of e-health technologies to improve care delivery processes as well as health outcomes for populations like DM patients.

2   Methods

2.1   System Description

The primary system of interest is a dashboard (Figure-1) used by clinicians (e.g., physicians, nurses, pharmacists) in the context of routine primary care. Clinicians review the information on the dashboard either before or during a patient visit to understand the patient's current adherence to their medication regimen for DM2.

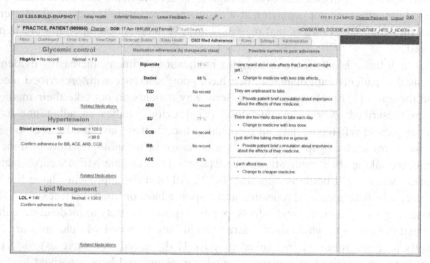

Fig. 1. Screenshot of clinical dashboard designed to integrate medication adherence information from multiple sources into electronic health record (EHR) system

The clinical dashboard is a Java-based module designed to plug into the Regenstrief CareWeb™ framework, an open-source electronic health record (EHR) platform developed by the Regenstrief Institute's Center for Biomedical Informatics. CareWeb is a web-based version of the Regenstrief Medical Record System (RMRS) [16], providing primary care clinicians in Eskenazi Health facilities access to patients' medical records. The framework provides all plugins with a common data retrieval and display interface, which the dashboard uses to access and visualize patient information. The framework also allows the dashboard to receive notification of and react to various events, including when a patient is selected by the user.

The dashboard was explicitly designed to be passive, or non-interruptive. When the clinician selects a patient, the dashboard refreshes with content from multiple sources: the electronic health record (RMRS) providing recent physiological data, pharmacy data detailing which medications have been dispensed to the patient, and patient-entered information on their personal challenges in taking their medication as prescribed. System users have the option to view the dashboard or ignore it.

When information is displayed, the dashboard uses several visual techniques to highlight normal as well as abnormal patient information. When a patient's blood pressure or glycosylated hemoglobin (HbA1c) is elevated, is it highlighted in red;

normal values are shown in black. When the patient is believed, based on pharmacy claims information, to be non-adherent to a class of DM medications, the information is highlighted in red; acceptable levels are highlighted in green; potentially problematic values are shown in yellow. Such color differentiation enables quick review of the dashboard contents by clinician users.

Electronic Health Record Data. The left panel of the dashboard displays information extracted from the patient's EHR. Three types of EHR data are displayed: blood pressure, HbA1c, and cholesterol. These data were targeted because they are relevant to DM patient populations. Clinicians routinely measure and analyze HbA1c levels to determine how well DM patients keep their disease under control. High blood pressure and poor lipid management are also commonly co-related with DM2, leading to medications that treat multiple conditions. Therefore clinicians can conveniently review common physiologic data for DM patients in one location.

Medication Adherence Data. Adherence to DM medications and cardiovascular risk factors is displayed in the middle panel of the dashboard. The information originates from the Medication (Med) Hub, an independent web service within the Regenstrief technology infrastructure [17]. The Med Hub serves as a central source of medication data for all CareWeb applications. Two sources of information currently feed the Med Hub: the Wishard Health Services pharmacy system, an internal database of medications dispensed to Wishard patients many of whom do not have insurance, and SureScripts, a national dataset of medications dispensed from independent chain and mail-order pharmacies.

Using the pharmacy data available from the Med Hub, we calculate the proportion of days covered (PDC), a ratio representing whether the patient possessed a drug or a class of drugs (e.g., all oral DM medications) during a defined measurement period. The PDC has been shown in numerous studies to accurately identify patients who fail to fill or refill their medications as directed by their physician or pharmacist [18]. We use a dichotomized 6-month (180-day) PDC with a cut-off point of 80%, which we have found to provide the strongest and most reliable correlation with patient glycemic control [19].

Patient Feedback. The right panel of the dashboard displays feedback from patients on their challenges in taking their medications. Patients interact with a personal health record (PHR) system to answer questions about their medication regimen. The data are then available for query by the DM application for display.

The PHR was developed using the Open Medical Record System (OpenMRS) platform [20], an open-source EHR that originated at Regenstrief but is now implemented and supported by a worldwide collaborative involving individuals from numerous counties involved in EHR, PHR, and m-Health initiatives [21]. Although OpenMRS was selected for our project, the dashboard could be integrated with any other PHR.

OpenMRS includes a forms module that allows collection of standardized data from patients. Using the forms module, we implemented a 5-point Likert style, validated questionnaire developed by researchers at the Diabetes Translational Research Center affiliated with the Indiana University School of Medicine [22, 23]. The questionnaire uses 20 items to assess possible barriers to medication adherence. For example, valid responses as to why one may not take his or her prescribed medications include "I can't afford them" and "I just forget to take them." Individual items are grouped into categories and ranked based on aggregate scores from patient responses. The highest ranking three categories are stored for retrieval by the dashboard.

The 20 items in the patient survey are factor analyzed with varimax rotation and correlated with perceived health status as well as satisfaction measures. Five factors or subscales can be identified and displayed to clinical users: poor access to medications; poor communication with providers; poor understanding of medications and/or difficulty in taking them; presence of side effects; and system-level barriers to use. Previous analysis suggests that persons with poor CVD risk factor control have more reported barriers that may inhibit medication adherence than do persons with good risk factor control [23].

2.2   Information Flow

Physiologic and medication adherence data are captured routinely from health care delivery processes and electronically sent to the RMRS. Patient feedback on medication adherence requires manual completion of the questionnaire within the PHR. Patients are asked every 2-3 months to complete a survey as previous studies found adherence to be fairly consistent over time.

The information needed for the dashboard is queried in parallel with other Care-Web processes when a clinician opens the electronic medical record for a patient (Figure-2). First, the CareWeb server notifies the DM2 module that a patient record has been selected. The module then, in parallel, requests the three sets of data from the EHR, PHR, and CDS web service. The EHR returns physiologic data for the selected patient. The PHR returns the highest ranking categories identified by the patient from their responses to the questionnaire. The CDS service retrieves the pharmacy data from the Med Hub service and calculates the PDC. The PDC is returned to the DM module. All three data sets are stored in the server's cache until the clinician selects the DM tab within the CareWeb application. Upon selection, the data sets are rendered into their respective columns for review by the clinician.

2.3   System Pilot

We completed development and implementation of the dashboard, DM module, and PHR in late 2012. In early 2013, we enrolled 15 primary care clinicians (Medical Doctors and Nurse Practitioners) at three community health centers part of Eskenazi Health, a publically funded health system that serves primarily the uninsured and underinsured population of the Indianapolis metropolitan area. Following enrollment of physicians, we enrolled 96 diabetic patients under the care of one participating clinicians. The pilot ran through the end of 2013.

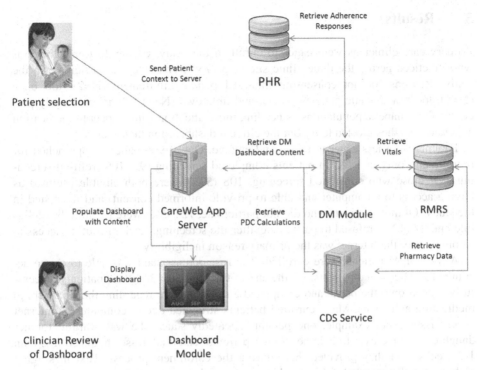

Fig. 2. Information flow diagram depicting the architecture of the DM clinical information system module and its integration with existing electronic health record, clinical decision support, and personal health record system components

2.4 Study Design

We collected baseline perceptions of providers regarding medication adherence discussions between them and their patients. Baseline perceptions of patients regarding current conversations occurring about medication adherence were also captured. In addition, we collected demographic information about patients and providers to enable comparison across health center locations and socioeconomic data, which has been shown to effect patient access to the Internet impacting PHR usage [24, 25].

Following enrollment, a research assistant created PHR user accounts for each of the enrolled patients. Account information was emailed to the patients, and they were asked to complete a baseline questionnaire regarding medication adherence. Patients who did not complete a baseline questionnaire were reminded via email or text message, based on patient preferences. Patients were then asked to complete a questionnaire every 2-3 months after baseline. Reminders were sent to unresponsive participants. After successful completion of each questionnaire, patients were mailed a $10 gift card to a local grocery store, gas station, or restaurant.

3   Results

Primary care clinicians were eager to enroll in the study. Of the 20 total clinicians who practiced across the three clinic sites, 15 (75%) consented to participate in the study. Reasons for not consenting included pending retirement (N=2), too busy (N=1), too few diabetic patients (N=1), and unknown (N=1). Clinicians largely perceived their diabetic populations as needing more attention with respect to medication adherence, so they elected to try out the clinical dashboard in their practice.

Patients were less eager to enroll and engage. Out of 906 patients approached for recruitment, only 203 (22%) patients completed screening (92; 10% refused screening). Of those who completed screening, 108 (53%) were both eligible (defined as having access to a computer and able to provide informed consent) and interested in the study. Of those patients who did not participate, 72 (35%) were found to be ineligible and 27 (13%) refused to participate after the screening. Lack of routine access to a computer or the Internet was the primary reason ineligibility.

A total of 96 patients were enrolled. The research assistant was able to create accounts for 92 enrolled patients. By the end of the pilot, just 24 (26%) patients successfully logged onto the portal and completed a questionnaire regarding their barriers to medication adherence. Many enrolled patients struggled due to computer or Internet access issues. For example, one patient repeatedly stated she was waiting for her daughter to come over to help her. Other patients' email addresses bounced less than 1-2 weeks after they provided them during the enrollment process. Text messaging and phone calls were helpful in reaching some of these patients, but access challenges remained for a significant number of study subjects.

4   Discussion

To fully realize the potential of health information technologies to impact population health outcomes, information and systems need to be integrated. Prior studies to improve adherence have focused on singular modalities to change provider or patient behavior. For example, in Vollmer et al [26] an interactive voice response system called patients who appeared to have gaps in refilling their asthma medication. The system was statistically significant in changing adherence, but the mean change was not clinically meaningful. Similarly, a recent systematic review of patient portals identified just one study that demonstrated an effect on diabetes care delivery [27]. However, in the one identified study, the portal was found to be associated with a change in medication regimen but had no impact on clinical outcomes as measured by HbA1c and blood pressure [28]. Our DM module integrates multiple information tools to address medication adherence in a coordinated fashion. While our approach may not be the only method to stimulate better adherence for patients with chronic illness, we believe that future approaches need to draw upon the power of EHR, PHR, and CDS systems to make adherence easier in the context of routine clinical care.

To be effective, 'routine clinical care' must include environments where patients exist (e.g., home, work, bus stop). Integrated informations solutions therefore must incorporate technologies that can be integrated into daily routines of people. Our efforts were hampered by system barriers that remain a challenge for many people, especially those who are elderly or of low socioeconomic status [29]. Therefore a digital divide still exists, even if it may be shrinking in populations burdened by multiple co-morbid diseases requiring complex drug regimens.

Finally, it is possible that patients may be resistant to describing barriers they experience to taking medications as prescribed by their providers. These may include embarrassment over non-compliance, their economic status, or failure to disclose secondary problems such as side effects. Resistance may also reflect a fear that disclosing issues may result in having to take additional medications. Furthermore, resistance could suggest there is simply a lack of interest in logging onto a portal to communicate. Future research will need to explore the factors that impact patients' willingness to use a portal to communicate with their providers about medication adherence.

Some of the challenges we describe, however, might be overcome with a smart phone app that integrates better into daily routine over an Internet-based app that must be used on a computer. Yet singular mobile apps that focus on just one aspect of health or wellness may not be usable in large populations. Multi-functional apps may be, or at least apps that cover multiple aspects of a chronic disease. For example, management of DM involves not only medication adherence but also changes to diet, exercise, and co-morbid conditions such as hypertension. Therefore technologies that engage patients will likely be those which can address multiple concerns in an integrated fashion (e.g., one-stop shop) rather than require multiple apps or interfaces. In addition, it will become critical that future applications include appropriate education that emphasizes the importance of patient-provider communication to enable shared decision making that will achieve optimal therapeutic outcomes.

5 Conclusions

We engaged a small number of physicians and patients in using novel e-health technologies to improve medication adherence by combining patient medication history data from a combination of electronic data sources with patient-reported barriers. Engagement of providers and patients was challenging. While providers were eager to enroll and try out the clinical dashboard, many patients experienced challenges in gaining routine access to the Internet to use a portal designed for patient engagement. Limited usage prevents integrated e-health technologies from impacting outcomes as providers continue to only see a partial picture of health. Further, digital divide issues remain important to address so that all patients can access and use e-health technologies, especially those who are vulnerable and at risk of serious complications from poor medication management.

Acknowledgements. This work was supported by a grant (R34DK092769) from the National Institute for Diabetes and Digestive and Kidney Diseases and by the Department of Veterans Affairs, Veterans Health Administration, Health Services

Research and Development Service CIN 13-416. Dr. Dixon is a Health Research Scientist at the Richard L. Roudebush Veterans Affairs Medical Center in Indianapolis, Indiana, USA. Dr. Dixon also receives funding from a Robert Wood Johnson Foundation Mentored Research Scientist Development Award (71596). The content is solely the responsibility of the authors and does not necessarily represent the official views of the National Institutes of Diabetes and Digestive and Kidney Diseases, the National Institutes of Health, the Department of Veterans Affairs, the Robert Wood Johnson Foundation, or the United States Government.

References

1. George, B., Cebioglu, M., Yeghiazaryan, K.: Inadequate diabetic care: global figures cry for preventive measures and personalized treatment. The EPMA Journal 1, 13–18 (2010)
2. Kim, C., Williamson, D.F., Herman, W.H., Safford, M.M., Selby, J.V., Marrero, D.G., Curb, J.D., Thompson, T.J., Narayan, K., Mangione, C.M.: Referral management and the care of patients with diabetes: the Translating Research Into Action for Diabetes (TRIAD) study. The American Journal of Managed Care 10, 137 (2004)
3. Kim, C., Williamson, D.F., Mangione, C.M., Safford, M.M., Selby, J.V., Marrero, D.G., Curb, J.D., Thompson, T.J., Narayan, K.V., Herman, W.H.: Managed Care Organization and the Quality of Diabetes Care The Translating Research Into Action for Diabetes (TRIAD) study. Diabetes Care 27, 1529–1534 (2004)
4. Levit, K., Smith, C., Cowan, C., Lazenby, H., Sensenig, A., Catlin, A.: Trends in US health care spending, 2001. Health Affairs 22, 154–164 (2003)
5. Kerr, E.A., Gerzoff, R.B., Krein, S.L., Selby, J.V., Piette, J.D., Curb, J.D., Herman, W.H., Marrero, D.G., Narayan, K.V., Safford, M.M.: Diabetes care quality in the Veterans Affairs Health Care System and commercial managed care: the TRIAD study. Annals of Internal Medicine 141, 272–281 (2004)
6. Mangione, C.M., Gerzoff, R.B., Williamson, D.F., Steers, W.N., Kerr, E.A., Brown, A.F., Waitzfelder, B.E., Marrero, D.G., Dudley, R.A., Kim, C.: The association between quality of care and the intensity of diabetes disease management programs. Annals of Internal Medicine 145, 107–116 (2006)
7. Hanlon, J.T., Schmader, K.E., Ruby, C.M., Weinberger, M.: Suboptimal prescribing in older inpatients and outpatients. Journal of the American Geriatrics Society 49, 200–209 (2001)
8. Vik, S.A., Maxwell, C.J., Hogan, D.B.: Measurement, correlates, and health outcomes of medication adherence among seniors. The Annals of Pharmacotherapy 38, 303–312 (2004)
9. Benson, J., Britten, N.: Patients' decisions about whether or not to take antihypertensive drugs: qualitative study. BMJ 325, 873 (2002)
10. Cramer, J.A.: Microelectronic systems for monitoring and enhancing patient compliance with medication regimens. Drugs 49, 321–327 (1995)
11. Cramer, J.A.: Enhancing patient compliance in the elderly. Drugs & Aging 12, 7–15 (1998)
12. Cramer, J.A.: A systematic review of adherence with medications for diabetes. Diabetes Care 27, 1218–1224 (2004)
13. Farmer, K.C.: Methods for measuring and monitoring medication regimen adherence in clinical trials and clinical practice. Clinical Therapeutics 21, 1074–1090 (1999)

14. Brown, M.T., Bussell, J.K.: Medication adherence: WHO cares? Mayo Clin Proc. 86, 304–314 (2011)
15. Dixon, B.E., Jabour, A.M., Phillips, E.O., Marrero, D.G.: An informatics approach to medication adherence assessment and improvement using clinical, billing, and patient-entered data. J. Am. Med. Inform. Assoc. 21, 517–521 (2014)
16. McDonald, C.J., Overhage, J.M., Tierney, W.M., Dexter, P.R., Martin, D.K., Suico, J.G., Zafar, A., Schadow, G., Blevins, L., Glazener, T., Meeks-Johnson, J., Lemmon, L., Warvel, J., Porterfield, B., Cassidy, P., Lindbergh, D., Belsito, A., Tucker, M., Williams, B., Wodniak, C.: The Regenstrief Medical Record System: a quarter century experience. Int. J. Med. Inform. 54, 225–253 (1999)
17. Simonaitis, L., Belsito, A., Overhage, J.M.: Enhancing an ePrescribing system by adding medication histories and formularies: the Regenstrief Medication Hub. In: AMIA Annu. Symp. Proc., pp. 677–681 (2008)
18. Sikka, R., Xia, F., Aubert, R.E.: Estimating medication persistency using administrative claims data. The American Journal of Managed Care 11, 449–457 (2005)
19. Zhu, V.J., Tu, W., Rosenman, M.B., Overhage, J.M.: Facilitating Clinical Research through the Health Information Exchange: Lipid Control as an Example. In: AMIA Annu Symp Proc. 2010, pp. 947–951 (2010)
20. Mamlin, B.W., Biondich, P.G., Wolfe, B.A., Fraser, H., Jazayeri, D., Allen, C., Miranda, J., Tierney, W.M.: Cooking up an open source EMR for developing countries: OpenMRS - a recipe for successful collaboration. In: AMIA Annu. Symp. Proc., pp. 529–533 (2006)
21. Mohammed-Rajput, N.A., Smith, D.C., Mamlin, B., Biondich, P., Doebbeling, B.N.: OpenMRS, a global medical records system collaborative: factors influencing successful implementation. In: AMIA Annu. Symp. Proc. 2011, pp. 960–968 (2011)
22. Monahan, P., Lane, K., Hayes, R., McHorney, C., Marrero, D.: Reliability and validity of an instrument for assessing patients' perceptions about medications for diabetes: the PAM-D. Qual. Life Res. 18, 941–952 (2009)
23. Marrero, D., Monahan, P., Lane, K., Hayes, R.: Validation of a scale to measure patient-perceived barriers to medication use. 2006 International Society for Quality of Life Research meeting abstracts. Qual. Life Res. 15, A34–A35, Abstract #1223 (2006)
24. Tang, P.C., Ash, J.S., Bates, D.W., Overhage, J.M., Sands, D.Z.: Personal health records: definitions, benefits, and strategies for overcoming barriers to adoption. J. Am. Med. Inform. Assoc. 13, 121–126 (2006)
25. Yamin, C.K., Emani, S., Williams, D.H., Lipsitz, S.R., Karson, A.S., Wald, J.S., Bates, D.W.: The digital divide in adoption and use of a personal health record. Arch. Intern. Med. 171, 568–574 (2011)
26. Vollmer, W.M., Feldstein, A., Smith, D.H., Dubanoski, J.P., Waterbury, A., Schneider, J.L., Clark, S.A., Rand, C.: Use of health information technology to improve medication adherence. Am. J. Manag. Care 17, SP79–SP87 (2011)
27. Ammenwerth, E., Schnell-Inderst, P., Hoerbst, A.: The impact of electronic patient portals on patient care: a systematic review of controlled trials. Journal of Medical Internet Research 14 (2012)
28. Grant, R.W., Wald, J.S., Schnipper, J.L., Gandhi, T.K., Poon, E.G., Orav, E.J., Williams, D.H., Volk, L.A., Middleton, B.: Practice-linked online personal health records for type 2 diabetes mellitus: a randomized controlled trial. Archives of Internal Medicine 168, 1776 (2008)
29. Pew Research Center http://pewinternet.org/~/media//Files/Reports/2013/PIP_Offline%20adults_092513_PDF.pdf

Mobile Healthcare

Miwako Doi and Kazushige Ouchi

Corporate Research & Development Center, Toshiba Corporation
1, Komukai Toshiba-cho, Saiwai-ku, Kawasaki 212-8582, Japan
{miwako.doi,kazushige.ouchi}@toshiba.co.jp

Abstract. It is important to easily and cheaply monitor elderly person's activities of daily living in order to allay the anxiety of their relatives and caregivers. We developed a smartphone-based monitoring system. A smartphone of the elderly person continuously recognizes indoor-outdoor activities by using only built-in sensors and uploads the activity log to a web server. By accessing the server, relatives etc. at remote locations can browse the log to make sure the elderly person is safe and sound. The evaluation experiment showed that the proposed system had practical recognition accuracy and satisfied the users' needs.

Keywords: Activity recognition, Smartphone, Accelerometer, Microphone.

1 Introduction

The developed countries face the aging problems. After 30 years, emerging countries also will face the aging problems. The monitoring of the activities of daily living of elderly people is increasingly important not only for the elderly people but also for their relatives, friends and caregivers. Various activities have become recognizable by wearing accelerometers on several parts of the body [1], or wearing a dedicated device on the wrist [2]. However, it is impractical for users to continuously wear many accelerometers in daily life or, from the viewpoint of the cost, to use a special device. On the other hand, outdoor activities such as migration have become recognizable by using built-in sensors on a mobile phone [3]. Although activity recognition by commonly used devices has an advantage over the solutions envisaged in the abovementioned studies in terms of practicality, it is difficult to recognize various indoor activities.

We proposed an indoor-outdoor activity recognition system on a smartphone which switches two engines based on GPS signal. The indoor engine recognizes various activities of daily living based on accelerometer data and environment sound. The outdoor engine recognizes the behavior based on accelerometer data and GPS data.

2 Related Works

Activity recognition researches are categorized into two types; embedded type and wearable type. Georgia Tech's Aware Home [4], Microsoft Research's EasyLiving

C. Stephanidis and M. Antona (Eds.): UAHCI/HCII 2014, Part III, LNCS 8515, pp. 248–255, 2014.

Project [5], NiCT's UKARI Project[6] are works of the embedded types activity recognition. The embedded type activity recognition needs many sensors, to be installed in the environment in order to get the accurate activity recognition. In the result, the cost is high and the installation to the legacy home is difficult. Intelligent distribution panel is one of the embedded type commercialized examples. It realizes the power use visualization. Intelligent distribution panel only recognizes whether householders is or not at home and cannot recognize the daily activities because the sensor information is only poser usage.

The wearable type activity recognition uses wearable sensors such accelerometers, GPS, and other sensors. Early many researchers developed the special wearable devices. LifeMinder^{TM}[7] is an example of the wearable device. LifeMinder^{TM} is able to collect two axis accelerometer, temperature, blood wave data and sends them to a cell phone in order to analyze and recognize behavior, such as walking, running, eating meals and so on. The prototyped healthcare application gives advices to the user; taking drug, exercising, and so on. LifeMinder^{TM} was commercialized as a body motion sensor with sleep monitoring software [8] in 2004.

Nowadays, mobile phones equipped with a 3-axis accelerometer are becoming popular [9]. Studies on activity recognition using an accelerometer on mobile phones have also been reported. For example, [10] recognizes 5 migration activities—walking, fast walking, climbing up stairs, climbing down stairs, and running—with about 80% accuracy. In such studies, several migration activities are detectable by a mobile phone. It is difficult, however, to precisely recognize our target activities—in-home living activities, including not only migration but also housework and so on—by using an accelerometer and GPS.

A mobile phone naturally has a microphone for its primary function and it can also be used as an acoustic sensor. [11] recognized 19 sounds of 4 groups such as Kitchen, Office, Workshop and Outdoor, with more than 80% accuracy by using acoustic features. However, acoustic analysis needs higher sampling frequency than acceleration sensing and needs to compute a large amount of data. So, considering processing power and power consumption, it is undesirable to continuously execute acoustic analysis. Thus we propose a low-throughput in-home living activity recognition method combined with acceleration sensing and acoustic sensing that firstly estimates a user's movement condition roughly by acceleration sensing and then classifies the working condition in detail by acoustic sensing based on the estimated condition.

3   System Overview

We developed an indoor living-activity recognition engine and an outdoor migration activity recognition engine, and combined them into an Android^{TM} application. By switching between the two engines depending on the acquisition condition of GPS satellites, the system enables users to continuously monitor indoor-outdoor activities.

Indoor Living-Activity Recognition
It consists of a two-step classification process [12] as shown in Figure 1. Firstly, it roughly classifies the user's movement into "Resting," "Walking," and "Performing

an activity" by using variances of 1-sec data series from the 3-axis accelerometer. When it classifies "Performing an activity," it activates the microphone and calculates MFCC (Mel-Frequency Cepstral Coefficient), RMS (Root Mean Square) and ZCR (Zero-Crossing Rate) as acoustic features. Then it classifies the nature of the activity by SVM (Support Vector Machine) every 1 second. Then, it smoothes the classification results through an additional recognition scheme by majority voting for each task.

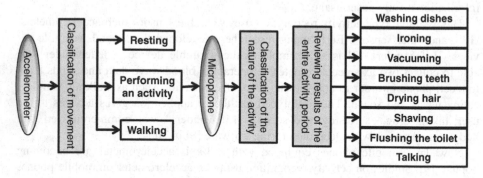

Fig. 1. Processing flow of indoor living-activity recognition

Outdoor Migration Activity Recognition

It works according to the following steps [13] as shown in Figure 2. It calculates device direction-independent feature quantities, namely, "Length of the acceleration vector," "Inner product of the acceleration vector and the gravity vector," and "Their cross product." Then, it calculates statistics of the 3 quantities, namely, average, minimum, maximum and variance of these quantities in a certain time window. It classifies these quantities into 4 migration classes by a neural network using back-propagation learning. Finally, it smoothes the fluctuating result by using a stochastic model generated by several heuristics.

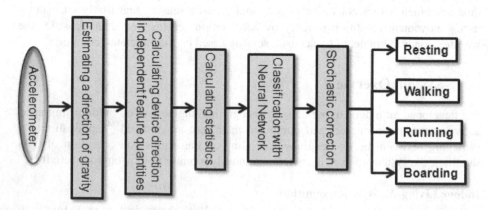

Fig. 2. Processing flow of outdoor migration activity recognition

Monitoring Server

The monitoring server is built on a web server. It is composed of an activity log data-base, an HTML5 generator, an anomaly detector and an e-mail generator. The activity log database stores the results of activity recognition from the smartphone in the el-derly person's home. Figure 4 shows an example of a one-week activity log generated in HTML5 format by the HTML5 generator. It allows observers, such as care manag-ers and relatives, at remote locations to browse the log data on most browsers of vari-ous information devices. Additionally, we also created a biological database to collect biological information such as ECG, pulse wave from a wearable vital sensor in

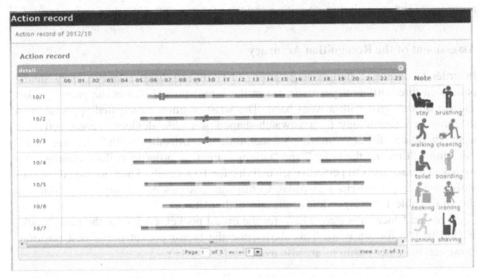

Fig. 3. An example of one-week activity log

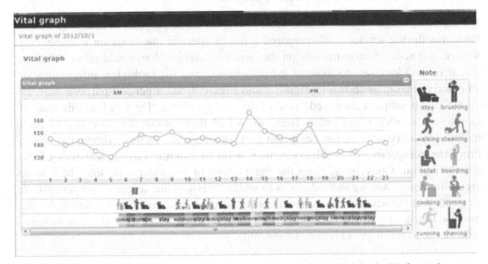

Fig. 4. An example of simultaneous monitoring of activity and biological information

cooperation with the smartphone [14]. Simultaneous monitoring of activity and bio-logical information enables users to analyze their health condition in detail as shown in Figure 4. It is also equipped with an anomaly detector and an e-mail generator to notify them of anomalous conditions.

4   Evaluation Experiment

An evaluation experiment was held with 22 subjects (6 men and 6 women in their 60s, and 5 men and 5 women in their 20s to 40s) at a mock living room to assess the accuracy of indoor activity recognition and the requirements for a monitoring service.

Assessment of the Recognition Accuracy

In order to contrast smartphone positions, the subjects were asked to carry smart-phones in three different positions, (a) in the breast pocket, (b) in the pants' pocket and (c) on the wrist with a wrist band. The wrist position anticipated application of the proposed technology to wristwatch-shaped wearable devices. Target activities were "washing dishes," "ironing," "vacuuming," "brushing teeth," "drying hair," "shaving," "flushing the toilet," and "talking." First, in order to collect training data, we asked the subjects to perform each activity for 10 seconds. Then, we asked them to perform all target activities as usual. Confusion matrices of activity recognition are shown in Table 1 corresponding to the attached position.

Averaged f-measures were 93.8% for the breast pocket, 89.5% for the pants' pock-et, and 91.0% for the wrist. This shows that the breast pocket is the best position. However, the other positions are also available.

Assessment of Needs for a Monitoring Service

We also conducted a questionnaire survey with the same subjects to assess the needs for a monitoring service. We prepared a list of specific questions on a monitoring service and some demonstrations on the assumed service that would allow relatives etc. at remote locations to monitor the activity log and the biological information of an elderly person, as shown in Figure 3 and Figure 4, via a general-purpose browser on a TV. All subjects answered 'Yes' to the first question, "Do you find this kind of monitoring service beneficial?" Then, we asked them about the necessity of each monitoring activity from the perspective of an observer. Table 2 shows the result. From the perspective of an observer, they want to monitor various activities of the elderly person. Conversely, from the perspective of the elderly person, there were great differences among individuals as to which activities are acceptable to monitor. It suggests that the activities to be monitored should be customizable. Although, for the proposed technology, it is necessary to train each target activity for 10 seconds befo-rehand, the technology is highly customizable.

Table 1. Confusion matrices of activity recognition results corresponding to the attached position

(a) Breast pocket

Actual \ Classified as	Washing dishes	Ironing	Vacuuming	Brushing teeth	Shaving	Drying hair	Flushing the toilet	Talking	Untrained task	Recall (%)
Washing dishes	20			1					1	90.9
Ironing		19						1	2	86.4
Vacuuming			22							100.0
Brushing teeth				19				1	2	86.4
Shaving					20				2	90.9
Drying hair			1			21				95.5
Flushing the toilet							21		1	95.5
Talking		1						18	3	81.8
Precision (%)	100.0	95.0	95.7	95.0	100.0	100.0	100.0	90.0		F-measure 93.8

(b) Pants' pocket

Actual \ Classified as	Washing dishes	Ironing	Vacuuming	Brushing teeth	Shaving	Drying hair	Flushing the toilet	Talking	Untrained task	Recall (%)
Washing dishes	19			2					1	86.4
Ironing		19	1					1	1	86.4
Vacuuming			22							100.0
Brushing teeth	1			17				2	2	77.3
Shaving		1			18			1	2	81.8
Drying hair			1			21				95.5
Flushing the toilet							21		1	95.5
Talking		2		1				16	3	72.7
Precision (%)	95.0	86.4	95.7	81.0	100.0	100.0	100.0	80.0		F-measure 89.5

(c) Wrist

Actual \ Classified as	Washing dishes	Ironing	Vacuuming	Brushing teeth	Shaving	Drying hair	Flushing the toilet	Talking	Untrained task	Recall (%)
Washing dishes	19			1				1	1	86.4
Ironing		18						2	2	81.8
Vacuuming			22							100.0
Brushing teeth	1			18				1	2	81.8
Shaving					18			1	3	81.8
Drying hair			1			21				95.5
Flushing the toilet							22		0	100.0
Talking		2						17	3	77.3
Precision (%)	95.0	90.0	95.7	94.7	100.0	100.0	100.0	77.3		F-measure 91.0

Table 2. The result of the questionnaire survey on the necessity of each monitoring activity

Activity	Yes (%)	No (%)
Brushing teeth	100	0
Drying hair	82	18
Shaving	93	7
Toileting	100	0
Washing dishes	75	25
Vacuuming	89	11
Talking	100	0
Walking	95	5
Running	65	35
Going outside	100	0

Future Direction of Medical Electronics

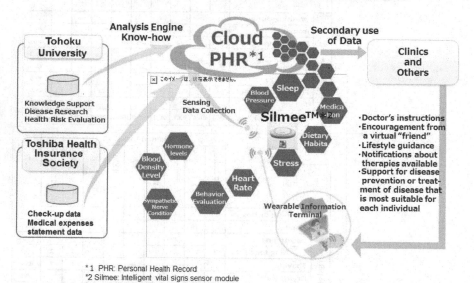

Tohoku University

Analysis Engine Know-how

Cloud PHR*1

Secondary use of Data

Clinics and Others

Knowledge Support Disease Research Health Risk Evaluation

Sensing Data Collection

Silmee™*2on

Blood Pressure | Sleep

Medica

Hormone levels

Dietary Habits

·Doctor's instructions
·Encouragement from a virtual "friend"
·Lifestyle guidance
·Notifications about therapies available
·Support for disease prevention or treatment of disease that is most suitable for each individual

Toshiba Health Insurance Society

Blood Density Level

Stress

Heart Rate

Check-up data Medical expenses statement data

Sympathetic Nerve Condition

Behavior Evaluation

Wearable Information Terminal

*1 PHR: Personal Health Record
*2 Silmee: Intelligent vital signs sensor module

Fig. 5. Toshiba's direction of medical electronics

Conclusion and Future Work

We developed a smartphone-based living-activity monitoring system to allay the anxiety of elderly people and that of their relatives, friends and caregivers by unobtrusively monitoring activities of daily living.

Toshiba continues to focus on the scheme of easy access to electronic medical records and sensing data concerning individuals' health in order to improve overall healthcare shown in Figure 5.

Acknowledgements. This research was partly supported by the Ministry of Internal Affairs and Communications, Japan.

References

1. Bao, L., Intille, S.S.: Activity Recognition from User-Annotated Acceleration Data. In: Ferscha, A., Mattern, F. (eds.) PERVASIVE 2004. LNCS, vol. 3001, pp. 1–17. Springer, Heidelberg (2004)
2. Maekawa, T., Yanagisawa, Y., Kishino, Y., Ishiguro, K., Kamei, K., Sakurai, Y., Oka-dome, T.: Object-Based Activity Recognition with Heterogeneous Sensors on Wrist. In: Floréen, P., Krüger, A., Spasojevic, M. (eds.) Pervasive 2010. LNCS, vol. 6030, pp. 246–264. Springer, Heidelberg (2010)
3. Miluzzo, E., et al.: Sensing Meets Mobile Social Networks: The Design, Implementation and Evaluation of the CenceMe Application. In: Proc. SenSys 2008, pp. 337–350 (2008)
4. http://www.cc.gatech.edu/fce/ahri/projects/
5. http://research.microsoft.com/apps/pubs/?id=68393
6. Yamazaki, T., et al.: Real-life Supporting Services by Distributed and Cooperative Service Platform "UKARI-Core": Development and Implementation at NICT Ubiquitous Home, UBI, IPSJ, 2004-11-10, pp. 71–77 (2004)
7. Ouchi, K., Suzuki, T., Doi, M.: LifeMinder A Wearable Healthcare Support System Using User's context. In: Proc. ICDCS Workshop 2002, pp. 791–792 (2002)
8. Suzuki, T., Ouchi, K., Kameyama, K.-I., Takahashi, M.: Development of a Sleep Monitoring System with Wearable Vital Sensor for Home Use. In: Proc. BIODEVICES 2009, pp. 326–331 (2009)
9. iSuppli Press Release (July 9, 2009)
10. http://www.isuppli.com/MEMS-and-Sensors/News/Pages/One-Third-of-Mobile-Phones-to-Use-Accelerometers-by-2010-Spurred-by-iPhone-and-Palm-Pre.aspx
11. Iso, T., Yamazaki, K.: Gait Analyzer based on a Cell Phone with a Single Three-axis Accelerometer. In: Proc. MobileHCI 2006, pp. 141–144 (2006)
12. Peltonen, V., Tuomi, J., Klapuri, A., Huopaniemi, J., Sorsa, T.: Computational auditory scene recognition. In: Proc. ICASSP 2002, pp. 1941–1944 (2002)
13. Ouchi, K., Doi, M.: Living activity recognition using off-the-shelf sensors on mobile phones. Annals of Telecommunications 67(7-8), 387–395 (2012)
14. Cho, K., et al.: Human Activity Recognizer for Mobile Devices with Multiple Sensors. In: Proc. UIC-ATC 2009, pp. 114–119 (2009)
15. Suzuki, T., et al.: Wearable wireless vital monitoring technology for smart health care. In: Proc. ISMICT 2013, pp. 1–4 (2013)

Recovery Prediction in the Framework of Cloud-Based Rehabilitation Exergame

Mohamad Hoda[1], Haiwei Dong[1,2], and Abdulmotaleb El Saddik[1,2]

[1] School of Electrical Engineering and Computer Science,
University of Ottawa
Ottawa, Ontario K1N 6N5, Canada
[2] Division of Engineering, New York University Abu Dhabi
Abu Dhabi, UAE
{mhoda053,hdong,elsaddik}@uottawa.ca

Abstract. In this paper, we propose a framework of a cost-effective, entertaining, and motivating home-based upper limb rehabilitation system which consists of a cloud system and a client interface. The framework provides real-time feedback to the patient subject, summarizes the feedback after each session, and predicts the rehabilitation performance. As an implementation of the framework, a Kinect sensor is used to collect real-time data for upper limb joints of the subjects while they are participating in rehabilitation exergames. The Dynamic Time Warping (DTW) algorithm is then applied to compare the movement pattern of a patient subject with the movement pattern of a healthy subject. Next, the Auto-Regressive Integrated Moving Average (ARIMA) is utilized to forecast the rehabilitation progress of the patients based on their performance history. The prototype of this system is tested on six healthy individuals and one patient. The results show that the patients' movement patterns have a similar curve shape to the healthy individuals' movement patterns and, hence, the DTW algorithm can be used as an effective index to describe the rehabilitation statuses of the subjects. The forecasting method is briefly tested by feeding the rehabilitation status history.

Keywords: Home-based Rehabilitation Framework, Model Matching, ARIMA Prediction, Virtual Reality.

1 Introduction

According to the World Health Organization (WHO), there are about ten million people who are injured in traffic accidents and fifteen million people who suffer from strokes every year. Of those, six million of those suffering from traffic-related injuries and five million of the stroke patients are permanently disabled [1,2]. These people need a special rehabilitation program that starts when the patient is admitted to the hospital and does not end, even after the patient has been discharged from the hospital. Also, in many cases, stroke patients suffer from depression, which leaves family members and caregivers to wonder how

C. Stephanidis and M. Antona (Eds.): UAHCI/HCII 2014, Part III, LNCS 8515, pp. 256–265, 2014.
© Springer International Publishing Switzerland 2014

they can motivate the patients and better engage them in the rehabilitation program.

Arm rehabilitation is a restorative process that aims to hasten and maximize the recovery of the patients in order to get them as close as possible to pre- injury levels. Researchers have revealed that duration, capacity, and intensity of the training session have a huge impact on the rate of rehabilitation improvement [3]. However, adhering to the strict guidelines of a long-term rehabilitation process might be cumbersome for many patients who do not have access to rehabilitation es in their communities. Consequently, those people are required to travel a long distance to get treatment. In addition, a long-term rehabilitation process can be expensive and unaffordable for patients who do not have adequate public or private health insurance.

Many therapists recommend that patients perform a daily life activity, such as making coffee, in order to improve their upper limb movements. Since such tasks may be dangerous for a patient with an arm injury, researchers have developed virtual and augmented reality systems where tangible objects are associated with a virtual object that simulates the real object [4,5]. The current technological advancements have brought new perspectives to the rehabilitation process. Researchers have designed computerized rehabilitation robotic tools associated with virtual environments and games which are meant to be used at home. Therapists use these tools to track the progress of patients. However, two of the common inconveniences for many of these rehabilitation devices are related to their bulky shape and the complexity of their deployment. Consequently, these shortcomings make them impractical for home training because they require the presence of an expert. Cost is also an important factor for many patients when acquiring such devices. For these reasons, most of the robotic-assisted therapy devices are commonly used in clinic centers or hospitals.

Besides informing family and close friends, showing the real progress to the patients is another significant motivating factor. This can increase the self-satisfaction, engagement, and enjoyment levels of patients [6]. Many time-series matching algorithms have been used to compare kinematics data obtained from patients with the data from healthy people [7,8]. However, those algorithms are used in systems where the user is required to wear a garment (which is a difficult task for many stroke patients.)

In this paper, we propose the framework of a cost-effective, entertaining, and motivating home-based upper limb rehabilitation system which consists of a cloud system and client interface. The framework provides real-time feedback to the patient subject, summarizes the feedback after each session, and predicts the rehabilitation performance. In addition, this framework shows a new style of home-based rehabilitation system that motivates the patients by engaging family and friends in the rehabilitation process, and allowing therapists to remotely assess the progress of the patients and adjust the training strategy accordingly. As an implementation of the framework, a Kinect sensor is used to collect real-time data from the upper limb joints of the subjects while they are participating in rehabilitation exergames [9,10]. The Dynamic Time Warping (DTW) algorithm is then applied to compare the movement pattern of a patient subject with the movement pattern of a healthy subject. Next, the Auto-Regressive Integrated Moving Average (ARIMA) is utilized to forecast the rehabilitation progress of the patients based on their performance history. The prototype of this system is tested on six healthy individuals and one patient. Results show that the patients' movements have a similar curve shape to that of the healthy individuals and hence the DTW algorithm can be used as an effective index to describe the rehabilitation status. The forecasting method is briefly tested by feeding the rehabilitation status history.

2   Framework Architecture

The high level architecture of the proposed cloud-based rehabilitation exergame is shown in Figure 1. The aim of this framework is to motivate patients through social engagement and provide doctors with a tool for continuous observation and rehabilitation strategy predictions. The major components of the proposed framework are briefly explained as follows:

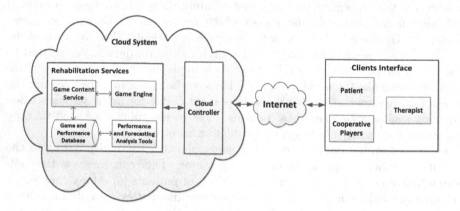

Fig. 1. The cloud-based rehabilitation exergame framework

Client Interface: Stroke patients and therapists are the users of the rehabilitation game system. The cooperative gamers (e.g., family members of the patient) are engaged in the rehabilitation exergames in order to motivate the patient subject in their rehabilitation process. A Kinect sensor is used to connect the system's users with each other through a cloud environment. Therapists guide the patients and monitor their progress through the rehabilitation course. Additionally, therapists can change the difficulty level of the rehabilitation exercises for both the patients and the cooperative players whenever it is needed.

Rehabilitation Services: Services needed by the users are provided through this module. It consists of game content services, game engine services, and performance assessment and rehabilitation forecasting services. The game content service is responsible for monitoring all the game-related logic by the help of the game and performance database. Moreover, it manages the connection between different system users and provides them with the necessary data. It should be noted that the game engine also performs logical operations and is responsible for synchronization. The difficulty level of the game is automatically adjusted at real-time to adapt to the patient's performance. As an implementation, a cloud-based rehabilitation exergame that has been developed for stroke rehabilitation is the Basketball game, which can be played by single or multiple users. The physical setup of the game is shown in Figure 2. The Basketball game is designed to measure the kinematics of the upper limb of the patient in the vertical direction. The performance evaluation module provides the clients with real-time feedback about the performance of the patients. The rehabilitation prediction module gives the doctors a prediction about the prospective recovery of the patients, depending on their rehabilitation history.

Cloud Controller: This component is responsible for instantiating a game session. Like a facilitator, this enables the communication between the gamers and the exergame servers. The cloud controller provides several services (including authentication, profile and activity management, game statistics, and notification management) to manage the whole exergame framework.

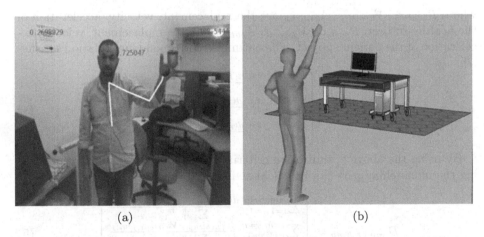

(a)   (b)

Fig. 2. Physical Environment of the Basketball game. (a) Experiment view. (b) Avatar view.

3 Forecasting of Rehabilitation Performance

We consider the movement pattern of a healthy subject (replacement, velocity, and acceleration) as a template, and the differences between the patient's movement pattern. This template indicates the recovery status of the patient. Specifically, a healthy subject's movement pattern is given as:

$$\text{Healthy Subject's Pattern} : \begin{cases} R_{healthy} = \begin{bmatrix} R_{healthy,1} & R_{healthy,2} & \cdots & R_{healthy,m} \end{bmatrix}^T \\ V_{healthy} = \begin{bmatrix} V_{healthy,1} & V_{healthy,2} & \cdots & V_{healthy,m} \end{bmatrix}^T \\ A_{healthy} = \begin{bmatrix} A_{healthy,1} & A_{healthy,2} & \cdots & A_{healthy,m} \end{bmatrix}^T \end{cases}$$

(1)

and a patient's movement pattern as:

$$\text{Patient's Pattern} : \begin{cases} R_{patient} = \begin{bmatrix} R_{patient,1} & R_{patient,2} & \cdots & R_{patient,n} \end{bmatrix}^T \\ V_{patient} = \begin{bmatrix} V_{patient,1} & V_{patient,2} & \cdots & V_{patient,n} \end{bmatrix}^T \\ A_{patient} = \begin{bmatrix} A_{patient,1} & A_{patient,2} & \cdots & A_{patient,n} \end{bmatrix}^T \end{cases}$$

(2)

To quantify the movement pattern between a healthy subject and a patient subject, we find a correspondence matching between these two patterns

$$\Theta \left(Healthy \ Subject's \ Pattern, \ Patient's \ Pattern \right) =$$

$$\begin{bmatrix} \Theta \left(R_{healthy}, R_{patient} \right) & \Theta \left(V_{healthy}, V_{patient} \right) & \Theta \left(A_{healthy}, A_{patient} \right) \end{bmatrix}^T$$

(3)

where $R_{healthy}$, $V_{healthy}$, $A_{healthy}$ are the replacement, velocity, acceleration of the healthy subject. $R_{patient}$, $V_{patient}$, $A_{patient}$ are the replacement, velocity, acceleration of the patient subject. The optimized correspondence relation satisfies [7]

$$\hat{\Theta} = arg \ min \begin{bmatrix} \sum_{i=1,j=1}^{i=m,j=n} \frac{d(R_{healthy,i}, R_{patient,j})p_{i,j}}{\sum_{i=1,j=1}^{i=m,j=n} p_{i,j}} \\ \sum_{i=1,j=1}^{i=m,j=n} \frac{d(V_{healthy,i}, V_{patient,j})q_{i,j}}{\sum_{i=1,j=1}^{i=m,j=n} q_{i,j}} \\ \sum_{i=1,j=1}^{i=m,j=n} \frac{d(A_{healthy,i}, A_{patient,j})r_{i,j}}{\sum_{i=1,j=1}^{i=m,j=n} r_{i,j}} \end{bmatrix}$$

(4)

By using the above optimization criteria, the cumulative distance representing the unmatching part can be calculated as

$$D_{unmatching} = \begin{bmatrix} \sum_{i=1,j=1}^{i=m,j=n} \frac{d(R_{healthy,i}, R_{patient,j})p_{i,j}}{\sum_{i=1,j=1}^{i=m,j=n} p_{i,j}} \\ \sum_{i=1,j=1}^{i=m,j=n} \frac{d(V_{healthy,i}, V_{patient,j})q_{i,j}}{\sum_{i=1,j=1}^{i=m,j=n} q_{i,j}} \\ \sum_{i=1,j=1}^{i=m,j=n} \frac{d(A_{healthy,i}, A_{patient,j})r_{i,j}}{\sum_{i=1,j=1}^{i=m,j=n} r_{i,j}} \end{bmatrix}$$

(5)

Then the patient's rehabilitation status is modeled as a combination of the elements of $D_{unmatching}$, i.e.,

$$\begin{cases} S_{rehabilitation} = w_1 \cdot D_{unmatching}[1] + w_2 \cdot D_{unmatching}[2] + w_3 \cdot D_{unmatching}[3] \\ w_1 + w_2 + w_3 = 1 \end{cases}$$

(6)

Although the patient's rehabilitation status ($S_{rehabilitation}$) at a given time gives the doctors an indication about the current situation of the patient, it does not help them to answer a simple, yet important question that patients and family members usually ask: what is the timetable for the recovery process? To answer this question, researchers have proposed statistical theories that are based on specific achievements by the patients [11,12]. However, these achievements may differ from one patient to another, and hence the prediction results have individual differences. In this paper, we forecast the recovery of the patients depending on their initial conditions and their progress rate. We use the Auto-Regressive Integrated Moving Average (ARIMA) model to forecast the future progress of the patients depending on their rehabilitation status $S_{rehabilitation}$ [13].

4   Results and Discussion

4.1   Model Matching

The reference dataset samples are obtained from six healthy people. The sets consist of ninety time series of kinematics values, i.e., the replacement, the velocity, and the acceleration (thirty series for each value). Two types of model matching approaches are applied: (1) real-time model matching that is used when the patient competes against a healthy subject, and (2) off-line model matching that is used when the patient competes with another patient, or he/she is performing the rehabilitation exergame alone. In the first approach, we compare the time series of the patient and the healthy subject in real-time and adjust the difficulty level of the game for both according to the patient's performance. In some cases, when the patient subject has difficulty completing the exergame task, a message is sent to the healthy subject asking them to slow down. In the second approach, the performance of the patient is compared to the reference movement pattern of a healthy subject that has already been stored in the system. The rehabilitation status ($S_{rehabilitation}$) is calculated and the difficulty level of the game changes accordingly.

The model matching result (between the healthy subjects and a patient subject) is shown in Figure 3 where (a), (b) and (c) correspond to the model matching results of replacement, velocity, and acceleration, respectively. The unit we use is: time in s, replacement in cm, velocity in cm/s, and acceleration in cm/s^2. We conclude that while the patient's movement pattern has a similar curve shape to the healthy subject's movement pattern, there are more isolations. The model matching differences (i.e., dynamic time warping distance) are 0.17, 0.11, and 0.13 respectively, corresponding with the replacement, velocity, and acceleration's case. In this paper, for simplicity, we choose $w_1 = w_2 = w_3 = \frac{1}{3}$ in the calculation of rehabilitation status (Equation 6) and thus $S_{rehabiltation} = 0.41$.

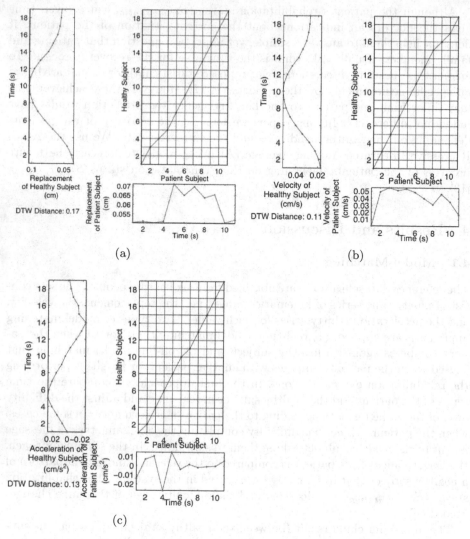

Fig. 3. Model matching between patient and healthy subject. (a) Replacement. (b) Velocity. (c) Acceleration.

4.2 Rehabilitation Prediction

The values of the rehabilitation status $S_{rehabilitation}$ are applied in the ARIMA predication model. Four rehabilitation sessions are conducted on one patient each week for seven weeks. The data obtained from the first six weeks is used for the model training, while the rest of the data is used for prediction. In this paper, we provide a simulation for short-term rehabilitation status prediction. To test the method used in creating rehabilitation prediction models, we suppose the measured rehabilitation status obtained in a continuous seven weeks as 0.41,

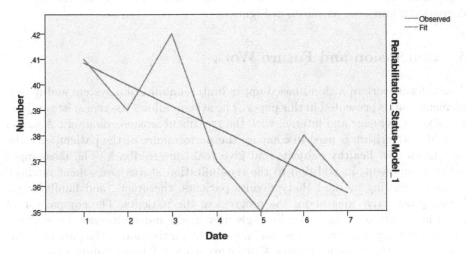

Fig. 4. Rehabilitation status prediction

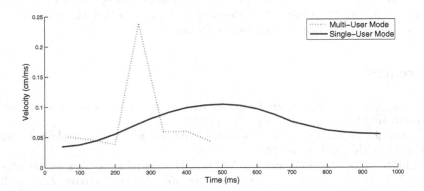

Fig. 5. The velocity comparison of the arm in reaching the final target under single-player mode and multi-player mode

0.39, 0.42, 0.37, 0.35, 0.38, 0.36, and we give the prediction model by our method in Figure 4. Here, the model type we used is ARIMA (0,0,0). The number of predictors is 1 and stationary R^2 is 0.522.

4.3 Multi-player's Benefit

The measurement of the hand velocities under single-user mode and multi-user mode are compared in Figure 5. As many previous studies have shown [14], the trajectory of the hand velocity is a bell-shaped curve. In addition, the results are consistent with what we expected: in the multi-user environment the players were competing with each other and thus, the time needed to complete the exercise decreased about 50% as shown in Figure 5.

5   Conclusion and Future Work

A new framework of a cloud-based upper limb rehabilitation system and its implementation is presented in this paper. The system allows the therapists and the caregivers to engage and interact with the treatment sessions remotely. A model matching algorithm is used to compare the performance of the patient with the performance of healthy subjects and give real-time feedback. The most innovative component, in addition to the rehabilitation status assessment method, is the forecasting method that provides patients, therapists, and family members a prospective idea about the progress of the patients. The comparison of the rehabilitation performance in single-user mode and multi-user mode shows that the multi-player exergames can increase the motivation of the patient to engage more in the training sessions. Our future work will be including a long-term study with ten patients to determine the accuracy of the system in predicting the progress of the patients. Moreover, we are planning to involve other kinematics parameters in the rehabilitation evaluation and test whether these parameters increase the accuracy of rehabilitation assessment.

References

1. Elsohairy, Y.: Fatal and injury fatigue-related crashes on Ontario's roads: A 5-year review. In: Driver Fatigue Symposium (2007)
2. Mackay, J., Mensah, G.: The atlas of heart disease and stroke. Technical report, World Health Organization (2004)
3. Nudo, R., Wise, B., SiFuentes, F., Milliken, G.: Neural substrates for the effects of rehabilitative training on motor recovery after ischemic infarct. Science 272, 1791–1794 (1996)
4. Hilton, D., Cobb, S., Pridmore, T., Gladman, J.: Virtual reality and stroke rehabilitation: A tangible interface to an every day task. In: Proceedings of the 4th International Conference on Disability, VirtualReality and Associated Technologies (2002)
5. Jack, D., Boian, R., Merians, A.S., Tremaine, M., Burdea, G.C., Adamovich, S.V., Recce, M., Poizner, H.: Virtual reality-enhanced stroke rehabilitation. IEEE Transactions on Neural Systems and Rehabilitation Engineering 9, 308–318 (2001)
6. Deci, E., Ryan, R.: Handbook of Self-Determination Research. University of Rochester Press (2002)
7. Tormene, P., Giorgino, T., Quaglini, S., Stefanelli, M.: Matching incomplete time series with dynamic time warping: an algorithm and an application to post-stroke rehabiltation. Artificial Intelligence in Medicine 45, 11–34 (2009)
8. Giorgino, T., Tormene, P., Maggioni, G., Pistarini, C., Quaglini, S.: Wireless support to poststroke rehabilitation: Myheart's neurological rehabilitation concept. IEEE Transactions on Information Technology in Biomedicine 13, 1012–1018 (2009)

9. Alamri, A., Cha, J., El Saddik, A.: Ar-rehab: An augmented reality framework for poststroke-patient rehabilitation. IEEE Transactions on Instrumentation and Measurement 59, 2554–2563 (2010)

10. Karime, A., Al-Osman, H., Aljaam, J.M., Gueaieb, W., El Saddik, A.: Tele-wobble: A tele-rehabilitation wobble board for lower extremity therapy. IEEE Transactions on Instrumentation and Measurement 61, 1816–1824 (2012)

11. Dong, H.W., Ugalde, I., Figueroa, N., El Saddik, A.: Towards whole body fatigue assessment of human movement: A fatigue-tracking system based on combined semg and accelerometer signals. Sensors 14, 2052–2070 (2014)

12. Dong, H.W., Luo, Z.W., Nagano, A., Mavridis, N.: An adaptive treadmill-style locomotion interface and its application in 3-d interactive virtual market system. Intelligent Service Robotics 5, 159–167 (2012)

13. Box, G.E.P., Jenkins, G.M., Reinsel, G.C.: Time Series Analysis: Forcasting and Control. Prentice Hall (1994)

14. Morasso, P.: Spatial control of arm movements. Experimental Brain Research 42, 223–227 (1981)

A Study on Effect of Media Therapy for the Elderly with Dementia to Nursing Care Quality

Miyuki Iwamoto[1], Noriaki Kuwahara[1], Kazunari Morimoto[1], Yoshihiro Niki[2], Doi Teruko[3], Yuka Kato[4], and Jin Narumoto[4]

[1] Kyoto Institute of Technology, Japan
cabotine.six.stars@gmail.com
[2] Vision Ace Co., Ltd., Japan
[3] T M Medical Service Co., Ltd., Japan
[4] Kyoto Prefectural University of Medicine, Japan

Abstract. Japanese society contains an extremely large elderly population, unprecedented elsewhere in the world. In fact, the elderly make up about 23.3% of the Japanese population. Consequently, the number of elderly people with dementia is also increasing at an unexpectedly rapid pace, with 10% of Japanese citizens over 65 diagnosed with dementia. While group homes are covered by the Japanese "Long-term Care Insurance System," and offer people with dementia a better quality of life, the behavioral and psychological symptoms of dementia, (BPSD,) often place a great burden on care staff. Many facilities now suffer from a shortage of care staff .Drug therapies have limited effects on BPSD, so non-pharmacological therapies, like reminiscence therapy, are sometimes used. However, the effects of these techniques are often not medically confirmed. In this study, we introduce a media therapy technique, which enhances reminiscence therapy by using media and information technologies, and report promising results for mitigating BPSD. Also, we investigate the keys to our success. So far, we have conducted our proposed media therapy on two residents in the nursing home. Both cases showed significant improvements, but due to space limitations, we only show the effects on the ability of the care staff to see to the patient's needs. The therapy session allowed care staff to distract the patient from her BPSD and calm her down by offering her topics from her past. For further investigation, we analyzed videos recorded during therapy sessions, with interesting results. Sharing a resident's good memories with care staff is key to quality care, and media and information technologies can facilitate this process. While we only examine one case here, we would like to note that the results of our other resident case indicated similar effects.

Keywords: elderly, reminiscence videos, senior care home, dementia.

1   Introduction

According to world population reports, in 2001, it was estimated that there were 24.3 million people with dementia. In developed regions, dementia rates for people over the age of 60 were reported between 4 and 6%. This number increases to 20-33% in

C. Stephanidis and M. Antona (Eds.): UAHCI/HCII 2014, Part III, LNCS 8515, pp. 266–277, 2014.
© Springer International Publishing Switzerland 2014

people over 85. Estimates suggest that the number of people diagnosed with dementia continues to grow at a rate of 4.6 million people annually, reaching 81.1 million people in 2040.

Population aging has accelerated rapidly in Japan, and now the aging rate is very high. There are 1.5 million people with dementia over the age of 65 in Japan today, but it is estimated that they will be over three million people in the 2020s, approaching 10 percent of the population over the age of 65. The increased number of people diagnosed with dementia is a major social problem that will only grow more serious in the future, as life expectancies continue to rise.

Dementia is quite varied in its symptoms, severity, and extent. We extracted the overview of the definition, types and symptoms of dementia from the dementia text book published by Japan Society of Dementia Research and described below [2].

Several definitions have been proposed, including in the World Health Organization's ICD-10, the DSM-III-R, and the DSM-IV-TR. Here, we provide an overview of dementia for those unfamiliar, largely taken from the Japan Society for Dementia Research's "Dementia Textbook." Differences aside, the concept remains the same. Dementia is a collection of impairments of previously normal intellectual function, caused by acquired brain dysfunction, which decreases mental performance. This includes such symptoms as memory loss, aphasia, and executive function disorder. For a symptom to be an "acquired dysfunction," it must involve a change in the organic material of the brain and lower the patient's intelligence. The ICD-10 states that this fault must be sustained for more than six months. The intellectual disability thus creates a strong effect on the patient's daily life and social behavior. It is not intended to be acute or temporary, and the above symptoms are also found in the absence of consciousness disturbances

Due to the damage to higher brain functions such as memory, orientation, knowledge, action, cognition, language, emotion, and personality, people with dementia become antagonistic towards situations in which they've placed themselves. Dementia can be induced by a variety of causes. Its pathology and symptoms are very diverse. Symptoms can be divided into core symptoms and peripheral symptoms. The core symptoms include memory impairment, executive function disorder, apraxia, aphasia, and agnosia. Patients with dementia may exhibit execution dysfunction, difficulty in initiating action, reduction of spontaneity, behavioral conversion dysfunction, impulsive behaviors, and disinhibition. Apraxia is a degradation of motor skills or coordination without any link to sensory impairment. Patients may be unable to put on clothes or use tools properly. Agnosia is an inability to recognize objects through use of the senses, including physical landmarks or other visual stimuli, as in visuospatial agnosia. It may also apply to sounds. "Peripheral symptoms" refers to various behavioral disorders and psychiatric symptoms that appear to be affected by the patient's environment and physical condition. This category includes delusions, hallucinations, anxiety, impatience, depression, wandering, aggressive behavior, sleep disorders, eating disorders, including binge eating and pica, and resistance to care, among others.

The Symptoms of "BPSD". The Behavioral and Psychological Symptoms of Dementia, or BPSD, are the "core symptoms" of dementia. It occurs in conjunction with memory loss, psychiatric symptoms, and a decline in comprehension ability, and was previously referred to as "problematic behavior" or "nuisance behavior". The symptoms are divided into behavioral and psychological symptoms, with more symptoms appearing as the dementia progresses from mild to moderate. Behavioral symptoms may include violence, verbal abuse, wandering, rejection, and unsanitary acts. As the manifestation of symptoms differs from person to person, all symptoms may not always appear. These symptoms appear frequently as dementia progresses from mild to moderate, leading to a rapid decrease in quality of life accordingly, and an increased burden on caregivers.

As symptoms develop and progress, dementia patients often become apathetic, entering a lethargic state. They lose the desire to do things themselves, and eventually lose interest in everything, even daily life. Patients with vascular dementia, often caused by repeated mild strokes, often become apathetic. Uninterested even in getting dressed or washing their faces, patients with apathy cause great mental stress for family members and caregivers. Apathy can also lead to a patient becoming bedridden, due to disuse of physical and mental functions. Drug therapy is often unsuccessful in treating apathy. As drug therapy is often ineffective, caregivers reach out to patients with touch and eye contact, and address the patient by name. Getting close to patients is thought to help them maintain their bodily functions and cognitive functions.

Also, the frequency of sleep disorders is very high in elderly patients with organic brain diseases, such as dementia. In fact, the symptoms which are most frequently observed in limbic dementia are insomnia, irregular sleep patterns, (such as day-night reversal,) and sleep-related disorders, such as delirium. In many insomnia cases, patients do not remain in bed, which leads to behavioral disorders such as wandering, agitation, excitement, and even violence. Caregivers and family members often become exhausted before the patient tires. As a result, it is difficult for some elderly people with dementia and behavioral disorders like night wandering to receive home care. This has become one of the biggest reasons leading to their institutionalization [1].

Drug therapy for dementia is presently limited to therapeutic medication, but these medicines are basically for Alzheimer's disease. In Alzheimer's disease, anticholinesterase inhibitors such as donepezil hydrochloride are effective, but these are symptomatic drugs, which only suppress its progress to a certain extent [2].

As drug therapy to eradicate dementia does not currently exist, it is necessary to increase the therapeutic effects of non-drug therapy.

Currently, reminiscence therapy is a well-known non-drug psychological and social therapy for dementia. Reminiscence therapy is a form of psychotherapy used mainly for the elderly, first used in the early 1960s by Dr. Robert Butler. Butler believed that elderly people's talk about memories is meaningful, though it had previously been regarded as the "tedious talk of old age." Simply put, reminiscence therapy asks patients to talk about their memories, either one-on-one or in small groups.

This is part of daily life, and perhaps nothing special, but the act serves several different psychological functions. The conversation is not used strictly as psychotherapy, but also as an activity in intergenerational exchanges or community activities.

At the moment, reminiscence therapy is gaining attention as a non-drug therapy in both clinical psychology and medical institutions, such as nursing care facilities and long-term care facilities. With the increase in number of the elderly requiring care and assistance, preventive care has become an important part of welfare. Additionally, research has suggested that reminiscence, including conversation with people, is effective at preventing or slowing the onset of dementia. This method draws attention to respecting the feelings and experiences of each individual. Non-drug treatments such as day care are also essential, but some regard for the caregivers, who exhaust themselves physically and mentally caring for their patients, is also important. In many cases, patients do not get enough conversation partners due to the decreasing staff-to-patient ratio. Enhancing the support for both caregivers and patients is thus an important issue. Various methods have been proposed to help improve for patients and their families so far. In this study, we created an interactive digital photo album using old photos of the patient, and showed it to the patient, her family, and nursing staff together over a large screen. We then conducted media-based reminiscence therapy, enjoying the conversation with the patient. Reminiscence therapy is believed to stabilize the mental condition of elderly people suffering from dementia, and reduce behavioral disorders. This therapy was also conducted using old tools, toys, or photos, in a group led by experienced listening staff. Our reminiscence therapy is different from general cases, since the patient, her family, and the nursing staff became a therapy group while using the photo album. Using photographs and visual stimuli to aid memory recall is considered effective in reducing the psychological disorders and behavioral disturbances of dementia.

In this study, we focused on the content and photographic images when the patient, family, and staff engaged in conversation using media therapy, and hope to quantify those images effective at promoting stable actions and mental condition in the patient.

The process of the media treatment is as follows.

First, the family of the patient provided old photographs of the patient's life. In order to make the media therapy "album of memories" [2], the editor listened to stories about the patient associated with old photos, selected a portion of the patient's history, then copied the selected photos to an iPad as a digital photo album. The photos were arranged in chronological order and categorized by story. After that, the patient had six weekly media therapy sessions, each lasting 60 minutes. Family and staff were present for all sessions, and the photos were displayed on a large screen.

2   Experiment

2.1   Experiment Abstract

In this study, for the patient, her family members, and nursing staff participating in the media therapy, we quantified the effects of the therapy and to what degree it elicited mental and behavioral changes in the patient.

This experiment was conducted with the assumption that all those present for the therapy participated in group sessions actively and had a positive relationship. The purpose of the experiment was to verify what kinds of images produced a positive response, and associate the images with their effects after the session, by recording the sessions with a video camera. We analyzed the patient's expression and speech during therapy. We also carried out interviews with the patient's family and close nursing staff.

2.2   Contents of Experiment

In the experiment, we allowed the patient, her family, and care staff to freely talk about the memories associated with the photographs presented. This process is referred to as media therapy, which is a type of reminiscence therapy. Reminiscence therapy is said to be an effective conversational support in suppressing dementia. It often helps stabilize individuals with dementia and reduces behavioral disorders. Normally, It is done in groups led by experienced staff using items such as old tools, toys, photos, and paintings. Media therapy is quite different from standard reminiscence therapy in that we create a digital photo album using photographs from the patient's life, and the therapy is carried out using that album, with family and care staff who are close to the patient.

2.3   Experiment Environment

Figure 1 shows the state of the experiment. Figure 2 shows the equipment used in the experiment. Figure 3 shows the layout of the experimental environment. This experiment was carried out using the multi-purpose room of the nursing facility. As shown in Figure 3, conversation was conducted with the patient's family sitting next to her, and the nursing staff further away. Images were displayed on a large screen as shown in Figure 1, and an iPad was used as shown in Figure 2. The iPad was put at the patient's side, and experiment staff was waiting behind the patient in order to change to the next photo. The experiment staff changed to the next slide whenever they got the signal from the family member, or when too much time was taken on any particular slide. As shown in the environment layout in Figure 3, we set three video cameras to capture the change in the patient's expression. One was placed in position to capture the patient's reactions; the second was placed to capture all participants; the third was placed to capture the large screen at the front.

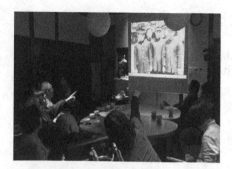

Fig. 1. The state of the experiment

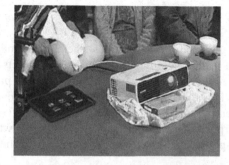

Fig. 2. The equipment used in the experiment

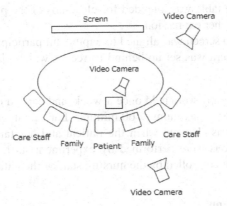

Fig. 3. The layout of the experimental environment

2.4   Experiment Participants

Our participants for this experiment were one elderly resident of a nursing home, one member of her family, and several members of the nursing home staff.

Nursing Home Resident

Age: 80s

Difficulty of daily life due to dementia: Moderate

Symptoms of dementia: Moderate

Diagnosis: Alzheimer's with mild memory failure

Problem in care assistance: Habitual of delusion and wandering (BPSD)

The resident participating in our study had developed a wandering habit and a delusion habit consisting of a distrust of familiar people, such as nursing staff and family.

2.5   Experimental Methods

The media therapy was performed as follows.

— Acquire photographs from the nursing home resident's life from her family.

— Interview family members about episodes associated with the photo in advance.

— - Choose the most memorable episodes in the patient's life as content for each session.

— Create an interactive digital photo album on the iPad using the photos that have been selected. Photos are classified according to the event or story, and sorted in chronological order.

— In each session, the resident, her family, and nursing staff discussed the photos presented in the multipurpose room freely, as the photos were presented on the screen.

— Each session was recorded with cameras, positioned as shown in Figure 3.
— The camera on the table was intended for close-ups of the patient's face during the session, to monitor her expression.
— The camera next to screen was aligned to capture all participants in the session.
— A third video camera was set up behind to record which photo is being displayed on the screen.

Sessions of media therapy were held once a week, and carried out a total of six times. Each session lasted for a maximum of 60 minutes. Each photograph was displayed for several minutes, or was changed when the patient and her family wanted a change. The first few transitions were performed by experiment staff, but further transitions between pictures were controlled by the nursing staff or the patient's family.

2.6   Evaluation Items

Three cameras were used to capture the resident's expressions and actions throughout the sessions. In addition, we recorded the conversation, and used it as a guide to help gauge the strength of her responses. We compared it to her expression to see which photographs brought her pleasure or joy. Facial expressions were correlated with emotions in a previous study [2]. In addition, after the session, changes observed in the patient during and after therapy were discussed and recorded in interviews with her family and care staff.

2.7   Analysis of Expression

The expressions of the patient were analyzed from the video recordings. Analysis was carried out using the major literature "expression analysis" techniques, to understand which photos made her look happier or more joyful [3]. This document defines expressions of happiness as follows.

— Lower eyelids rise, eyes narrow
— Pupils dilate
— Wrinkles appear in the outer corners and beneath the eyes
— The mouth opens to expose the teeth as the upper lip rises and the lower lip lowers.
— Grooves or wrinkles appear over the corners of the mouth from the sides of the nose

These conditions, usually in conjunction, characterized a "happy" or "joyful" expression.

In this expression analysis, we expressed the degree of smile on a frame-by-frame basis. We defined 0% as an expressionless state that does not laugh at all, and 100% as a state of highest laughter. We used the highest degree of smile expressed as the result for each photograph displayed.

3   Results

The results of the experiment described in section 2.5 are shown below.

In Figure 4, we show the results of the expression analysis from the content of the video recorded during the experiment. As the photograph was changed roughly every 2 minutes, the average smile time was about 2 minutes per photo. Figure 4 places the contents of the video on the horizontal axis, and the degree of the patient's smile on the vertical axis.

The alphabet of the horizontal axis indicates the following.

A: Images from the patient's time as a nursing student (16 pieces)
B: Images of the patient's newlywed days (25 pieces)
C: Images of the patient's marriage and child-rearing days (17 pictures)
D: Images of the patient's family and home during her middle age (23 pictures)
E: Images of the patient's time as a nurse (21 pieces)

In this expression analysis, we expressed the degree of smile on a frame-by-frame basis. We defined 0% as an expressionless state that does not laugh at all, and 100% as a state of highest laughter. We used the highest degree of smile expressed as the result for each photograph displayed.

From the results of the session shown in Figure 4, we can see that the patient's smile became more pronounced when we were talking about her time as a nurse and as a nursing student, (letters A and E.) The photographs for sessions B to D are from her life after working as a nurse, covering the time from her marriage through her middle age. We found that there tended to be more smiles when the topic of her time as a nurse arose. In addition, as a result of the (significance level 5%) t-test of the degree of smile in each video, we recognized a significant difference between the smiles related to her time as a nurse and the others.

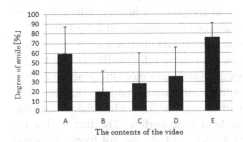

Fig. 4. Degree of smile

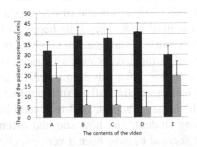

Fig. 5. Time of not smile and smile

Figure 5 shows the average time that the smiled for each type of image during the 60 minutes session. The vertical axis represents the degree of the patient's expression. The horizontal axis shows the contents of the video. The labels A to E are the same as in Figure 4. The left side of the bar in the graph indicates no expression, the right indicates a smile. Figure 5 shows more smiles for photos related to topics A and E. We also observed a low tendency towards lack of smile for topics B to D. In addition, due to the onset of BPSD before starting the fourth session, the patient's mental state before the session was worse than usual. However, the session started with a story from the patient's time as a nurse, so there was no significant difference compared to two other times when we talked about her family. We believe that when we talk about her time working as a nurse, her emotions are more changeable and more apparent. The graph shows that the amount of time unsmiling is longer than the time spent smiling. This is because the patient concentrated on the image for a long time to find a particular person or herself in the photo. Thus, she tended to smile less while concentrating. Also, as a result of the (significance level 5%) t-test on each video, we recognized a significant difference between the subject's time as a nurse and other topics. Considering the general positive response of the patient and the reports of care staff, the results of this experiment showed that the patient tended to look happier to talk with her family and nursing staff during therapy than at other times. It is possible that the patient herself felt special to have so many people gathered about her just to take part in her reminiscence. During second session, the conversation turned to a time when the patient's family suffered misfortune. When the patient discussed this period, the care staff honestly felt that the patient had been through a hard time and struggled, but the family members participating in the session had doubts as to the content of the conversation. It is considered possible that the patient's story was not necessarily true in some parts.

In the fourth session, emotional incontinence had been observed in the patient before the session began. At the start of the session, we used photographs from when the patient was working as a nurse at a university hospital. This seemed to cause a change in the patient's feelings. After that, there was no significant change in sentiment even after a story of her home and family. From this, we believe that it was the content of her memories from when she was working as a nurse that made her feelings milder.

From about the fourth therapy session, changes also appeared in the patient's family. Gradually, they began to show understanding towards the patient's caregivers. We believe this change was due to learning more of the patient's history, which they did not know until now. They thus began to understand the patient, little by little. Also, one of the nursing staff made a notable comment during an interview after completing the media therapy. After media therapy, when the patient fell into BPSD, the burden of calming her down was dramatically reduced, as staff had more clues about how to let the feelings of the patient subside. For example, in case the patient tries to escape from the nursing facility, staff reminded her of an episode from when the patient was a nursing student, and how she had often defeated the curfew. The fact is that the patient seemed to have been a very excellent student, but she did not forget the sense of fun she had felt during the therapy. Staff and family felt that this story was told with a touch of pride. This episode struck a sympathetic chord with the patient. After that, she did not attempt to escape.

4   Differences from before and after Therapy

The following three points from the patient's care record indicate changes brought about as a result of therapy. First, Figure 6 shows the hours the staff spent sharing

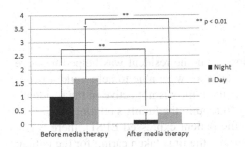
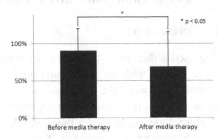

Fig. 6. The hours the staff spent sharing with the patient

Fig. 7. The time that the patient appealed to nursing staff

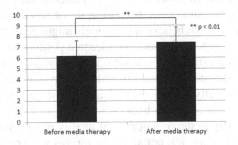

Fig. 8. Sleep time

with the patient night and day. Figure 7 shows the time that the patient appealed to nursing staff. Figure 8 shows the patient's sleep times.

Figure 6 shows the time on the vertical axis, before and after therapy on the horizontal axis. The left side of the graph shows daytime, and the right shows night. After therapy, the time spent with the patient was significantly reduced to less than 30 minutes both at night and during the daytime, while before therapy that time was about one hour at night and over one hour during the day. When the patient spoke to nursing staff before therapy, staff had difficulty understanding how to calm her down, but after therapy, they had a better understanding of what topics to use. We believe this is why care time decreased so significantly after therapy. In addition, we compared the patient's complaints to nursing staff before and after therapy. We found that the patient complained nearly 90% of the time, almost every day, before therapy, but only 70% of the time after the therapy. We believe the nursing staff were able to make a conversation with the patient, and use what they learned during therapy to help make the patient happy. We examined the patient's sleep time before and after therapy.

The sleep time is on the vertical axis, before and after therapy on the horizontal axis. We found that after therapy, the patient was able to sleep longer than before.

5   Conclusion and Future Topics

5.1   Discussion

Using media therapy, wherein an elderly nursing home resident was helped to share her life history with her family and nursing staff, we were able to help build a better relationship between the three parties. Even if the family is not active in the resident's care, we believe this provides an opportunity to rebuild the family's relationship.

Before undergoing media therapy, when the patient expressed BPSD, there was a serious burden on the nursing staff. After therapy, the time taken caring for the patient and subsequent stress on care staff was significantly reduced, as staff had better knowledge of the patient's personality and emotional triggers.

After several sessions of therapy, the patient felt more able to talk about her past. Furthermore, even if the patient's mental state is agitated at the beginning of a session, gradually, she was able to calm down, because a lot of people were paying attention and listening to her stories. We believe that patients might be able to forget their misgivings about the future by talking about the pleasant portions of the past. Thus, even if the patient experienced extreme emotional ups and downs, or BPSD, by participating in media therapy, other people would be able to help stabilize the patient and provide better care. Additionally, media therapy allows the patient to return to normal spirits in a short time, rather than be trapped in feelings of discord. We believe this approach might be the key to improving patient quality of life. While all images used were tied to the patient's memories, not all of the images were necessarily tied to positive memories. We believe it best to work to identify those images and experiences that bring the patient happiness. These images and memories provide better tools with which to calm the patient down, and can be discovered during therapy.

5.2   Summary and Future Challenges

The media therapy that we have proposed is a potential treatment, part of dementia care for elderly people who have been placed in long-term care facilities.

By providing a case study, we have shown the improvements that can be expected: the quality of services can be improved, family ties can be rebuilt, and the burden on care staff can be reduced.

In analyzing the patient's facial expressions, we found that the freest smiles came from memories that made the patient want to boast the most, when she talked about the times she most enjoyed. We found that the patient examined the pictures related to these memories more seriously.

We regard the fact that the family participated in the session together, and were able to know a side of the patient that did not know before, as a great achievement. However, if family members talk more than the patient, the patient would often nod, occasionally agreeing or prompting the conversation forward, saying little other than, "Yes," "No," or, "Is that so?" In the future, when family members participate, we will need to encourage the patient to speak more freely about others' remarks. For this reason, it may be necessary to set up a system to signal the family members without the patient noticing if the patient seems to be growing bored or restless.

To enable longer conversations, this time, staff created the digital photo album manually. However, it would be more convenient to have a database of photos relevant to the patient, and construct the photo albums that way. These are our challenges for the future.

We would like to consider a system that can search videos and images easily using a touch panel, so that it can be easily manipulated without special staff, with media categorized in different folders. While we were able to conduct these sessions in one location, we would also like to consider more difficult situations, as when the family and resident are separated by a long distance. In these cases, some manner of PC or tablet PC software would allow therapy to take place, provided care staff could be trained in its use.

Lastly, we would like this system to be usable as a remote interactive system, but also serve as a way for families, local residents, medical staff, or volunteers to monitor elderly people who live independently.

Acknowledgement. This work was supported by KAKENHI 24650037.

References

1. Kazuo, M.: Sleep Disorders and Sleep Medicine in Demented Patients. Psychiatria et Neurologia Japonica 114(2) (2012)
2. Noriaki, K., Kazuhiro, K., Shinji, A., Kenji, S., Kiyoshi, Y.: Video memories that utilize annotation of photo–Application and evaluation to persons with dementia - - making support. Artificial Intelligence Journal 20(6), 396–405 (2005)
3. Tomomi, O., Mariko, T., Mariko, A., Naoko, K., Yukikazu, S.: Expression analysis- Comparison of the characteristics of the facial expression. Proposed by Ekman (2010)

Neurological Disorders and Publication Abstracts Follow Elements of Social Network Patterns when Indexed Using Ontology Tree-Based Key Term Search

Anand Kulanthaivel[1,2,*], Robert P. Light[1], Katy Börner[1],
Chin Hua Kong[1], and Josette F. Jones[2]

[1] Indiana University Bloomington (Cyberinfrastructure for Network Science,
Information & Library Science), Bloomington 47405 USA
[2] Indiana University-Purdue University Indianapolis (BioHealth Informatics),
Indianapolis 46202 USA
{akulanth,lightr,katy,kongch}@indiana.edu,
jofjones@iupui.edu

Abstract. Disorders of the Central Nervous System (CNS) are worldwide causes of morbidity and mortality. In order to further investigate the nature of the CNS research, we generate from an initial reference a controlled vocabulary of CNS disorder-related terms and ontological tree structure for this vocabulary, and then apply the vocabulary in an analysis of the past ten years of abstracts (N = 10,488) from a major neuroscience journal. Using literal search methodology with our terminology tree, we find over 5,200 relationships between abstracts and clinical diagnostic topics. After generating a network graph of these document-topic relationships, we find that this network graph contains characteristics of document-author and other human social networks, including evidence of scale-free and power law-like node distributions. However, we also found qualitative evidence for Z-normal-type (albeit logarithmically skewed) distributions within disorder popularity. Lastly, we discuss potential consumer-centered as well as clinic-centered uses for our ontology and search methodology.

Keywords: Ontology, information retrieval, neuroscience, networks, indexing, knowledge gaps, semantic medicine, translational medicine, knowledge discovery, neurology, psychiatry.

1   Introduction

Research in the field of biomedical science associating publications with explicit clinical diagnostic terms is lacking. While central nervous system (CNS) disorders are a major cause of morbidity and mortality worldwide, there have been no studies to date on correlates between clinical and basic neuroscience terminology.

---

* Corresponding author.

C. Stephanidis and M. Antona (Eds.): UAHCI/HCII 2014, Part III, LNCS 8515, pp. 278–288, 2014.
© Springer International Publishing Switzerland 2014

Given a controlled vocabulary (CV) whose members are organized into a tree-structured ontology, it is possible to search for biomedical or clinical meaning in a corpus of abstracts or other publication identifiers [1, 2]. If such an analysis is performed, one result may be the return of another ontology (this time, document-to-topic). The properties of such a network, as with any network, may be explored using basic social graph metrics [3].

Degree-based centrality (connectedness) is one measure of the influence of a node. Distributions of node centralities (including node degrees) have been postulated to allow conclusions to be drawn about a network in general given its centrality distributions [4]; Barabasi [5] in particular states that social-like network distributions, such as the power law distribution, are seen in a variety of situations that extend beyond sociology. Milojevic [6] proposes that modifications of power laws are allowed, including modification resulting in a Pareto Type-2 distribution. Finally, ranks among degree centralities of entities are proposed by Frasco et al [7] to have a geographic-social basis, possibly one laid on the foundations of individual-level interactions.

Therefore, a computational study of neuroscience publications with respect to clinical topics is likely to yield useful clues as to the *aboutness* of these publications and also reveal any topic bias(es). In particular, *Brain Research*, one particularly influential neuroscience journal with over 55,000 publications to date [8], provides an exemplar for a publication network of CNS-related topics. In this study, the past ten years (2004-2013) of abstracts written for *Brain Research* are analyzed against clinical terms from the Merck Manual for Professionals (in particular, the sections on neurological [9] and psychiatric [10] disorders).

2   Materials and Methods

2.1   Ontology Construction

The ontology and controlled vocabulary used in this study was derived from the Merck Manual for Professionals, particularly the sections on CNS pathologies [9, 10]. From this source, we found ninety-six (96) unique disorders. Each disorder super-heading was made into one diagnostic entity. Using the discretion of the authors, discrete and exclusive key words and key terms were mapped to each diagnostic entity. Therefore, a structure of disorder-to-keywords was created for each disorder. One example of a disorder-keywords tree as used here is seen in Figure 1.

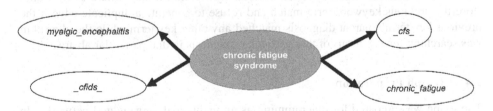

Fig. 1. Ontology map visualized (example; one of 96). Chronic fatigue syndrome is the diagnosis, and the entities it points to are the machine-searchable key terms that this diagnosis maps to.

2.2   Querying and Basic Information Retrieval

Information retrieval was performed by using the query term Brain Research[journal] in PubMed [11]. In order to represent the most recent cohort of documents, the search was filtered to only include articles published from 2004-2013. The result set was downloaded in XML format, and a raw corpus data file created using the Python scripting language. The output generated by the Python script formatted the corpus as PMID,abstract where PMID is the PubMed Identifier (PMID) for each article and abstract represents the abstract text of the article. Furthermore, in order to enhance machine parsing, all punctuation within abstract texts was removed and replaced with the underscore (_) symbol.

A separate file was created in order to contain the ontology trees. The format for each individual disorder tree was *disorder:key_term_1,key_term_2*, with each disorder having one or more key terms. For example, the ontology tree visualized in the above Figure 1 would have been represented in our search word file as *chronic_fatigue_syndrome: _cfs_, _cfids_,chronic_fatigue,myalgic_encephalitis*. Note the underscores surrounding acronyms; these are used to exclude words that might contain these strings as substrings. Underscores were also utilized to facilitate disambiguation of actual words that were less than four characters in length.

2.3   Parsing and Knowledge Synthesis

In order to create a graph-like representation of our subject-object construction (and in turn, discover which abstracts were related to which disorders), the PMID/abstract output file was searched against the ontology tree file, and positive matches sent to output in a network tool-readable edge list.

For this purpose, we wrote a custom program in Java (Virtual Machine; JVM) using the Eclipse IDE software tool [12]. The search algorithm utilized was literal, searching explicitly through the corpus file for disorder key words. As output, the algorithm generated an edge list file, with each line being an edge, the left node being the PMID, and the right node being the disorder topic that the matching key term was mapped to in the ontology tree file.

Of remark is that our algorithm was able to avoid parallel edges while constructing an edge list: Should the above document have contained cfs, cfids, and chronic fatigue, our algorithm will only output the pair 99999999,chronic_fatigue_syndrome once. This referential integrity was enforced by creating a step where JVM would store the previous keyword term match and refuse to generate a duplicate edge if the previous key term's parent diagnosis matched any other key term while the algorithm was searching for key terms of that particular diagnosis in that particular abstract.

2.4   Graph Preparation

The graph was prepared for diagramming as an undirected, unweighted network. In addition, the graph, while not explicitly bipartite as stated in the edge list, was of a bipartite topology (refer to Figures 2 and 3 for details).

2.5   Graph Visualization and Metrics

The Sci2 software tool (v1.1b) [13] was utilized for initial visualization and metrics computing. Specifically, the DrL layout within Sci2 [14] was used in order to gravitate the node positions for better viewing. Sci2 was then used to compute degree centrality measures for publications and disorders.

Correlations between degree measures were performed by exporting Sci2-generated data tables into Microsoft Excel [15] and analyzing and plotting the data in Excel for the histograms as well as for the disorder degree-rank scatter plot. Power analysis and regressions were performed in SAS v9.4 [16].

3   Results and Conclusions

3.1   Match Rates

Match Rate of Publications. Recall from our abstract that we searched 10,488 papers (i.e., the result set returned from Brain Research as [journal] term in PubMed, with the range set to past 10 years, and papers that only have available abstracts). 5,269 relationships were established between topics and publications. We noted that 4,163 papers (39.7%) had abstracts that matched the key terms in our ontology, yielding a corresponding miss rate of 60.3%. However, due to the limited terminology set of the current ontology tree, we chose to use graph analysis for the sub-corpus of publications whose abstracts did match our tree.

One must nonetheless realize that the low match rate, despite our best efforts in engineering the ontology for matching documents, may point to a disconnect (or knowledge gap) between science and medicine. On the other hand, there exists the possibility that many studies are carried out in order to study the normal functioning in the CNS (as opposed to disorder or pathology).

Disorder-Terminology Match Rate. Out of the 96 disorders found in the CNS section of the Merck Manual, 68 of these matched with publications via our ontology tree, yielding a disorder match rate of 70.8%.

3.2   Network Visualization

Network visualization yielded 9 graph components, with the giant component holding 99.6% of all nodes. Therefore, only the giant component is visualized in Figure 2.

Remarks on Visual Topology. In our network graph (Figure 2), it is visually clear that a relatively small proportion of disorders studied held a wide amount of publication attention, while most disorders held relatively little attention. Some disorders in this layout appear to cluster via having many shared publications. For example, it is clearly visible in Figure 2 that the entity stroke is well linked with tbi (traumatic brain injury). This particular linkage is viewed more closely in Figure 3.

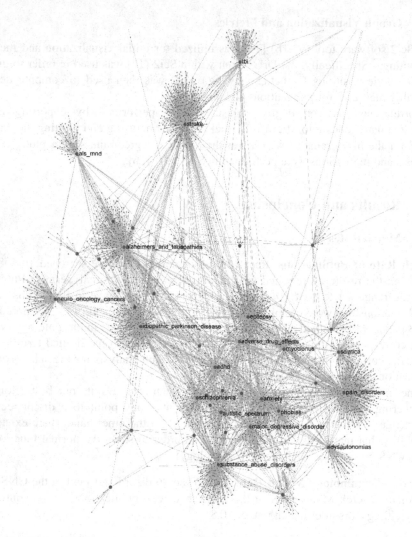

Fig. 2. Graph visualization of a majority of network giant component, performed using the DrL algorithm in the Sci2 Tool. Some high-profile disorders (Degree Centrality > 100) are highlighted by visible text labels. Most remaining disorders are highlighted by slightly larger node circles.

Nonetheless, the linkage model must be viewed with some degree of suspicion, as stroke was found to be linked to 482 publications and TBI to 143. Therefore, while it was possible in theory to have 143 mutual matches between the two disorders, only 12 were observed, as seen in Figure 3.

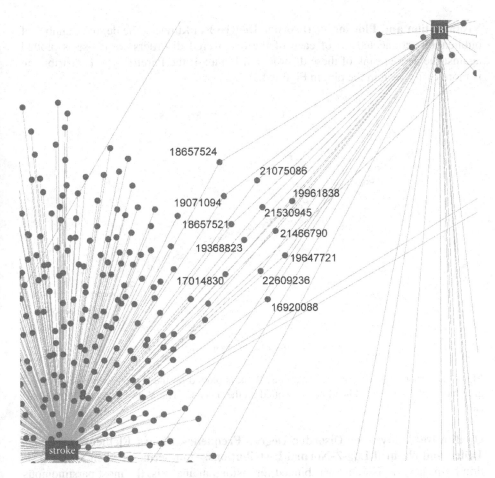

Fig. 3. Close-up view of two disorders our visualization and algorithm imply to be closely related. In this example, we see the entities *stroke* and *tbi* (traumatic brain injury) linked to each other by multiple publications, noted by their PMIDs.

3.3   Results of Graph Analysis

Regression of Ranking: Disorder Degree Centrality.   In order to confirm the hypothesis of logarithmic distribution upon disorder degree rank, we transformed degree by log (base 10) function and then regressed against degree rank.

SAS returned a single variable power of disorder degree of > 0.999 at a = 0.05 for the series of disorder degrees.   Single-factor ANOVA resulted in an F-value of 6710.15 (df = 66), and Pr > F was < 0.0001.   The R-squared (RSQ) value for the regression was 0.990.   P values for the slope and intercept of regression were both < 0.0001 (t stat = 132.19 for intercept and t stat = -81.92 for slope, respectively).   Such a strong fit in the context of this linear-logarithmic transformation suggests a Pareto Type-2 distribution [6] and elements of Barabasi's theory of scale-free deterministic distributions [5] within the knowledge domain (neuroscience) at study.

Visualization and Plotting of Disorder Degree Rankings. The degree (number of publications connected to) of each of the discovered disorders we chose is plotted against the degree rank of these disorders in Figure 4; the Pareto-Type II distribution is more easily seen in the plot in Figure 4.

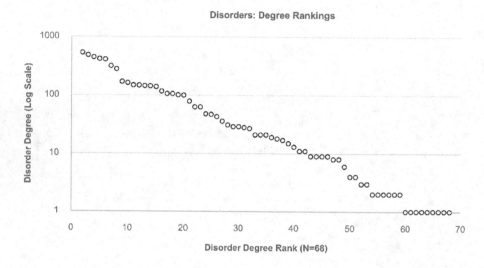

Fig. 4. Disorder degree-to-rank correlations. Rank is plotted on the X-axis, while disorder degree (connectedness to publications) is plotted on the Y-axis. The Y-axis is scaled logarithmically.

Qualitative Analysis of Disorder Degree Frequency Shows Elements of Long-Tailed and Natural Log-Z-Normal Distributions. Furthermore, when the publication frequency of disorders was binned for histogram analysis, the most parsimonious fit to a typical Z-type distribution appearance was obtained not by using linearly-sized bins, but instead, bins sized to powers of e (Euler's number; i.e., exponential binning was used). However, in our e-power histogram, there is still a peak of papers in bins corresponding to zero and one matches. This relationship is visualized in Figure 5. Topics of unusually high degree included pain disorders (D = 530 publications), stroke (D = 482 publications), and anxiety disorders (D = 279 publications).

Qualitative Analysis of Publication Degree Frequency. Shows a Logarithmic-Linear Distribution. Similarly, degree for each publication was analyzed (i.e., how many disorders each publication would connect to). It appears that most publications were connected to only one disorder, while a few yielded matches with several disorders. The highest number of disorders matched for any abstract was six, with three abstracts matching six disorders each. A logarithmically-scaled histogram shows the linear-logarithmic trend in decreasing frequency of publications with respect to increasing topic degrees (Figure 6).

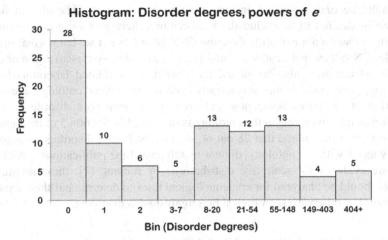

Fig. 5. Exponentially-binned histogram (powers of Euler's number) of disorder-to-publication degree distribution, shown on a linear frequency axis. Powers are rounded to the nearest whole number(s). A bin for unmatched disorders (degree = 0) is also included for reference on the far left of this figure.

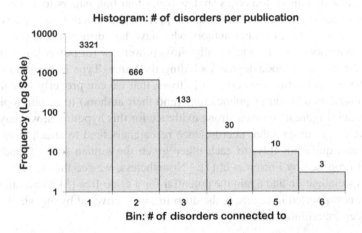

Fig. 6. Histogram of publication-to-disorder degrees (linear bin scale, logarithmic frequency scale). If non-matches were included in this histogram as they were included in Figure 5, another bin of magnitude 6,315 would be present to the left of the first bin.

4   Analysis and Discussion

4.1   Potential Reasons for Low Match Rate

Of great concern is that our model failed to match 60.3% of Brain Research abstracts. At this stage, we can only hypothesize upon the reasons for the lack of matching; a relatively small ontology (with only 260 base terms representing 96 disorders) could be of fault; the ontology must, in our opinions, be widened. The idea of full-text searching is also not to be excluded. Furthermore, there may exist large number of publications that do not explicitly describe CNS disorders per se, but normal functioning of the CNS; these publications would therefore evade any classification of disorders. Knowledge may also be gained by searching for related laboratory-to-clinic terminology; one example that was already used in the authors' ontology tree was the association of the terms nociceptor and nociception with pain disorders. Further discussion of improvements to the ontology is discussed in Section 5 of this report.

It also cannot be ignored that 28 out of 96 (i.e., 29.2%) of disorders, as mapped to their key terms with our ontology, did not match any of the publications. Along with the strong evidence for scale-free distributions by ranking [7], these non-matched disorders should be analyzed for epidemiological rates to determine if there exists true author-based or otherwise sociological bias against such disorders.

4.2   Distorted Distributions and Social Phenomenon

We required non-linear regression in topic ranking studies and exponential binning for frequencies in our publication topic distribution models; thus, our data supports some aspects of supporting social network patterning [5-7].

Classic co-authorship infometrics studies (ones that link papers to authors in similar networks) have shown that there exists` preferential attachment, that is, authors will preferentially attach to other authors who have had prior success publishing [6, 17]. Such co-authorship networks usually show power law (or power law-type) distributions and rankings of node degree, including the Pareto Type II distribution seen in our disorder-to-publication network. It follows, that we can properly speculate there is a preferential attachment of publications (and their authors) to certain topics. The ranking model (Figure 4) showed strong evidence for this hypothesis; we may certainly postulate from our data that neuroscience researchers tend to attach to established disorders, and quite possibly, to each other given the human-social foundations of attachment proposed by Frasco et al [7]. Nonetheless, we see that there was a great degree of specialization and again the potential for a scale-free [5] distribution. Such conclusion is supported in Figure 6, the drop in topics covered by any single publication is a steep logarithmic curve.

Ramifications of a Partial Log-Z-Normal Distribution in Disorder Degree. However, the explicit frequency model of disorder degree analysis (Figure 5) showed elements of both a log-Z-normal distribution (with peaks coinciding with values of 8 to 148 publications per disorder forming a bell curve-type shape in the exponential distribution in Figure 5) and a long-tailed [6] distribution, with the initial peak consisting zero and one matched publications. The former bell-like peak shows that there is a concentration of disorder study in more modest disorders, particularly given that the frequencies are scaled in a linear-normal fashion despite exponential binning.

5   Future Directions

5.1   Planned Studies: This Network; Improvements to Controlled Vocabulary

It is very important to note that the ontology (specifically, that of disorder-key term(s)) has not been curated by medical practitioners who deal with the CNS. We wish to subject the aforementioned ontology to validation by a panel of expert clinicians and researchers, possibly with a classical expert index card sort [18]. Such validation is likely to result in modest but significant modifications to this network based on explicit search terminology used.

   We then wish to evaluate the ability of the revised network to draw conclusions on the interactions of humans with clinical information using a human survey project that will record the opinions of clinicians and researchers as they pertain to their beliefs on the importance of their own sub-fields of neuroscience and neurology. Finally, we intend on allowing consumers of healthcare (i.e., the lay public) to interact with this network map and discover how it changes (or reinforces) their perceptions of particular CNS disorders.

5.2   Study of Non-pathological CNS Function

A high non-match rate between our controlled vocabulary and the corpus of abstracts warrants further searching; we may in the future create a node entity of non-pathological, assign it key terms as we did with the 96 disorders, and re-perform our network visualization and analyses.

5.3   Recommendations: Use of Ontology and Algorithm as a Framework

With various ontologies commonly used as a framework in various information science applications, it is clear that this ontology (or a revised version thereof) ought to be used as a framework for the future study of CNS disorders. While we have only applied our ontology to relatively recent articles from *Brain Research*, studies of the resulting network over time (e.g., by comparison to similar networks generated for other publication time periods) would be of great interest. Furthermore, the ontology may be applied outside of *Brain Research* for the purpose of engineering knowledge from any corpus of documents that are CNS-related.

Potential for a Disorder Similarity Network. By viewing the links of publications between two given disorders, one may speculate as to how closely they are related (please refer back to Figure 4). For such similarity scores to be valid, however, we would require more disorder terminology (i.e., a higher N) for better publication match rates.

Creating Frameworks for Consumer Studies and Consumer Applications. As implied in Section 5.1, this ontology may help create a framework specifically for health consumer studies, engineering consumer-centered knowledge of the basic research sciences. It is also possible that such ontology may be useful in the context of electronic medical records (EMRs) for semantic analysis of consumers' self-reported health information in order to extract information regarding potential disorders that may be of concern to the consumers and their clinicians.

References

1. Skusa, A., Ruegg, A., Koehler, J.: Extraction of Biological Interaction Networks From Scientific Literature. Briefings in Bioinformatics 6(3), 264–276 (2005)
2. Spasic, I., Ananiadous, S., McNaught, J., Kumar, A.: Text Mining and Ontologies in Bio-medicine: Making Sense of Raw Text. Briefings in Bioinformatics 6(3), 239–251 (2005)
3. Yan, E., Ding, Y., Milojevic, S., Sugimoto, C.R.: Topics in Dynamic Research Communi-ties: An Exploratory Story for the Field of Information Retrieval. Journal of Informe-trics 6(1), 140–153 (2012)
4. Newman, M.E.J.: Power Laws, Pareto Distributions, and Zipf's Law. Contemporary Phys-ics 46(5), 323–351 (2005)
5. Barabasi, A.L., Erzsebet, R., Vicsek, T.: Deterministic Scale-Free Networks. Physica Ac-ta 299, 559–564 (2001)
6. Milojevic, S.: Power-Law Distributions in Information Science – Making the Case for Lo-garithmic Binning. Journal of the American Society for Information Science and Technol-ogy 61(12), 2417–2425 (2010)
7. Frasco, G.F., Sun, J., Rozenfeld, H.D., Ben-Avraham, D.: Spatially-Distributed Social Complex Networks. Physical Review X 4(011008) (2014)
8. Brain Research (Journal). Information retrieved from
   http://journals.elsevier.com/brain-research/ (December 19, 2013)
9. Merck & Co., Inc.: Neurological Disorders (Section). In The Merck Manual of Diagnosis and Therapy for Professionals (2013-2014),
   http://www.merckmanuals.com/professional/
   neurologic_disorders.html (August 9, 2013) (retrieved)
10. Merck & Co., Inc.: Psychiatric Disorders (Section). In The Merck Manual of Diagnosis and Therapy for Professionals (2013-2014),
    http://www.merckmanuals.com/professional/
    psychiatric_disorders.html (August 9, 2013) (retrieved)
11. United States Government, National Institutes of Health, National Library of Medicine (n.d.-2014): PubMed (Database Website), http://www.pubmed.gov/ (n.d.) (retrieved)
12. Eclipse Foundation, Inc.: Eclipse IDE for Java EE Developers (Software),
    http://www.eclipse.org/downloads/ (retrieved)
13. Sci2 Team: Sci2 Tool (Software) (2009), http://sci2.cns.iu.edu/ (retrieved)
14. Martin, S., Brown, W.M., Klavans, R., Boyack, K.W.: DrL: Distributed Recursive (Graph) Layout. SAND Reports 2936, 1–10 (2008)
15. Excel 2014 (Software). Microsoft Corporation (Redmond/Seattle, Washington),
    http://www.microsoft.com/ (retrieved)
16. SAS 9.4 (Software). SAS Institute (Cary, North Carolina)
17. Milojevic, S., Sugimoto, C.R., Yan, E., Ding, Y.: The Cognitive Structure of Library and Information Science: Analysis of Article Title Words. Journal of the American Society for Information Science and Technology 62(10), 1933–1953 (2011)
18. Smith-Jentsch, K.A., Cannon-Bowers, J.A., Tannenbaum, S.I., Salas, E.: Guided Team Self-Correction: Impacts on Team Mental Models, Processes, and Effectiveness. Small Group Research 39(3), 303–327 (2008)

Identifying Mobile Application Design to Enhance the Subjective Wellbeing among Middle-Aged Adults

Shu-Chun Lee, Yu-Hsiu Hung*, and Fong-Gong Wu

Department of Industrial Design,
National Cheng Kung University, Tainan, Taiwan
{P36011113,idhfhung,fonggong}@mail.ncku.edu.tw

Abstract. Faced with life stress and peer competition, middle-aged adults increasingly are lacking happiness and well-being. The address this problem, this research studied current mobile applications for wellbeing and perceptions of Subjective Wellbeing (SWB) among middle-aged adults. In this study, questionnaires were administered with 100 middle-aged adults (aged 35-55) to understand their status quo of SWB, including the element of positive/negative affect, life satisfaction, as well as flourishing (i.e., overall life wellbeing). In the questionnaire, events that influenced the positive/negative affect were also investigated. Results of the study showed that the ratings for all SWB elements were at the average level and that they were positively correlated. Results also indicated that current wellbeing mobile applications did not have much effect on enhancing SWB. Results revealed that family relationships and job and life achievements were the key drivers for positive and negative affect. The outcome of the study made design recommendations for mobile applications for improving the SWB of middle-aged adults.

Keywords: Subjective wellbeing, middle-aged adults, mobile application.

1 Introduction

The Subjective Well-being (SWB) of middle-aged adults is generally low, which might be due to the breeding of children and parents, job and pressure from peer competition, etc. Middle-aged adults aged 35-50 stay at the lowest level of satisfaction [1]. Middle-aged adults are also in a state of "loss" (e.g., decline of physiological condition) and "gain" (e.g., enhancement in self-control capability) [2]. Jaques is the first person coining the term, "midlife crisis," happening among people in the middle age period [3]. Middle-aged adults generally are not satisfied with their current life situations [4]. The world happiness report found that among all ages, the subjective well-being of the middle-aged adults is the lowest [5].

Middle-aged adults have an important role in the entire social economy. Their well-being is therefore becoming critical to the status of economy. In fact, the suicide rate of middle-aged Americans increased 28% from 1999 to 2010 [6]. Research showed that large living pressure and depressive symptoms are probably the leading factors [7]. Meanwhile, economists start to investigate the correlation between

C. Stephanidis and M. Antona (Eds.): UAHCI/HCII 2014, Part III, LNCS 8515, pp. 289–299, 2014.
© Springer International Publishing Switzerland 2014

national policy and indicators for happiness [8] [9] [10]. Additionally, from the point of view of psychological and social science, a correlation exists between children's success and parents' well-being [11].To summarize, it is clear that the issue of low subjective well-being of middle-aged adults needs to be solved urgently.

With the advances of the mobile technology, people, including middle-aged adults use the Internet and smartphones to share their feeling and things they encountered with their relatives and friends. In fact, the need for improving the wellbeing/happiness of the public had got the attention from the industry and the academia. Studies were conducted and products were developed. For example, it was shown that using gaming and virtual reality could enhance wellbeing and happiness. Software and mobile applications (apps) were developed to make wellbeing/happiness happen among the users (e.g., *Happiness Quotes*, *Well-Being Plus*, and *Happiness Live Wallpaper, etc.*) [12].

SWB is a multi-dimensional concept, formed by affective components, cognitive components [13] [14], and flourishing (FS) [16]. In the literature, SWB and happiness are used interchangeably as they carried similar meanings. Little research has been done to verify the effectiveness of the mobile wellbeing apps in enhancing an individual's well-being from the perspective of user experience. Moreover, most of the wellbeing apps are not developed based on scientific evidence. Thus, the aim of this study was threefold:

(1) Examine the effectiveness of current mobile wellbeing apps with positive psychology literature.
(2) Evaluate the effectiveness of the current mobile wellbeing apps with middle-aged users
(3) Explore design possibilities for mobile wellbeing apps for the middle-aged adults.

2   Literature Review

2.1   Measurement of Enduring Happiness

Happiness (enduring happiness) = S + C + V [16]. S represents gene and cannot be changed by an individual. C represents an individual's living environment (the external environment), which includes social economic status, marital status, health, income and sex life, etc. V represents voluntary control factors. This is psychological strength that can be controlled actively, for example, concept and action, things related value, a view of life your life, habit of thinking social connection, understanding on things and capability to face and handle things, etc. From the view point of this equation, it is clear that for SWB, S in the equation cannot be changed. C is circumstance of life, which might fluctuate from time to time and vary from people to people. To enable the well-being of middle-aged adults, V might be the component that designers can leverage in the design of mobile apps.

2.2   Measurement of Subjective Well-Being

Wellbeing is defined as the state of being comfortable, healthy, or happy. Seligman [28] indicated that the best measurement standard of well-being is flourishing. Flourishing briefly defines that a psychologically healthy adult will own a high level of emotion well-being [18] and thus feeling happy and satisfied, and is purposive in viewing his/her own life. With respect to SWB, according to Diener [14] [15], it refers to how people experience the quality of their lives and includes both emotional reactions and cognitive judgments. SWB is consisted of positive affect (PA)/negative affective (NA), life satisfaction (LS), and flourishing (FS). From research, SWB equations developed with the adding of the concept of flourishing (FS). In this present study, Diener's definition of SWB was adopted to guide the evaluation of current mobile apps as it explains SWB more broadly.

2.3   Wellbeing and Middle-Aged Adults

Well-being is very important for middle-aged adults. From the physiological perspective, individuals with low cortisol content always have high-level positive affect [21]. Adults males have an increasing NA and high cortisol in the morning while low cortisol and relatively high PA in the afternoon. On the contrary, adult females show a decreased NA and an increased PA in the morning [22]. In addition, Gomez et al [23] showed that there is a strong correlation (one kind of personality trait, the trait will be more NA) between neuroticism and SWB. Among different age levels, middle-aged adults are more affected by negative life event for their SWB as compared to the old-aged adults. Fortunately, with regard to relevance between age of middle-aged people and Well-being, NA declines along with increase in age. The average correlation coefficient very low between the PA and NA (PA $r = -0.03$, NA $r = -0.01$), the age factor represents only explain less than 1% of the difference [24].

2.4   Recent Studies on Enhancing Wellbeing

In recent years, lots of studies were conducted on how to enhance Well-being. For instance, investigate possibility of influence of technology-mediated reflection (MRT) on well-being, establish an Echo, as well as use a Smartphone application to record everyday well-being and then make response by the system [12]. Some use therapeutic writing intervention method to ask to incubate sacred moments within three weeks, and the result shows that significant effect can be achieved in SWB related assessment [26]. In addition, for PA among elements of well-being and in the perspective of how the mental state affects the physiological health, the pain of Ankylosing Spondylitis [27] can be surmounted through 10 minutes of laughing.

3   Methodology

3.1   Research Approach

The purpose of this study was to propose design recommendations for mobile applications. It was achieved by the following four steps (Figure 1):

(1) Identify the relationships among the wellbeing elements (PA/NA, LS, and FS) existing in the middle-aged adult population.
(2) Investigate the events leading to PA and NA from the viewpoint of middle-aged adults
(3) Analyze the effectiveness of current mobile wellbeing apps with the literature.
(4) Investigate users' perceptions of PA/NA, LS, and FS after using the current mobile wellbeing apps.

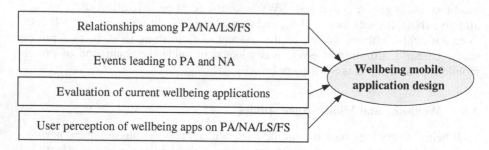

Fig. 1. Research approach

3.2   Participants

Convenience sampling was used in this study. One hundred middle-aged adults (50 males, and 50 females) were recruited to fill out the questionnaire the (with the PA/NA, LS, and FS scales). The mean age of the male participants was 42.74 (SD = 5.5). The mean age of the female participants was 42.55 (SD = 5.38). The proportion distribution of the age was 35-39 (29%), 40-44 (37%), 45-49 (18%) and 50-55 (16%). The questionnaire was administered in public space, such as train stations, shops and fast-food restaurants in the Tainan and Chiayi cities in Taiwan. In addition, snowball sampling was used to recruit participants. Eight volunteered married middle-aged adults agreed to evaluate our selected wellbeing mobile apps. The age range is 35 to 55 years old.

3.3   Procedure

This research contains Part A, the questionnaire (including open-ended and close-ended questions) and Part B, the selection process of mobile apps, and Part C, the user evaluation of mobile apps.

• **Session 1:** Investigations of the wellbeing status (close-ended questions) and events leading to the PA and NA (open-ended questions). The researcher sent paper questionnaires (including electronic questionnaires, http://www.mysurvey.tw/) to people in public space. Through two-week data collection, 112 samples were recruited. After removing invalid samples, 100 effective samples are left.

• **Session 2 (the selection of mobile apps):** Mobile apps related to well-being were search in the Android play store. Only popular mobile apps were included in this study. The selection criteria were (1) key word search (wellbeing and happiness), and the number of application downloads and user ratings. The mobile apps used in this study were shown in Table 1.

• **Session 3 (user feedback on current welling apps):** The selected mobile apps were installed into a smart phone, each of which was demonstrated to the participants. Participants were allowed to use as much time as they needed to manipulate the apps. After the manipulation of every app, participants were asked to provide a score (1 to 5, low to high) for PA, LS, and FS, individually. Participants were also required to provide simple explanations on their ratings.

Table 1. Six well-being apps receiving the highest reviews and # of download (Source: the Android play store)

Type/ Category	App Name	Description	Review (out of 5) (# of downloads)
Recording	Secret of Happiness	Enter 3 good things into the app right after you get up in the morning and just before you hit the bed in the night. Repeating it for 30 days will train your brain to think positively.	4.3 (50,000 - 100,000)
Planning	Happy Habits: Choose Happiness	This app uses the techniques of cognitive-behavioral therapy (CBT) and provides you with detailed results and suggestions to affect happiness.	4.4 (10,000 - 50,000)
Quotes	Happiness Quotes	Save your favorite quotes for later viewing. Share via Facebook, Twitter, SMS, email and all your social apps.	4.4 (10,000 - 50,000)
Meditation	Simply Being Guided Meditation	It allows you to choose from 4 meditation times and gives you to option to listen with/without music/nature sounds.	4.3 (10,000 - 50,000)
Tips	101 How To Be Happy Tips	The simple solution is these 101 quick, easy and free happiness ways to make you feel happy right now.	4.4 (100,000 - 500,000)
Moments Share	Moments - Making You Happier	Use photos, voice and/or text to capture beautiful happy moments as they happen.	4.7 (1,000 - 5,000)

3.4 Instrument

Open-ended and close-ended type questions were used:

• **Events leading to positive/negative affect (open-ended questions):** There were 2 questions included in the questionnaire, one asking participants to list 2 events leading to positive affect, and the other asking participants to list 2 events leading to negative affect in the past 4 weeks.

- **Measurements of PA/NA/LS/FS (close-ended questions):** The close-ended questions included questions from: (1) the scale of Positive/Negative Experience (SPANE) [19], to know middle-age people's past experiences in positive affect and negative affect of SWB; (2) the satisfaction with life scale (LS) [20], designed to measure individual life satisfaction. This score represents the level of satisfaction of an individual on his/her own life; (3) the flourishing scale [19], designed to measure the individual self-perceived success in differing area. This score represents the number of psychological resources and strengths available for an individual.

3.5   Data Analysis

- **Events leading to positive/negative affect (open-ended questions):** In this research, Affinity Diagram is used for categorization and analysis in an attempt to understand what events lead to the PA and NA of middle-aged adults.
- **Measurements of PA/NA/LS/FS (close-ended questions):** For close-ended questions, Pearson correlation analysis of SPSS software is used to understand the correlation among key elements of PA, NA, LS and FS for well-being of middle-aged adults.

4   Results

4.1   The Wellbeing Status Quo: PA/NA/ FS/LS

The average scores for PA/NA/LS/FS are as following: SPANE: The mean score is 1.104 (SD=6.69), close to the mean zero. Such result indicates middle-aged group is in a moderate state of affect. Overall, their affect was neither too positive nor too negative in the past four weeks. LS: All items score M=4.88, SD=6.85. FS: Every participant scores M=43.22.

The correlation among Gender and FS, Marriage and FS, Marriage and Age, SPANE and Age is very low or of non-existence, for the detailed score, please see Table2. SPANE and LS were moderate positive correlation, $r=.526$, $p<0.01$. SPANE and FS were moderate positive correlation, $r=.539$, $p<0.01$. LS and FS were high positive correlation, $r=.680$, $p<0.01$. Therefore, the key elements PA/NA, LS and FS of SWB are of high or middle correlation to each other.

Table 2. Results of the correlation analysis of the questionnaire

Variable	Gender	Marriage	Age	SPANE	LS	FS
Gender	1	-.173	-.010	-.126	-.147	-.234*
Marriage		1	.168	.154	.185	.293*
Age			1	.205*	.103	.122
SPANE				1	.526*	.539*
LS					1	.680*
FS						1

* denotes $p < .05$.

4.2   Affinity Diagrams of PA/NA

Open-Ended Question Items: after summarizing participants' answers and implementing affinity diagram, following results are obtained (Table 3):

180 events resulting in positive affect and 157events resulting in negative affect are collected. The following includes top three positive and negative events ranked in terms of percentage in the table3. Other events leading to positive affect are: Stay and interaction with friends (7.6%), help or serve for others (6.5%), accomplishment of something, and the feeling of achievement in the work (5.9%), full of hope to the future (1.8%), unexpected happiness (1.8%) and others (8.8%). Other events leading to negative affect are: Unfortunate things on relatives and friends (7.6%), friction with others or displeasure (7%), illness on the body (6.3%), others (including dissatisfaction on politics and policy, viewing of negative news, dissatisfaction on unfair things in the society, 22.9%).

Table 3. Top three positive and negative event categories

Positive events	Percentage	Negative events	Percentage
Family relation	38.8%	Family relation	30.0%
Relaxation & satisfaction from leisure activities	17.6%	Work problem	14.7%
Security sense from stable economy, job & income	11.2%	Pressure from environment/self	11.5%

4.3   User Feedback on Current Mobile Apps

Apps with the highest number of download and the highest review scores among all categories were selected and shown in front of 8 middle-aged adults. Questions for the level of PA, LS, as well as FS after using the given apps were asked. The ratings are shown in the following (Table 4):

Table 4. User feedback on six popular mobile apps

App Name	Average score results (out of 5)			Rank
	PA	LS	FS	
Secret Of Happiness	3.9(SD=0.62)	3.8(SD=0.64)	3.9(SD=0.64)	1
Happy Habits: Choose Happiness	3.3(SD=0.43)	3.5(SD=0.62)	3.9(SD=0.53)	2
Simply Being Guided Meditation	3.3(SD=1.10)	3.3(SD=1.06)	3.5(SD=0.89)	3
Moments - Making you happier!	3.2(SD=0.58)	3.3(SD=0.64)	3.4(SD=0.71)	4
101 How To Be Happy Tips	3.0(SD=0.62)	3.4(SD=0.71)	3.2(SD=0.71)	5
Happiness Quotes	2.9(SD=0.57)	2.9(SD=0.69)	2.8(SD=0.34)	6
Average scores	3.3(SD=0.35)	3.4(SD=0.29)	3.5(SD=0.42)	

5   Discussion

There are lots of rooms in PA/NA, LS and FS for improvement. In this research, it was understood that middle-aged adults has medium value of SPANE (M=1.104, SD=6.69), and the emotion of middle-aged adults is not so positive. For LS, the score of all items M=4.88, SD=6.85, which represents that our participants feel slightly satisfied on their life. Finally, the result of FS issues (M=5.4, SD=7.9) shows that middle-aged adults have some psychological resources and strengths.

According to the result of Pearson correlation analysis that we can find elements of SWB (PA / NA, LS and FS) showed moderate or high positive correlation with each other. That is; when middle-aged adults have more positive affect, FS within them will be expected to be higher. If FS is high, LS will not be low either. If the middle-aged adults have more positive affect in their daily life, their life satisfaction will be higher.

5.1   Affinity Diagram for Events Leading to Positive and Negative Affect

Affinity diagram analysis results lead us to the events leading to positive and negative affect. In the family and family member items (38.8%) among the events leading to positive affect, "things related to children" occupy a percentage about 22.5%, and such data shows that for middle-aged adults, family is the major source affecting the positive affect, and it is especially true in children. After summarizing events leading to the negative affect of middle-aged adults, some belong to external environment (The part of circumstance of your life in the equation), for example, economic recession, expectation of stable job and the pressure causing by low income and high expense, since they are not within self-controllable range because they involve too many variables, hence, they will not be investigated for design direction in this research.

5.2   User Perceptions on Mobile Wellbeing Applications

In addition, after real operation test performed on well-being application currently available in the market, it was found that the real effectiveness of apps is low. Besides, current apps are more or less of indirect type. Among the SWB key elements, PA/NA (M=3.3, SD=0.35), LS (M=3.4, SD=0.29) and FS (M=3.5, SD=0.42) have very uniform score, that is, no single element showed high or low scores. It was also found that the apps (ranked from #1 to #3 in Table 1) have relatively higher score in the FS element, showing that the middle-aged participants concerned with self-development, work, life, fulfillment, purpose, and meaning, rather than short-term happiness. In addition, some participants mentioned that they did not have high intention or motivation using the apps that simply provide tips and happiness quotes. Some indicated that these tips and quotes were too general and did not reflect and fit their life situations. Some participants suggested that mobile apps should help them keep track on their children's status and show relationships growing among family members, etc. Some participants cared more about their work pressure and suggested that mobile apps should help them relieve from work pressure.

5.3   Recommendations for the Mobile Application Design for Wellbeing

According to the results and the analysis of the questionnaire, the following mobile application design recommendations for middle-aged adults are summarized:

- Mobile apps for wellbeing do not necessarily need to address the differences of gender, age, and marital status.
- Family connections/communications should be emphasized, especially building relationships with children.
- Mobile apps designed to help manage/fulfill leisure activities are likely to make positive affect happen.
- Mobile apps designed to demonstrate or reflect work/job achievement would enable positive affect and sense of wellbeing.
- Mobile apps that help enable interactions and maintain relationships with close friends are expected to be appreciated by the middle-aged adults.
- Mobile apps that provide flexibilities to store family moments and events would help the middle-aged adults develop a sense of wellbeing.
- Mobile apps that are designed to help relieve life pressure are desired.
- Old school quotes/tips were not generally appreciated. Mobile apps could provide hands-on tips that help middle-aged adults manage/develop family/friend relationships, or work achievements, or options to build leisure activities.
- Mobile apps that attempt to demonstrate an individual's wellbeing status quo should use easy questions or criteria to collect user data.

6   Conclusions

The purpose of this study was to (1) examine the effectiveness of current mobile wellbeing apps with positive psychology literature, (2) evaluate the effectiveness of the current mobile wellbeing apps with middle-aged users, and (3) explore design possibilities for mobile wellbeing apps for the middle-aged adults. Questionnaires were distributed and administered with 100 middle-aged adults in the public space. The wellbeing status (consisting of scores of PA/NA, LS, and FS) and the life events leading to positive and negative affect were investigated. User evaluations of 6 popular wellbeing mobile apps were also conducted. Results of the questionnaire indicated that the average scores for PA, NA, LS and FS for the middle-aged participants were around the medium level, meaning that their wellbeing status may be merely acceptable, thus, having room for improvement. In addition, our study also found that middle-aged adults generally had pressure from differing sources, e.g., family, work, economy, life achievement/fulfillment, and deteriorations of body and physical capabilities, etc. The user evaluation for six popular mobile apps for wellbeing showed that providing old school tips to users was considered inappropriate in leading people to wellbeing; guiding people to develop good habits was also considered an indirect way to enhance wellbeing as it deviate from the major life concerns of middle-aged adults. Thus, to improve the wellbeing/happiness status quo of middle-aged adults, pressure management or psychologically relief from the tension of family relationships and workload becomes design directions and also a challenge for mobile app designers. Future research is required on the motivation and adoption issues of wellbeing mobile apps. The outcomes of this study may be limited by the small sample size. It is our expectation that the wellbeing mobile design communities can benefit from our research outcomes.

References

1. Frijters, P., Beatton, T.: The mystery of the U-shaped relationship between happiness and age. Journal of Economic Behavior & Organization 82(2), 525–542 (2012)
2. Lachman, M.E., Lewkowicz, C., Marcus, A., Peng, Y.: Images of midlife development among young, middle-aged, and older adults. Journal of Adults Development 1(4), 201–211 (1994)
3. Jaques, E.: Death and the mid-life crisis. The International Journal of Psychoanalysis 46, 502–514 (1965)
4. Hermans, H.J.M., Oles, P.K.: Midlife crisis in men: affective organization of personal meanings. Human Relations 52(11), 1403–1426 (1999)
5. Helliwell, J.F., Layard, R., Sachs, J. (eds.): World happiness report 2013. Sustainable Development Solutions Network (2013)
6. Centers for Disease Control and Prevention (CDC):Suicide among adults aged 35-64 years-United States, 1999-2010. MMWR. Morbidity and Mortality Weekly Report 62(17), 321 (2013)
7. Casey, P.R., Dunn, G., Kelly, B.D., Birkbeck, G., Dalgard, O.S., Lehtinen, V.: Factors associated with suicidal ideation in the general population. British Journal of Psychiatry 189, 410–415 (2006)
8. Diener, E., Lucas, R., Schimmack, U., Helliwell, J.: Wellbeing for public policy. Oxford University Press, New York (2009), doi:10.1093/acprof:oso/9780195334074.001.0001
9. Layard, R.: Happiness: Lessons from a new science. Penguin, New York (2005)
10. Stutz, J.: The role of well-being in a great transition. GTI Paper Series No. 10. Tellus Institute (2006)
11. Fingerman, K.L., Cheng, Y.P., Birditt, K., Zarit, S.: Only as Happy as the Least Happy Child: Multiple Grown Children's Problems and Successes and Middle-aged Parents' Well-being. The Journals of Gerontology Series B: Psychological Sciences and Social Sciences 67(2), 184–193 (2012)
12. Isaacs, E., Konrad, A., Walendowski, A., Lennig, T., Hollis, V., Whittaker, S.: Echoes from the past: how technology mediated reflection improves well-being. In: Proceedings of the SIGCHI Conference on Human Factors in Computing Systems, pp. 1071–1080. ACM (April 2013)
13. Diener, E., Emmons, R.A.: The independence of positive and negative affect. Journal of Personality and Social Psychology 47, 1105–1117 (1984)
14. Diener, E., Suh, E.M., Lucas, R.E., Smith, H.L.: Subjective well-being: Three decades of progress. Psychological Bulletin 125(2), 276 (1999)
15. Diener, E., Biswas-Diener, R.: Happiness: Unlocking the mysteries of psychological wealth. John Wiley & Sons (2008)
16. Seligman, M.E.: Authentic happiness: Using the new positive psychology to realize your potential for lasting fulfillment. Simon and Schuster (2002)

17. Keyes, C.L.: The mental health continuum: From languishing to flourishing in life. Journal of Health and Social Behavior, 207–222 (2002)
18. Diener, E., Wirtz, D., Tov, W., Kim-Prieto, C., Choi, D., Oishi, S., Biswas-Diener, R.: New measures of well-being: Flourishing and positive and negative feelings. Social Indicators Research 39, 247–266 (2009)
19. Diener, E., Emmons, R.A., Larsen, R.J., Griffin, S.: The Satisfaction with Life Scale. Journal of Personality Assessment 49, 71–75 (1985)
20. Dockray, S., Steptoe, A.: Positive affect and psychobiological processes. Neuroscience & Biobehavioral Reviews 35(1), 69–75 (2010)
21. Polk, D.E., Cohen, S., Doyle, W.J., Skoner, D.P., Kirschbaum, C.: State and trait affect as predictors of salivary cortisol in healthy adults. Psychoneuroendocrinology 30(3), 261–272 (2005)
22. Gomez, V., Krings, F., Bangerter, A., Grob, A.: The influence of personality and life events on subjective well-being from a life span perspective. Journal of Research in Personality 43(3), 345–354 (2009)
23. Mroczek, D.K., Almeida, D.M.: The effect of daily stress, personality, and age on daily negative affect. Journal of Personality 72(2), 355–378 (2004)
24. Pinquart, M.: Age differences in perceived positive affect, negative affect, and affect balance in middle and old age. Journal of Happiness Studies 2(4), 375–405 (2001)
25. Goldstein, E.D.: Sacred moments: Implications on well‐being and stress. Journal of Clinical Psychology 63(10), 1001–1019 (2007)
26. Cousins, N.: Anatomy of an illness (as perceived by the patient). The New England Journal of Medicine 295(26), 1458 (1976)
27. Seligman, M.E.: Flourish: A visionary new understanding of happiness and well-being. Simon and Schuster (2012)

A Virtual Trainer by Natural User Interface for Cognitive Rehabilitation in Dementia

Alessandro Leone, Andrea Caroppo, and Pietro Siciliano

CNR-IMM, via Monteroni presso Campus Universitario – Lecce, Italy
{alessandro.leone,andrea.caroppo,
pietro.siciliano}@le.imm.cnr.it

Abstract. The aim of this work is the design and the development of an ICT platform integrating advanced Natural User Interface technologies for multi-domain Cognitive Rehabilitation without the direct physician involvement to the rehabilitation session. The platform is made up of a set-top-box connected to a TV monitor, a Microsoft Kinect RGB-D sensor and a (optional) WWS Smartex e-shirt for clinical signs monitoring.

Customized algorithms for calibration, people segmentation, body skeletonization and hands tracking through the RGB-D sensor have been implemented in order to infer knowledge about the reaction of the end-user to the Graphical User Interface designed for specific cognitive domains. For proper interaction, gestures of Alzheimer Disease's patients are acquired by Microsoft Kinect in the nominal functioning range, allowing 100% hands detection rate, useful for an error free human-machine interaction.

Keywords: Natural User Interface, Active Vision System, Cognitive Rehabilitation.

1 Introduction

In the recent years, the phenomenon of ageing population is receiving increasing attention mainly for healthcare and social impacts, so a great effort has been addressed by the scientific community in order to provide specific enabling solutions. Alzheimer's Disease (AD) is a chronic neuro-degenerative disease (dementia) in which the first symptom is a slowly increasing memory loss. As the disease progresses, the brain deteriorates more rapidly with apparent cognitive limits.

Several scientific publications [1-5] highlight the usefulness and importance of Cognitive Rehabilitation (CR) in the treatment of patients with dementia. In order to increase the chances of an appropriate care, the development of a cost-effective home-care service with CR functionalities could be very useful. Moreover, although education and ICT skills level among the elderly is often low, various pilot studies on small samples show that ICT tools are accepted improving quality of life and increasing the permanence at home. In the field of healthcare, technologies such as virtual reality,

C. Stephanidis and M. Antona (Eds.): UAHCI/HCII 2014, Part III, LNCS 8515, pp. 300–309, 2014.
© Springer International Publishing Switzerland 2014

augmented reality and serious games have being applied for long time, including cognitive training and rehabilitation [6-8].

Virtual reality offers training environments in which human cognitive and functional performance can be accurately assessed and rehabilitated [9-10]. On the other hand, augmented reality provides safer and more intuitive interaction techniques allowing interaction with 3D objects in real world [11-12]. In this scenario social communication channels (natural speech, para-language, etc.) are not blocked, breaking down mental barriers applying such a technology to specific problems or disabilities. New solutions for cognitive assistance based on serious games have been implemented: in the field of CR commercial products (Nintendo's Brain Age, Big Brain Academy, etc.) have been tuned as educational tools helping to slow the decline of AD [13-16].

More recently, the large diffusion of interaction devices enabling body movements to control systems have been investigated, with specific focus on ICT technologies for natural interaction. Microsoft Kinect is the state-of-the-art [17] as device for body movements acquisition and gesture recognition; the effects of this kind of technology for rehabilitation purposes is widely investigated [18,19].

In this paper, a Natural User Interace (NUI) platform for remote CR has been designed with the aim to support AD patients during the rehabilitation pratice without the presence of any caregiver. A new hands tracking filter has been implemented with the aim to overcome the well-known limitations of the royalties-free NUI middleware architecture used in the platform.

The paper is organized as follows. Section 2 presents the overall implemented platform with specific focus on the rehabilitation practice in a cognitive multi-domain scenario. Section 3 presents the HCI methodology in which the customized hand tracking filter is described. Section 4 presents the evaluation of the proposed system on real data in different scenarios.

2   Platform Overview

The developed ICT platform provides a system for Cognitive Home Rehabilitation (called AL.TR.U.I.S.M.) through a customized Virtual Personal Trainer (VPT) allowing the patients to perform the rehabilitation practice at home. The platform gives the opportunity to perform the cognitive therapy without the presence of a caregiver. Details about the platform are in the following.

2.1   AL.TR.U.I.S.M. Platform Architecture

The CR platform is made up of a set-top-box connected to a TV monitor with Internet connection, a Microsoft Kinect RGB-D sensor for human body tracking and gesture recognition and a (optional) WWS Smartex e-shirt [20] with textile electrodes for clinical signs monitoring (Fig. 1).

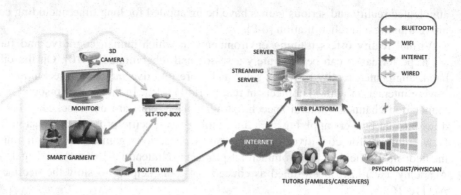

Fig. 1. AL.TR.U.I.S.M. platform overview

The left hand side part of the Fig. 1 shows the hardware equipments in which the set-top-box (a commercial embedded pc) is the gateway able to automatically downloads sequences of exercises from a remote server through the internet connection. The system provides a web-based platform that allows the physician to customize directly the therapy: this process is a highly innovative compared to existing systems [21-22] as the caregiver/physician defines a specific sequence of exercises (the therapeutic session) according to the residual abilities of the patient.

In order to infer more knowledge during the rehabilitation activities, the main clinical parameters (heart-rate, breathe-rate, electrocardiogram, etc.) are monitored by wearing the WWS Smartex e-shirt that integrates several sensing devices for biomedical applications. Through a Bluetooth radio link with the platform, each useful clinical parameter provided by the WWS device is stored on the set-top-box and, then sent to the physician with a multi-modal paradigm for clinical evaluations. Moreover, the platform integrates streaming functionalities allowing visual/audio recording for post-verification or online feedback to the physician which is able to follows the execution of the exercises from a remote architecture. From this perspective, the physician/psychologist of the reference center could communicate to the patients through a remote connection and then monitor the progress or trouble in the execution of the different required tasks. At the end of the rehabilitation session, the central platform collects different kinds of data locally stored on the set-top-box. An ad-hoc multi-modal messaging procedure (e-mail, SMS, App, ...) is performed and relevant data are sent to the physician allowing instant verification of the performance through an easy-to-use Graphical User Interface (GUI).

2.2 Multi-domain Cognitive Rehabilitation Practice

On the basis of the severity of cognitive impairment and residual skills of the target, the CR program provides specific categories of exercises, in order to assess specific domains of deficits. In order to make the system reliable, flexible and compliant with the international evaluation scales (Mini Mental State Examination [23]), few input

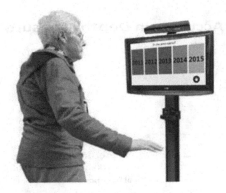

Fig. 2. Rehabilitation approach by gesture as Natural User Interface

parameters need to be defined a-priori (execution time, maximum numbers of allowed errors, movement sensitivity). The platform provides sixteen different exercises belonging to the following cognitive domains:

- Orientation (temporal, personnel and spatial)
- Memory (topographic, verbal and visual)
- Attention (hearing and visual)
- Categorization
- Verbal fluency
- Logic

In order to allow an appropriate display of every exercise and become independent from the specific output device (digital monitor, HD TV, …) a software module for the best video rendering is implemented. The definition of graphics objects displayed on the GUI has been designed according to the principles of ergonomics, usability and acceptability as referred in ISO/IEC 2001a [24].

3   Contact-Less Natural User Interface for Cognitive Rehabilitation

Each exercise is performed via a multi-modal contact-less NUI (Fig. 2) available through the use of both the Microsoft Kinect device for gesture recognition and Microsoft Text-To-Speech engine (TTS) [25] for human voice synthesis (italian language). The platform allows the user to interact with the GUI in a natural way without the use of a mouse or any kind of controller. The interaction is achieved by hand gestures performed by the patient according to the ad-hoc designed GUI, compliant the specific CR exercise. From the functioning principle point of view, the Kinect device is a RGB-D camera integrating both a high resolution RGB camera (640×480 at 30 fps) and an infrared depth sensor (640×480 at 30 fps), providing a metric reconstruction of a scene. The RGB-D device allows to capture mid-resolution depth and

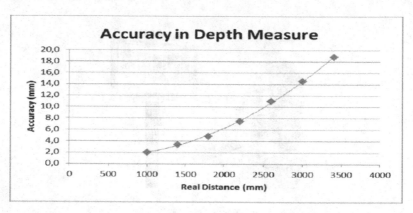

Fig. 3. Accuracy of Microsoft Kinect by varing the distance between target and the optical centre of the device

appearance information at high data rates (up to 30fps) for real-time functioning. The space resolution along the x and y axis is 3 mm at a depth of 2 meters, whereas the resolution of z-depth is 1 cm at the same depth. While increasing distance from the sensor, the accuracy decreases remaining within an acceptable range for people and hands tracking (Fig. 3).

3.1   Gesture Recognition by Hand Tracking for Human Computer Interaction

For the considered CR scenario, the upper part of the human body needs to be completely visible, avoiding situations in which large occlusions occur. As AD patient may have troubles moving the own hands, the procedure for hand tracking and gesture recognition provided by the Microsoft Kinect SDK [26] may be affected by critical issues, for example when hands and body torso are overlapped. In particular, AD patient may not be able to move hands in a spatially extensive environment, so that the interaction with objects belonging to the GUI could be hard and the CR practice could be dramatically affected. In this context graphical objects are codified as "hidden buttons" able to discover the hovering time for specific end-user choices. The NUI procedure is depicted in Fig. 4.

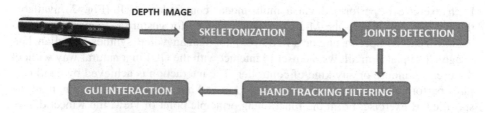

Fig. 4. Hand tracking procedure for contact-less natural user interaction

The skeletonization procedure provided by Microsoft Kinect SDK can be affected due to noise in the acquisition process so that the joint positions estimations can fail and the interaction with the GUI could be sometimes hard to handle. In order to overcome this kind of issue, a noise reduction filter has been designed removing as much as possible noise from raw data. The suggested filter operates as a smoothing filter that overcome the performaces of the Holt Double Exponential Smoothing Filter (HDESF) [27] built in Microsoft Kinect SDK. The HDESF procedure reduces the jitters from skeletal joint data providing a smoothing effect with lower latency than other smoothing filter algorithms. The main issue with HDESF application is that Kinect sensor does not have sufficient resolution to ensure consistent accuracy of the tracked joints over time. Observing real data, the problem is apparent when different joints are overlapped.

An improved smoothing algorithm has been designed, overcoming the performance of HDESF. From the analysis of the state of the art, the Exponential Weighted Moving Average Filter (EWMAF) [28] appears as the best trade-off between smoothing effect and jitter control. The EWMAF is given by the following formula:

$$S_t = \alpha X_{t-1} + (1 - \alpha) S_{t-1} \qquad t > 1 \qquad (1)$$

where X_t is the 2D coordinate sample at a time period t, S_t is the smoothed statistic as simple weighted average of the previous observation X_{t-1} and the previous smoothed statistic S_{t-1}. Generally, the setting of the initial smoothed value S_1 is performed by averaging the first six samples, limiting the delay of the interaction. The coefficient α is constant smoothing factor between 0 and 1 and it represents the decreasing weighting degree. Values of α close to 1 represents a lower smoothing effect, whereas values of α closer to 0 make a greater smoothing effect. Details about the best value of α are reported in Section 4. The last step of the hand tracking procedure involves the use of a function that allows to scale a joint's position to the maximum width and height specified (in our case the maximum screen resolution). Moreover, the setting of specific scaling factors simplifies the interaction of the end-user with the GUI, according the residual movement hands abilities of the end-user. For this purpose, three different combinations of scaling values (corresponding to different movement hands abilities) are set as reported in Tab. 1. High values of scaling require a wider real movement of the hand to cover the entire spatial resolution of the GUI, while low values of scaling allow the natural interaction of the end-user that may not be able to move the hand in a spatially extensive.

Table 1. Scaling parameters along the x axis and y axis of the screen

Level of Accuracy	Scale X	Scale Y
Low	0.6	0.4
Medium	0.3	0.2
High	0.15	0.1

4   Experimental Results and Discussion

The experimental evaluation of the proposed platform was based on real-world se-
quences obtained during the execution of specific movements acquired by Microsoft
Kinect operating in the range 1.5 m - 4.0 m. The platform is hosted on an embedded
PC equipped with an Intel® Core i5 CPU.

Since ground truth data for real-world image sequences is hard to obtain, according
to the experimental section proposed in [29], the evaluation of hand tracking procedure was made analyzing the hand trajectory on the "Visual Attention" exercise GUI.
The hand trajectory is reported in Fig. 5 in which a loop gesture is represented: the blu
line is referred to the hand movement by using HDESF, while the red line is referred
to the trajectory achieved by applying the proposed EWMAF. By comparing the two
trajectories, it is apparent that EWMAF reduces the jittering of the signal, removing
spikes presented in the hand tracking returned by HDESF. The analysis of the trajectories highlights the problems in some critical situations (yellow circle in Fig. 5):
HDESF returns false paths that invalidate the process of graphic element selection,
while the application of EWMAF allows the correct item selection by the end-user.
The aforementioned issue may be negligible in gaming context, whereas in the considered CR scenario the consequences are apparent affecting the CR practice. A quantitative measurement of the performances can be carried out analyzing the difference
between values calculated by a model (e.g. an ideal trajectory over the numbers
placed on the board) and the tracked values recorded in the two previous cases.

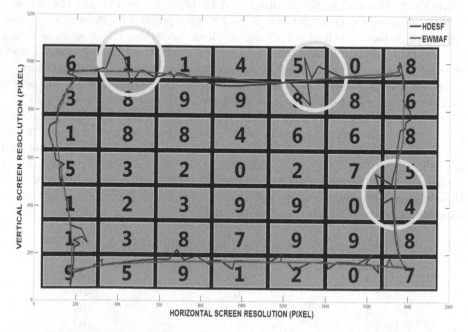

Fig. 5. Hand Trajectory obtained with HDESF (blu line) and EWMAF (red line) applications in
"Visual Attention" exercise

For this purpose, a frequently used measure is the Root-Mean-Square Deviation (RMSD), that represents the sample standard deviation of the difference between predicted and observed values.

Table 2. RMSD values at different distance for HDESF and EWMAF on 500 samples

Distance from Kinect	RMSD (HDESF, in pixel)	RMSD (EWMAF, in pixel)
1,5 m.	60,30	22,87
2,5 m.	61,06	23,36
3 m.	68,12	25,67
4 m.	87,98	28,32

Table 2 shows the results obtained at four different distances, selected in the operating range of Microsoft Kinect; the sample number used to estimate RMSD is approximately 500. RMSD values for EWMAF demonstrate the validity of the proposed solution: the average deviation never exceeds the value of 30 pixel, allowing greater precision in the selection of a graphic element. Instead, HDESF performs an average error always greater than 60 pixels, so that the gap in some cases affects the correct selection of a graphic element belonging to the GUI.

EWMAF presents the issue of introducing a lag relative to the input data. In real time application latency is a critical factor, therefore it is essential to tune up in the rigth way the parameters of the fiter, with the aim of obtaining the best performance with the lowest latency.

Table 3. RMSD values by evaluating EWMAF for different α smoothing factor and amount of observations

# of observations	$\alpha = 0.1$	$\alpha = 0.3$	$\alpha = 0.7$	$\alpha = 0.9$
5	34,3212	29,1258	25,3427	23,0045
10	33,5662	28,9083	24,9980	22,6754
15	32,0113	28,3397	24,6548	22,3359
20	32,9675	28,0989	24,1765	21,8675
30	31,3444	27,5674	23,8413	21,6754

As mentioned in Section 3.1, values of α close to 1 presents a lower smoothing effect, since greater weight to recent changes in data is considered. A choice of $\alpha = 0.9$ allows EWMAF to reduce significantly the RMSD compared to the result obtained with $\alpha = 0.1$ and $\alpha = 0.3$ (see Table 3). On the other hand, when the number of past observations grows in size results are better but a latency effect is introduced in the tracking procedure. For all considered scenarios, the best tradeoff is achieved for $\alpha = 0.9$ and the amount of past observations equal to 10 (as 300 ms).

4.1   Computational Load Evaluation

The computational workload, referred to the three main steps of Fig.4 (hand tracking methodology), is evaluated in terms of processing time. The skeletonization and Joint detection algorithms require exactly the same time on the target machine (2.5 ms). On the other hand, the time spent for EWMAF application is invariant to the amount of past observation used for the evaluation of the hand position, requiring an average processing time of 1.4 ms. These average values do not affect the frame rate of the application and consequently the overall computational load allows the execution of every exercise at 30fps.

5   Conclusions

The main idea of the proposed system is to promote multi-domain cognitive rehabilitation of Alzheimer Disease patient at home through an ICT platform integrating low-cost contact-less Natural User Interface devices.

As a patient with Alzheimer's disorder may have trouble moving the own hands, a new filter for hand tracking has been implemented, overcoming the performances of the built-in filter of Microsoft Kinect SDK. The improvement allows an easy and accurate interaction of the end-user and the platform, even in the presence of complex ad-hoc designed GUI. The proposed platform allows both the evalutation of the progress of the dementia (useful for the caregiver) and the cognitive stimulation of the end-user in several domains. Future works are addressed to deploy the platform to a wide class of Alzheimer's disease patients in order to have the feedback (validation) during the technological tool usage. This will allow to tune up each component of the platform (GUI, knowledge discovery logic, filter parameters) in order to make it highly compliant with the needs and the requirements of the patients, according to the recent User Centered Design paradigm.

Acknowledgements. This work has been carried out within AL.TR.U.I.S.M. project, funded by Apulia Region under the Health-care call for the promotion of regional partnerships for innovation.

References

1. Clare, L., et al.: Cognitive Rehabilitation in Dementia. In: Neuropsychologistical Rehabilitation, pp. 193–196. Psychology Press Ltd. (2001)
2. Neal, M., Briggs, M.: Validation therapy for dementia (Cochrane Review). The Cochrane Library, Chichester, UK, vol. (2) (2004)
3. Spector, A., Orrell, M., Davies, S., Woods, B.: Reality orientation for Dementia. Cochrane Database Syst. Rev. (4): CD001119. Review (2000)
4. Woods, R.T., Bruce, E., Edwards, R.T., Hounsome, B., Keady, J., Moniz-Cook, E.D., Orrell, M., Russell, I.T.: Reminiscence groups for people with dementia and their family carers: pragmatic eight-center randomised trial of joint reminiscence and maintenance versus usual treatment: a protocol. Trials 10, 64–74 (2009)
5. Clare, L., Woods, R.T., Moniz Cook, E.D., Orrel, M., Spector, A.: Cognitive Rehabilitation in Alzheimer's Disease. Aging Clin. Exp. Res. 18, 141–143 (2006)
6. Richard, E., et al.: Augmented Reality for Rehabilitation of Cognitive Disable Children: A preliminary Study. Virtual Rehabilitation, 102–108 (2007)

7. Standen, P., Brown, D.: Virtual reality and its role in removing the barriers that turn cognitive impairments into intellectual disability. Virtual Reality 10(3), 241–252 (2006)
8. Taylor, M.J.D., et al.: Activity-promoting gaming systems in exercise and rehabilitation. Journal of Rehabilitation Research 48(10), 1171–1186 (2011)
9. Pugnetti, L., Mendozzi, L., Barbieri, E., Motta, A.: VR experience with neurological patients: basic cost/benefit issues. Stud. Health Technol. Inform. 58, 243–248 (1998)
10. Rizzo, A.A., Buckwalter, J.G.: The status of virtual reality for the cognitive rehabilitation of persons with neurological disorders and acquired brain injury. Stud. Health Technol. Inform. 39, 22–33 (1997)
11. Azuma, R., Baillot, Y., Behringer, R., Feiner, S., Julier, S., MacIntyre, B.: Recent advances in augmented reality. IEEE Comput. Graph. 21(6), 34–47 (2001)
12. Azuma, R.T.: A survey of augmented reality. Presence: Teleoperators and Virtual Environments 6(4), 355–385 (1997)
13. Nacke, L.E., et al.: Brain training for silver aged gamers: effects of age and game form on effectiveness, self-assessment, and gameplay. Cyberpsychology & Behavior 12(5), 493–499 (2009)
14. Imbeault, F., et al.: Serious Games in Cognitive Training for Alzheimer's Patients. In: IEEE Int. Conference on Serious Games and Applications for Health, pp. 122–129 (2011)
15. Jiang, C.F., Chen, D.K., Li, Y.S., Kuo, J.L.: Development of a computer-aided tool for evaluation and training in 3d spatial cognitive function. In: 19th IEEE Symposium on Computer-Based Medical Systems, pp. 241–244 (2006)
16. Tremblay, J.B., Bouchard, A., Bouzouane, A.: Adaptive game mechanics for learning purposes: making serious games playable and fun. In: Proc. Int. Conf. on Computer Supported Education, vol. 2, pp. 465–470 (April 2010)
17. http://www.microsoft.com/en-us/kinectforwindows
18. Da Gama, A., et al.: Improving Motor Rehabilitation Process through a Natural Interaction Based System Using Kinect Sensor. In: Proceedings of IEEE Symposium on 3D User Interfaces, pp. 145–146 (2012)
19. Lange, B., et al.: Development and evaluation of low cost game based balance rehabilitation tool using the Microsoft Kinect Sensor. In: 33rd IEEE International Conference on Engineering in Medicine and Biology Society (2011)
20. http://www.smartex.it
21. Soong, Y.L.W., Man Way, K.D.: A Tele-cognitive Rehabilitation Platform for Persons with Brain Injuries. In: TENCON IEEE Region 10 Conference (2006)
22. Solana, J., et al.: PREVIRNEC, A new platform for cognitive tele-rehabilitation. In: The Third Int. Conference on Advanced Cognitive Technologies and Applications (2011)
23. Folstein, M., Folstein, S., McHugh, P.: Mini-mental state: a practical method of grading the cognitive state of patients for the clinician. J. Psychiat. Res. 12, 189–198 (1975)
24. ISO/IEC. 2001. International Standard ISO/IEC 9126 – 1. Software engineering - Product quality - Part 1: Quality model. International Organization for Standardization/ International Electrotechnical Commision, Geneva (2001)
25. http://msdn.microsoft.com/en-us/library/hh361572%28v=office.14%29.aspx
26. http://www.microsoft.com/en-us/kinectforwindowsdev/start.aspx
27. Holt, C.C.: Forecasting seasonals and trends by exponentially weighted moving averages, ONR Memorandum, vol. 52. Carnegie Institute of Technology, Pittsburgh (1957), available from the Engineering Library, University of Texas at Austin
28. Roberts, S.W.: Control Chart Tests Based on Geometric Moving Averages. Technometrics (1959)
29. Sangheon, P., Sunjin, Y., Joongrock, K., Sungjin, K., Sangyoun, L.: 3D hand tracking using Kalman Filter in depth space. EURASIP Journal on Advances in Signal Processing 2012, 36 (2012)

Encouraging Brain Injury Rehabilitation through Ludic Engagement

Rachel McCrindle[1], Stephen Simmons[1], Richard Case[1], Malcolm Sperrin[2], Andy Smith[3], and Carol Lock[4]

[1] School of Systems Engineering, University of Reading, Reading, UK
[2] Department of Medical Physics, Royal Berkshire Hospital, Berkshire, UK
[3] Department of Clinical Engineering, Royal Berkshire Hospital, Berkshire, UK
[4] Headway Brain Injury Association, Thames Valley, UK
r.j.mccrindle@reading.ac.uk

Abstract. Whilst in hospital immediately following a stroke or other acquired brain injury, patients receive, and engage in, a structured, concentrated and supervised programme of rehabilitation. However, once they leave hospital patients frequently fail to engage in the rehabilitation exercises provided for them. This paper describes how the Microsoft Kinect sensor has been used with computer games to engage patients with their rehabilitation following stroke and other brain trauma injuries. Initially off-the-shelf games were used, the ludic nature of the games, masking the treatment element of the exercises. However, whilst this approach was a great success in terms of patient engagement it was found that off-the-shelf games were frequently too fast or too complex for some patients to play and set-up due to the extent of their brain traumas. To address these issues, a system, PURR (Prescription Software for Use in Recovery and Rehabilitation), has been developed that uses the same ludic principles to enagage patients whilst allowing games to be tailored to a patients condition, requirements and interests.

Keywords: Ludic engagement, Kinect, brain trauma, stroke, recovery and rehabilitation, case study, personalization, usability.

1   Introduction

Acquired brain injury refers to all circumstances in which brain injury has occurred since birth, and includes traumatic brain injuries caused by incidents such as road traffic accidents, assaults and falls, as well as injuries acquired through conditions such as tumor, stroke, brain hemorrhage and encephalitis. The effects of a brain injury can be wide ranging, and depend on a number of factors such as the type, location and severity of injury. Every person's injury is unique, so they will experience any number of symptoms, which can range from mild to severe [1]. The resulting damage caused by a stroke or other types of acquired brain injury can be very widespread and long-lasting often requiring rehabilitation both in the hospital and after discharge. Statistics indicate that there are in excess of 1 million people in the UK and 5.3 million people

C. Stephanidis and M. Antona (Eds.): UAHCI/HCII 2014, Part III, LNCS 8515, pp. 310–320, 2014.
© Springer International Publishing Switzerland 2014

in the US living with long-term effects of brain injury [2, 3]. Putting these figures further into perspective 558 per 100,000 UK residents will sustain a brain injury, with someone in the UK being admitted to hospital with an acquired brain injury every 90 seconds. Nor is brain injury restricted to older adults. Whilst over 80 year olds are a major risk group, anyone can acquire a brain injury, with for example, one of the groups most at risk groups being 15-24 year old males [2]. The need to find ways of cost effectively and engagingly providing routes to recovery and rehabilitation that can be continued after discharge from hospital is a pressing one. The work described in this paper is collaboration between the University of Reading, the Royal Berkshire Hospital and Headway Brain Injury Association. It has focused on the use of the Kinect as a supplementary treatment to traditional rehabilitation and continued assessment of patients following a stroke or other serious brain injury, initially using off-the-shelf games and subsequently a system that can deliver bespoke rehabilitation programmes tailored to a patient's interests, condition and abilities, both in the hospital and after patients are released.

2   Games for Therapy

The use of games and/or gamification for therapy and rehabilitation has been gaining momentum over the past decade. Not only has there been a realization of the power of games to engage and motivate players, but the advent of social networking and causal gaming has broadened the market for and acceptance of gaming in general [4]. The plethora of gaming devices now available and the play anytime, play anywhere, nature of many games has made gaming a ubiquitous pass-time. More natural and accessible ways of interacting with games coupled with more affordable pricing structures has led to a mass uptake of gaming technology by the general population. Games are no longer just for children or young adults they can be played and enjoyed by all age groups [4].

Games and their ludic elements have been used in many health-related practices including pain distraction, cyberpsychology, disease management, health education and rehabilitation [5, 6]. Ludic engagement may be considered as a way of blurring the distinctions between 'work' and play [7] such that participants are motivated by curiosity, exploration, and reflection rather than the externally-defined tasks [8]. In a health context this is seen as patients interacting with and becoming so engrossed in the gameplay that they perceive it to be a fun and inclusive experience, rather than a set of repetitive exercises. This encourages them to participate more regularly and to engage for longer periods of time with their therapy especially when they leave the hospital environment and continue therapy at home.

The application of entertainment technology to stroke and brain injury rehabilitation has been boosted by the invention of home based gaming technologies such as the Nintendo Wii [9], PlayStation Move [10] and Microsoft's Kinect [11] which, with their natural user interfaces (NUIs), have made it easier for people of all ages and with varying health conditions, disabilities and technical know-how to interact with computer games. The Kinect, a motion sensing input device capable of tracking the whole human body without the need for the user to hold any physical device, together with its ability to collect a vast amount of data about skeletal positioning, motor control and game play interaction has become of particular interest for use in brain injury rehabilitation and recovery [12, 13, 14, 15].

In this paper we report on a study into how concepts of gamification and ludic engagement [8] have been combined with more traditional physio/occupational therapy exercises in order to engage patients in brain injury recovery and rehabilitation at the Royal Berkshire Hospital and Headway Brain Injury Association. How this approach has aided one patient is described in detail in the paper. Analysis of their experience together with feedback from other patients and physio/occupational therapy staff regarding the use of off-the-shelf games for rehabilitation purposes has led to the development of a system, PURR (Prescription Software for Use in Recovery and Rehabilitation), which can deliver treatment programmes tailored to an individual patient's condition, requirements and interests.

3   Study to Assess Engagement of Brain Injury Patients with the Kinect

In the summer of 2012, the Royal Berkshire Hospital (RBH) initiated a study which used 'off-the-shelf' Xbox games as a supplementary treatment to traditional rehabilitation for stroke patients, both in the hospital and after patients were released (Fig.1).

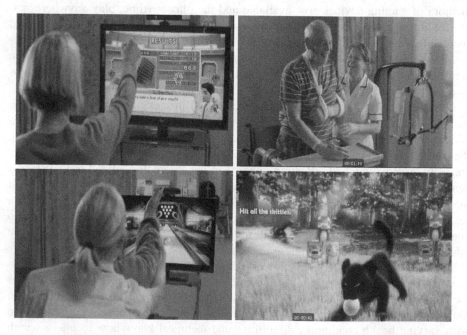

Fig. 1. Patients engaging with off-the-shelf Kinect games during study [17]

This approach to rehabilitation proved to be highly effective with regards to patients' engagement in and enjoyment of therapy [17]:

> *"... a very big part of rehabilitation is trying to enjoy what you do and a sense of achievement gives you that sensation ..."* Vipal Thaker, Patient Royal Berkshire Hospital

It was also seen to have the effect of making therapy more inclusive by involving other members of the family in the same activities:

> *"... at home it can be a good family gathering and at the same time helping you regain your mobility and balance ..."* Vipal Thaker, Patient Royal Berkshire Hospital.

Therapists also saw the value of including Kinect-based games within their therapy sessions:

> *"... can note the improvement in their score and how that translates into what they can do for themselves in terms of their standing balance and arm strength ... and how this translates into them becoming more independent ..."* Vicky Morris, Occupational Therapist, Royal Berkshire Hospital.

As part of the same study the Kinect and Xbox 360 were also used extensively with the clients of Thames Valley Headway Brain Injury Association, who had varying symptoms resulting from acquired brain injuries. As indicated, the nature of brain injuries and their impact is different for every person, however the case study reported in Section 4 is typical of patient interaction with, and responses, to the introduction of off-the-shelf Kinect games as part of their treatment.

4   Case Study – Therapy Utilising the Kinect

In order to determine if the ludic nature of the Xbox and Kinect sensor can engage a patient and encourage them to follow a post-hospital rehabilitation programme, a number of follow up interviews were undertaken with patients who had been given a Kinect/Xbox to use in their own homes. One such case is described below.

4.1   Description/Pathology

The patient is a gentleman in his mid thirties, married with two young children. For the purpose of this paper he will be referred to as Mr P. Due to this patient's communication difficulties, all the following information has been gathered from his spouse.

Mr P. sustained a traumatic head injury some eight years ago which resulted in a lengthy hospital stay followed by nine months as an inpatient on the Putney Rehabilitation Unit. Previous to his injury, Mr P. was in full time employment and his leisure activities included walking, going to the gym and playing computer games.

As a direct consequence of his head injury Mr P was left with the following residual deficits:

- Dense right sided hemiplegia
- Neglect of right upper limb
- Flexed deformity to his right elbow
- Extensor pattern in right lower limb
- Poor gait pattern
- Reduced mid line awareness
- Receptive and expressive disphagia causing significantly problematic communication
- Impulsivity
- Lack of initiation
- Lack of motivation
- Reduced confidence

4.2   Formal Rehabilitation

Whilst on the brain injury rehabilitation unit in Putney, Mr P. received both occupational therapy and physiotherapy input. Occupational therapy was on a daily basis and physiotherapy two to three sessions per week.

Although he engaged well with occupational therapy (as it had immediate meaning to him in his activities of daily life) Mr P. was difficult to engage in the physiotherapy sessions due to his cognitive changes. He found it a challenge to understand their significance, as to him, the exercises were 'just exercise' and bore little relevance to everyday life. Post injury, he was unable to appreciate that the programmes were designed to physically enable him to achieve independence with his ordinary daily needs. Mr P. would only engage in physical activity when instructed to do so and had no carryover of information to enable him to undertake exercises independently. Lack of motivation would appear to be another of the significant issues in his reluctance to participate as the exercises he was required to practise were presented in a manner that was too abstract for him to appreciate.

4.3   Post Structured Rehabilitation

Although Mr. P. was discharged home with a physiotherapy programme to undertake with family members, engagement was difficult due to already mentioned factors. Despite much effort from the family, Mr P's wife believes that for him to engage in formal physiotherapy exercises they would need to be undertaken within a rehabilitation setting as this was where he would associate some relevance. As a direct consequence, Mr P. would not do his physiotherapy exercises within the home unprompted

4.4   Introduction of the Xbox in the Home Environment

Mr P. was introduced to the Xbox Kinect approximately 6 months ago, when, on a typical day would spend 99% of his waking day sat in a chair, unchallenged and unmotivated to partake in any physical activity.

Initially he would begin a game but would fatigue and rest again after 5-10 minutes, as although enjoying the participation he was unused to physical exertion. His stamina has now greatly improved and nowadays he is able to play for up to 2 hours before tiring. Although, due to his cognitive and physical limitations he is unable to set up to play, he will ask for someone to set up for him, this is one of a very few things Mr P. will initiate.

In a direct comparison to his formal physiotherapy regime, Mr P never needs reminding to use the Xbox Kinect and his engagement has shown many positive benefits. He is now able to socialise. As Mr P. has very limited speech and has physical limitations, he was unable to engage in meaningful discussion with the family nor was he motivated to play with his children. Since the introduction of the Kinect system he has demonstrated vocal improvements as he's having to teach the children certain things about the games. It has given him a new role. Mr P. is now able to fully share an interest with other members of the family that doesn't make him feel 'different', as they all share the same experience with each other.

There have also been improvements made in his ability to sustain and switch his attention. Whilst playing, he is constantly having to maintain and adapt his focus to achieve better scores.

Confidence is another area of improvement. This has grown out of teaching his children how to play the games and them looking to him for advice and guidance.

Both sitting and standing balance ability has increased, Mr P now has improved mid line awareness and can self correct when prompted whereas, before the introduction of the Xbox Kinect he would always favour his unaffected left side. Mr P. now engages the use both of his upper limbs to play the games and his right lower limb has increased in strength, enough to rely upon it in dynamic standing.

The question of engagement with the Xbox Kinect within the hospital setting was put to the spouse of Mr. P. As he sustained his injury 8 years previously, the console was not available, however, she interestingly reported that, had Mr P. used the Xbox within the acute setting, he would have associated its use at home with his hospital stay. She felt that this would have had a negative bearing on Mr P.'s acceptance and use of it within the home.

4.5   What Modifications Could Be Made to Make the X Box Kinect More User Friendly to the Study Group?

This client, as others, has difficulty with the setting up of the console and individual games. He is unable to type in names as he can't maintain a steady upper limb and finds it too difficult to use his hand in the correct position to select options. Thus far, he only tends to play when his wife is present to set up a programme on his behalf, if this was made easier for him to achieve independently she is confident that he would learn how to do this for himself. Mrs P. also fed back that the whole set up process at present is too lengthy, by the time Mr P. had gone through all of the separate stages he would probably give up on playing the game itself.

At present, there are only a limited number of games that Mr P. can participate in fully, his main difficulty with the more 'active' games such as Rapids is that he is unable to jump or move quickly enough to gain scores. It was suggested that perhaps the speed of the games could be adjustable to suit varying physical abilities, increasing as the player was able.

Although Mr P. is able to stand, it was also suggested that there could be games designed around wheelchair users who are only able to use their upper bodies.

4.6   Discussion

Mr P. is unable to fully appreciate the physical and cognitive improvements he has made in this relatively short time since his introduction to the Xbox Kinect, therefore, as before, we have gathered the summary of information from his wife.

Mrs P. reports that her husband has become better able to communicate and connect with his children and members of his extended family since being able to use the console. He is re engaging in aspects of family life and has a new, positive role to play as a father. In her own words: 'It is a joy to see'.

His ability to concentrate on tasks has improved and he is making efforts to verbally communicate. His physical improvements are various and positive. He is able to use his upper limbs bilaterally when playing the games, he doesn't need to think about trying to do this, he just does it. Awareness of his mid line is more automatic, the strength in both upper and lower limbs has increased and both his sitting and standing balance has improved.

Mr P. regards the Xbox Kinect as a recreational pursuit and does not perceive the exercise he is undertaking to be an alien concept as he does the formal physiotherapy programmes. He is having fun, improving his ability to concentrate, becoming fitter and is motivated to engage in something that involves a physical challenge.

5   PURR System

Despite receiving a positive response from many patients especially with regards to making their treatment more fun and engaging, feedback, like that from Mr P., also showed that off-the-shelf games were frequently too complex and 'fast' to play for many patients, and were difficult to set up.

Additionally, whilst the scoring system of an off-the-shelf game provides a goal for patients to exceed, from a clinical point of view off-the-shelf games can only provide subjective results, as scores are not truly representative of improvement and therefore have limited medical benefit for healthcare professionals in assessment of patient progress.

In order to address these issues, the PURR (Prescription Software for Use in Recovery and Rehabilitation) system has been developed in consultation with occupational therapists and physiotherapists who defined the metrics they need collected from the system in order to assess patient progress, and with potential users of the system, who had suffered different types and severity of brain injuries, with regards to developing games tailored to their abilities, interests and rates of recovery. PURR can be used with patients at all stages of their neurological injury rehabilitation, in hospital and at home. It comprises two key components [18]:

1. A games development platform utilizing the Microsoft Kinect that can be used to create engaging and clinically relevant Patient Rehabilitation Experiences (PREs) tailored to a patients abilities and improvement of their clinical symptoms, as well as to their personal interests (Fig 2 left).
2. A metrics and monitoring engine for collecting data that can be used to track and assess the progress a patient is making as a result of their rehabilitation programme, and for adjusting in real-time game play to a level that suits their capabilities (Fig 2 right).

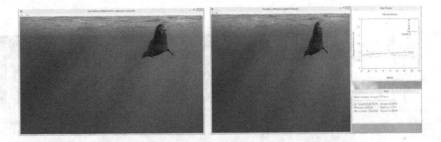

Fig. 2. Example of Patient's view (left) and Therapist's view (right) of screens

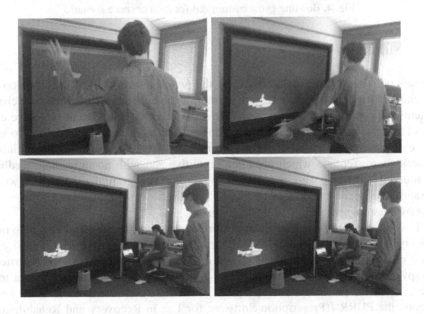

Fig. 3. Interacting with the game

The PREs operate as mini-games, challenging the patient to perform activities normally limited by their injuries encouraging them to perform better than they had previously thought possible and facilitating recovery (Fig 3). Feedback is given instantly for exceeding goals. Each experience dynamically alters to the abilities of a patient such that if a patient struggles to complete an action in a timely manner the next similar iteration will be simplified, thereby providing challenges that scale with ability and progress. Additionally, as the demographic of patients with brain injuries is wide, ranging across ages, backgrounds and interests, the PREs can be configured to be visually appealing and engaging to a specific patient and can be played whether standing or sitting. The ability for the software to self-adjust gameplay parameters based on a person's abilities means that rehabilitation can become a family-centred activity, something that was seen to be very important by many patients including Mr P (Fig 4).

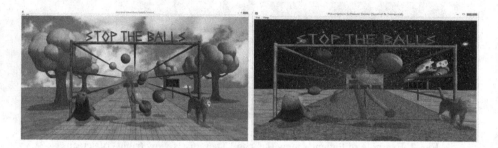

Fig. 4. Bowling game customized for field or space scenario

6   Summary

In trials utilizing off-the-shelf games and the personalised Patient Rehabilitation Experiences (PREs) we have consistently seen how the ludic nature of games can change patients' perceptions of the treatments they are receiving from being repetitive exercises to entertaining experiences. By making the recovery and rehabilitation process a fun, engaging, personalised and family-centric activity, in comparison to traditional rehabilitation exercises which are often repetitive and with no immediate feedback, we found that patients were more likely to not only engage in their treatment when a therapist was present, but also to initiate therapy sessions themselves when within their own homes and outside of therapist visits.

However, whilst off-the-shelf games were considered to be fun and engaging many patients were unable to make full use of the game features due to their complexity and speed of play, as well as the need for more tailored gameplay to suit their particular therapy needs. Additionally off-the-shelf games did not provide enough data to be able to clinically assess patients' progress. With these considerations in mind we developed the PURR ((Prescription Software for Use in Recovery and Rehabilitation) system.

Use of the PURR system to date has been well received by patients and health professions. The system is currently being enhanced and expanded to encompass further PREs, personalization, metrics collection and medical conditions. Larger scale trials are underway, as are trials with particular individuals over longer periods of their rehabilitation. The new Kinect 2 sensor is also being integrated into the PURR system in order to exploit its greater sensitivity and features with regards to providing more accurate tracking and a larger data set that can be analyzed to provide therapists with more precise assessments of patient progress.

Acknowledgements. We are very grateful for the contributions made and evaluations undertaken by the staff and patients of the RBH and Headway.

References

1. Headway, About Brain Injury (2014),
   https://www.headway.org.uk/About-Brain-Injury.aspx
2. Headway, Brain Injury Statistics (2014),
   https://www.headway.org.uk/key-facts-and-statistics.aspx
3. Brain Injury Association of America, Brain Injury Facts (2014),
   http://www.biausa.org/LiteratureRetrieve.aspx?ID=104992
4. McCallum, S.: Gamification and Serious Games for Personalilised Health. In: Blobel, B., et al. (eds.) pHealth 2012, pp. 85–95. IOS Press (2012)
5. Sawyer, B.: From Cells to Cell Processors: The Integration of Health and Video Games. IEEE Computer Graphics and Applications 28(6), 83–85 (2008)
6. Peterson Brooks, E.: Non-formal Learning through Ludic Engagement within Interactive Environments. Doctoral Thesis, Malmo University Electronic Publishing (2006),
   http://dspace.mah.se/handle/2043/7970
7. Lindley, C.A.: Ludic Engagement and Immersion as a Generic Paradigm for Human-Computer Interaction Design. In: Rauterberg, M. (ed.) ICEC 2004. LNCS, vol. 3166, pp. 3–13. Springer, Heidelberg (2004)
8. Gaver, W.W., Boucher, A., Bowers, B., et al.: The Drift Table: Designing for Ludic Engagement. In: CHI 2004, April 24-29. ACM 1-58113-703-6/04/0004, Vienna (2004)
9. Nintendo, Nintendo Wii,
   http://www.nintendo.co.uk/Wii/Wii-94559.html
10. Sony, PlayStationMove, Motion Controller,
    http://uk.playstation.com/psmove/
11. Microsoft, Kinect for Xbox, http://www.xbox.com/en-GB/Kinect
12. Broeren, J., Jalminger, J., Johansson, L.-Å., Parmerud, A., Pareto, L., Rydmark, M.: Information and communication technology - a person-centered approach to stroke care. In: Proc. 9th Intl Conf. Disability, Virtual Reality & Associated Technologies, Laval, France (2012)
13. Chang, Y.-J., Chen, S.-F., Huang, J.-D.: A Kinect-based system for physical rehabilitation: a pilot study for young adults with motor disabilities. J. Research in Developmental Disabilities 32(6), 2566–2570 (2011)
14. Lange, B., Chang, C.Y., Suma, E., Newman, B., Rizzo, A.S., Bolas, M.: Development and evaluation of low cost game-based balance rehabilitation tool using the Microsoft Kinect sensor. In: Proc. IEEE Conf. Eng. Med. Biol. Soc., pp. 2011:1831–2011:1834 (2011)
15. Shires, L., Battersby, S., Lewis, J., Brown, D., Sherkat, N., Standen, P.: Enhancing the tracking capabilities of the Microsoft Kinect for Stroke Rehabilitation. In: IEEE 2nd International Serious Games and Applications for Health (SeGAH), Portugal, pp. 1–8 (May 2013)

16. Deterding, S., Dixon, D., Khaled, R., Nacke, L.: From Game Design Elements to gameful-ness: Defining "Gamification". In: MindTrex 2011, Tampere, Finland (September 28030, 2011)
17. Microsoft, Kinect Effect – Rehabilitating with Kinect | Royal Berkshire Hospital, England, XboxViewTV, http://www.youtube.com/watch?v=5sv3nKPeM9g
18. Simmons, S., McCrindle, R., Sperrin, M., Smith, A.: Prescription Software for Recovery and Rehabilitation using Microsoft Kinect. In: Proc. 7th International Conference on Per-vasive Computing Technologies for Healthcare (Pervasive Health), Venice, pp. 323–326 (May 2013)

A Design-led Research Approach
to Contextual Evaluation of Socio-psychological Factors
in the Development of Telehealth Devices

Anna Mieczakowski, James King, and Ben Fehnert

Science Practice Ltd. & Eclipse Experience Ltd. (SPEE Ltd.)
83-85 Paul Street, London, EC2A 4NQ, UK
{anna,ben}@eclipse-experience.com,
james@science-practice.com

Abstract. Well-designed medical devices that embrace the socio-psychological needs of patients lead to increased customer acceptance, sustained use, improved safety and cost-effectiveness for both the professional and lay users. This paper proposes a new iterative design-led research approach for collecting and evaluating socio-psychological contextual user experience of patients and care providers in the telehealth development process. This approach, which has been applied to a multi-country development of a medical device, is based around the usage of a telehealth prototype from early stages of the design process. This allows for 'mini' elements of all design stages to be addressed in each individual stage to ensure the capture of contextual data from users about usage patterns, feelings and impact on the patient-clinician care relationship.

Keywords: Medical Devices, User Experience, Design-led Research Process, Contextual Inquiry, Socio-psychological Contextual Factors, Telehealth.

1 Introduction

The acceptance and seamless regular use of medical devices by end-users is a complex process, demanding the alignment of four layers of contextual factors: (1) characteristics of the environment in which the device is used; (2) knowledge and supplies required for the efficient operation of the device; (3) expectations about the performance and possible results reached with the device; and (4) demands placed by the device on the organisational structure of the healthcare delivery system [1].

Healthcare devices are typically subjected to safety evaluations [2], as well as clinical efficiency and related cost-effectiveness assessments [3]. However, although the International Organization for Standardization (ISO) 62366 [4] guidance emphasises the need to address wider usability issues in medical device development, the US Food and Drug Administration (FDA) [5] has recently identified a poor fit between healthcare devices and the home environment.

While there is a growing interest in the design of accessible and usable home-use medical devices, influenced by increased life expectancy and the accompanying

C. Stephanidis and M. Antona (Eds.): UAHCI/HCII 2014, Part III, LNCS 8515, pp. 321–332, 2014.
© Springer International Publishing Switzerland 2014

prevalence of chronic conditions, such as diabetes, heart disease, hypertension, COPD, arthritis and depression [6], systematic evaluations of users' contextual socio-psychological factors – which are critical to successful adoption and adequate sustained use of self-care systems impacting long-term health, and overall patient safety – are still largely a rarity [7]. Sadly, it is also a sporadic occurrence to conduct contextual evaluations of the continuous collaborative interaction between patients and health care providers, both of which are inherent parts in the deployment and running of every self-care monitoring system, as well as the changes to the care relationship that a telehealth device is likely to bring about.

Part of the problem lies in constrained ability to develop and validate user-centered devices, brought about by restricted product quality within medical device design and manufacturing, which, in turn, is a result of increasing competition, tightening profit margins and cost reduction requirements. The other part of the problem stems from a lack of a coherent understanding of all user needs, especially the more subtle socio-psychological ones which are more difficult to capture than the physical requirements, which only a well-crafted user research and design process can address.

This paper complements previous studies in the fields of human factors and usability design, which highlighted the need for a carefully-crafted design-led research approach to telehealth development that takes account of users' socio-psychological contextual factors. Specifically, this paper provides experiential insight from constructing and applying a design-led research process (pioneered by SPEE Ltd.) in the creation of a telehealth device for the motoring and treatment of a long-term condition in a number of countries. The objectives of this paper are three-fold:

1. First, this paper reviews current legislative guidance and good-practice advice on conducting human factors and usability engineering research during medical device design in order to determine the extent to which it promotes exploration of socio-psychological contextual user factors;
2. Second, it explores human socio-psychological contextual factors, both positive and negative, impacting on medical device usage and the patient-clinician care relationship, but which remain largely unaddressed. It also discusses design challenges that telehealth providers face with a missing, or sometimes fragmented, picture of the socio-psychological requirements of lay and professional users;
3. Third, it describes a practical experience, and its benefits, of constructing and applying an iterative design-led research process in the design of a self-management healthcare system to elicit and address socio-psychological requirements of both lay and professional users.

2   Human Factors and Usability Regulations and Standards

Given that medical devices play a growing role in the care of millions of patients worldwide [8], they have to be designed to high-quality safety and usage effectiveness standards to ensure continual use. In order for a medical device to be approved for commercialisation, it requires adherence to specific regulations, with certain degrees of variability within the global regions in which they are to be launched [9, 10].

Recent greater focus on user safety and long-term usage effectiveness of the device has been triggered in the EU and the US due to a number of high-profile post-market surveillance device recalls, typically occurring as a result of quality or usability flaws [11, 12]. For example, Kramer et al. [13], who reviewed publicly available weekly enforcements report listings by FDA from January 2009 through May 2011, found 1,845 recalls. One recent recall case involved the *23andMe* company being requested by the FDA to stop marketing its genetic tests for healthcare purposes [14].

What these efforts and medical device research collectively indicate is that capturing the requirements of targeted users and incorporating these into design in an iterative manner is an essential component of the design process, and is widely advised by both the aforesaid regulatory bodies and standardisation organisations (e.g. International Organization for Standardization (ISO) and British Standards Institute (BSI)). In essence, human factors and usability techniques are critical to fulfilling the design control requirements for the FDA regulation so that medical devices are designed for safety, effectiveness and sustained usage of professional and lay users.

2.1 Differences between and Common Application of Human Factors Analyses

Recently, there have been numerous calls to increase the application of *human factors* (i.e. safety, effectiveness and human capability limits evaluations) and *usability engineering* (i.e. investigations of ease-of-use, system intuitiveness and task completion timing) assessments in healthcare and patient safety [15, 16]. In fact, most of the medical devices standards and regulations for the design of medical devices heavily promote the application of contextual inquiry and overall user-centred testing [10].

However, whilst *contextual inquiry* lies at the heart of these user-centred investigations, it is not always clear how to best conduct it. In particular, much good-practice guidance [17, 18] lists the different user methods (e.g. *focus groups, ethnography, task analysis*) for conducting contextual investigation, but it does not specify how to best choose the 'right' set of methods, nor does it explain their underlying linkages. For instance, the *contextual inquiry* method can potentially span and direct the usage of such research techniques as *task analysis, interviews* and *usability tests*.

On a related but separate note, there is a common tendency in the user research guidance to break up the application of research methods for three complementing tiers – *identifying user needs, ensuring that the device meets user needs* and *evaluating how well the user needs are met* – when it fact the methods used for one of these tiers can be best utilised when applied with others in one holistic process.

On top of this, little effort has been expended on performing in-depth evaluations of users' contextual socio-psychological needs in relation to sustained use. Instead, most contextual inquiry effort has been on uncovering the contextual factors of a household's physical environment, such as the impact that humidity, temperature, inappropriate illumination and glare, vibrations and magnetic interference of the environment might have on the device [e.g. 19], rather than subtle socially- and psychologically-induced feelings and behaviours towards the device adoption and use.

3   Socio-psychological Factors in Telehealth Design

Ultimately, good design must take into account both the physical and socio-psychological needs of patients and care providers. For example, May-Russell [20] stresses that "for users it is often not just a case of what the device does, but how it makes them feel that really matters". Martin et al. [21] warn that for any one device there will be a number of different users to consider, including doctors, nurses, patients and their carers, and the maintenance staff, and so it is important to consider the diverse environments in which it is to function. There is currently much postulation for undertaking human factors and ethnographic methodologies extensively.

Greater focus on users' physical needs is not a by-product of device developers not caring or not considering users' socio-psychological needs as important, but the problem likely lies in that most medical device developers have not necessarily been aware of how to best elicit information about users' social-psychological needs. This issue potentially stems from a number of human factors techniques in healthcare being relatively immature and in need of further scientific development [22].

This situation is slowly shifting, however. Psychological (i.e. emotional and cognitive) aspects of design are slowly gaining their rightful visibility in product creation, as more attention is being progressively given to the natural variability in the decomposition of and emotional response to products among generations and cultures [23].

Numerous studies have indicated that motivation, in particular, has a significant impact on the emotional experience and perseverance with a product. Specifically, Deci and Ryan's [24] Self-Determination Theory (SDT) stipulates that three underlying core psychological needs are required to ensure that a user actively engages with products, services and environments: *competence*, *autonomy* and *relatedness*. For example, the acquisition of feelings of competence (i.e. feeling effective) early in an experience can prevent later negative reactions to errors and promote perseverance in the face of challenge [25]. Importantly, individuals must have many early successes and positive feedback to increase intrinsic motivation and to lessen the negative impact of future failures [25, 26]. The feelings of competence can be enhanced by both rewards and feedback, among other factors such as an optimal level of challenge, but only if there are sufficient feelings of autonomy (i.e. feeling a full sense of choice and endorsement of an activity [e.g. 27]). Evidence shows that having a sense of autonomy over one's activity is associated with: alertness and well-being [28], positive effects on patient outcomes [29] and enhanced object attractiveness [30]. The optimal levels of both competence and autonomy are, in turn, affected by sufficient feelings of relatedness (i.e. feeling connected to others).

Furthermore, an optimal user experience can be achieved when *task challenge* levels are matched to the skill set of the user, an activity has *clear and bounded goals* and *immediate feedback* is provided so that the user knows how they are doing [31]. A separate but important feature of this optimal user experience (called *Flow* by Csikszentmihályi [31]) is a sense of *control*, which is a major component of autonomy, the sufficient levels of which lead to more exploratory behaviour in users.

A previous body of work has also indicated that other psychological factors, such as personality traits, influence the degree to which the manipulation of challenge level affects motivation [32]. In particular, goal-setting, directly linked to increased motivation, has been reported to be more effective for certain personality types. Generally, human behaviour is affected by three sets of factors: *personal* (i.e. self-esteem, personality traits, locus of control, emotions, health concern); (2) *demographic* (i.e. age, gender, race, ethnicity, education, income, religion); and (3) *environmental* (i.e. diagnosis, stress, media exposure) [33]. What these studies collectively show is that that any artifact adoption and usage is influenced by subtle, multi-faceted, and often early formed, socio-psychological factors, which are largely non-trivial to elicit.

The importance of balanced socio-psychological aspects of interaction with medical devices has been discussed by Thomson et al. [34]. In particular, this study, which investigated the integration of home use medical devices into the lives of 12 older people over 65 with chronic conditions and five of their partners, identified areas of tension between users in general and the medical devices they used. In essence, this investigation showed that the studied devices generally did not slot into people's lives and required adjustments and alternations to fit in. There were also problems with people feeling that they had little control over their devices as they entered their lives and feared the potentially fatal consequences of not using them. This led to the feelings of resignation, which, in turn, had a detrimental impact on users' self-esteem. Related studies by the Multidisciplinary Assessment of Technology Centre for Healthcare (MATCH) project [35] also showed that home-use medical devices have emotional consequences not just for the user, but also for their partner. In particular, the build-up of negative emotions, including anxiety and annoyance, in both the user and their partner were said to be triggered by the device constantly reminding of the illness in the house, as well as the high-noise levels that such devices can produce. This negativity often led users to use the device in isolation, for example in the bathroom which is not always an ideal usage setting. Moreover, especially for older individual with grandchildren, a proper set-up and operation of the device was compromised after becoming a central focus of play during grandchildren's visits.

The key tensions uncovered by Thomson et al. [34], which span all levels of human affect towards the device, fall within two overarching themes:

1. *Striving to maintain self-esteem*, which highlights the importance of co-design co-research attendance to users' *psychological* factors such as: *feeling powerless*; *experiencing personal control* over illness; *mastering the device* which generates self-esteem and a sense of pride; and *comparing oneself to others* (i.e. deriving a sense of confidence from own regular skilled usage, as compared to others with a less robust device interaction).

   All of these factors are, of course, interwoven – feelings of personal control motivate device usage and subsequent mastery and vice versa, feelings of pride about own regular and skilled device usage and obtainment of positive feedback from others also impact on feelings of mastery and control, and collectively these factors significantly reduce feelings of powerlessness.

2. *The social device*, which highlights the importance of co-design co-research attendance to the impact medical devices have on their users' *social* interactions. Important social factors to address in medical device design include: *feelings of disrupted social harmony* (i.e. the negative impact the devices can have on the

users' partners and the overall household organisation, as well as interactions with visitors and the wider community); and ability of *bringing people together* (i.e. the device triggering a realisation of the illness in a family, leading to an increase of time spent together and greater interest in how the device operates, and creation of a joint ownership and responsibility for the device within a family).

In comparison, while it is certainly important to investigate the contextual needs of professional users (clinicians), previous research [19] argues that healthcare environments are very precise, controlled settings where integration of devices happens continuously and thus faster. In particular, users of medical devices in health care settings are likely to be experienced, trained, healthy professionals operating in standardised and regulated environments, and whilst devices likely have a big impact of their work outcomes, they would not generally generate similar levels of affective response toward their devices as home-use device users would.

While it is beyond the bounds of this paper to discuss the specific socio-psychological tensions found during the design-led research work on a telehealth device by the authors due to project confidentiality issues, it should be noted that careful attention was paid to the method selection for contextual inquiry in order to best elicit (through phased questioning) the subtlety of socio-psychological human factors of all system users as they learnt to use the device overtime. A great level of attention was also given to the attitude and behavioural change that the system brought out in patients and their healthcare providers overtime.

3.1 Problems with Elicitation of Socio-psychological Factors in Telehealth Design

As the abovementioned studies collectively show, there is an escalating need to increase the understanding of human socio-psychological user aspects by designers and healthcare professionals in order to better facilitate and support the integration of medical devices into the homes of lay users, and the overall monitoring of them in the clinical setting by professional users.

Thomson et al. [34], in particular, revealed the need for longitudinal qualitative study, utilising methods such as the Interpretative Phenomenological Analysis to describe the socio-psychological experience of device users before, during and after medical device acquisition for home use.

While it may not always be possible, or for other reasons feasible, to spend extensive amounts of time applying resource-heavy methods to elicit important contextual information as to how the device under development slots into people's lives, whether it requires further alternations to fit in and how it affects the patient's overall attitude toward their illness and long-term self-care, it is critical to consider the alternative methods for stimulating and simulating the gathering of user-focused contextual experience. Importantly, since people's initial response is driven by instincts, only then by often unpredictable pre-conceptions, the use of physical cues, such as a high-fidelity (i.e. three-dimensional design) telehealth prototype, to trigger human instinctual response is believed to be a powerful elicitation tool and a much stronger driver than spoken or printed words [20].

The new iterative contextual design-led research approach to telehealth design, which early on embedded an elaborate prototype in patients' homes and clinicians' work settings, is described in the following sections. This approach aids in the collection of rich contextual user information about professional and lay users' attitudes, behaviours and usage patterns, and the care relationship between them.

4   Proposed Iterative Design-led Research Process

The new contextual design-led research process proposed herein (see Figure 1) is a mindful user-focused aggregation of leading healthcare medical device design processes (as advised by the regulatory and standardisation bodies) and other user-centred iterative design methodologies [e.g. 17].

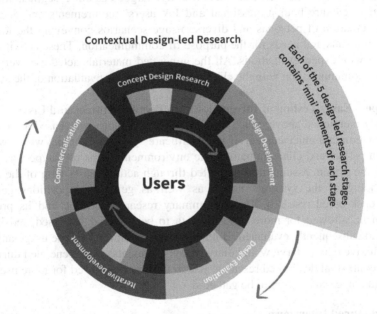

Fig. 1. Visualisation of the new iterative design-led research process for telehealth design (applicable also to development in other sectors)

While it is composed of the same design stages that are typical in the medical device development, its key innovation is greater focus on users' needs through an early usage of a system prototype that enables application of 'mini' elements of all stages with each of the five stages of telehealth design (i.e. *concept design research, design development, design evaluation, iterative development* and *commercialisation*).

The following sections describe the key contextual inquiry activities aimed at eliciting rich socio-psychological contextual factors, carried out during each of the iterative miniturised process activities within each of the macro design stages.

4.1   Types of Materials Used in Socio-psychological Contextual Inquiry

The contextual inquiry method is generally advised by different regulatory and stan-dardisation bodies (e.g. FDA, ISO) as the key approach to investigation and evalua-tion of user requirements and needs as operating within a given environment. While this approach is widely promoted, the application of specific methods and materials that it encompasses is rarely explained in sufficient depth, allowing plenty of room for interpretation, and more importantly misinterpretation. This section, therefore, de-scribes the different methods, together with their specific iterative application, that were used within the contextual inquiry part of the healthcare system design.

The project adopted a continual questioning approach throughout the whole design process. In the initial stage, a design rationale document was constructed by question-ing the knowledge and assumptions of the client and devising key assumptions as to the system's inputs and outputs. Subsequently, target customer segmentation was generated to capture both professional and lay users' requirements and needs, fol-lowed by creation of personas and diverse usage scenarios conveying the identified user requirements and needs for the purpose of communication. These activities were interfaced with expert evaluations. All the generated materials acted as a very useful trigger for communication with the client and collaborative evaluation of the system.

Prototype – Early Testing of Integration into People's Homes and Lives

As already mentioned above, much of the contextual inquiry was based around itera-tive evaluation and enhancement of the healthcare system prototype, which was em-bedded in patient and clinician naturalistic environments. This prototype was built in line with the system assumptions compiled through active questioning of the client's understanding of the system's needs, as well as general suppositions generated through desk-based research. This preliminary research activity, and its prototype embodiment, allowed for more research data to be gathered, analysed, fed into the design and subsequently evaluated. Both quantitative data (prototype usage analytics) and qualitative data (interview and diary study statements) were generated during this iterative contextual design-led research, which ultimately allowed for more user expe-rience and contextual factors to be gathered.

Semi-structured Interviews

In-depth *semi-structured interviews* with target patients and clinicians were carried out at four-weekly intervals to elicit and re-evaluate the requirements and needs of the professional and lay users of the healthcare system. Overall, each patient and clinician participated in three interviews, ranging between one-two hours. All the interviews were carried out in the naturalistic home or work setting of the patients and clinicians, and focused around discussing the usage of the prototype (i.e. ease of set-up, adoption and use, regularity of use, general feelings toward the device and how it fitted within life, and changes in patient-clinician care relationship). Apart from discussing general usage and the feelings it generated, the interviews also focused around showcasing new, often more advanced, illustrations of system features (through a paper-based prototype) and eliciting participants' response to them. Before being implemented, each set of new features had to be first discussed with the patient and clinician users.

The interviews were recorded through notes and videos, transcribed and analysed thematically, and then immediately updated in the system's requirements document. Given that the whole contextual inquiry approach was of an iterative nature, both higher-level and lower-level requirements, user feature lists and functional requirements were constantly addressed and re-addressed during the system design.

Structured Discussion Guides

Although the interviews were of a semi-structured nature, structured discussion guides broken into two parts – discussing existing usage and new use through illustrated paper prototypes – were created for each interview to facilitate participatory design and to ensure that all necessary topics relating to the usage of the system and users' feelings, as perceived by the researchers and the client, were covered, whilst also allowing the freedom for the participants to express any other insights and feelings that they observed and wanted to share. Each discussion guide was built on the findings of the previous set of patient and clinician interviews and the extent to which they helped to answer the project questions.

Interestingly, two of the second interval interviews had to be conducted in the hospital, rather than the home, setting as two patients suffered periods of ill health requiring hospitalisation. This allowed for additional rich data to be gathered about the emotional experience of patients relating to the 'failed' expectation of the system, as they believed it would keep them out of the hospital. In addition, the hospitalisation experience allowed the researchers to observe direct interaction between the patient and hospital clinicians and provided additional insight into the management of the health condition by both parties concerned.

Diary Study and Multimedia Personas Simulations

The design-led research process also employed a diary study to capture patient and clinician insights about system usage and the change it has brought about in their care relationship during the four-week break in meetings with the researchers. This was an important part of the research as it captured insights about usage patterns and feelings when participants were relaxed in their natural environment, as opposed to being potentially less relaxed during the interview visits.

In addition, the communication of key contextual findings regarding usage and its environment from the point of view of both professional and lay users was performed by the use of multimedia personas and their contextual life/work scenarios.

5   Evaluation of Proposed Design-led Research Process

Overall, the design-led research process described in this paper yielded rich and nuanced socio-psychological contextual data about medial device usage that was continually re-addressed in each design iteration phase. To this extent, this context-focused design-led research process provided a very good fit and sufficient depth for answering the key questions around user needs posed in this telehealth design project. Ultimately, this process allowed to generate design content that involved all project stakeholders and device users at both ends of the healthcare provision system.

This section aims to evaluate the efficacy of the proposed design-led research process to fulfilling the World Health Organization [1] guidance regarding the alignment of four layers of contextual factors in healthcare design outlined earlier in this paper.

The iterative nature of the twinned co-design co-research activities and its focus on usage of a system prototype by sampled target users (patients and clinicians) in their naturalistic usage environments from early stages allowed to gather and address intended users' lifestyle needs (also in relation to other household members), usage motivation, underlying feelings that the illness and the device bring about, and diverse levels of technological competence. In relation to clinicians, this process also enabled the design team to gather and address important workload management needs and, in particular, the coping with technology-induced instantaneous information, reminders and warning signals, as well as the relationships between co-clinicians and the individuals they cared for. In addition, it allowed to investigate how better patient condition visibility would increase rapidity of responses and the transmission of information between healthcare resources and departments, and changes in the care provision.

6   Discussion and Conclusions

In a much-needed search for a new approach to design of medical devices that would embrace the important socio-psychological contextual needs of users, this paper reviewed the extent to which current legislative guidance and good-practice advice promotes exploration of contextual user factors. It also explored existing evidence on the influence that socio-psychological factors, both positive and negative, have on medical device usage. Lastly, it described a practical experience, and its benefits, of constructing and applying an iterative design-led research process in the design of a home-use medical device to be used internationally in order to elicit and address socio-psychological requirements of both lay and professional users.

Overall, this paper has demonstrated the value of applying a mindfully crafted contextual design-led research in order to elicit socio-psychological factors of healthcare device users during medical device design. This new process builds on the existing design practice from a highly regulated medical device sector, but, unlike the current design approach, it drives all research activities through an early embedding of a telehealth prototype in natural user environments to generate continuous design embodiment of the identified needs for constant user evaluation. To achieve this, miniturised versions of all stages' activities are addressed in each of the five formal design stages. The highly positive feedback from users and the project client demonstrated a strong business case for the application of this iterative design-led research process.

While the application of the new design-led research process proved invaluable during the authors' project in the elicitation of rich contextual data regarding device usage and the impact of human affective state on it, it is also understood that this approach requires further verification. Thus, future work will focus on further evaluating the proposed process during telehealth device realisation.

References

1. World Health Organization (WHO): Medical Devices: Managing the Mismatch: An Outcome of the Priority Medical Devices Project. World Health Organization Report (2010)
2. International Organization for Standardization (ISO) 14971: Medical Devices: Application of Risk Management to Medical Devices, Geneva, Switzerland (2007)
3. Tice, J.A., Helfand, M., Feldman, M.D.: Clinical Evidence for Medical Devices: Regulatory Processes Focusing on Europe and the United States of America. The World Health Organization Report, Geneva (2010)
4. International Organization for Standardization (ISO) 62366: Medical Devices: Application of Usability Engineering to Medical Devices, Geneva, Switzerland (2008)
5. US Food and Drug Administration (FDA): Medical Devices: Home Use Devices, US Food and Drug Administration (2012)
6. World Health Organization (WHO): Primary Health Care (Now More Than Ever). The WHO Report (2009)
7. Lang, A.R., Martin, J.L., Sharples, S., Crowe, J.A.: The effect of design on the usability and real world effectiveness of medical devices: A case study with adolescent users. Applied Ergonomics 44, 799–810 (2013)
8. Curfman, G.D., Redberg, R.F.: Medical devices: Balancing regulation and innovation. The New England Journal of Medicine 365, 975–977 (2011)
9. Medical Devices Directive: Council Directive 93/42/EEC of 14 June 1993 concerning medical devices. European Commission (1993)
10. US Food and Drug Administration (FDA) 21CFR 820.30: Quality System Regulation: Design Controls (2013)
11. European Commission: Proposal for a Regulation of the European Parliament and of the Council on Medical Devices, and Amending Directive 2001/83/EC, Regulation (EC) No 178/2002 and Regulation (EC) No 1223/2009 (2012)
12. US Food and Drug Administration (FDA): Understanding Barriers to Medical Device Quality. FDA (2011)
13. Kramer, D.B., Baker, M., Ransford, B., Molina-Markham, A., Stewart, Q., Fu, K., Reynolds, M.R.: Security and Privacy Qualities of Medical Devices: An Analysis of FDA Postmarket Surveillance. PLoS ONE 7, e40200 (2012)
14. US Food and Drug Administration (FDA): "23andMe, Inc. 11/22/13" (2012),
   http://www.fda.gov/iceci/enforcementactions/warningletters/
   2013/ucm376296.htm
15. Gurses, A.P., Ozok, A.A., Pronovost, P.J.: Time to accelerate integration of human factors and ergonomics in patient safety. BMJ Quality and Satefy 21, 347–351 (2012)
16. US Food and Drug Administration (FDA): General Human Factors Information and Resources: What is Human Factors/Usability Engineering? (2013)
17. NHS National Patient Safety Agency: Design for patient safety: User testing in the development of medical devices (2010) ISBN: 978-1-906624-11-8
18. US Food and Drug Administration (FDA): Applying Human Factors and Usability Engineering to Optimise Medical Device Design. US Department of Health and Human Services (2011)
19. Bitterman, N.: Design of medical devices: A home perspective. European Journal of Internal Medicine 22, 39–42 (2011)
20. May-Russell, S.: Medical devices designed with patients in mind. European Industrial Pharmacy 14, 13–15 (2012)

21. Martin, J.L., Norris, B.J., Murphy, E., Crowe, J.A.: Medical device development: The challenge for ergonomics. Applied Ergonomics 39, 271–283 (2008)
22. Waterson, P.E., Anderson, J.: Bridging the Research Practice Gap in Healthcare Human Factors and Ergonomics. In: Ergonomics & Human Factors Conference, Cambridge, UK, April 15-18, pp. 15–18 (2013)
23. Demirbilek, O., Sener, B.: Product design, semantics and emotional response. Ergonomics 46 (2003)
24. Deci, E.L., Ryan, R.M.: Self-determination theory: A macrotheory of human motivation, development, and health. Canadian Psychology-Psychologie Canadienne 49, 182–185 (2008)
25. Bandura, A.: Self-efficacy: Toward a unifying theory of behavioral change. Psychological Review 84, 191–215 (1977)
26. Vallerand, R.J., Reid, G.: On the causal effects of perceived competence on intrinsic motivation: A test of cognitive evaluation theory. Journal of Sport Psychology 6, 94–102 (1984)
27. The Marmot Review: Fair Society Healthy Lives. Strategic Review of Health Inequalities in England post-2010 (2010)
28. Langer, E.J., Rodin, J.: The effects of choice and enhanced personal responsibility for the aged: A field experiment in an institutional setting. Journal of Personality and Social Psychology 34, 191–198 (1976)
29. Ogden, J., Daniells, E., Barnett, J.: When is choice a good thing? An experimental study of the impact of choice on patient outcomes. Psychology, Health & Medicine 14, 34–47 (2009)
30. Huang, Y.H., Lei, W., Junqi, S.: When do objects become more attractive? The individual and interactive effects of choice and ownership on object evaluation. Personality and Social Psychology Bulletin 35, 713–722 (2009)
31. Csikszentmihályi, M.: Flow: The Psychology of Optimal Experience. Harper Perennial, New York (1991)
32. Durik, A.M., Harackiewicz, J.M.: Achievement goals and intrinsic motivation: Coherence, concordance, and achievement orientation. Journal of Experimental Social Psychology 39, 378–385 (2003)
33. Ajzen, I.: The theory of planned behavior. Organizational Behavior and Human Decision Processes 50, 179–211 (1991)
34. Thomson, R., Martin, J.L., Sharples, S.: The psychosocial impact of home use medical devices on the lives of older people: A qualitative study. BMC Health Services Research 13, 1–8 (2013)
35. Multidisciplinary Assessment of Technology Centre for Healthcare (MATCH) (2014), http://www.match.ac.uk/

Memory Box: A Personalised Multimedia Device for Individuals with Dementia

Kanvar Nayer[1], Arthur de Bono[1], Selby Coxon[1],
Eva van der Ploeg[2], and Daniel O'Connor[2]

[1] Department of Art Design & Architecture, Monash University, Melbourne, Australia
{kanvar.nayer,arthur.debono,selby.coxon}@monash.edu
[2] Department of Psychological Medicine,
Monash University, Melbourne, Australia
esvdploeg@gmail.com, daniel.oconnor@monash.edu

Abstract. A significant percentage of those aged 65 and over live with a group of disorders known collectively as dementia, an irreversible and progressive decline in cognitive function beyond that expected from normal ageing. In 2013, 44 million people worldwide were affected, and this figure is projected to reach 135 million by the year 2050. However, due to busy schedules, caregivers are unable to provide everyone in their charge with as much personal attention as they would like. This reduction in stimulation and social contact can result in monotony and concomitant boredom, loneliness, agitation and even aggression. This paper provides information on the progress and process of research conducted between 2011 and early 2014, directed at developing 'Memory Box'; a personalised multimedia device, which can be used independently by individuals with dementia, to access their favourite music, videos, photographs and pre-recorded messages from family members.

Keywords: Dementia, Multimedia, Touch-screen, Interface.

1 Introduction

Since the beginning of recorded history, the global population has been ageing, and this trend shows no sign of abating. On the contrary, according to a 2002 United Nations report (UN), the rate of global population ageing in the 21st century is expected to exceed that of the previous century; those over 80 are currently the fastest growing age-group (UN, 2002). Although largely the result of positive factors (such as increased life expectancy) one of the unfortunate side-effects of global ageing is a higher prevalence of dementia, as the condition is far more common in the elderly. Global incidence is expected to rise from 44 million in 2013 to 135 million by the year 2050 (BBC, 2013). The UN report also predicts that the same year will mark the reversal of the global ratio of young (under 15) to old (over 60) for the first time in human history, and warns of the socio-economic stress that current trends portend. The 'global disaster waiting to happen' is predicted to be 'the biggest health and care problem of our generation' (BBC, 2013). This paper will summarise the development

C. Stephanidis and M. Antona (Eds.): UAHCI/HCII 2014, Part III, LNCS 8515, pp. 333–341, 2014.

of a multimedia device called 'Memory Box' that aims to treat the Behavioral and Psychological Symptoms of Dementia (BPSD) and improve the quality of life of its users.

1.1   What is Dementia?

The term dementia describes a collection of conditions caused by a progressive decline in cognitive function beyond that expected from normal ageing (Disabled World, 2013). These conditions include amnesia, changes in personality, language attrition, loss of perception and cognitive dysfunction (AIHW, 2007) which may affect one's intellect, sociability, rationality and normal emotional reactions (Alzheimer's Australia, 2009). In summary, the condition makes day to day life very difficult for those affected (Alzheimer's Australia, 2012).

Although it can occur at any stage of adulthood, dementia is far more common in the geriatric population (Disabled World, 2013). Unfortunately, the effects are both degenerative and irreversible. There is currently no cure for dementia (Access Economics, 2009).

1.2   Non-medicinal Interventions

Data from numerous trials indicate that medication is still used as the primary form of treating BPSD despite there being frequent evidence from clinical trials of high placebo response rates (Ballard & O'Brien, 1999). In the developed world, more than 40% of people with dementia are taking inappropriate and unnecessary prescribed medication (Margallo-Lana et al, 2001) which can lead to negative side-effects such as sedation, concomitant falls, reduced well-being and quality of life (Ballard et al, 2001) and even a decline in cognition (McShane et al, 1997).

These and other negative side-effects encourage the development of effective non-medicinal forms of treatment that would address the causes of psychological distress, which include boredom, loneliness, loss of intimacy, diminished self-esteem, curtailed opportunities for meaningful activity, and the like, without any adverse side-effects.

1.3   The Problem

As O' Connor et al. (1990) observe, carer burden is proportional to the severity of BPSD and is usually the main reason for the placement of those afflicted into aged-care facilities. The result is a high prevalence of BPSD in the interned population (Schultz & Williamson, 1991 and Haupt and Kurz, 1993).

Research suggests that due to busy schedules, caregivers at aged-care facilities may not always have the opportunity to provide persons with dementia with an ideal amount of attention (Cohen-Mansfield, 2001). As BPSD exacerbate, it is more difficult for family members and caregivers to communicate with and handle those exhibiting them (O'Connor et al., 1990). Individuals with dementia therefore spend much of their time in isolation, which can cause boredom, loneliness, agitation or even aggression (as well as other common symptoms) (Alm et al. 2003).

2   Literature Review Summary

To date, there are hundreds if not thousands of studies that have looked at interventions for the reduction of BPSD. Since non-medicinal interventions have been reported to be effective in reducing BPSD, it is on this basis that a literature review was conducted in 2011 by the authors of this paper. Some positive results reported that:

- audio-visual stimulation is an effective intervention for the reduction of BPSD, especially if tailored to suit their personal tastes (Cohen-Mansfield and Werner, 1997; Thomas et al., 1997; Clark et al., 1998; Gerdner, 2000; Sherratt et al., 2004; Garland et al., 2007)
- the use of touch-screen technology works well in allowing a degree of independence to residents at aged-care facilities, without the presence of a caregiver (Astell et al., 2008).

3   The Gaps

Because individuals with dementia responded well to personalised audio-visual stimulation (Cohen-Mansfield and Werner, 1997; Thomas et al., 1997; Clark et al., 1998; Gerdner, 2000; Sherratt et al., 2004; Garland et al., 2007) and since the intensity of one-on-one interaction with caregivers had practical limitations due to the busy schedules of the caregivers (Cohen-Mansfield, 2001), it followed, therefore, that there was a need to design a digital device that can serve as a means of making such audio-visual stimulation available to individuals with dementia in the most effective and most convenient way possible.

A question that is often asked is, "...so why, then, isn't everyone with dementia walking around with an iPod, or an iPad?" Unfortunately, it's not that simple. Owing to the nature of their impairment, individuals with dementia would require a highly specialised multimedia interface, if they are to operate it independently.

4   The Challenges

Between 2011 and early 2014, positive non-medicinal interventions have been tested on 7 individuals with mild dementia at Chelsea Manor, an aged-care facility in Melbourne.

Information from caregivers at Chelsea Manor reported that people with dementia possess certain characteristics that we must take into account during the design process:

- they are increasingly more forgetful as their impairment exacerbates, and they may misplace things, so the device can be neither too small nor portable
- they sometimes become agitated and aggressive, and may vent their anger at the equipment, so it has to be sturdy and durable, and made of material that will not cause them injury

- they may easily be distracted, so it has to offer variety to keep them continually interested, and riveted to the device
- they should be able to operate the interface easily, and independently, over a considerable period of time, irrespective of the decline in their level of impairment; so it has to adapt to their condition
- caregivers or family members should be able to update the content easily and as often as needed.

With these challenges in mind, we realised our device should not just be another generic computer, but a multimedia device dedicated to the use of our target group. It is from this information that we began to develop 'Memory Box'.

5   'Memory Box' (Summary)

This chapter summarises the key features of 'Memory Box' and briefly touches on test results from Chelsea Manor. In 2011, we introduced our project to residents at Chelsea Manor which resulted in the compilation of a Product Design Specification (P.D.S.) to establish usability requirements. Results demonstrated that:

- residents had their own personal media preferences. This brought about the design of individual devices or units for their bedrooms (rather than having a single device located in a hallway for everyone to share)
- the incorporation of a visual display, interface and media storage device of some sort would be necessary
- the product would need to be both accessible to people in wheel-chairs and on walkers, and capable of being mounted securely on a wall, table or at a bed-side

These constraints together with the valuable information from caregivers at Chelsea Manor narrowed down the amount of research we had to consider and led to the development of concepts, some of which have been simulated (figures 1, 2, and 3).

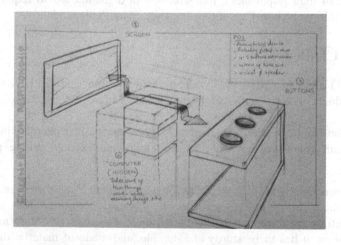

Fig. 1. Concepts (Nayer, K et al., 2011)

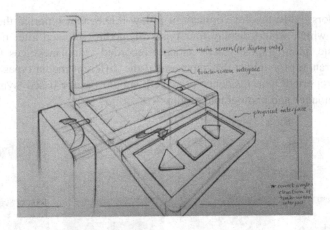

Fig. 2. Concepts (Nayer, K et al., 2011)

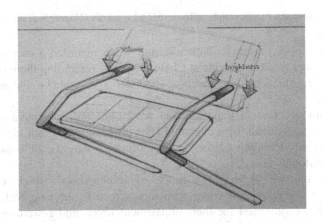

Fig. 3. Concepts (Nayer, K et al., 2011)

A few months later, ideation followed, resulting in a range of interface concepts, from physical buttons to icons on a touch-screen. Several of these concepts were built, tested, and evaluated during visits to Chelsea Manor.

Consultation and usability-testing revealed that although the novelty of touch-screen technology prolonged interest in use of the product, physical controls may be necessary for moderately and severely impaired users. Some users with mild impairment were unable to operate a touch-screen and preferred pushing the physical buttons as they were more familiar with these types of interfaces.

Our literature review reported that muted colours were preferred to bright colours; however, tests at Chelsea Manor proved otherwise. Accordingly, we selected and tested these bright colours which contrasted one another and received positive feedback. One resident was still able to identify the different colours despite being colour-blind. A black background offered the best contrast for our media buttons.

These factors led to the development of a new P.D.S. that reported the need for a touch-screen which would display four types of media (selected after our literature review): music, photographs, videos and pre-recorded video messages from family members. A range of symbols that represented the different media types were tested and results reported that residents preferred simple vector-based symbols to 3-dimensional images and photographs (figure 4).

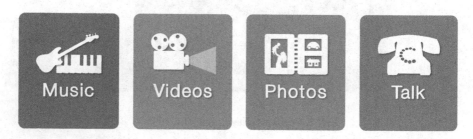

Fig. 4. Our selected media, colour selections and symbols (Nayer, K et al., 2011-12)

We then developed our first simulation, and video recorded a user operating the device. This was played to residents at Chelsea Manor, reminding them of the aim of our project. All residents enjoyed watching the video and wanted to try out the device for themselves.

An important observation indicated that we would not only have to design an interface for the individuals with dementia (our primary users), but also one for the caregivers or family members (secondary users), which would enable them to easily upload media onto the device.

From there on, we developed a range of screen-shots[1] which would allow individuals with dementia to navigate from one screen to the next with ease, using simple interfaces customised for their impairment level, and rewarding them with their favourite media (figure 5).

On our next visit to Chelsea Manor, we presented residents with a touch-screen (iPad) which none of them had ever used before. Residents were asked to play a simple game of Solitaire that would test the ease with which they could use the touch-screen. Results reported that residents preferred double-tapping the screen to sliding their fingers from one point to another. Some residents found the screen to be too bright, while others said it was too sensitive and too small to notice the numbers on the playing cards.

Further insight led to a solution that incorporated a larger touch-screen, physical buttons and the ability to select one of two interfaces to suit the different levels of dementia (mild, moderate and severe). Aspects of this design have undergone several rounds of usability tests and revision, with several simulations tested at Chelsea Manor. All users were able to navigate independently from one page to another using

---

[1] An image taken by a computer to record the visible items displayed on the monitor, television, or other visual output device.

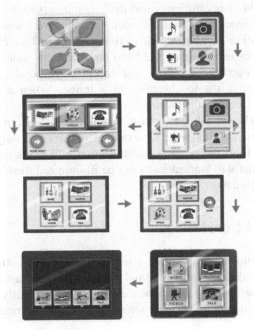

Fig. 5. The development of our screen-shots (Nayer, K et al., 2011-13)

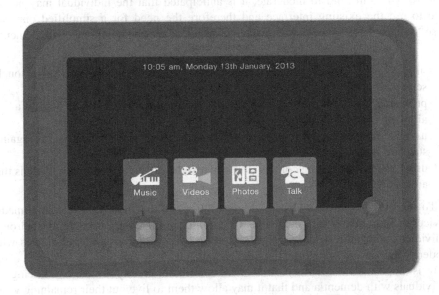

Fig. 6. 'Memory Box' (Nayer, K et al., 2013-14)

the touch-screen without any difficulty and made comments such as: "easy and fun to use", "incredible", "something I could get used to" and "now I won't get bored!"

Our latest simulation of Memory Box comprises of a 23 inch, infra-red touch-screen. This allows for users to navigate from one screen to another using the digital buttons on the touch-screen as well as translucent corresponding physical buttons, which are placed above the touch-screen in a frame. When a physical button is pushed, it makes contact with the touch-screen and activates it.

Our physical translucent Silicone buttons capture the light from the screen beneath it allowing it to glow. In this way, for example if there are only 3 media options available instead of four, the missing fourth section will black out creating a 'dead button' or a button that will automatically not be illuminated thereby not drawing any attention to itself (figure 6).

6   Results and Conclusions

Tests at Chelsea Manor confirmed that a touch-screen device offering personalised multimedia (music, videos, photographs and pre-recorded messages) can be used and enjoyed by individuals with mild dementia. However, for fully autonomous use, digital buttons / selections on the touch-screen should be accompanied by redundant physical counterparts.

Other tests indicated that if the impairment level of an individual with dementia exacerbated from mild to moderate, it is anticipated that the individual may not be able to use the existing interface and therefore the need for a simplified one will arise. 'Memory Box' aims at optimising independent use by individuals with dementia by:

- implementing physical buttons that correspond to digital buttons on a touch-screen
- providing interfaces that cater for the different impairment levels of dementia
- allowing for customisation; uploading an individual's favourite media
- using symbols that are familiar to an individual with dementia (as against standard international symbols)
- using bright contrasting colours (that can also be distinguished by individuals that are colour-blind)

To the best of our knowledge, 'Memory box' is the first dedicated multimedia device for individuals with dementia. To date, testing has only been conducted on 7 individuals with mild dementia. Further testing by psychologists on individuals with moderate and severe impairment is soon anticipated.

It is hoped that 'Memory Box' will contribute greatly to the well-being of individuals with dementia and that it may allow them to live out their remaining years with active minds and an improved quality of life, which would restore a sense of joy and contentment in them, their caregivers and family members.

References

1. AIHW (Australian Institute of Health and Welfare), 2007. Keeping Dementia Front of Mind: Incidence and Prevalence 2009-2050. Report by Access Economics Pty Limited for Alzheimer's Australia, p. 2 (2009)
2. Alm, N., Astell, A., Gowans, G., Ellis, M., Dye, R., Campbell, J.: Designing an Interface Usable by People with Dementia (2003)
3. Alzheimer's Australia. Keeping Dementia Front of Mind: Incidence and Prevalence 2009-2050. Report by Access Economics Pty Limited, p. 2 (2009)
4. Alzheimer's Australia. What is Dementia (2012)
5. Astell, A., Alm, N., Gowans, G., Ellis, M., Dye, R., Campbell, J., Vaughan, P.: Working with people with dementia to develop technology. PSIGE Newsletter (105) (October 2008)
6. Ballard, C.G., O'Brien, J.T.: Pharmacological treatment of behavioural and psychological signs in Alzheimer's disease: how good is the evidence for current pharmacological treatments? BMJ 319, 138–139 (1999)
7. Ballard, C.G., O'Brien, J., James, I., et al.: Dementia: Management of Behavioural and Psychological Symptoms. Oxford University Press, Oxford (2001)
8. Clark, M.E., Lipe, A.W., Bilbrey, M.: The use of music to decrease aggressive behaviours in people with dementia (1998)
9. Cohen-Mansfield, J., Werner, P.: The management of verbally disruptive behaviours in nursing home residents. Journal of Gerontology 52A, M369–M377 (1997)
10. Garland, K., Beer, E., Eppingstall, B., O'Connor, D.W.: A comparison of two treatments of agitated behaviour in nursing home residents with dementia: simulated presence and preferred music. American Journal of Geriatric Psychiatry 15, 514–521 (2007)
11. Gerdner, L.A.: The effects of individualised versus classical 'relaxation' music on the frequency of agitation in elderly persons with Alzheimer's disease and related disorders. International Psychogeriatrics 12, 49–65 (2000)
12. Haupt, M., Kurz, A.: Predictors of nursing home placement in patients with Alzheimer's disease. International Journal of Geriatric Psychiatry 8, 741–746 (1993)
13. Margallo-Lana, M., Swann, A., O'Brien, J., et al.: Prevalence and pharmacological management of behavioural and psychological symptoms amongst dementia sufferers living in care environments. International Journal of Geriatric Psychiatry 16, 39–44 (2001)
14. McShane, R., Keene, J., Gedling, K., et al.: Do neuroleptic drugs hasten cognitive decline in dementia? Prospective study with necropsy follow-up. BMJ 314, 211–212 (1997)
15. O'Connor, D.W., Pollitt, P.A., Roth, M., Brook, C.P.B., Reiss, B.B.: Problems reported by relatives in a community study of dementia. British Journal of Psychiatry 156, 835–841 (1990)
16. Sherratt, K., Thornton, A., Hatton, C.: Emotional and behavioural responses to music in people with dementia: an observational study. Aging and Mental Health 8, 233–241 (2004)
17. Schultz, R., Williamson, G.H.: A 2-year longitudinal study of depression among Alzheimer's caregivers. Psychology and Aging 6, 569–578 (1991)
18. Thomas, D.W., Heitman, R.J., Alexander, T.: The effects of music on bathing cooperation for residents with dementia. Journal of Music Therapy 34, 246–259 (1997)
19. UN (United Nations). World Population Ageing: 1950-2050. Executive Summary (2002)
20. BBC (2013), http://www.bbc.co.uk/news/health-25263341 (accessed December 11, 2013)
21. Disabled World. Dementia Facts and Information on Decline in Seniors Cognitive Function (2013), http://www.disabled-world.com/health/aging/dementia/ (accessed December 11, 2013)

Haptic AR Dental Simulator Using Z-buffer
for Object Deformation

Katsuhiko Onishi[1], Kiminori Mizushino[2], Hiroshi Noborio[1], and Masanao Koeda[1]

[1] Osaka Electro-Communication University
1130-70 Kiyotaki, Shijonawate, Osaka 5750063 Japan
`{onishi,nobori,koeda}@oecu.jp`
[2] Embedded Wings Co. Ltd, Japan
`k_mizushino@ewings.biz`

Abstract. Dental surgical simulator could be one of the efficient tools to learning and practicing dental surgical skills. To these simulators, the visual and tactile feedback is desirable to be processed in real time. And, in the dental operation, the hand position during operations is one of the skills to learn and practice. Therefore, we develop the dental surgical simulator which use virtual tooth surface model for processing real time rendering. And we develop a display system which allow users to training dental operation by a right hand position.. The tooth model is deformed by cutting and drilling operation using haptic device. And the display is set close to user's hand position and shows combined image with virtual tooth model as a surgical target and a real tooth model as other parts of the patient dental model. The system uses a collision detection and deformation method by using Z-buffer for virtual objects. This method enables users to view the complex shape of virtual tooth model by the surgical operation tasks and practicing dental surgical tasks. We developed prototype system and confirmed about the capability of our system.

Keywords: Collision detection, dental surgical simulator, augmented reality, GPU.

1   Introduction

In dental surgery, most surgical training methods use plastic tooth or live patients. These methods are good for improving surgical skills, for example, the use of surgical tools and surgical procedures. But it is difficult to do repetitive practice, because of the need for new plastic tooth or patients for each task. Therefore, several types of dental surgical simulator have been proposed [1], [2]. These simulators allow users to training dental surgical methods by using visual and haptic rendering [3], [4]. Most of systems use the volumetric implicit surface model for simulating dental surgical operation, such as cutting and drilling a tooth. Therefore, to reducing the rendering cost is one of the challenging issues. And to training complex tasks, some of the dental simulators use unique interfaces [5], [6], [7], [8]. However, most of these simulators use a typical computing display system. Therefore, the user cannot experience the actual hand positions or body posture required during dental surgery.

C. Stephanidis and M. Antona (Eds.): UAHCI/HCII 2014, Part III, LNCS 8515, pp. 342–348, 2014.
© Springer International Publishing Switzerland 2014

In this paper, we describe about our preliminary work of a dental surgical training system. Our system allows users to operate the surgical tasks by using haptic device. The system uses surface polygon model as a tooth model. And the deformation of a tooth model is generated by using GPU architecture. And our system set a display screen close to user's hand position for learning about real hand position and the body posture. The display screen shows combined image with virtual tooth model as a surgical target and a real tooth model as other parts of the patient dental model. In order to adapt to any head position of the user, the system measured the head position of the user and the position of the real tooth model. We make a prototype system which is implemented our deformation algorithm for dental tooth model on our display screen system.

2   Deformation Algorithm

Our system uses a deformation algorithm for rendering a tooth model to operating surgical tasks, cutting, drilling and so on. In order to reduce the computation time to rendering it, our system use a coordinate system organized the depth direction as a drilling direction. And our system use Z-buffer that is stored depth map in the coordinate system. Figure 1 shows the abstract of our algorithm.

2.1   Generating Depth Map

Generally, Z-buffer is used to rendering only the model showed from a viewpoint in 3D graphic scene. To use the Z-buffer, the system is enable to process many polygons simultaneously and reducing the rendering time. In our algorithm, it is used to measure the deforming volume by user's interaction. At first, the region of manipulation is defined by the virtual tool and the tooth model. And the coordinate system is defined in this region and stored the depth map. Figure 2 shows summary of this process.

2.2   Generating Depth Map within Collision Detection

In order to generate the depth map after the deformation by drilling with a virtual tool, it is stored amount of changing the depth map when the virtual tool drills it. This is used to change the shape of tooth model and calculate parameters to generate tactile feedback. This depth map is a simple two-dimensional array, and this process is executed by GPU.

2.3   Deforming Tooth Model by the Depth Map

The deformation tooth model is generated by the following process. At first, in order to be assigned vertex of the tooth model to Z-buffer, it uses a conversion method to change the vertex with world coordinate system, which constructs Z-buffer. And it acquires z value from the pixel, which contains the vertex in Z-buffer. The deformation volume is defined from this volume and it is reconverted to the vertex position in world coordinate system. All of this process is executed in the high-speed transaction by using the parallel processing in GPU.

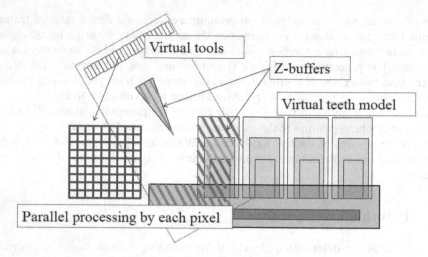

Fig. 1. The abstract of our algorithm

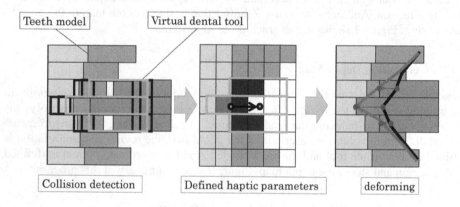

Fig. 2. Our deformation process

2.4   Subdivision Surface of a Tooth Model Deformation

To adapt this deformation process, our algorithm uses a method which changes the vertex point of a tooth model to deform it. In this algorithm, the surface of model is extended to a direction of deformed region and it is not enable to deform to other direction. To solve this problem, our system uses a subdivision surface algorithm to divide the extended surfaces. A summary of this method is that generates middle point to the edge between 2 vertexes with length more than a certain threshold.

Figure 3 shows this process. For example, in a case of adjacent surfaces, 1,2,3, and 1,3,4, it generates new vertex as index 5 on a side between index 1 and index 2. And it searches another surface which share the same vertex and side to generate same vertex, 5. Finally, these surface data is divided into 4 surfaces data. These data is stored only the index number of three vertex points. And the order of this three points is located in a clockwise direction.

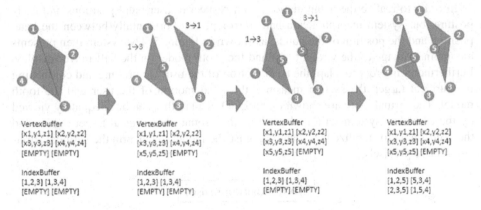

VertexBuffer
[x1,y1,z1] [x2,y2,z2]
[x3,y3,z3] [x4,y4,z4]
[EMPTY] [EMPTY]

VertexBuffer
[x1,y1,z1] [x2,y2,z2]
[x3,y3,z3] [x4,y4,z4]
[x5,y5,z5] [EMPTY]

VertexBuffer
[x1,y1,z1] [x2,y2,z2]
[x3,y3,z3] [x4,y4,z4]
[x5,y5,z5] [EMPTY]

VertexBuffer
[x1,y1,z1] [x2,y2,z2]
[x3,y3,z3] [x4,y4,z4]
[x5,y5,z5] [EMPTY]

IndexBuffer
[1,2,3] [1,3,4]
[EMPTY] [EMPTY]

IndexBuffer
[1,2,3] [1,3,4]
[EMPTY] [EMPTY]

IndexBuffer
[1,2,3] [1,3,4]
[EMPTY] [EMPTY]

IndexBuffer
[1,2,5] [5,3,4]
[2,3,5] [1,5,4]

Fig. 3. A process of subdivision surfaces

3   Display System

The real surgical environment is usually such that a patient is lying in front of a dentist while the dentist operates. In such a situation, the position of the dentist hands and the body posture of the dentist are different from those in traditional dental surgical simulation. For example, Figure 4 shows a typical hand position in dental surgical operation. It is needed strict movement to manipulate a dental tool for operating surgical tasks. The dentist put their hand on the patient teeth or gum as the fulcrum.

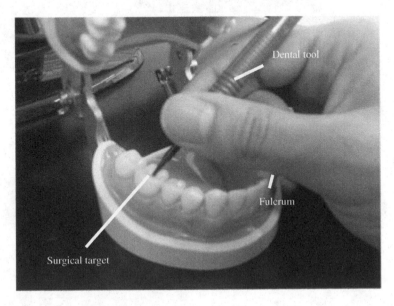

Fig. 4. An example of surgical hand position

In order to realize the manipulations with respect to user hand positions and body posture, our system incorporates a half mirror placed horizontally between the head position and the position of the hands, as shown in Figure 5. The system then presents a combined image of the virtual tooth and the tooth model on the half mirror display. Furthermore, in order to adapt the head motion of the user for probing and confirming the surgical target, the system measures the head motion of the user and the tooth model. The virtual tooth are shown on an LCD display that can be adequately viewed by the user. The system set a real tooth model around the surgical target tooth. And the user is able to stabilize their hands against the model to perform the surgical simulation tasks precisely.

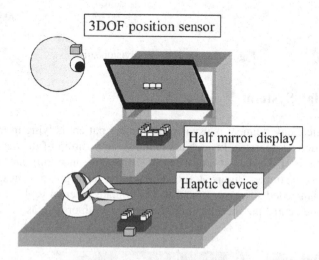

Fig. 5. Our dental surgical system

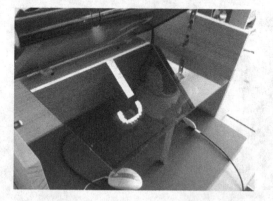

Fig. 6. Our prototype display

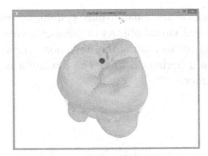

Fig. 7. Virtual tooth model

4   Prototype System

The prototype display is shown in Figure 6. The proposed system is implemented on a Windows PC, and the system measures the user's head position and real teeth model position using 3DOF magnetic sensors. It shows the users a tooth model and virtual tooth reflected onto the display from the half mirror. Figures 7 shows a virtual tooth model used in our system. This model is created as a surface model by each parts and the system check the collision detection in real time between surgical tools and the tooth model. And it is deformed the shape by user's surgical operation. A usage image of our system is shown in Figure 8. The system measures a viewing position of the user and shows the appropriate view based on that position. Then, the system allows the user to display the virtual and real tooth models simultaneously from any viewing position.

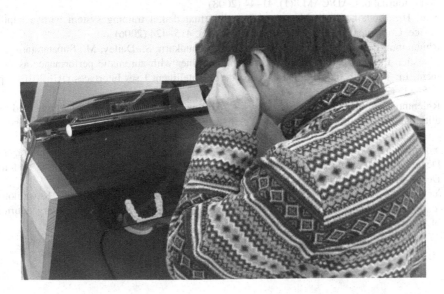

Fig. 8. An example of our display system

As a preliminary evaluation about the display system, we have measured the deviation between real objects and virtual objects in the user's view image. We use a cube model as the target model for measuring the deviation precisely. And it is measured from 8 view positions on a horizontal line. The deviation is about from 0.06cm to 1.00cm in these view positions.

5   Conclusion

We developed a dental surgical simulator system for learning and practicing dental surgical skills. The proposed system enables the user to view a combined image of virtual tooth and a tooth model. The user can see the combined image from any point of view by tracking his or her head position and the model position. We constructed a prototype system and confirmed the capability and the limitation of this system.

In future work, we will evaluate the haptic feedback module in this system. And we will improve the accuracy of the user's view image.

References

1. Jasinevicius, T.R., Michael, L., Suchitra, N., Alice, U.: An evaluation of two dental simulation systems: virtual reality versus contemporary non-computer-assisted. Journal of Dental Education 68(11), 1151–1162 (2004)
2. Dută, M., Amariei, C.: An overview of virtual and augmented reality in dental education. Oral Health and Dental Management 10(1), 42–49 (2011)
3. Kim, L., Park, S.: An efficient virtual teeth modeling for dental training system. International Journal of CAD/CAM 8(1), 41–44 (2008)
4. Yau, H., Tsou, L., Tsai, M.: Octree-based virtual dental training system with a haptic device. Computer-Aided Design & Applications 3, 415–424 (2006)
5. Rhienmora, P., Gajananan, K., Haddawy, P., Suebnukarn, S., Dailey, M., Supataratarn, E., Shrestha, P.: Haptic augmented reality dental trainer with automatic performance assessment. In: The 15th International Conference on Intelligent User Interfaces (IUI 2010), pp. 425–426 (2010)
6. Rhienmora, P., Gajananan, K., Haddawy, P., Dailey, M.N., Suebnukarn, S.: Augmented reality haptics system for dental surgical skills training. In: Proc: the 17th ACM Symposium on Virtual Reality Software and Technology, pp. 97–98 (2010)
7. Yoshida, Y., Yamaguchi, Y., Kawamoto, Y., Noborio, H., Murakami, S., Sohmura, T.: Development of a multi-layered virtual tooth model for the haptic dental training system. Dental Material Journal 30(1), 1–6 (2011)
8. Yoshida, Y., Yamaguchi, S., Wakabayashi, K., Nagashima, T., Takeshige, F., Kawamoto, Y., Noborio, H., Sohmura, T.: Virtual reality simulation training for dental surgery. Journal of Studies in Health Technology and Informatics, 435–437 (2009)

A Dialogue System for Ensuring Safe Rehabilitation

Alexandros Papangelis[1,2], Georgios Galatas[1,2], Konstantinos Tsiakas[1,2],
Alexandros Lioulemes[1,2], Dimitrios Zikos[1], and Fillia Makedon[1]

[1] Heracleia Human Centered Computing Lab,
Computer Science and Engineering Dept. University of Texas at Arlington, USA
[2] Institute of Informatics and Telecommunications, NCSR "Demokritos", Athens, Greece
{alexandros.papangelis,georgios.galatas,
konstantinos.tsiakas,alexandros.lioulemes}@mavs.uta.edu,
{zikos,makedon}@uta.edu

Abstract. Dialogue Systems (DS) are intelligent user interfaces, able to provide intuitive and natural interaction with their users, through a variety of modalities. We present, here, a DS whose purpose is to ensure that patients are consistently and correctly performing rehabilitative exercises, in a tele-rehabilitation scenario. More specifically, our DS operates in collaboration with a remote rehabilitation system, where users suffering from injuries, degenerative disorders and others, perform exercises at home under the (remote) supervision of a therapist. The DS interacts with the users and makes sure that they perform their prescribed exercises correctly and according to the specified, by the therapist, protocol. To this end, various sensors are utilized, such as Microsoft's Kinect, the Wi-Patch and others.

1   Introduction

To guarantee safe system access, we employ a secure log-in mechanism, which is being used for identification and personalization. As far as the identification is concerned, the system will be able to identify a subject by their biometric data. In related works, subject identification is achieved by speech or image [1,2]. In this work, we apply techniques for audio-visual data fusion in decision level. More specifically, after the identification, the user must verify his / her identity by saying a unique subject id which is assigned by the system. If the subject does not exist in the database, then the system adds the user into the database after collecting the required data. The system then can retrieve the user's profile and in this way, the session is personalized and adapted to this individual user, preventing injuries or harmful activities. We plan to evaluate our method against other proposed feature sets or similar methods, such as [3]. Regarding robust communication with the system, we employ state of the art Audio Visual Automatic Speech Recognition (AVASR) algorithms, paired with a Natural Language Understanding (NLU) component, responsible for making sure the subject's response is on-topic and satisfactory. AVASR utilizes the visual modality in addition to audio, in order to accomplish accurate and robust recognition of spoken words. More specifically, 3-dimensional visual speech articulation information is

C. Stephanidis and M. Antona (Eds.): UAHCI/HCII 2014, Part III, LNCS 8515, pp. 349–358, 2014.
© Springer International Publishing Switzerland 2014

extracted from the subject's mouth region using a Kinect sensor, and the data is fused with audio information. The output of the AVASR component is then fed to the NLU component. In case there is a misunderstanding (e.g. the user's response is off topic), the system will ask for clarification (e.g. explicit / implicit confirmation, repetition). The NLU component is also able to identify keywords indicating pain and rank them accordingly. Database attributes are vital for the system adaptation and important for personalization of each rehabilitation session. These attributes include user demographics, physical condition, history (chronic diseases, syndromes, previous rehabilitation) and physiological data (heart rate, respiration rate, blood pressure). This information is stored into a rule based backend server, which contains an evidence-based knowledge base on what is an appropriate rehabilitation activity for different demographics, clinical profiles, underlying physiological metrics and past performance. Data are either stored a-priori into the system (i.e. demographics) or dynamically acquired during the lifecycle of the system (i.e. rehabilitation history). The aforementioned information may be utilized for the adaptive personalization of the system, in an effort to maximise the benefits of the rehabilitation activities. When the subject completes a session, the system updates the database, storing useful information for future sessions (i.e. if a user gets easily tired, then the system should provide less intensive activities, or even switch to alternative exercises). To ensure correct execution of rehabilitative exercises and compliance with the current protocol (prescribed by the therapist), the DS analyzes data from Microsoft's Kinect and Wi-Patches (which monitor heart rate, blood pressure, and acceleration), in order to detect indicators of pain from facial expressions and speech as well as correct execution of exercises, within the prescribed acceptable boundaries. When the system detects unacceptable levels of pain, which may be explicitly stated by the user or inferred from sensor data, the exercise stops immediately and a report is issued to the therapist. When the system detects execution outside the prescribed boundaries (e.g. the subject raises their hand too high), it provides encouragement or warnings. Pain itself is not very informative regarding safety and compliance in exercise, so we use real-time monitoring of the rate of decline in exercise activity. Moreover, the DS prompts the subject at regular intervals, asking for comfort and pain levels, aiming to get an explicit answer. Responses are translated into a numeric value (0-11), according to the Numeric Rating Scale (NRS-11), an 11-point scale for patient self-reporting of pain. Sensor measurements have the added benefit of providing a ground truth, therefore enhancing the system's understanding, so for example, if the subject does not speak clearly, the system can infer pain levels by analyzing input from the sensors. To our knowledge, few related works combine audio-visual stimuli in order to extract human's feelings and the interest in these works has focused for example in emergency response systems, where the user cannot signal an emergency (e.g. by pressing a button) and in emotional expression recognition. In [8] a speech recognition interface has been developed that triggers a connection to an assistant when the users do not have access to an emergency signal button or to avoid unwanted and intrusive calls. In [9], the authors conducted experiments that combine facial and vocal expressions in order to infer the users' real emotions, through multi sensory interaction. Furthermore, rehabilitation systems researchers [10][11] have conducted experiments using 3D avatars and virtual environments that enable users to interact with the system and give force feedback to the therapist by analyzing the resistive forces from the body's movements and exercises [12][13][14][15]. However, these systems do not provide safe rehabilitation and to bridge this gap, we propose a multimodal system that ensures, to the extent possible, the users' correct execution of rehabilitative exercises.

2   Architecture

In this section we present the architecture of our system. We describe our novel user log-in method, as well as the AVASR technique we applied and present in detail how we model the interaction between the user and the dialogue system.

2.1   User Login and System Personalization

As already mentioned in the introduction, ensuring safe execution of the rehabilitation exercises is an essential part of our system. Users are required to follow a certain rehabilitation schedule, based on various criteria, decided by both the therapist and the user. The purpose of the login mechanism is twofold: it is used for automatic user recognition based on audiovisual features and also for personalization of the rehabilitation session. As far as the user recognition is concerned, the user can login to the system in an automatic way, without having to perform any specific action. This can be very useful for users that may suffer from kinesiology-related problems, or users that are unable to login to the system manually. On the other hand, the user, after the login process, connects to the user database. This database includes information about each user, describing their physical condition and other useful data regarding the rehabilitation session. During each session, the database is being updated, helping the system be better personalized for a user's future session.

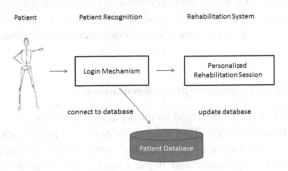

Fig. 1. Architecture of the proposed automatic log-in mechanism

2.2   Audio Visual User Recognition

User identification systems are very important for many applications, where the system must recognize a user's identity amongst many known users. Such systems mostly use speaker and face identification technologies, the most common being bio-metric identification. In this work, we implement an audiovisual user recognizer, combining speaker identification (or speaker recognition) and face recognition techniques. Speaker identification consists of recognizing a user based on the speech features of each user. It requires a prior enrollment phase, where the speech signal is processed extracting features to train an explicit model for each user.   Our system is a text- independent speaker recognition system that starts with an audio feature extraction module; for each speech signal, we extract the Mel Frequency Cepstral Coefficients (MFCC), which are being used extensively in such applications and have also been used for text- independent speaker recognition systems.   During our evaluation, we plan to compare a variety of classification methods, such as Euclidean distance, Nearest Neighbor and Gaussian Mixture Models (GMM). Face recognition is the procedure of identifying a person from a digital image. It has many applications on security systems and is another part of the biometric identification systems. It is based on comparing the user's facial features to a database of stored features and selecting the face that matches better, with respect to explicit facial features. A well-known facial feature extraction method is the Local Binary Patterns (LBP) method, a texture operator that is reliable and computationally efficient.   Shortly, it labels the pixels of an image by thresholding the neighborhood of each pixel and considers the result as a binary number.   LBP is widely used in face recognition systems, due to its simplicity and reliability, as well as robustness to illumination variations. After the facial feature extraction, we use specific classifiers (Euclidean Distance and Nearest Neighbor) to identify a test face image. In order to implement the audiovisual user recognition system, we perform data fusion at the decision level. To train the classifier, we create an audiovisual feature vector, unique for each user. Each vector consists of a unique user ID (UID), the LBP facial features and the MFCC speech features. We apply all the classification methods we referred to, and we classify each new entry (set of audiovisual features) to a UID. For the specific UID, we can retrieve all the useful information for each user. The user is thus automatically logged in the system and ready to perform any required exercises.   After the session, the user database can be updated for a future session. In this way, we achieve both user identification and system personalization.

2.3   Audio Visual Automatic Speech Recognition

The AVSR module that is integrated to the system is used to communicate with the user via recognition of speech. This module is based on prior work [4] and utilizes three distinct modalities captured by the Kinect, namely the audio signal of the speaker's voice and both color video and depth information from the mouth region of speaker's face. This approach ensures higher reliability for the system, since each stream captures correlated information from a different source, which can complement each other as well as account for different speech disorders expressed either in the vocal tract or the lip muscles. An important aspect of the effort is related to extracting speech informative features from the visual and depth streams. For this purpose, we employ appearance based features, obtained from the 2-D Discrete Cosine

Transform (DCT) of the mouth region-of-interest. A straightforward feature selection method of the resulting DCT coefficients is the use of feature energy and position as a measure of information content. The aforementioned approach is also applied to the depth data, after appropriate mapping of the tracked mouth region-of-interest from the traditional video data to the depth data stream. The features extracted from the audio stream are the well-known MFCCs. The statistical modeling is carried out by means of HMMs and the implementation is based on a modified version of HTK.

3   Dialogue System

Dialogue Systems (DS) are able to interact with their users in a natural manner, typically using spoken natural language input and output. Figure 2 shows the overview of our architecture, including the DS, where the user's input is processed and analysed, then forwarded to the Dialogue Manager (DM), which is the decision making component of the DS and decides how to respond to the user. This response is then forwarded to the appropriate modules, such as Natural Language Generation or Text to Speech.

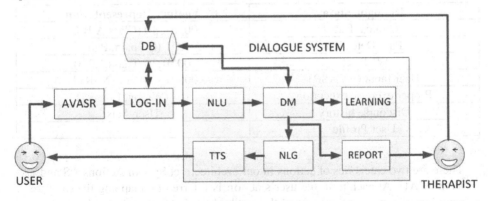

Fig. 2. The architecture of our proposed safe tele-rehabilitation system

To model the dialogue problem, we follow the Information State Update (ISU) paradigm [5]. According to this model, there is a current system state, called the dialogue state, typically represented as a vector that contains information of interest (such as user name, medical history, etc.). The dialogue state is updated according to a set of rules that are triggered during the interaction. In order to achieve adaptation to various user types and circumstances, we apply Machine Learning methods and specifically Reinforcement Learning (RL). Before applying such techniques, we need to define the dialogue problem as an optimization problem. We therefore use a Markov Decision Process (MDP) to model the interaction, which is defined as a tuple $\{S,A,T,R,\pi\}$, where S is the (dialogue) state space, A is the available actions the system can take, T is a transition probability matrix $SxA{\rightarrow}S$, $R:SxA{\rightarrow}Re$ is a reward function, π is a (dialogue) policy and is defined as a mapping between state-action pairs and probabilities, π: SxA→[0,1]. RL techniques, such as SARSA [6] or Natural Actor Critic (NAC) [7] are able to find, in an online fashion, an optimal policy π^*, i.e. a policy that yields maximum rewards. RL algorithms typically suffer from the curse of dimensionality and in an attempt to alleviate this problem, DS usually operate in feature space φ. Dialogue states are then mapped into this feature space and the Reward function as well as the dialogue policy are defined in φxA. Our system receives continuous feedback from both the user and the sensors (Kinect, Wi-patch). More specifically, we process input from these sensors to extract features that can be used by the dialogue system to determine the best possible action at each moment. These features are concatenated to a feature vector that determines the next dialogue state, as shown in Table 1. An algorithm that uses metrics to decide if each exercise is performed correctly by the user is also employed by the DS. Based on the user actions and the current dialogue state, the RL algorithm determines the next system action.

Table 1. class A: the user can perform all exercises based on clinical data, class B: the user can perform most of exercises, class C: the user can perform certain exercises, class 1: normal blood pressure, class 2: warning, class 3: high blood pressure

Dialogue State	Feature Representation
Clinical Data	00, 01, 10 (Class A,B,C)
Pain Detection	0, 1 (No pain, Pain)
WI-Patch	00,01,10 (Class 1,2,3)
User input (AVASR)	00001 – 01011 (NSR11)
Proper exercise execution	0,1 (Wrong, Correct)
Discourse history	User Acts
User Profile	

There are two categories of actions in our architecture, System Actions AS and User Actions AU. At each turn, the user's action is inferred by mapping the input (e.g. speech, facial expression) into one of the available AU. AS are selected by the system with the goal of making the user perform the prescribed exercises correctly, while simultaneously maximizing the effort of the exercise performance and the user's commitment. For example, if the user feels tired, the system will not move to an easier exercise at the first time, but will try to encourage the user continue the exercise. If the user is not able to do the specific exercise, the system moves on an easier exercise. AU allow the users to personalize their session, based on their needs and physical condition. They are always able to provide the system with information about their pain level, the exercise difficulty, or even stop the current exercise. Moreover, using our novel AVASR system, the users are able to interact reliably with the system in spoken natural language. Table 2 shows the available AS and AU.

We define the reward function as follows:

$R(\varphi(s),a) = 100$, upon successful completion of exercise
$R(\varphi(s),a) = -100$ upon unsuccessful completion of exercise
$R(\varphi(s),a) = -1$, otherwise (dialogue turn penalty)

Table 2. Available System and User Actions

System Actions	User Actions
GREET_USER	LOGIN
REQUEST_LOGIN	GREET
EASIER_EXERCISE	REQUEST_STOP
HARDER_EXERCISE	PROVIDE_PAIN_LEVEL
NEXT_EXERCISE	REQ_NEXT_EXERCISE
STOP_EXERCISE	REQ_INSTRUCTIONS
ENCOURAGE_USER	
PROVIDE_INSTRUCTIONS	

4   Clinical Data

Clinical attributes stored into the database are vital for the system adaptation and the personalization of each rehabilitation session. The required information is stored by the therapist who uses a backend server and addresses critical aspects of the rehabilitation therapy process. This information falls into two different categories: (i) the user related and (ii) the exercise related attributes. Important user related information includes the demographics, profile information (height, weight) medications, user history and chronic conditions. Exercise related information includes the specification of appropriate exercises, their duration and frequency, the performance during previous rehabilitation sessions and physiological data (heart rate, respiration rate, blood pressure) during performance.

These data will be sent to an expert system, which is a rule based backend suggesting appropriate exercises based on the input from the database. We are here describing an evidence based knowledge base on what is an appropriate rehabilitation activity for different demographics, clinical profiles, underlying physiological metrics and past performance. By using a priori information stored into the system (i.e. rehabilitation history), automated reasoning will provide recommendations about the appropriate exercises. This recommendation is then stored into our database and the therapist is given the opportunity to fine-tune the prescription, in favor of his/her patient.

The aforementioned information system (database and expert knowledge base) may be utilized for the adaptive personalization of the system, in an effort to maximise the benefits of the rehabilitation activities. When the subject completes a session, the system updates the database. New information for future sessions (i.e. if a patient gets easily tired, then the system should provide less intensive activities, or even switch to alternative exercises) will then be taken into consideration when a new session starts.

In order to assess the level of exercise, out of the three levels we propose, we have to be certain that the clinical input itself is enough for such a decision. For example, a patient with diabetes mellitus may or may not be able to undergo a level 1 exercise, and this is something to be decided based on the severity of his condition. There are though specific conditions which restrict the patient from performing intensive exercises, most typical one being the ischemic disease. Based on this, we can use the following input as an assessment for exercise level variability:

- Patient is older than 65 years
- Patient suffers from
  - Specific cardiovascular diseases (ie congestive heart disease)
  - Specific chronic diseases, i.e. in asthma, activities that involve long periods of exertion, such as soccer, distance running, may be less well tolerated. Another example is arthritis, and can cause great pain in the hips, knees and wrists. Mobility and physical exercise can be impossible or intensely painful for those people
  - Other conditions like inguinal which has not been operated
  - Auto-immune diseases: some of these diseases can affect balance, movement and coordination, affecting the sufferer's ability to move about and exercise freely
  - Pregnancy
- Users with a high body mass index may be classed as morbidly obese. Moving around with so much excessive weight on the body can cause exhaustion and breathlessness, because of the workload on the heart.

Based on the above information, here are four scenarios for the assessment of potential patients:

Case 1. A 35 year old man with no prior diseases has recently been diagnosed with rheumatoid arthritis and the pain levels are well controlled: the system may suggest level 2 (medium) or level 3 (intense) exercises, based upon other data, like exercise history, which is collected and stored into the system.

Case 2. A 67 year old man who is healthy and has no clinical conditions may undergo level 2 exercises

Case 3. A 40 year old woman in the 20th week of her pregnancy would only be allowed to undergo very light exercising (level 1)

Case 4. A 60 year old, obese male (BMI = 33) who has been diagnosed with ischemic heart disease will undergo light to medium exercise (level 1 or 2), also based upon other data, like exercise history, which is collected and stored into the system.

5   Evaluation Plans and Concluding Remarks

In order to train the adaptive DM, we plan to first conduct Wizard of Oz (WoZ) experiments with human users. In such a setting, there is an initial version of the system (where only the interface is implemented) and the DS is controlled by a human operator. The human users are unaware of this and believe they are interacting with an automatic system. Data will be recorded during these interactions and will be then used as training data for the learning algorithms. After the algorithms have been trained, we will conduct a second round of experiments in order to evaluate our system with human users who are not patients as well as with trained therapists to gain intuition from their perspective. In this work, we have proposed an initial prototype of a tele-rehabilitation platform, able to interact in spoken natural language with users and ensure safe execution of the exercises. In the future we plan to evaluate our system with patients in need for rehabilitation using televisions as the primary interface, as well as the necessary sensors, all of which are inexpensive.

References

1. Parmar, H.: Control System with Speech Recognition Using MFCC and Euclidian Distance Algorithm. International Journal of Engineering 2(1) (2013)
2. Jha, A.K., Gupta, R., Saini, D.: Face Recognition: A Fourier Transform and SVD Based Approach. In: 2013 5th International Conference on Computational Intelligence and Communication Networks (CICN). IEEE (2013)
3. Alam, M.R., et al.: Linear Regression-based Classifier for audio visual person identification. In: 2013 1st International Conference on Communications, Signal Processing, and their Applications (ICCSPA). IEEE (2013)
4. Galatas, G., Potamianos, G., Makedon, F.: Audio-visual speech recognition incorporating facial depth information captured by the Kinect. In: 2012 Proceedings of the 20th European Signal Processing Conference (EUSIPCO), pp. 2714–2717. IEEE (August 2012)
5. Traum, D.R., Larsson, S.: The information state approach to dialogue management. In: Current and New Directions in Discourse and Dialogue, pp. 325–353. Springer, Netherlands (2003)
6. Sutton, R.S., Barto, A.G.: Reinforcement learning: An introduction, vol. 1(1). MIT Press, Cambridge (1998)
7. Peters, J., Vijayakumar, S., Schaal, S.: Natural actor-critic. In: Gama, J., Camacho, R., Brazdil, P.B., Jorge, A.M., Torgo, L. (eds.) ECML 2005. LNCS (LNAI), vol. 3720, pp. 280–291. Springer, Heidelberg (2005)
8. Hamill, M., Young, V., Boger, J., Mihailidis, A.: Development of an automated speech recognition interface for personal emergency response systems. Journal of NeuroEngineering and Rehabilitation, 6–26 (2009)
9. Collignon, O., Girard, S., Gosselin, F., Roy, S., Saint-Amour, D., Lassonde, M., Lepore, F.: Audio-visual integration of emotion expression. Brain Research 1242, 126–135 (2008)
10. Kurillo, G., Koritnik, T., Bajd, T., Bajcsy, R.: Real-Time 3D Avatars for Tele-rehabilitation in Virtual Reality. Stud. Health Technol. Inform. 163, 290–296 (2011)
11. Holden, M.K., Dyar, T.A., Dayan-Cimadoro, L.: Telerehabilitation Using a Virtual Environment Improves Upper Extremity Function in Patients With Stroke. IEEE Transactions on Neural Systems and Rehabilitation 15(1) (2007)
12. Popescu, V.G., Burdea, G.C., Bouzit, M., Hentz, V.R.: A virtual-reality-based telerehabilitation system with force feedback. IEEE Transactions on Information Technology in Biomedicine 4(1) (2000)

13. Burdea, G., Popescu, V., Hentz, V., Colbert, K.: Virtual reality-based orthopedic telereha-
    bilitation. IEEE Transactions on Rehabilitations Engineering 8(3) (2000)
14. Deutsch, J.E., Lewis, J.A., Burdea, G.: Technical and Patient Performance Using a Virtual
    Reality-Integrated Telerehabilitation System: Preliminary Finding. IEEE Transactions on
    Neural Systems and Rehabilitation Engineering 15(1), 30–35 (2007)
15. Holden, M.K., Dyar, T.A., Schwamm, L., Bizzi, E.: Virtual-Environment-Based Telereha-
    bilitation in Patients with Stroke. Teleoperators and Virtual Environments 14(2), 214–233
    (2005)

Engagement in Game-Based Rehabilitation for Women with Fibromyalgia Syndrome

Eva Petersson Brooks and Anthony Lewis Brooks

Centre for Design, Learning and Innovation / SensoramaLab Department of Architecture, Design and Media Technology Aalborg University, Niels Bohrs Vej 8, 6700 Esbjerg, Denmark
{ep,tb}@create.aau.dk

Abstract. This paper reports on two linked studies exploring the general potentials, with foci on constraints and facilitators, of engagement in rehabilitation during motion-controlled video gameplay (MCVG). 17 female participants diagnosed with fibromyalgia syndrome (FMS) took part in the studies, wherein three different MCVGs were used, which were conducted by session leaders having different profiles. This investigation demonstrates the potentials of how MCVGs can act as an effective healthcare intervention for women with FMS with regards to offering activity structured around their interest, goals and choices. These aspects were found to be empowering as well as encouraging the participants to take on an active role in the activity. The analysis identified four main themes relative to the perception of constraints and facilitators to engagement in FMS gameplay-based rehabilitation: goal setting, facilitator approach, personalized gameplay and feedback and achievement. These are further elaborated and discussed in the paper. Conclusions are that deeper understanding of engagement within the FMS community, in particular related to rehabilitation using MCVGs, can be useful to enhance rehabilitation processes and better dress rehabilitation providers to better facilitate engagement and enhance the effectiveness of rehabilitation interventions.

Keywords: Fibromyalgia syndrome (FMS), Rehabilitation, Habilitation, Motion-controlled video gameplay (MCVG).

1   Introduction

This paper reports on two linked studies (programmes) exploring general potentials, with foci on constraints and facilitators, of engagement in rehabilitation during motion-controlled video gameplay (MCVG). 17 female participants diagnosed with fibromyalgia syndrome (FMS) completed the two programmes consisting of sessions using different motion-controlled video gameplay (MCVG) – namely the Nintendo Wii (Wii) using the Wii Remote handset (the Wii Nunchuk – i.e. the additional handset – was not used), the PlayStation 3 Move (PS3 Move) with two handsets, and the Microsoft Xbox Kinect (Xbox Kinect) without any handset or tangible peripheral (held, worn, or manipulated) – only torso/limbs. The consoles and handsets are shown in figures 1-3 respectively). Figure 4 shows the size of the two handsets when held in an adult's hand.

C. Stephanidis and M. Antona (Eds.): UAHCI/HCII 2014, Part III, LNCS 8515, pp. 359–367, 2014.
© Springer International Publishing Switzerland 2014

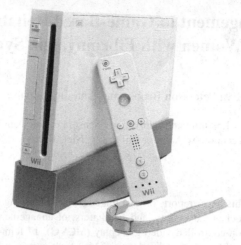

Fig. 1. Nintendo Wii with handset as used in our study. (image http://en.wikipedia.org/wiki/File:Wii-Console.png).

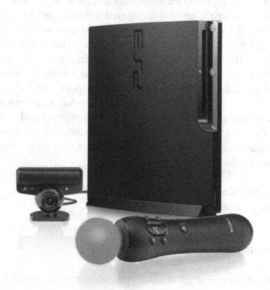

Fig. 2. PS3 MOVE showing console, camera and a single handset (image http://us.playstation.com)

Facilitators that had differing profiles led the sessions: a mature games/technical oriented PhD student led the first study sessions (only using the Wii), and two medical-oriented students (occupational therapists) led the second study sessions (using all three MCVGs.

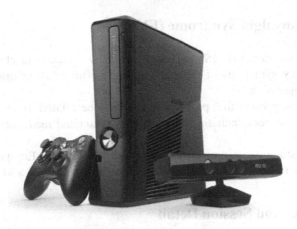

Fig. 3. X-Box console (gamepad not-used in this study) and Kinect camera-based sensor device (image www.microsoftstore.com)

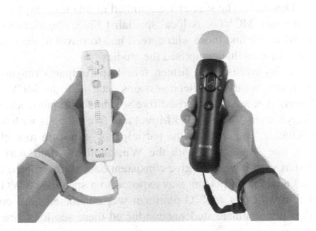

Fig. 4. Wiimote and PS3 MOVE handsets (image http://ps3maven.com)

The design of different session facilitator profiles was to assess the difference that the facilitator's input made to the sessions of each program. The difference of MCVGs was to assess if the participants' engagement differed according to the platforms and the difference in peripherals that capture the motion input.

Completion of the studies was problematic - as is typical in FMS research. However, those who complied gave sufficient input to the studies that is considered indicative of the goal at outset, and this is discussed and concluded at the end of the paper. The next section introduces the FMS condition. The following section outlines the studies including details of the MCVGs.

2 Fibromyalgia Syndrome (FMS)

Fibromyalgia syndrome (FMS) is characterized by widespread chronic pain; often accompanied by symptoms of fatigue; morning stiffness; sleep disorder; headache; anxiety and depression [1].

It has been suggested that pain symptoms may be related to abnormalities in the central nervous system, including central sensitization and inadequate pain inhibition [2].

In a recent study, the estimated prevalence of FMS in five European countries varied from 1.4% to 3.7%, with overrepresentation of women aged >30 years [3].

3 Studies and Session Detail

3.1 Studies Overview

Two studies were conducted in the SensoramaLab research complex at Aalborg University Esbjerg, Denmark. The studies were linked in that they explored FMS and the affect of contemporary MCVGs. A local specialist FMS/Rheumatism doctor invited his patients to participate and those who agreed had to travel to the university outside of the city for the sessions that comprised the studies.

One of the studies consisted of fifteen female participants diagnosed with FMS who completed a programme of fifteen sessions each with the MCVGs (i.e. 15 subjects x 15 sessions). The study comprised five sessions with Nintendo Wii (Wii), five sessions with PlayStation 3 Move (PS3 Move) and five sessions with Microsoft Xbox Kinect (Xbox Kinect). The order of the participants' exposure to each MCVG platform varied (i.e. one would start with the Wii, another would start with PS3 and another would start with Kinect) to give consistent data not corrupted by any ordered learning aspect. Once the participant was exposed to a specific MCVG platform then the full set of five with that MCVG platform was conducted until completed. Two occupational therapist graduate students conducted these sessions, one male and one female.

The second of the studies included two female participants who were also diagnosed with FMS. These were the only participants who completed the programme of 10 sessions with the Wii only. A PhD student in Medialogy focusing on the use of games technology and gameplay for therapeutic purposes from a media and technology perspective rather than a medical/physiological conducted the sessions.

3.2 Motion-Controlled Video Game (MCVG)

A Motion-Controlled Video Game (MCVG) is a non-immersive variation of VR, which is enhanced by use of gesture recognition [4]. Such MCVGs are commercially available via the game consoles Nintendo Wii (Wii), Sony PlayStation 3 Move (PS3 Move) and Microsoft Xbox Kinect (Xbox Kinect). According to Taylor et al. [5], MCVGs offer new opportunities in therapeutic rehabilitation as they make it possible for people with impairments to participate in simulated sports and game-based activities. Furthermore, it is possible that pain distraction from playing MCVGs can result in a more enjoyable experience and thereby enhances the participant's interest and engagement with a gameplay-based exercise program [5].

Engagement is acknowledged as an important ingredient in improving rehabilitation outcomes. For example, engagement has shown enhanced attendance, adherence and functional improvement [cf. 6]. However, few studies have investigated the complexities of individual's engagement within the FMS community. This study focuses in particular on the aspects of (1) game attributes, (2) participant's gameplay (inter)actions, and (3) facilitator intervention as key factors influencing the participant's engagement in rehabilitation sessions in order to offer insight into the constraints and facilitators of engagement during motion-controlled video gameplay. This requires that investigations look beyond what traditional training systems have to offer in order to consider wider scenarios for rehabilitation.

The present studies used a qualitative approach supported by the Test of Playfulness (ToP) as an observational tool for assessment of gameplay experience [cf. 7].

The study of engagement is relative to the need of a more holistic view on a complex situation. In order to consider this complexity, we used interaction analysis [8].

All data were treated confidentially. The Regional Scientific Ethical Committee for Southern Denmark approved the study.

Interviews with each participant were conducted at baseline and post intervention and followed a semi-structured interview guide with pre-selected topics.

Participants played for 30 minutes at each session and had at least two days rest before the next session. During each session, a facilitator was present, using an observational tool for assessment of play experience and giving instructions if participants had game difficulties.

Interviews were administered pre/post intervention and the facilitators used ToP as an in-session observational tool. Participants reported on ADL, pain level and fatigue pre-intervention as well as their responses to each session, which was gathered post intervention.

At baseline and post-intervention, information on ADL, pain level and fatigue was gathered using an ADL Questionnaire (ADL-Q), Visual Analogue Scale (VAS) and Brief Fatigue Inventory (BFI) respectively[1,2,3]. ADL-Q was used self-administered and the rheumatologist at Reumaklinik Danmark administered VAS and BFI. Baseline Interview questioning goals and expectations was conducted on the first day of

---

[1] ADL-Q is a questionnaire used to illustrate how well a person performs ADL (19). It consist of a number of daily and weekly activities. Each item can be answered from 0 (cannot perform) to 6 (performs without any assistance).

[2] VAS is a scale that allows the participant to quantify pain level with numbers from 1 to 10. BFI is a questionnaire concerning fatigue and encompasses nine questions with an overall score, ranging from 0 (no impact) to 90 (big impact).

[3] ToP is an observational tool used to evaluate how much a person engages in play. It encompasses 18 items, each with three subcategories; (1) Extent: To what extent is the person engaged, (2) Intensity: With what intensity is the person engaged, and (3) Skill: How skilful is the person. Each of these items can be answered from 0 (not at all) to 3 (highly).

the studies together with an introduction of the first console that the participant would engage with.

Interview analysis was done using qualitative content analysis.

Selected games were consistent to a "sports" theme with participants choosing their own favorite on each MCVG platform.

Following completion of the studies it was planned to re-contact the participants after one-year via a telephone interview to hear if the participants had bought a console for themselves or played elsewhere, and if yes, if it had an impact on their symptoms and daily living.

4   Results

Participants enjoyed playing the games and stated that they were able to distract from pain symptoms while playing. To some the participation in the sessions had an impact on their daily living and to others it did not.

All participants stated that they did not take notice of pain symptoms while playing and they enjoyed playing the games. Several participants explained that it was a good way to be physical active. However, following the exercise sessions the participants reported that participation did not contribute to a feeling of general reduction in pain or fatigue and did not increase independence in performing Activities of Daily Living (ADL)

5   Discussion

The linked studies demonstrate the potentials of how MCVGs can act as an effective healthcare intervention for women with FMS with regards to offering activity structured around their interest, goals and choices.

These aspects, interest, goals and choices, were empowering as well as encouraging the participants to take on an active role in the activity.

It was identified that the participants enjoyed the slow pace and familiarity of Wii, while some considered PS3 Move to be too fast paced. Xbox Kinect was reported as the best console for exercise because of full body involvement, but was almost too demanding for some of the participants.

The analysis identified four main themes relative to the perception of constraints and facilitators to engagement in FMS gameplay-based rehabilitation: goal setting, facilitator approach, personalized gameplay feedback and achievement.

6   Conclusions

Chronic widespread musculoskeletal pain is the main symptom of people with the diagnosis of fibromyalgia. Other symptoms are typically including chronic fatigue and lethargy as well as sleep disturbance, fatigue, irritable bowel syndrome, headache, and mood disorders. Mease in [9] reviewed FMS concluding it as a condition that affects at least 2% of the adult population in the USA and other regions in the world where FM is studied. In Denmark prevalence is reported as 0.7% and this ranges to a European high of 3.7% in Italy.

Prevalence rates in some regions have not been ascertained and may be influenced by differences in cultural norms regarding the definition and attribution of chronic pain states. A unifying hypothesis is that FM results from sensitization of the central nervous system. A range of medical treatments, including antidepressants, opioids, non-steroidal anti-inflammatory drugs, sedatives, muscle relaxants, and anti-epileptics, have been used to treat FM. Non-pharmaceutical treatment modalities, including exercise, physical therapy, massage, acupuncture, and cognitive behavioral therapy, can be helpful. Few of these approaches have been demonstrated to have clear-cut benefits in randomized controlled trials [9].

Some in the medical profession consider the condition psychosomatic, believed to have a mental component derived from the stresses and strains of everyday living. Distinguishing somatoform disorders (disorders in which mental factors are the sole cause of a physical illness) from psychosomatic disorders (disorders in which mental factors play a significant role in the development, expression, or resolution of a physical illness) is problematic [e.g. 10, 11]. Studies of fibromyalgia pain characteristics, muscle function, and impact on daily activities have been conducted (e.g. 12) with aberrations of pain experience literature subject of review [13].

According to Melzack and Wall in [14], pain signals can be controlled, modified and inhibited by distraction. They presented the Gate Control Theory, which proposes that the level of attention given to the pain sensation, emotions associated with the pain sensation and past experiences with the pain sensation are elements that contribute to how the pain sensation is perceived. Wismejler and Vingerhoest in [15] suggest that a good distractor involves multiple sensory modalities, emotional engagement and participation. According to Taylor et al. [5], it is possible that the enjoyment of playing VR games distract the player so that he/she will focus on the gameplay rather than pain sensations. This can result in a more enjoyable experience and thereby improve motivation to comply with the training.

Sarzi-Puttini, et al. [16], in examining treatment strategies in FMS sufferers concluded that exercise does benefit sufferers as well as psychophysiologically based therapy, such as electromyography biofeedback, and interventions based on cognitive–behavioral therapy. Summing up the team suggest 'an individually tailored multidisciplinary pharmacologic, rehabilitative, and cognitive–behavioral approach currently seems to be the most effective'.

The specialist doctor (Reumaklinik Danmark) involved in our studies believes exercise and drugs as a best treatment. In a review titled "Exercise for treating fibromyalgia syndrome" [17], Busch et al., detail related work, strategies, and outcomes that was informative for our design.

Little is known about the impact playing with Virtual Reality gaming consoles have on this group of patients. The aim of this study was to explore the experience, women with fibromyalgia had, using movement-based gaming consoles and to investigate the impact on their daily living. In line with other research it is problematic to generalize and to conclude anything other than some enjoyed the experience and felt benefit. On the follow-up after one-year some had purchased a MCVG, while others believed the benefit to not be worth the investment.

In summing up this limited investigation, which exhibited severe drop outs and thus lack of compliance, we find that a deeper understanding of engagement within the FMS community, in particular related to rehabilitation using MCVGs, can be useful to enhance rehabilitation processes and better dress rehabilitation providers to better facilitate engagement and enhance the effectiveness of rehabilitation interventions.

Acknowledgements. The authors wish to thank the women who participated in this study and rheumatologist Dr. Hans-Jacob Haga (Reumaklinik Danmark). The Danish Association of Occupational Therapists supported the studies. The Danish Fibromyalgia union also contributed to assess and eventually evaluate aspects of the studies.

References

1. Wolfe, F., Clauw, D., Fitzcharles, M., Goldenberg, D., Katz, R., Mease, P., et al.: The American College of Rheumatology preliminary diagnostic criteria for fibromyalgia and measurement of symptom severity. Arthritis Care Res. (Hoboken) 62, 600–610 (2010)
2. Staud, R.: Biology and therapy of fibromyalgia: pain in fibromyalgia syndrome. Arthritis Res. Ther. 8, 208 (2006)
3. Branco, J.C., Bannwarth, B., Failde, I., Abello Carbonell, J., Blotman, F., Spaeth, M., et al.: Prevalence of fibromyalgia: a survey in five European countries. Semin. Arthritis Rheum. 39, 448–453 (2010)
4. Robertson, G., Card, S., Mackinlay, J.: Nonimmersive virtual reality. IEEE Computer 26 (1993)
5. Taylor, M.J., McCormick, D., Shawis, T., Impson, R., Griffin, M.: Activity-promoting gaming systems in exercise and rehabilitation. J. Rehabil. Res. Dev. 48, 1171–1186 (2011)
6. Kortte, K.B., Falk, L.D., Castillo, R.C., Johnson-Greene, D., Wegener, S.T.: The Hopkins Rehabilitation Engagement Rating Scale: development and psychometric properties. Archives of Physical Medicie and Rehabilitation 88, 877–884 (2007)
7. Bundy, A., Nelson, L., Metzger, M., Bingaman, K.: Validity and reliability of a test of playfulness. OTJR TS Occupation, Participation and Health 21, 276 (2001)
8. Jordan, B., Henderson, A.: Interaction Analysis: Foundations and Practice. The Journal of the Learning Sciences 4(1), 39–103 (1995)
9. Mease, P.: Fibromyalgia syndrome: review of clinical presentation, pathogenesis, outcome measures, and treatment. The Journal of Rheumatology 75, 6–21 (2005)
10. Kaplan, H.I., Sadock, B.J.: Synopsis of psychiatry: Behavioral sciences clinical psychiatry. Williams & Wilkins Co. (1988)
11. Kellner, R.: Psychosomatic syndromes, somatization and somatoform disorders. Psychotherapy and Psychosomatics 61(1-2), 4–24 (1994)
12. Imbierowicz, K., Egle, U.T.: Childhood adversities in patients with fibromyalgia and somatoform pain disorder. European Journal of Pain 7(2), 113–119 (2003)
13. Lautenbacher, S., Krieg, J.C.: Pain perception in psychiatric disorders: a review of the literature. Journal of Psychiatric Research 28(2), 109–122 (1994)
14. Melzack, R., Wall, P.D.: Pain mechanisms: a new theory. Science 150, 971–979 (1965)

15. Wismeijer, A.A., Vingerhoets, A.J.: The use of virtual reality and audiovisual eyeglass systems as adjunct analgesic techniques: a review of the literature. Ann. Behav. Med. 30, 268–278 (2005)
16. Sarzi-Puttini, P., Buskila, D., Carrabba, M., Doria, A., Atzeni, F.: Treatment strategy in fibromyalgia syndrome: where are we now? Seminars in Arthritis and Rheumatism 37(6), 353–365 (2008)
17. Busch, A.J., Barber, K.A., Overend, T.J., Peloso, P.M., Schachter, C.L.: Exercise for treating fibromyalgia syndrome. Cochrane Database Syst. Rev. 4(4) (2007)

Tapology: A Game-Based Platform
to Facilitate E-Health and E-Inclusion

Kenneth C. Scott-Brown[1], Julie Harris[2], Anita Simmers[3], Mhairi Thurston[1],
Malath Abbas[4], Tom de Majo[4], Ian Reynolds[4], Gareth Robinson[4], Iain Mitchell[1],
Dan Gilmour[5], Santiago Martinez[6] , and John Isaacs[5,*]

[1] School of Social and Health Sciences, Abertay University, Dundee, UK
[2] School of Psychology and Neuroscience, University of St Andrews, Fife, UK
[3] Vision Sciences Department, Glasgow Caledonian University, Glasgow, UK
[4] Quartic Llama, Bannerman House, 27 South Tay Street, Dundee, UK
[5] School of Science, Engineering & Technology,
Abertay University, Dundee, UK
[6] Center for eHealth and Healthcare Technology,
University of Agder, Grimstad, Norway
{k.scott-brown,M.Thurston,d.gilmour,j.isaacs}@abertay.ac.uk,
jh81@st-andrews.ac.uk,
Anita.Simmers@gcu.ac.uk,
{mal,gaz,ian,tom}@quarticllama.com,
izmitchell@dundee.ac.uk,
santiago.martinez@uia.no

Abstract. We have developed a tablet computer game app for low vision users
that can be used to introduce a platform for gaming, internet and visual rehabilitation to older users who have not had prior experience with information communication technology (ICT). Our target user group is people diagnosed with
Age Related Macular Degeneration (AMD). The primary goal of the app is to
present a fun and engaging means for participants to engage with Information
Communication Technology (ICT). A long-term goal of the project is to build a
platform to gather data on current and on-going visual function by creating a
suite of games that could generate sufficient regular visual engagement to enable perceptual learning in the preserved peripheral retina that is spared in AMD.
The inclusive design process took into consideration the perceptual and cognitive constraints of the user group in. The 'Tapology©' app was formally
launched at a large computer games festival where we gathered data from a
range of users to inform the development of the gameplay. The initial results
and feedback inform the ultimate goal of creating a suite of applications that
have a wide social and geographic reach to promote and inform e-inclusion and
e-health.

Keywords: E-Health; E-Inclusion, Games, co-design, accessible design,
Mobile HCI.

---

* Corresponding author.

C. Stephanidis and M. Antona (Eds.): UAHCI/HCII 2014, Part III, LNCS 8515, pp. 368–377, 2014.
© Springer International Publishing Switzerland 2014

1   Introduction

Few of us can imagine the impact and sense of loss associated with a diagnosis of an irreversible sight-loss condition such as Age-Related Macular Degeneration (AMD). Recently, one of the authors [1] has documented the social and emotional impact of making the transition from sightedness to blindness using to a series of interviews with clients who have undergone such a journey. It transpires that there is often a temporal disconnect between diagnosis, the behavioural 'point of impact' of sight loss, and the point of clinical intervention. In this gap, there is an opportunity to develop interventions designed to address the dramatic changes imminent in life prior to the 'point of impact' of blindness (where dramatic changes in lifestyle become unavoidable). Although treatments are developing, as yet conditions such as AMD have no 'cure', this should not prevent clinicians and the third sector from being able to offer a constructive set of interventions. A wide variety of assistive technology is available, yet Thurston [1] has identified that there is often reluctance to take on board such technology early in the disease trajectory since this would be an outward sign of defeat.

In view of the reluctance of newly diagnosed clients to move to overt and potentially stigmatising assistive technologies, the current project is aimed at providing an inclusive and engaging intervention that can promote e-inclusion and adoption of assistive technologies. This need is amplified by the well-documented lack of uptake of Information Communication Technology (ICT) in older groups [2]. The resulting intervention is based on an interactive tablet computer 'app' designed to challenge different cognitive and visual components of the users visual system in a fun and engaging way that can facilitate interaction with ICT and indirectly engender a broader awareness of the assistive technologies embedded in tablet computers. There is a longer term goal to use this intervention to develop a specific vision training protocol to test the hypothesis that peripheral vision in AMD patients might be subject to visual training to improve visual function [3]. This would first require a palatable non-clinical vehicle for regular interaction.

The visual experience of AMD is one of loss of central visual acuity. Initially this is not subject to conscious awareness, but it progresses, meaning that items must be scaled up in size and effectively presented in periphery in order to be visible. Our peripheral vision is not as good as central vision, but tantalising results from video games research suggest that it might be possible to 'train up' peripheral vision to improve visual function [4,5]. These experiments indicate that in experienced video games players, the so-called Useful Field of View is increased compared to non-video gamers. These results are typically found with players of military-based first-person 'shooter' games. However, such combat based titles do not fit the demographic of the target patient group which is the over 60s. However, one of us has shown that in the case of Amblyopia, much simpler games such as Tetris can have beneficial effects on visual performance [6]

The crucial skill in developing the AMD patients' transition to reading with low vision is their ability to recruit peripheral vision using their so-called Preferred Retinal Locus (PRL), the region of spared vision [7]. This skill requires the ability to fixate steadily in one location, yet attend to a peripheral one. It is precisely these sorts of skills that characterize modern video game play, and this indicates the potential of developing a games based approach to fixation training. Previously it has been argued that the recognition of users personal goals is crucial for accessible development for occasional users or users with no prior experience of ICT [8]. For example, the primary goals for the users in the ICT contexts discussed may not be primarily of a clinical nature. Rather, the ability to communicate with friends and family or to share activities would likely be a primary goal. With this in mind, an assistive app will still benefit from its ability to address primary goals of the user rather than secondary goals. This is the justification for the game-based approach: to make the experience enjoyable.

2   Development

As pointed out by Keates [9] the profile of users must be considered during the design of accessible apps. Thus, in collaboration with the clients from Fife Society for the Blind, initial research and development led to a design project with a number of patients at various stages of AMD. During the meeting, the co-design methodology [10] was used to incorporate user feedback to help shape the game. By meeting and listening to the target audience it helped the design team to understand their particular needs, gain insight into AMD and helped us to gather information based on habits and daily life, which ultimately helped us design an appropriate game. During the design meeting basic paper prototypes were built to help visualise the design and user feedback was recorded to help steer the process. Additional immersive techniques, such as sight simulation spectacles were used by the team to assist in the development of the prototypes in line with previous recommendations [11] for inclusive design.

The initial step was to work out what form the app would take, with the original plan being some sort of sight based game. Approximately a week was spent making a number of very quick, simple, prototypes; this would serve as a platform to test internally and provide a clearer path forward. The prototypes were analysed based on visual aesthetic, usability, and data collection potential to help further analysis on user behaviour and playing patterns. Around nine simple prototypes were made, but due to the potential complexity of AMD none of these prototypes on their own were thought to cover the range of impairments. Instead, the five prototypes with the most potential were collated into a mini-game collection. Together they would better cover the different aspects and issues of e-inclusion and engagement.

The suite of mini-games suite was developed using the Unity game engine (© Unity Technologies). Team roles ranged from project management and game design to development and testing. This decision to use the Unity development environment came down to past experience of working with the game engine developing rapid prototypes and its porting ability making it easy to deploy to a range of different platforms. The suite was named 'Tapology' (© Abertay University) (Fig. 1) and was designed for the iPad (© Apple Corporation) due to its large screen size and touch interface. By focusing on a single device it was possible to develop a robust prototype. By using the Unity game engine the app can easily be deployed on other tablet or touch screen devices currently available on the market.

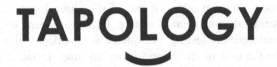

Fig. 1. The 'Tapology' branding allows for the addition of additional minigames, all based around the concept of tap based gesture interaction

Five mini-games were developed: Reaction, Target Tap, Colour Change, Card Match, and Pouring. Each of the mini-games is backed by a unique colour, to differentiate it from the others. Throughout each game, bright colours and strong contrasts are used to make all the presented information as clear as possible for any user.

The 'Pouring' mini-game illustration (Fig 2) shows how the game developers brought to life the concept from one of the co-design groups. In essence, the game involves collecting rain from the increasingly rapidly moving clouds to develop the garden. By focusing on a relevant, skill, the training aspects of visually guided action can be developed in a manner relevant and engaging for the user group. It is worth noting that the game 'mechanic' is in essence a reverse 'space invaders' game. In discussion, there was a strong sense that mainstream video games did not identify the appropriate demographic touchstones, nor did they address required skills for low-vision users. Nevertheless, older users regularly play games such as Scrabble, Cards, Mah Jong etc., despite not seeing themselves as 'gamers' in the modern sense.

The mini-games are kept short, and most increase in difficulty over the course of the game. Once the user finishes a game, they are awarded a score out of three stars, similar to a number of popular mobile games depending on how well they performed. This score, along with other relevant statistics are sent to a cloud-based data account so that they can be later reviewed. Data to be tracked includes the player's score, their reaction times and the current difficulty settings. Importantly for the player, this helped to add replay value to the experience and a sense of competition, which helped to make the experience social – a priority that was identified in the co-design meetings.

A key goal of the app is visual assessment of clients, and this is provided by a 'Target Tap' mini-game. In this game, the user must as quickly as possible touch the centre of a circular target. This is the clearest link to visual assessment that forms the backbone of the long-term goal of patient ownership concept of the app. By personalising visual assessment and taking it out of the clinical setting, it becomes possible to reduce the stressful component of testing. Further, it opens up the possibility for a longitudinal component of testing, not otherwise practical with fixed clinical testing locations due to the cost of travel and clinician time. In the context of the North Sea Region of Europe, this mobile aspect of testing is particularly useful since distances to travel to clinics in Scotland, Norway and Sweden become prohibitively obstructive.

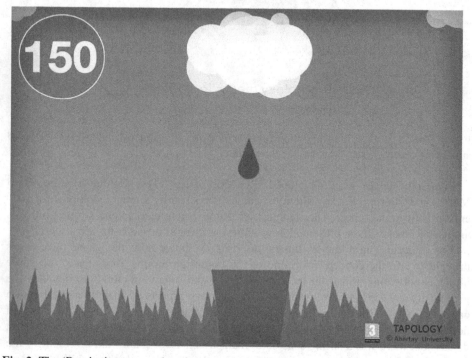

Fig. 2. The 'Pouring' game requires the user to use their finger to drag the bucket left and right and catch the rain drops. The bucket moves more quickly at each level to increase playability.

In the mini-game 'Card Match' (Fig. 3) where participants must fixate the central card during an exposure of an array of cards, and then subsequently locate and tap the correct peripheral card. This game involves steady gaze fixation and good short-term memory.

'Reaction' is a game requiring the user to respond with the appropriate interface gesture, the targets appear randomly on the screen requiring distributed attention. The aim is to reinforce the tactile skills required to operate a capacitive touch screen – an effective 'tap'.

'Colour Change', requires the user to focus on the centre of the screen to identify a central objective colour, and then 'tag' similarly coloured elements as they approach the centre. Loosely based on the concept of radar, the objective is sustained vigilance with visually guided action.

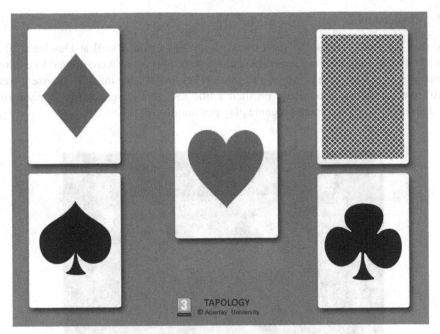

Fig. 3. Development still from 'Card Match' Memory and stable fixation are required for the Card Match game

3   First User Trial

3.1   Participants

User trials involved 60 participants, 37 male, 23 female (age range 7-66, average 28.22) who agreed to take part in a formal evaluation of the app. The procedure was approved by the University of Abertay, Social and Health Sciences Research Ethics Committee.

3.2   Apparatus

The software comprises the Tapology suite of 5 mini-games, each designed to challenge a different part of the visuo-motor control of the participants.

The app makes use of the Flurry (© Flurry) analytics API to keep track of player information in the cloud during testing. Flurry is designed to keep track of thousands of users for company analytics and marketing, and by using the event tracking system it provides, it serves the purpose of information gathering. When a player starts the app it logs them as a new player and assigns them a unique identifier for the iPad they are using. As they complete the different mini-games, they trigger events which are sent to Flurry with information regarding what just happened. For example, in the card matching game, once they make the first match, the time taken is sent to Flurry to give an idea of the user's reaction time. With the data being stored in the cloud this made analysis easy to access.

3.3　Procedure

For the user trials, visitors to the official 'Tapology' launch stall at Dundee's 2013 DareProtoplay Indiefest national video games festival (Fig. 4) were invited to explore the app to assess the ease of use of the game. Those who gave informed consent were then given a short questionnaire on their game use, including number of platforms used and length of time spent on game play per month.

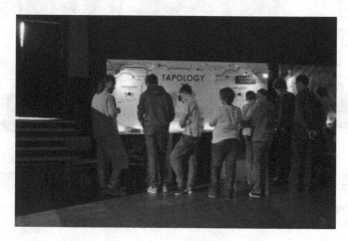

Fig. 4. Users recruited at the 'Tapology' stall at Dare Protoplay Indiefest, video games festival in Dundee

4　Results

Average App completion time was found to be 4.88 minutes with a mean of 3 and a max of 8 minutes (SD 1.09). Age of tester accounted for 25% of the variance in the app completion time. These durations are appropriate for a repeated regular casual game app. The key is to create a short burst of engagement that can be used on a daily basis.

Inspection of the open prompt questionnaire responses also revealed the positive reaction from users of all age groups, with over 50 individual positive statements and 25 suggestions for additional apps or improved gameplay. In addition to approving of the game play, on debrief, the users were particularly receptive to the idea of an e-inclusion based assistive app. An insight from this communication with users was that the app was of potential use, not just to elderly users, but also to other users with educational special needs.

Further informal acceptance testing was done with the original co-design client group and other clients from Fife Society for the Blind (Fig 5). This enabled the team to close the loop with the co-design group with the intention of fostering a sense of ownership of the project with the client group.

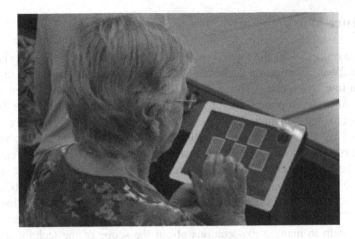

Fig. 5. Fife Society for the Blind User testing the card match app

5   Summary

We have co-designed a group of 5 mini-games, all designed to challenge different parts of visual cognitive function. The 'Tapology' app is an attempt to bridge the gap that can occur between diagnosis and point of impact of sight loss [1] in a constructive engaging manner. This was achieved thanks to a coordinated sequence of design events including a co-design session; conference calls; user test sessions at Dare Protoplay and at 'Road Map' meetings. Further user trials have been conducted with clients from the Fife Society for the Blind and with members of the public and the DareProtoplay video games festival. The information gained from this feedback reinforce the original concept of an assistive suite of apps with the capacity to monitor and in the longer term, rehabilitate visual function in a group of users with impaired vision and no prior experience of ICT. However, the need for social 'scaffolding' of the interactions is acknowledged, since the long term ownership and maintenance of ICT devices remains not fully accessible to low vision users.

Using pervasive, low-cost computing devices such as tablet computers for patient driven visual rehabilitation and monitoring offers health care professionals a chance to completely reorient the ownership of self-assessment of health using an engaging platform. By making the assessment protocol game-based, and delivering it in a standard household device that has additional functions and purposes beyond clinical ones, the scope of Tapology is focused on a broad e-inclusion goal. In the long term, this is to personalise healthcare assessment and to contextualise it within a wider accessibility function to enable users to gradually access communication, internet and accessibility functions associated with tablet based systems. Digital exclusion is a problem across both rural and urban Scotland [2], but low cost, easy to use tablet computers offer a pervasive solution suitable for ice breaking sessions in ways that standalone PC computers cannot deliver. In particular, the multi-touch capacity of modern tablets has brought the written word to low vision users by enabling intuitive, pinch-based scaling of text with capacitive multi-touch gestures.

6   Future Work

The ultimate objective for the team is to create fully working and testable visual rehabilitation software application embedded in a more general vehicle to facilitate e-
inclusion in low vision users. This will be achieved through a two-pronged approach.
The first goal is develop the Tapology 'app' as an enabling tool for care-based and
voluntary sector led e-inclusion outreach work. With a series of collaborative workshops hosted by Fife Society for the Blind and involving their clients, we aim to
assess the extent to which group based activity, supported by specialists, can demonstrate how the introduction of ICT in the form of tablet computers can raise awareness
about a wide range of assistive functions. Facilitation of introduction to ICT prior to
adoption is critical, and the role of a trusted source in the introduction of new
processes. These 'meet the ipad' sessions, facilitated by support workers and specialists will help to manage expectations about the scope of the technology and the
requirements for adoption. The workshops can promote awareness of the built-in
accessible features in devices such as the iPad. The ability to use Siri (© Apple Corporation) to talk to the device and command actions, coupled with its ability to read
back to the user is not widely publicized in minority end user groups, yet is of high
value.

The second element of the project involves refining the gameplay and demonstrating peripheral vision improvement using the perceptual learning tasks previously
shown to have potential benefit in AMD (e.g. [3]). As a complex intervention, this
application will benefit from the proof of feasibility of Tapology as a vehicle for behavioural engagement in game-based studies of visual function [e.g., 12].

Acknowledgement. This project was part funded by a grant to K. Scott-Brown from
Scottish Crucible, and further supported by the iAge Project (*iAge:e-inclusion in ageing Europe*; www.iageproject.eu). We are grateful to Alan Suttie and his colleagues
and clients at the Fife Society for the Blind for facilitating co-design and evaluation
sessions. We are also grateful to Caroline MacEwen from NHS Tayside for advice on
the direction of focus for the application development. We are also grateful to Bela
Havasreti, Mark Adams, Pauline Mack, Lesley Parker-Hamilton for facilitating the
User Trial.

References

1. Thurston, M.: An enquiry into the emotional impact of sight loss and the counselling experiences and needs of blind and partially sighted adults. Counselling and Psychotherapy
Research 10(1), 3–12 (2010)
2. White, D.: Across the Divide. Tackling digital exclusion. Carnegie UK Trust Report
(2013),
http://www.carnegieuktrust.org.uk/publications/2013/
across-the-divide—full-report

3. Yu, D., Cheung, S.-H., Gordon, E., Legge, G.E., Chung, S.: Reading speed in the peripheral visual field of older adults: Does it benefit from perceptual learning? Vision Research 50(9), 860–869 (2010)
4. Green, C.S., Bavelier, D.: Action video game experience alters the spatial resolution of attention. Psychological Science 18, 88–94 (2007)
5. Dye, M.W.G., Green, C.S., Bavelier, D.: Increasing speed of processing with action video games. Current Directions in Psychological Science 18(6), 321–326 (2009)
6. Knox, P.J., Simmers, A.J., Gray, L.S.: An exploratory study: Prolonged periods of binocular stimulation can provide an effective treatment in childhood amblyopia. Investigative Ophthalmology and Visual Science 3, 817–824 (2012)
7. Chung, S.T., Mansfield, J.S., Legge, G.E.: Psychophysics of reading. XVIII. The effect of print size on reading speed in normal peripheral vision. Vision Res. 38, 2949–2962 (1998)
8. Martinez, S., Carrillo, A.L., Scott-Brown, K., Falgueras, J.: AGILE Interface for 'No-Learning nor Experience required' Interaction. In: Martín, E., Haya, P.A., Carro, R.M. (eds.) User Modeling and Adaptation for Daily Routines. Human-Computer Interaction Series, pp. 119–151. Springer (2013)
9. Keates, S.: Pragmatic research issues confronting HCI practitioners when designing for universal access. Int. J. on Universal Access in the Information Society 5(3), 269–278 (2006)
10. Albinsson, L., Lind, M., Forsgren, O.: Co-Design: An Approach to Border Crossing, Network Innovation (2007)
11. Isaacs, J., Martinez, S., Scott-Brown, K., Milne, A., Evans, A., Gilmour, D.: Mobile Technology and E-Inclusion. In: Stephanidis, C., Antona, M. (eds.) UAHCI 2013, Part III. LNCS, vol. 8011, pp. 626–635. Springer, Heidelberg (2013)
12. Li, R., Polat, U., Makous, W., Bavelier, D.: Enhancing the contrast sensitivity function through action video game playing. Nature Neuroscience 12, 549–551 (2009)

User Experience Considerations
for Patient-Centered Handoffs in Surgical Oncology

Nancy Staggers[1,2], Marge Benham-Hutchins[3], and Laura Heermann Langford[2,4]

[1] School of Nursing, University of Maryland, USA
[2] University of Utah, USA
[3] Texas Woman's University, USA
[4] Intermountain Healthcare, USA
nancystaggers@sisna.com

Abstract. Handoffs, the transfer of care responsibility from one provider to another, commonly occur in intra-disciplinary silos that exclude patients. Little is known about patient preferences about handoff participation in surgical oncology and key information needs including user experience (UX) considerations. This exploratory, descriptive study was conducted at a cancer center in the western United States using a purposeful sampling technique to select 20 surgical oncology in-patients. The team used methodological pluralism for data collection: naturalistic observations, interviews, field notes, and artifact capture. Data analysis included systematic steps and content analysis consistent with accepted qualitative research methods. The analysis resulted in 356 codes synthesized into 15 categories and 3 themes: Depends Upon How Sick I Am, I Want To Know Everything, and My Life Is In Their Hands. Fifteen participants expressed varying levels of interest in participating in handoffs, and 18 of the 20 wanted to know "everything" about themselves. Initial categories of patients' information needs were developed. An opportunity exists to expand health informatics tools to inpatients and their families and design them from patients' perspectives. UX considerations are outlined to expand informatics tools for collaborative decision making to inpatient activities and include person-centered applications, electronic white boards to consider user diversity and tasks as well as context-sensitive information design.

Keywords: Handoffs, user experience, qualitative research.

1 Background

Communication breakdowns between providers are recognized as a predisposing factor in medical error. [1] Standardized information exchange protocols, such as SBAR (situation-background-assessment-recommendation), are viewed as a solution for these kinds of communication breakdowns that include patient care handoffs. Unfortunately, the complex, interruption-filled, healthcare environment is not conducive to providers focusing on a single event even with a tool such as SBAR. This has

C. Stephanidis and M. Antona (Eds.): UAHCI/HCII 2014, Part III, LNCS 8515, pp. 378–386, 2014.
© Springer International Publishing Switzerland 2014

led to workarounds and limited adoption of standardized methods of information exchange during patient care handoffs and other communication activities.

The patient is, arguably, the most vested member of all involved in the process of patient care. This recognition has resulted in a move toward patient-centered care and has become the focus of many healthcare safety and quality improvement initiatives. [2] Despite the recent acknowledgement of patient engagement needs, handoffs or the transfer of patient care responsibility from one provider to another commonly exclude patients and occur in intra-disciplinary silos. Yet, including patients in handoff processes would support shared decision making while respecting patient autonomy. Patient participation in handoffs also would reflect the right for them to partner in their own care as well as having the potential to improve care outcomes, communication accuracy and informed decision-making. [3]

Family-centered multidisciplinary rounds [4] and bedside nursing shift change report [5,6] have been implemented in many hospitals as a way to include patients and family members in the information exchange process. In the United States, government initiatives have mandated the adoption of electronic health records (EHR) and patient access to their health information. [7] An important component of these initiatives is commonly referred to as the Meaningful Use mandate. This mandate addresses specific uses of EHRs and electronic access to health information by patients. Although these mandates currently focus on the outpatient setting, a natural next step is developing tools to assist with patient access to clinical information in the inpatient environment. These tools are needed to enhance patient involvement during the provider handoff process.

Appropriate information content for collaborative handoffs, where patients are active participants, has not been determined. [8] Social roles, demographic factors such as age, physician authority and the fear of being labeled "difficult" have been shown to be obstacles for patient participation. [9] Little is known about patient preferences regarding handoff participation in surgical oncology and key information needs including user experience (UX) considerations. The purpose of this qualitative study was to determine patients' preferences about handoffs, identify current tool use and specifications for patient-centered information tools including UX requirements.

2   Methods

This exploratory, descriptive study was conducted on a 25-bed patient care unit at a cancer center in the western U.S. Using a purposeful sampling technique across demographics, levels of care, types of surgical procedures and recovery course, 20 adult surgical oncology patients were selected and agreed to participate.

Institutional Review Board approval was obtained. The team used methodological pluralism for data collection: naturalistic observations, interviews, field notes, and artifact capture. The scripted interviews used standardized questions with probes. Three areas were the focus for the interviews: preferences about participating in handoffs, patients' information requirements and tools patients or families currently used to track care. Interviews were transcribed by a professional transcription company, checked for accuracy and uploaded into Atlas titm for analysis. The team analyzed data using systematic steps [10] and content analysis. [11] First cycle coding, completed jointly, allowed definitions and boundaries to be created. Second cycle coding was completed by defined pairs of coders across all transcripts, and third cycle coding consolidated the generated categories into themes.

3   Results

The mean age of the 20 participants was 58.4 with a range from 28-85, and both genders were equally represented. One-half of the sample completed at least some college-level coursework although two had not graduated from high school. The patients underwent a variety of surgical procedures typically seen on this patient care unit.

The analyses resulted in 356 codes synthesized into 15 categories and 3 themes: Depends Upon How Sick I Am, I Want To Know Everything, and My Life Is In Their Hands. [8] This paper focuses on the first two themes because they are more relevant for user experience considerations. For the first theme, 15 participants expressed varying levels of interest in participating in handoffs. Six were neutral about their participation with statements such as, "Yes, I might." A small subset saw handoffs as the sole purview of providers while as many others had strong sentiments about participating, saying "It's my body and my health." The types of handoff participation patients wanted varied from just listening to being very active in the handoff process. Most participants wanted to be invited into the handoff process by being asked questions.

For the second theme, five categories were identified: patient tools, shared electronic health record information, information needs, discharge information and patient preferences. None of the participants currently used electronic tools or had EHR information shared with them while they were in-patients. Most tracked information in their heads or had family members act as information managers.

Ten of the 20 used hospital provided in-room white boards to track information (names of their nurses, family contact information and/or medications). Examples of whiteboards are in Figures 1 and 2 below. As may be seen in the figures, the whiteboards had a variety of uses from minimal (caregiver names or family contact information) to more information including scheduled medication times or the number of times the patient ambulated during a shift. One patient tracked his stated daily goals and his progress toward those goals on the whiteboard. None of the patients used the pain scale available on these artifacts. Four participants/families used hand-written records of varying depths. These records spanned in-patient, home and out-patient settings.

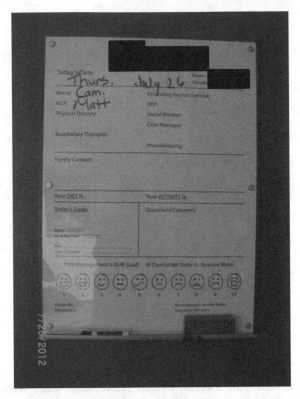

Fig. 1. An Example of a Whiteboard with Minimal Information

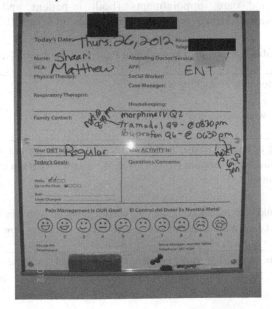

Fig. 2. Examples of Whiteboards with More Information

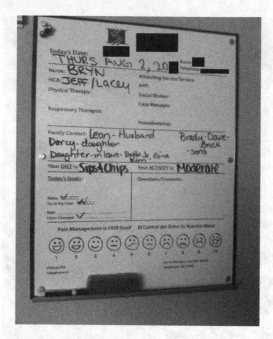

Fig. 2. (*continued*)

Sample information needs from the participant interviews are represented in Table 1. From the variety of sources, overall information needs were identified including initial categories of patients' information needs. Common categories were: medications, wound care, appointments (both in-patient and out-patient) and discharge information. However, most participants (18 of 20) wanted to know

Table 1. Exemplar Quotes about Patients' Information Needs

"I would love to know everything about me." "I want to hear what's going on. This is my life."
"What's going to happen to me, about my incision? When are the staples supposed to come out? What time am I supposed to meet with the doctor? What doctor am I supposed to meet with? Everything." "I think it would help me understand more what's going on with me. More of what I can do for myself. Make me more aware of how severe my problem is or how not so severe."
"I have a notebook that I keep. I have people, pain control…and the things that I should and shouldn't eat. The different type of chemo treatment they're supposed to give, different medications."

"everything" about themselves including their prognosis, saying for example, "I think you should be aware of everything," and "This is my body and I want to be aware of what's going on..."

Participants were evenly divided on the need for an electronic in-patient tool for oncology. Quotes on this topic ranged from "I know what's going on. It's nothing I have to write down..." to "...I need to be aware of everything."

4   Discussion

No patients used electronic tools, not even to take simple notes or write questions for providers to answer. This was surprising given the general public's use of smart phones and mobile devices such as iPADs. In contrast to this lack of tools, the vast majority of participants wanted to know everything about themselves, which would imply tool usage to track information. Therefore, an opportunity exists to expand health informatics tools to inpatients and their families and to design them from patients' perspectives. Most important, these tools need to support collaborative decision-making in the inpatient setting. User experience (UX) considerations need to be created even before initial prototyping begins.

A long-term goal would be to create person-centered health records that manage health data in a longitudinal manner, beyond the current notions about personal health records (PHRs) or episodic, inpatient personal health records. These new longitudinal electronic tools could provide support for collaborative activities that include, for example, patient-centered handoffs and facilitated participative information management in other settings including the ambulatory care or home care arenas. While it may be tempting to create inpatient records tethered to acute care EHRs as a more permanent solution, this move would be short-sighted. Much like current personal-health records with limited data availability and requirements to manually enter information, [12] tethered person-centered health records would include only limited data and information centered on organizations or a subset of providers instead of more person-centered data and information.

Long-term, these new tools would follow precepts outlined by Cortese [13] about a "keep you well" health system: (1) care wherever the person is (home, work, school), (b) by an integrated, multidisciplinary team, (c) with whatever device, (d) providing information at the point of care. The longer-term focus would shift to home or work while allowing collaborative decision making activities such as handoffs in an acute care setting. Most important, individuals need health records that allow interoperability and data access across settings, i.e., records centered on them versus providers and organizations as is the current method. With the individual as the center of data and information management instead of organizations, supporting informatics tools would need to be redesigned. This vision would require years of development. In the meantime, other options may be fruitful.

5   Context-Sensitive Information Design and Tools

First steps may include a patient-centered tool tethered to the EHR and to expand the use of the whiteboards in patients' rooms. A tethered, person-centered healthcare record would include pertinent data from the EHR related to the current course of stay but would need to be robust enough also to allow data input by patients and their families, e.g., preferences, family contact information, questions for providers. This represents a change from current capabilities as patients are not allowed access to in-patient EHRs. These could be designed using either the patient care summary or the multidisciplinary plan of care to push information to an application useful for handoffs in surgical oncology. This kind of summary could guide shared decision-making among providers, patients and family members. Pertinent information could be sent to other devices such as electronic white boards in patients' rooms to display key information as discussed below.

Typical information would be available to the patient as well as the patient and nurse collaborations during handoffs: medication information, daily care goals such as ambulation or pulmonary activities, test results, and discharge planning. Handoff content would include collaboratively-set care goals for discharge and for the day or shift, information related to the problems with interventions and progress toward these goals and/or problem resolution. At discharge, a summary of care, home care requirements such as medications and wound care, would be electronically sent and/or printed for patients. Portions of this record could allow data entry by patients to update emergency contact information, care preferences or restrictions such as a do not resuscitate order or to pose questions to nurses or physicians.

Another promising method may be to expand white boards to an electronic means that allow information input as well as viewing by patients/family members and providers. The whiteboards could include basic information such as collaboratively set care goals including collaborative pain management goals, medication times with patient response and next dose information as well as patient progress toward shift or daily goals. Specific interventions, such as wound care every eight hours, and scheduled inpatient procedures, such as MRIs, could be listed. For both of these options, interoperability with the local electronic health record would be an obvious requirement. Ideally, inpatients and families would be able to bring their own devices such as iPADs to use. Clearly using mobile devices would offer an optimal method for the opportunity to participate in care and flexibility for patients and family members.

5.1   Users and Tasks

Potential surgical oncology inpatient users will have diverse characteristics so designs would be similar to mHealth applications targeted for use by the general public. Because inpatients may not feel well enough to participate in collaborative activities, defined users must be expanded to include family members as well as the inpatients themselves. Both inpatients and their families will be diverse in technology experience and education levels as exemplified in our exploratory research. Thus, future devices and applications need to be targeted to accommodate individual characteristics representative of the general public. Using mHealth design considerations may be helpful. [14,15]

Task-related information for surgical oncology inpatient records includes: ability to access information about the specific type of cancer including educational material, the type of surgery performed with diagrams or illustrations, length of time since surgery, ability to access medication information such as time of last dose, next dose and a pain effectiveness rating. These last two could be trended over time and plotted against each other. Certain fields should allow patient input as discussed above.

Task representation for whiteboards may be more limited: time and name of last pain medication, time next pain med is due, patient care goals for the day such as number of times to ambulate or an intake goal of, say, 2000 cc's, family or emergency contact information and patients' progress toward daily and discharge goals. If space is available, including any scheduled appointments or activities would also be useful.

6   Conclusions

Inpatient tools and their HCI considerations represent a new area of inquiry. A potential exists to improve patient outcomes, care satisfaction and smooth transitions from acute care to ambulatory and home care especially when the user experience is considered as these new tools emerge.

This exploratory study is, to our knowledge, the first to outline initial information content and UX considerations for patient-centered handoffs. This initial study showed patients' willingness to participate in handoffs, outlined information needs and uncovered potential tools for person-centered applications of the future. Inpatients typically want access to robust information about themselves. UX considerations are multiple. Stakeholders need to include family members and any designs need to be targeted to use by the general public with varying education levels, technology experience and abilities. Tasks are designed based upon patient care goals/problems, interventions and progress toward goals. Context-specific information for surgical oncology specifically includes pain management, wound information, follow-up cancer care and appointment schedules.

6.1   Limitations and Future Research

Limitations to this study include: (1) the sample was slightly more well educated overall than most and (2) the study was completed in a cancer specialty hospital, potentially limiting the generalizability of the findings. Future research may be to develop user experience requirements in more depth, to create a pilot project for electronic white boards and to expand decision aids to the inpatient arena and handoff activities. The user experience requirements could be validated using an initial prototype electronic whiteboard or handoff tool that is interoperable with the institution's electronic health record. A diverse set of inpatients and their families could be tested for the feasibility and design of this new tool in oncology.

References

1. Abraham, J., Kannampallil, T., Patel, B., Almoosa, K., Patel, V.: Ensuring patient safety in care transitions: an empirical evaluation of a handoff intervention tool. In: AMIA Symposium on American Medical Informatics Association (AMIA) Annual Symposium Proceedings, pp. 17–26 (2012)
2. Osborn, R., Squires, D.: International perspectives on patient engagement: results from the 2011 Commonwealth Fund Survey. The Journal of Ambulatory Care Management 35(2), 118–128 (2012)
3. McMurray, A., Chaboyer, W., Wallis, M., Johnson, J., Gehrke, T.: Patients' perspectives of bedside nursing handover. Collegian 18(1), 19–26 (2011)
4. Rappaport, D.I., Ketterer, T.A., Nilforoshan, V., Sharif, I.: Family-centered rounds: views of families, nurses, trainees, and attending physicians. Clinical Pediatriatrics (Phila) 51(3), 260–266 (2012)
5. Flink, M., Hesselink, G., Pijnenborg, L., et al.: The key actor: a qualitative study of patient participation in the handover process in Europe. BMJ Quality & Safety 21(suppl. 1), i89–i96 (2012)
6. Chaboyer, W., McMurray, A., Johnson, J., Hardy, L., Wallis, M., Sylvia Chu, F.: Bedside handover: quality improvement strategy to transform care at the bedside. Journal of Nursing Care Quality 24(2), 136–142 (2009)
7. Wilson, M.L., Murphy, L.S., Newhouse, R.: Patients' access to their health information: a meaningful-use mandate. The Journal of Nursing Administration 42(11), 493–496 (2012)
8. Staggers, N., Benham-Hutchins, M.B., Heermann-Langford, L.: Exploring patient-centered handoffs in surgical oncology. Journal of Participatory Medicine 5 (2013)
9. Frosch, D.L., May, S.G., Rendle, K.A., Tietbohl, C., Elwyn, G.: Authoritarian physicians and patients' fear of being labeled 'difficult' among key obstacles to shared decision making. Health Affairs 31(5), 1030–1038 (2012)
10. Bernard, R., Ryan, G.: Analyzing Qualitative Data: Systematic Approaches. Sage, Thousand Oaks (2010)
11. Hsieh, H.F., Shannon, S.: Three approaches to qualitative content analysis. Qualitative Health Research 15(9), 1277–1288 (2005)
12. Gibson, B.: Personal Health Records. In: Nelson, R., Staggers, N. (eds.) Health Informatics: An Interprofessional Approach, pp. 244–257. Elsevier, Louis (2014)
13. Cortese, D.: A health care encounter of the 21st century. JAMA 310(18), 1937–1938 (2013)
14. Brown, W., Yen, P.Y., Rojas, M., Schnall, R.: Assessment of the Health IT Usability Evaluation Model (Health-ITUEM) for evaluating mobile health (mHealth) technology. Journal of Biomedical Informatics 46(6), 1080–1087 (2013)
15. Sheehan, B., Lee, Y., Rodriguez, M., Tiase, V., Schnall, R.: A comparison of usability factors of four mobile devices for accessing healthcare information by adolescents. Applied Clinical Informatics 3(4), 356–366 (2012)

A Pilot Study in Using a Smart Voice Messaging System to Create a Reflection-in-Caregiving Workshop

Taro Sugihara[1], Yuji Hirabayashi[2,4], Kentaro Torii[3],
Tetsuro Chino[3], and Naoshi Uchihira[4]

[1] Okayama University, Tsushimanaka 3-1-1, Kita-ku, Okayama 700-8530, Japan
[2] Shimizu Corporation, Chuo-ku, Tokyo, Japan
[3] Toshiba Corpration, Kawasaki, Kanagawa, Japan
[4] Japan Advanced Institute of Science and Technology, Nomi, Ishikawa, Japan
t-sugihara@okayama-u.ac.jp

Abstract. This paper describes a pilot study in terms of reflection-in-caregiving with an assistive technology employing smart messaging by Bluetooth for location identification and annotation for tweets. We conducted 3 sorts of investigations (i.e. questionnaire of role stress, semi-structured interview and reflection workshop) to explore potential for inducing caregiver's behavior change by the assistive technology. Thereafter, we concluded that the assistive technology shows the potential of reflection and behavior change.

Keywords: People with dementia, caregiving, reflection workshop, case study, massaging system with voice tweeting.

1 Introduction

In Japan, an increasing number of people are over sixty-five years of age. Consequently, the demand for qualified caregivers is increasing; however, most care centers for the elderly are short-staffed and caregiver workloads are increasing. This has resulted in numerous caregivers reaching a burnout state. Japan is not the only country facing this challenge; many other developed countries, such as Germany, Italy, and the Republic of Korea face similar problems. According to a United Nations report [1], many countries are expected to become "super-aged" societies by the year 2050, by then, there is a prediction that more than twenty percent of the population will be sixty-five years or older.

Technology can play an important role in helping caregivers of aging population. For example, several devices (such as sensors) and services have been developed to help locate a person with dementia who may be wandering aimlessly outdoors. Health and safety monitoring technologies aim to keep the elderly healthy and look after them in case their safety is at risk. These technologies are most effective for monitoring people who tend to go about unnoticed.

The devices include various sensors such as GPS-enabled mobile phones. Several monitoring systems have been developed to ensure the safety of people with dementia. Such systems focus on preventing residents from taking risky actions such as

C. Stephanidis and M. Antona (Eds.): UAHCI/HCII 2014, Part III, LNCS 8515, pp. 387–394, 2014.

wandering [2–5]. A smart home with a sensor network enables caregivers to monitor the whereabouts of residents. When a smart home is inhabited by people with dementia, the home can help caregivers identify the risks involved in any unusual behavior, such as wandering and agitation [6–9]. Although technology may be useful for assisting such people and their caregivers, these technologies have not been embedded into the job processes and workflows of caregivers.

We have therefore developed a workshop for reflection-in-caregiving with an assistive technology employing smart messaging and location identification via Bluetooth; and have developed the Bluetooth component in advance of this current study [10]. We conducted a series of investigations, which consisted of questionnaires regarding role stress, semi-structured interviews, and field trials of our proposed system at a care house, all in an effort to explore and identify the requirements of the workshop. With respect to care tasks, the investigations targeted meal assistance; further, 25 caregiver-days participated in this study.

2   Smart Voice Messaging System

Figures 1 and 2 show a smart voice messaging system that provides a hands-free communication method for temporal–spatial collaboration among caregivers and nurses. In our proposed smart voice messaging system, voice messages can be automatically distributed to the right person at the right time and place and in the right way without cumbersome input operations. To do so, as shown in Figure 2, the automatic voice message distribution engine uses tags appended to the voice messages. These voice message tags annotate the message and indicate contextual information about the message. These tags are generated from keywords (obtained via voice recognition) as well as location and acceleration (from sensor data) [11].

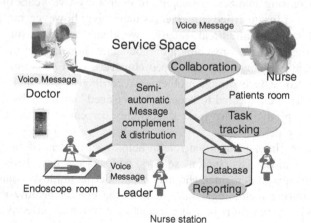

Fig. 1. An overview of our smart voice messaging system [10]

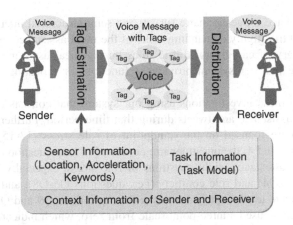

Fig. 2. Message distribution engine that tags and transmits messages from sender to receiver [10]

Nurses and caregivers record voice messages with information observed about patients and care recipients. A better awareness of care recipient conditions is recorded vocally with ease. Further, nurses and caregivers record voice messages of tasks to be performed. Next, a reminder about the task is given. The messages are then used at the shift-change meeting as triggers for reminding staff of incidents or pending tasks to be performed.

A caregiver's voice messages are transmitted to his or her colleague whenever he or she desires. Nurses and caregivers report and share their progress status, and appropriate actions and support can be adaptively implemented collaboratively. During his or her rounds, a nurse speaks with residents and records messages about each patient. These messages are then, for example, distributed to a bath caregiver at bath time. Similarly, other messages are distributed to other nurses during a shift meeting at the nursing station or other specified times. These messages are automatically classified and distributed without any smart phone operations. In traditional communication, information is shared with a sender's intentions and efforts (operations); therefore, only critical information is shared and most noncritical information is lost. While instructions and requests are often critical, other information regarding each client and process are often noncritical. The smart voice messaging system can handle the noncritical information without requiring a sender's strong intentions and efforts.

3   Study Design

In our study, we first obtained informed consent from the manager and caregivers of a care house, who were the participants in our study. Next, we explained to them how to use the system, what equipment each participant would need, and how to record messages in the system. We then operated our system throughout meal assistance for approximately one hour, fully transcribing all tweets regarding caregiving; we annotated the tweets with tags determined by another of our preliminary studies [12] as a Wizard of Oz experiment.

We also conducted a questionnaire survey and semi-structured interviews with the caregivers to identify highly demanding tasks of the meal assistance process; we also showed a summary of caregivers' traffic lines during meal assistance generated by our system. Note that our system provides a function for repeating all tweets with traffic lines.

We conducted these investigations using our system that consists of a traffic line viewer for meal assistance and tweets during that time period. Further, the questions of our questionnaire focused on the standpoint of role stress [13-15]. With results shown in Figures 3 and 4, the questionnaire consisted of one question regarding overall stress in meal assistance, eight questions of role stress, especially role ambiguity (i.e., questions Q1-Q4) and role conflicts (i.e., questions Q5-Q8), and two questions regarding knowledge levels matched to tasks (i.e., questions Q9 and Q10). The question regarding fatigue used a three-point scale from zero, which indicated no stress, to two, which indicated heavy stress; the other questions used a seven-point scale. Caregivers received a higher fatigue score for certain messages if he or she was faced with a burden during meal assistance or graded it without identification to a certain message (if the caregiver could not identify a specific occasion at the time). Next, the caregivers answered questions regarding role stress and their (self-assessed) knowledge levels.

Inherent to caregiving, the decision-making process of caregivers often becomes vague under the stress of multiple and simultaneous tasks. In the semi-structured interviews, we primarily focused on asking caregivers about the reasons they felt they received the aforementioned questionnaire scores; each interview took approximately 15 minutes.

Workshop requirements were determined based on the results of the questionnaires and interviews. As a result, a workshop for reflecting on the role of the caregiver was held in the same care house.

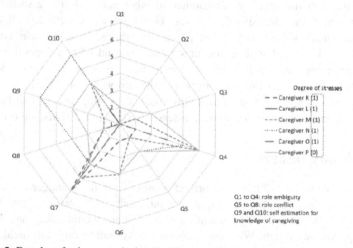

Fig. 3. Results of role stress during the daytime meal assistance process

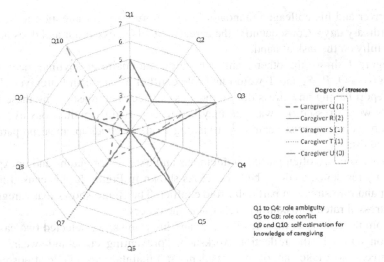

Fig. 4. Other results of role stress during the daytime meal assistance process

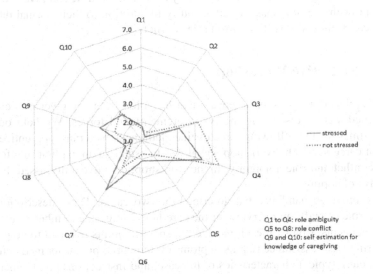

Fig. 5. Averages of role stress

4   Results

Figure 3 shows an example of results of the questionnaire given in regards to day meal assistance. Caregivers who felt high levels of stress scored higher on questions of role stress—especially question Q8—than others who did not feel such stress. For instance, Caregiver K, a competent caregiver, reported during her interview that a resident with dementia often becomes unquiet during lunch. This resident sometime yells at the other residents if she feels ignored by her caregivers. In response, the caregiver and his colleague mandatorily pay more frequent attention to her than that on ordinary days. Consequently, the caregiver feels stressed out and does not concentrate fully on the task at hand.

Figure 4 shows the other results of the questionnaire at daytime meal assistance. Caregivers Q, R, S, and T were rated role conflict higher than Caregiver U, who did not report having any stress during meal assistance. The reason why these four caregivers were stressed out was that they had to cope with simultaneous events in their day, including exercise, haircuts, a visiting medical checkup, meal preparation, and meal assistance.

Caregivers are often placed in dilemmas and experience claims and unexpected actions by residents, as described above. As shown in Figure 5, this caused mental anguish and role stress, in particular role conflict. The figure shows that caregivers who felt stressed rated role conflict higher than the others.

From the results of the questionnaire and interviews, we selected two cases as discussion topics in the reflection workshop: "preventing curse-and-swear," in which caregivers must take care of their residents and maintain a sociable atmosphere while providing quality care for everyone, in addition to ordinary meals; "preventing a domino effect," in which if there were many events in the day, caregivers were imposed to cope with multiple tasks simultaneously in addition to their normal daily tasks. In such cases, they also suffered from role conflict.

5   Reflective Workshop

We developed a workshop to ensure that the role of the caregiver was clear; and approached this by discussing the two aforementioned topics. We held our workshop three times for the following three distinct audiences: veterans, apprentices, and competent caregivers. The workshop's goal was to establish an explicit rule for mitigating role conflict and role ambiguity. In the workshop, caregivers discussed their individual ways of coping.

We provided handouts that described the two cases. These descriptions consisted of the role of staff, an overview of the care house (e.g., the number of caregivers and care recipients, times for each meal, etc.), specific points that had to be paid attention to during meal assistance (e.g., symptoms of dementia, preparing medication after the meal, etc.), typical characteristics of the case, and instructions and themes for discussion. Workshop members were selected based on their levels of expertise and position in the care house; we played the role of facilitator. Through multiple sessions, three or four caregivers participated in the workshop; more specifically, there was a veteran caregiver, one or two intermediate caregivers, and one or two novices. Workshop discussions were fully recorded and transcribed for detailed analysis.

We observed that caregivers actively conversed with each other throughout the workshop. They tried to confirm their colleagues' ways of detecting signs of curse-and-swear behavior and how to cope with it, including when to contact the chief. Likewise, they discussed how they handled dealing with simultaneous events. Veteran caregivers recognized the workshop as an opportunity to share their experiences and knowledge with younger caregivers. In each workshop, participants produced a set of instructions on how to cope with the domino effect. More specifically, they were able to externalize their implicit knowledge as an explicit explanation. We therefore conclude that our workshop has the potential to change a caregiver behavior and mindset in regards to our smart voice messaging system.

6   Conclusion

We conducted a pilot study in a care house with our smart voice messaging system with the goal of designing a workshop to discuss key issues in the role of caregiving. Caregiver tweets during meal assistance that are collected by our system and are stored to serve as triggers of the incidents along with their responses and actions to these triggers. They reported their degrees of fatigue and the role of stress in terms of meal assistance via a questionnaire on our system. We also carried out semi-structured interviews to reveal the relationship between fatigue and stress as well as the cause of them. Workshop requirements for reflection-in-caregiving were then determined after the investigation and the workshop was held thrice. From our results, we concluded that our workshop development in conjunction with our system has great potential to trigger behavioral change. In our future work, we plan to carry out follow-up studies to validate and extend the findings of this study.

Acknowledgement. This study was supported in part by the Grant-in-Aid for Scientific Research (22615017, 24616004) of JSPS and the Service Science, Solutions, and Foundation Integrated Research Program (S3FIRE) from JST. We also appreciate Professor Satoko Tsuru from the University of Tokyo for her thoughtful advice in regards to our study.

References

1. United Nations Population Division, World Population Prospects: The 2008 Revision Population Database (2008), http://esa.un.org/unpp/index.asp?panel=2 (accessed April 30, 2011)
2. Masuda, Y., Yoshimura, T., Nakajima, K., Nambu, M., Hayakawa, T., Tamura, T.: Unconstrained monitoring of prevention of wandering the elderly. In: Proceedings of the Second Joint EMBS/BMES Conference and the 24th Annual Conference and the Annual Fall Meeting of the Biomedical Engineering Society, vol. 3, pp. 1906–1907 (2002)
3. Miskelly, F.: A novel system of electronic tagging in patients with dementia and wandering. Age and Ageing 33(3), 304–306 (2004)
4. Lin, C.-C., Chiu, M.-J., Hsiao, C.-C., Lee, R.-G., Tsai, Y.-S.: Wireless health care service system for elderly with dementia. IEEE Transactions on Information Technology in Biomedicine 10(4), 696–704 (2006)
5. Chen, D., Bharucha, A.J., Wactlar, H.D.: Intelligent video monitoring to improve safety of older persons. In: Proceedings of 29th Annual International Conference of the IEEE EMBS, pp. 3814–3817 (2007)

6. Hope, K., Waterman, H.: Using multi-sensory environments with older people with dementia. Journal of Advanced Nursing 25(4), 780–785 (1997)
7. Helal, S., Giraldo, C., Kaddoura, Y., Lee, C., El Zabadani, H., Mann, W.: Smart phone based cognitive assistant. In: Proc. of the 2nd International Workshop on Ubiquitous Computing for Pervasive Healthcare Applications (UbiHealth 2003) (2003)
8. Arcelus, A., Jones, M., Goubran, R., Knoefel, F.: Integration of smart home technologies in a health monitoring system for the elderly. In: Proceedings of the 21st International Conference on Advanced Information Networking and Applications Workshops (AINAW 2007), vol. 2, pp. 820–825 (2007)
9. Zhang, D., Hariz, M., Mokhtari, M.: Assisting Elders with Mild Dementia Staying at Home. In: Proc. of the 6th Annual IEEE International Conference on Pervasive Computing and Communications, pp. 692–697 (2008)
10. Uchihira, N., Torii, K., Chino, T., Hiraishi, K., Choe, S., Hirabayashi, Y., Sugihara, T.: Temporal-Spatial Collaboration Support for Nursing and Caregiving Services. In: Spohrer, J.C., Kwan, S.K., Sawatani, Y. (eds.) Global Perspectives on Service Science: Japan. Springer (in press)
11. Torii, K., Uchihira, N., Chino, T., Iwata, K., Murakami, T., Tanaka, T.: Service Space Communication by Voice Tweets in Nursing. In: Freund, L.E. (ed.) Proc. of the 1st International Conference on Human Side of Service Engineering, also in Advances in the Human Side of Service Engineering, pp. 443–451. CRC Press (2012)
12. Chino, T., Torii, K., Uchihira, N., Hirabayashi, Y.: Speech Interaction Analysis on Collaborative Work at an Elderly Care Facility. International Journal of Sociotechnology and Knowledge Development 5(2), 18–33 (2013)
13. Kahn, R.L., Wolfe, D.M., Quinn, R.P., Snoek, J.D., Rosenthal, R.A.: Organizational stress: Studies in role conflict and ambiguity. John Wiley (1964)
14. Moniz-Cook, E., Clin, D., Millington, D., Silver, M.: Residential care for older people: job satisfaction and psychological health in care staff. Health & Social Care in the Community 5(2), 124–133 (1997)
15. Rizzo, J.R., House, R.J., Lirtzman, S.I.: Role Conflict and Ambiguity in Complex Organizations. Administrative Science Quarterly 15(2), 150–163 (1970)

Toward a Companion Agent for the Elderly – The Methods to Estimate At-Home and Outside-Home Daily Life Activities of the Elderly Who Live Alone

Yuma Takeda, Hung-Hsuan Huang*, and Kyoji Kawagoe

Graduate School of Information Science & Engineering, Ritsumeikan University, Japan
hhhuang@acm.org

Abstract. With advances in medical technology, people's life have been extended, and there are more and more older adults isolated. If they do not maintain social life with others, they may feel loneliness and anxiety. For their mental health, it is reported effective to keep their social relationship with others, for example, the conversation with their caregivers or other elderly people. Active listening is a communication technique that the volunteer listener listens to the speaker (the elderly) carefully and attentively by confirming or asking for more details about what they heard. This helps to make the elderly feel cared and to relieve their anxiety and loneliness. This paper presents our in-progress project aiming to develop a framework of a virtual companion agent who is always with the user and can engage active listening to maintain a long-term relationship with elderly users. In order to achieve the agent's companionship with the user for a longer period, we believe that it is essential to make the agent to understand the user as best as it can. This kind of user-fitted conversation is not addressed in previous companion agent work. The proposed approach is the acquisition of the "memory" of the user's daily life in two situations, at-home and outside-home. In the former one, multiple Microsoft Kinect depth sensors were adopted. The depth information is integrated to detect the user's position and posture and then to estimate the user's daily activity. In the outside-home configuration, the prototype application is an Android smartphone application that recognizes the user's moving status with the information from the on-board three-axis accelerometer as well as the location of the user from GPS information. These data are then used to estimate the user's outside-home activity. All estimated daily activities are recorded in an activity history database. Both the at-home and outside-home activity estimation methods have been developed and have been evaluated in a laboratory environment with student subjects at a moderate accuracy. The interface of the companion agent is being designed with the results from human-human and human-agent (driven by the data from the human listener condition) subject experiments. After the technologies are more matured, we would like to conduct real-world experiment with elderly subjects in near future.

1   Introduction

With advances in medical technology, the average life expectancy of world population is increasing. Since the probability of becoming cognitively impaired increases with age

---

* Corresponding author.

C. Stephanidis and M. Antona (Eds.): UAHCI/HCII 2014, Part III, LNCS 8515, pp. 395–402, 2014.
© Springer International Publishing Switzerland 2014

(roughly 10% of over 65 years old people), one side effect of increasing life expectancy is the emerging number of dementia patients. It is said that currently there are already around 40 million dementia patients all over the world. This is particularly severe in developed countries where the problem of aging population proceeds. Japan, probably is the country in most severe situation in the world. According to a recent statistical data, the number of dementia patients in Japan has already exceeded two million (1.6% of the population), and the number will keep increasing to 4.5 million (4.1% of the population) by 2035.

If they do not maintain social life with others, they may feel loneliness and anxiety. For their mental health, it is reported effective to keep their social relationship with others, for example, the conversation with their caregivers or other elderly people. Reminiscence or life review [1] is a well known method to slow the progress of the most prominent symptom of dementia, memory impairment. It is also reported in the literature [2,3] that repetitive stimuli on cognitive functions in the environment is also effective in suppressing the degradation of specific cognitive abilities.

Active listening is a communication technique that the listener listens to the speaker carefully and attentively by confirming or asking for more details about what they heard. This kind of support helps to make the elderly feel cared and to relieve their anxiety and loneliness. However, due to the lack of the number of volunteers comparing to that of the elderly who are living alone, the volunteers may not be always available when they are needed. In order to improve the effect, always-available and trustable conversational partners in enough number are demanded. This paper presents our in-progress project aiming to develop a virtual companion agent who can engage active listening and maintain a long-term relationship with elderly users.

This paper presents our approaches in acquiring the "memory" of the user's daily life in two situations, at-home and outside home. Because of the different level of constraints of the situations, we tried to maximize the richness of sensory information with different sensor technologies for each of them. Fig. 1 shows the conceptual diagram of this project, where the companion / listener agent can utilize the daily activities of the user and engage the conversation with him / her. The daily activity database are created from the information gathered by portable device (smartphone) and at-home sensors (Microsoft Kinect). These information can be further searched by medical institutions or the family of the users from remote.

2   Related Work

Various assistive technologies for dementia patients have been proposed so far. Since it is difficult to find a sufficient number of caregivers for dementia patients in many countries, besides providing physical assistance to those with physical impairments, it is important for assistive artifacts to provide communication functions [4]. An embodied conversational agent can effectively serve as a listener for people with dementia if it is accepted as a companion by the patients. Previous studies on the acceptance of such an agent by elderly people reported that it is important for the agent to display social signals, like smiling and head nods [5]; this enables the agent to gain the patient's trust and enhances intimacy [6].

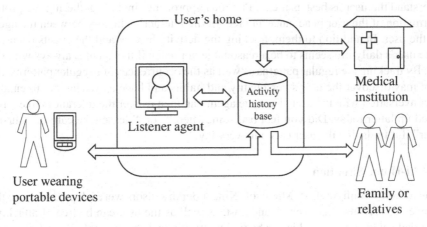

Fig. 1. Conceptual diagram of the project

In the aspect of conversational companion agents, most previous studies focused on user perception of empathy and affectiveness during the interaction with the agent. Kanoh et al. [7] investigated user acceptance of a robot in recreational use inside health care facilities for elderly people. Although the participants showed positive reactions to the robot, the interaction between the participants and the robot was seldom observed. Bickmore et al. [4] investigated the effects of verbal and non-verbal empathic behaviors of a 2D graphic agent and found that the subjects did rate the agent more caring if it shows those behaviors. Leite et al. [8] investigated a robot cat showing empathic behaviors (voice, facial expressions, and head movements) on the players of chess game. Smith et al. [9] proposed the integration of affective dialogue with a deliberative architecture. These studies showed that the display of empathic behaviors can usually make the conversational artifacts better accepted by users, which is a requirement of artificial companions. However, these proposed systems are neither equipped with the mechanism to keep long-term relationship with the users nor used in serious tasks.

Other studies try to model episodic memory which is essential to maintain the dialogue with users in long-term relationship. Sieber and Krenn [14] proposed a W3C RDF (resource description framework) based presentation of past interaction and user preferences. In order to achieve higher efficiency and more realistic dialogue, Lim et al. [10] integrated "forgetting" feature into their episodic memory model. Campos and Paiva [11] proposed a chat agent for assisting a teenager user on self-reflection about what happens in his / her life. The dialogue is pro-active and adapted to the main goals of a teenager user, school, love and play. These projects also do not aim serious use of companion agent, but the Campos' work shares similar general idea with us, i.e. store and acquire personal memory by the interaction with a companion agent.

3 Recording of Daily Activities

In order to achieve the agent's companionship with the user for a longer period from several months to several years, we believe that it is essential to make the agent to understand the user as best as it can. Previous approaches include gathering the profile information of the user in advance and record the interaction history between the agent and the user. In addition to them, tracking the activity history and the events occurred in the user's daily life seems to be a reasonable approach if the agent is always with the user. By tracking the regular patterns as well as the occurrences of irregular patterns, the agent may discover the user's personality and habits and have more chances to engage the conversation with the user. Then the agent can then trigger the utterances like "You waked up latter today. Did you feel bad somewhere?" or "Please take care of yourself better" if it finds that the user eats out everyday.

3.1 At-Home Situation

In the at-home configuration, Microsoft Kinect depth sensors were adopted because the balance between its effectiveness and cost, as well as the user can be free of attaching some dedicated sensors on his/her body. Due to the fact that a single Kinect can only detect the distance between itself and the objects within a range between 0.8 and 4 m, multiple Kinects are required to cover a typical one-room apartment (about 30 m^2) in Japan. The method to integrate the coordinate systems of two Kinects to the world coordinate system is evaluated to have a precision with errors less than 0.6 m in a simulated room. This should be enough to detect the locations of the user inside his/her home. From the location and prior knowledge of the room layout (the locations of TV, toilet, kitchen, etc), we expect that we can estimate the user's at-home activities. Fig. 2 shows the layout of the simulated room where we conducted the experiments. We measured the precision of the position estimation method at the preventative positions with a two-Kinect setup. Table 1 shows the results. The precision varies while the distance toward Kinects. The precision is only at moderate level but should be enough to distinguish the spaces where the user doing his / her activities.

Table 1. Measured precision of the position estimation method for at-home situation

ID	(X, Y)	estimated (X, Y)	error
1	(-2.000, -0.500)	(-1.121,-0.278)	1.136
2	(-0.500, -1.000)	(-0.331, -0.559)	0.471
3	(-1.000, -0.500)	(-0.580, -0.235)	0.496
4	(0.000, 0,000)	(0.591, -0.170)	0.524
5	(-0.500, 0.500)	(0.057, 0.084)	0.102
6	(-0.500, 0.500)	(-0.304, 0.323)	0.263
7	(0.500, 0.500)	(0.284, 0.333)	0.271
8	(-1.000, 1.000)	(-0.551, 0.473)	0.691
9	(1.500, 1.000)	(0.001, 0.004)	1.799
10	(0.000, 1.500)	(-0.024, 0.900)	0.600

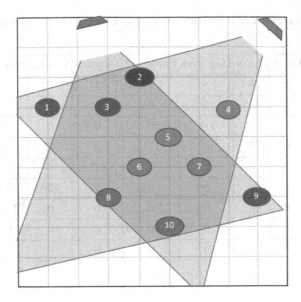

Fig. 2. Coordinations where the precision of position estimation was measured

3.2 Outside-Home Situation

In the outside home configuration, the prototype application is implemented on a Samsung Galaxy SII phone. This Android application recognizes the user's moving status (walking, running, bicycle, car, or train) with the information from the on-board three-axes accelerometer (sampling rate: 100 Hz). The recognition process uses a priorly trained C4.5 decision tree by Weka data mining tool [12] from 30-minute training data of each class. Since there should be no difference of feature values among different person on transport vehicles, those training data were collected from one person. On the other hand, the walking data were collected from five college students (three males and two females). The features used are the maximum, average, and deviation of each axis. The measurement is based on a 5-second sliding window in real-time, and a 92.2% 10-fold cross validation accuracy is achieved. Base on this mechanism, we further measure the activities in larger temporal granularity, i.e. 10 minutes, one hour, and one day. The preliminary experiment is done with one male college student's activities in one month. In addition to the features for detecting moving status, other features like time period and the types of facility where the subject is in were used. Table 2, 3, and 4 show the confusion matrices of the classification results of each granularity, respectively. The classification accuracy at 10-fold cross validation was shown in Table 5. Furthermore, these data were sent to a database where queries of the user activities is possible from Web interface (Fig. 3).

The application also logs the user's current position from the location information of on-board GPS sensor (sampling rate: 1 Hz). The moving status and position is sent to a back end server in trunks periodically (for example, once every 10 minutes). Our next

Table 2. Confusion matrix of 10-minutes activity estimation. The data in columns are the classification results

	Lunch	Dinner	Desk work	Restaurant	Shopping	Walking	Bicycle	Car	Train
Lunch	124	0	5	1	1	0	0	0	0
Dinner	0	127	5	0	1	0	0	0	0
Desk work	11	33	118	0	0	0	0	0	0
Restaurant	0	0	0	174	0	0	0	0	0
Shopping	0	0	0	0	173	0	0	0	0
Walking	0	0	0	0	0	150	0	0	0
Bicycle	0	0	0	0	0	0	156	0	0
Car	0	0	0	0	0	0	0	135	0
Train	0	0	0	0	0	0	0	0	138

Table 3. Confusion matrix of one-hour activity estimation. The data in columns are the classification results

	Meal	Shopping	Desk work	Moving
Meal	76	1	19	0
Shopping	16	91	5	0
Desk work	19	0	83	0
Moving	0	0	0	100

Table 4. Confusion matrix of one-day activity estimation. The data in columns are the classification results

	Study & Research	Meal	Recreation
Study & Research	10	0	0
Dinner with friends	0	8	2
Recreation	0	2	8

Table 5. Classification accuracy (10-fold cross validation) in different temporal granularities

Time Slice	Moving	10 minutes	One hour	One day
Accuracy	92.2%	95.9%	85.3%	86.6%

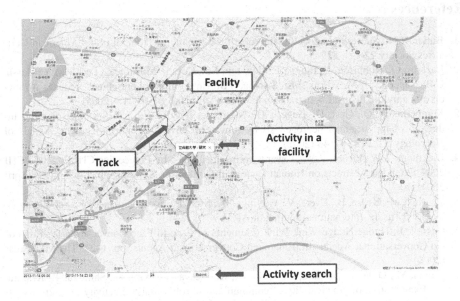

Fig. 3. Visualization of the activities of outside-home situation

step is to extend the companion agent interface to the smartphone. Considering safety issue, it is not necessary to include the graphical character. However, as the literature reports that the user can feel the agent migrate even its form changes [13], it would be easier to establish trustworthy relationship with the agent if the user can feel the agent is still with the user when (s)he is outside home. For example, using the same voice and the same personality model in both the at-home agent kiosk and the mobile phone.

4   Conclusions and Future Work

This paper presents a part of work of an ongoing project that aims to develop a virtual companion agent for the elderly. It is believed that the tracking and utilizing the daily life activity of the user for the agent's action decision-making can help to develop long-term relationship with the user. Kinect depth sensors were used in at-home situation while Android mobile phone is used in outside home situations to record the user's locations. These data are further used to estimate the user's activities. As future work, first of all, we would like to integrate the activity information from both the at-home and outside home situations and develop an uniformed memory representation for the agent. After that, we would like to complete the development of the interaction loop of user activity recognition and agent behavior generation. Finally, we would like to deploy the complete system in long-term practical use to evaluate its effectiveness.

References

1. Butler, R.N.: Successful aging and the role of the life review. Journal of the American Geriatrics Society 22(12), 529–535 (1974)
2. Lazarov, O., Robinson, J., Tang, Y.P., Hairston, I.S., Korade-Mirnics, Z., Lee, V.M.Y., Hersh, L.B., Sapolsky, R.M., Mirnics, K., Sisodia, S.S.: Environmental enrichment reduces Aβ levels and amyloid deposition in transgenic mice. Cell 120(5), 701–713 (2005)
3. Kempermann, G., Gast, D., Gage, F.H.: Neuroplasticity in old age: Sustained fivefold induction of hippocampal neurogenesis by long-term environmental enrichment. Annals of Neurology 52(2), 135–143 (2002)
4. Bickmore, T.W., Picard, R.W.: Towards caring machines. In: Proceeding CHI EA 2004 CHI 2004 Extended Abstracts on Human Factors in Computing Systems, pp. 1489–1492 (April 2004)
5. Heerink, M., Kröse, B., Evers, V., Wielinga, B.: Studying the acceptance of a robotic agent by elderly users. International Journal of ARM 7(3), 33–43 (2006)
6. Cassell, J.: Nudge Nudge Wink Wink: Elements of Face-to-Face Conversation for Embodied Conversational Agents. In: Embodied Conversational Agents, pp. 1–27. The MIT Press (2000)
7. Kanoh, M., Oida, Y., Nomura, Y., Araki, A., Konagaya, Y., Ihara, K., Shimizu, T., Kimura, K.: Examination of practicability of communication robot-assisted activity program for elderly people. Journal of Robotics and Mechatronics 23(1), 3–12 (2011)
8. Leite, I., Mascarenhas, S., Pereira, A., Martinho, C., Prada, R., Paiva, A.: "Why can't we be friends?" an empathic game companion for long-term interaction. In: Safonova, A. (ed.) IVA 2010. LNCS, vol. 6356, pp. 315–321. Springer, Heidelberg (2010)
9. Smith, C., Crook, N., Boye, J., Charlton, D., Dobnik, S., Pizzi, D., Cavazza, M., Pulman, S., de la Camara, R.S., Turunen, M.: Interaction strategies for an affective conversational agent. In: Safonova, A. (ed.) IVA 2010. LNCS, vol. 6356, pp. 301–314. Springer, Heidelberg (2010)
10. Lim, M.Y., Aylett, R., Ho, W.C., Enz, S., Vargas, P.: A socially-aware memory for companion agents. In: Ruttkay, Z., Kipp, M., Nijholt, A., Vilhjálmsson, H.H. (eds.) IVA 2009. LNCS, vol. 5773, pp. 20–26. Springer, Heidelberg (2009)
11. Campos, J., Paiva, A.: May: My memories are yours. In: Safonova, A. (ed.) IVA 2010. LNCS, vol. 6356, pp. 406–412. Springer, Heidelberg (2010)
12. Hall, M., Frank, E., Holmes, G., Pfahringer, B., Reutemann, P., Witten, I.H.: The weka data mining software: An update. ACM SIGKDD Explorations 11(1), 11–18 (2009)
13. Ogawa, K., Ono, T.: ITACO: Effects to interactions by relationships between humans and artifacts. In: Prendinger, H., Lester, J.C., Ishizuka, M. (eds.) IVA 2008. LNCS (LNAI), vol. 5208, pp. 296–307. Springer, Heidelberg (2008)
14. Sieber, G., Krenn, B.: Towards an episodic memory for companion dialogue. In: Safonova, A. (ed.) IVA 2010. LNCS, vol. 6356, pp. 322–328. Springer, Heidelberg (2010)

Age and Age-Related Differences in Internet Usage of Cancer Patients

Julia C.M. van Weert[1], Sifra Bolle[1], and Linda D. Muusses[2]

[1] Amsterdam School of Communication Research/ASCoR,
University of Amsterdam, Amsterdam, The Netherlands
j.c.m.vanweert@uva.nl
[2] Department of Social and Organisational Psychology,
VU University Amsterdam, The Netherlands

Abstract. This study investigates age and age-related differences in Internet usage of 952 cancer patients treated with chemotherapy. Older patients (≥ 65 years) reported significantly less Internet usage to find treatment-related information than younger ones (< 65 years). Still, 40.1% of the older patients used the internet regularly or often, as compared to 52.3% of the younger patients. About one quarter (26.4%) of the older patients and 14.6% of the younger patients didn't use the Internet at all during their chemotherapy treatment. In the younger age group, men, patients with a palliative treatment goal, a more monitoring coping style, more information preferences and higher fulfilled information and communication needs reported more Internet usage than their counterparts. In the older age group, only a monitoring coping style, being male and a higher education level predicted Internet usage. The results of this study provide guidance to improve Internet usage of older patients.

Keywords: Aging, Internet, Information Seeking, Cancer, Chemotherapy.

1 Introduction

Cancer is frequently a disease of older adults [1], [2]. Due to an aging population, the number of new cancer patients will rapidly increase in the coming years [3]. Fulfilling patients' information and communication needs can help them cope with their illness and improve their well-being [4]. Increasingly, health information is delivered on the Internet [5]. In The Netherlands, the vast majority of people aged 65 years and older have access to the Internet and more than half of these older Internet users, use the Internet to search for health related information [6]. This makes the Internet a strong medium to deliver health information to older people [7]. Little research has been conducted on Internet usage of older cancer patients and if, or to what extent, this differs from Internet usage of younger patients. As chemotherapy is in the top-three of most used treatments for cancer [8], our study focuses on Internet use to search for information about chemotherapy. Therefore, this study aims to investigate age differences in Internet usage of cancer patients treated with chemotherapy (from now on:

C. Stephanidis and M. Antona (Eds.): UAHCI/HCII 2014, Part III, LNCS 8515, pp. 403–414, 2014.
© Springer International Publishing Switzerland 2014

chemotherapy patients). According to the uses-and-gratifications theory, the use of media can be predicted by the needs for information of an individual [9-12]. Chemotherapy patients need information to cope with their illness and treatment. When healthcare providers are unable to fulfill the information needs of patients, they might turn to other sources, such as the Internet to fulfill their information needs. The second aim of our study is therefore to study the factors that might influence the level of Internet usage. To study these factors, we used a model, developed by Muusses et al. [13], that explains information source usage in chemotherapy patients. This model assumes that background characteristics (i.e., socio-demographic factors and medical background factors) and psychological factors (i.e., cancer-related stress reactions, coping style and information preferences) predict information needs, which subsequently predict information source usage, in this case Internet usage (see Figure 1).

This model was originally developed for patients of all ages. However, the factors in the model might be age-related. Regarding the psychological factors, older cancer patients are found to perceive less severe psychosocial problems than younger ones [14], [15]. Their cancer-related stress reactions might be lower because they have fewer competing demands on their time and resources than younger patients. This, along with different expectations, may mitigate the negative impact of the specific psychosocial consequences of the disease and its treatment [14]. This might also influence their information seeking behavior, possibly resulting in less Internet usage. Moreover, older cancer patients in general have a lower monitoring coping style than younger ones [16]. A monitoring coping style means that someone prefers high-information input when experiencing a stressful event to cope with the event, in this case chemotherapy treatment, and suffers less psycho-physiological arousal when receiving information [13], [17]. People with a lower monitoring coping style are expected to use the Internet less often. Last, it is suggested that older cancer patients have a slightly lower need for information than younger patients. They prefer to receive information about the most important aspects of the disease and treatment, but are less interested in detailed information in general [15], [18]. This might result in less Internet usage.

In addition, *background characteristics* might play a different role in older than in younger patients. Next to age, information seeking behavior can be explained by gender and education [13]. Because the education opportunities have increased over the years, older people are, on average, lower educated than younger people [19], and this particularly counts for older woman. In addition, both treatment goal (curative vs. palliative) and quality of life are expected to influence information seeking behavior. Older people receive palliative treatment (aiming to reduce the severity of disease symptoms) more often than younger ones [20]. They may also suffer from age related problems such as co-morbidity and functional problems [21], which might negatively influence their quality of life, and might result in less information seeking [13], [18].

By investigating the assumed predictors of Internet usage separately in a younger (< 65) and an older (≥ 65) age group, we aim to get more insight in the influence of the above-mentioned age-related factors on Internet usage of younger and older chemotherapy patients. We considered 65 years and older as the older age group, as this cut-point has been used in other studies on diseases or impairments in older patients [22], [23].

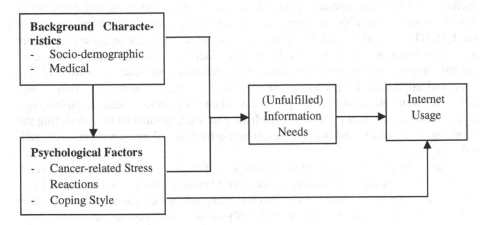

Fig. 1. Conceptual model of Internet usage by cancer patients

2   Method

Data was collected in the context of the national survey "Chemotherapie, Wat Weet u Ervan?" [Chemotherapy, What Do You Know about it?] [24]. Respondents were invited to complete an online questionnaire through several websites of cancer associations (e.g., the Dutch Federations of Breast Cancer, Colorectal Cancer, Gynecological Cancer, Urological Cancer and Leukemia), online cancer forums (e.g., www.de-amazones.nl, www.borstkankerforum.nl, www.iknl.nl) and hospitals. Special effort was made to reach older adults, e.g. using support of the ANBO, the largest Dutch association for older people. Furthermore, the questionnaire was advertised through media (e.g., newspapers, popular magazines, tabloids, radio, and websites) and presentations in walk-in centers for cancer patients, where older people could receive support in filling out the questionnaire.

In total, 1074 (former) chemotherapy patients completed the questionnaire at least partly. For the current study, data of 952 participants who answered the majority of the questions including the question about Internet usage, was used. Of these participants, 227 (23.8%) were aged 65 years or older. There were no significant differences in socio-demographic (age, gender, education) and medical background characteristics (diagnosis, treatment intent, infusion method, still in treatment, other treatments) between completers and non-completers.

Internet usage was measured on a 5-point Likert scale, ranging from 1 (*did not use*) to 5 (*used often*). Next to age, we measured the following socio-demographic and medical background information: gender, education level, quality of life (by using the two-item subscale 'Quality of Life' of the EORTC QLQ-30 [25]) and treatment goal (curative vs. palliative). Regarding psychological factors, the Impact of Event scale was used to measure cancer-related stress reactions [26], [27], the shortened Threatening Medical Situations Inventory (TMSI) to measure monitoring coping style [28], [29] and the Information Satisfaction Questionnaire to measure information preferences [30]. The amount of unfulfilled information and communication needs during consultations with caregivers was measured by using a shortened version of the QUOTE^{chemo}, existing of 28 items about information needs regarding treatment related information, rehabilitation information, discussing realistic expectations, coping information, interpersonal communication, tailored communication and affective communication [24], [31]. Participants indicated for each item whether they would have liked more attention to this topic or not. The total number of unfulfilled information and communication needs was established for each participant by calculating the sumscore of items that did not receive enough attention. All measurements were reliable and valid.

T-Tests and χ^2-tests were used to determine differences in background characteristics between completers and non-completers and between younger (< 65) and older (≥ 65) participants. Three multivariate regression analysis were conducted with Internet usage as dependent variable. In the first analysis the whole sample was used, in the second only the younger age group (< 65) was included and in the last only the older age group (≥ 65). The following three sets of independent variables were entered as separate blocks: (1) background characteristics, (2) psychological factors; and (3) unfulfilled information and communication needs.

3　Results

3.1　Participants

Table 1 presents socio-demographic and medical background characteristics about the respondents. The mean age of all participants was 56.9 years (range 23-82). On average, the majority of the respondents were female. Educational level was divided into lower, middle and higher. About one third of the sample had a lower (31.2%), one third a middle (32.2%) and one third a higher (36.6%) education level. The younger (< 65) and older (> 65) group differed significantly on almost all background characteristics, except for 'gynaecological tumour', 'melanoma', 'other cancer', 'injection', 'other infusion method', and whether the respondent was 'still in treatment'. Most of the differences are population-related. For instance, older people in general have a lower education level than younger ones [19] and receive more frequently a (palliative) chemotherapy treatment only or a chemotherapy treatment without, for instance, radiation [e.g., 32] or operation [e.g., 33]. Patients of 65 years and older have a gastro-enterological tumour, lung tumour or urological tumour more often than younger people, while breast cancer is the most common cancer among younger people [20].

Table 1. Socio-demographic and medical background characteristics ($n = 952$)

Characteristics	Younger (< 65) ($n = 725$)		Older ($\geq$ 65) ($n = 227$)	
	N	%	N	%
Age***				
Mean (SD)	53.0 (8.1)		69.4 (3.9)	
Range	23 – 64		65 – 82	
Gender***				
Female	615	84.8	129	56.8
Male	110	15.2	98	43.2
Education level***				
Low	195	26.9	102	44.9
Middle	251	34.6	56	24.7
High	279	38.5	69	30.4
Diagnosis				
Breast cancer***	430	59.3	56	24.7
Lung tumour***	33	4.6	26	11.5
Gastro-enterological tumour***	83	11.4	66	29.1
Gynaecological tumour	64	8.8	24	10.6
Hematological tumour*	106	14.6	46	20.3
Urological tumour***	20	2.8	20	8.8
Melanoma	15	2.1	7	3.1
Other	34	4.7	14	6.2
Treatment intent***				
Curative	585	80.7	153	67.4
Palliative	125	17.2	64	28.2
Don't know	15	2.1	10	4.4
Infusion method				
Intravenous**	683	94.2	202	89.0
Oral (pills)**	134	18.5	63	27.8
Injection	19	2.6	10	4.4
Other	8	1.1	9	4.0
Still in treatment?				
Yes	140	19.3	40	17.6
No	585	80.7	187	82.4

Table 1. (*continued*)

Characteristics	Younger (< 65) (n = 725)		Older (≥ 65) (n = 227)	
	N	%	N	%
Treatments in addition to chemotherapy #				
Only chemotherapy*	69	9.5	35	15.4
Operation*	542	74.8	150	66.1
Radiation***	399	55.0	90	39.6
Hormone treatment***	284	39.2	25	11.0
Immunotherapy*	93	12.8	15	6.6
Targeted therapy*	27	3.7	17	7.5

*=significant difference between younger and older patients at $p<.05$; **=significant at $p<.01$; ***=significant at $p<.001$.

percentages do not add up to 100 because patients can have received more than one additional treatment

3.2 Internet Usage of Older and Younger Chemotherapy Patients

Figure 2 shows how often younger (< 65) and older (≥ 65 years) chemotherapy patients used the Internet to find information about chemotherapy treatment.

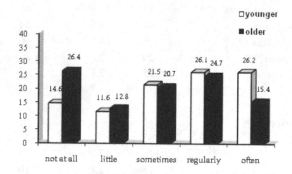

Fig. 2. Percentage of younger (< 65) and older (≥ 65) chemotherapy patients that used the Internet for information about chemotherapy (n = 952)

Older patients reported significantly (p < .001) less Internet usage to find information on chemotherapy treatment than younger ones. Still, 40.1% of the older patients used the internet regularly or often, as compared to 52.3% of the younger patients. About one quarter (26.4%) of the older patients and 14.6% of the younger patients did not use the Internet at all during their chemotherapy treatment. Comparable percentages, but in opposite direction, were found for very frequent Internet usage: about one quarter (26.2%) of the younger patients and 15.4% of the older patients used the Internet often for information about chemotherapy.

When making a further distinction between age groups, i.e., 23-44, 44-64, 65-74 and 75 years and older, we found no significant differences between the two youngest age groups nor between the two oldest age groups. However, both younger age groups differed significantly from both older age groups.

3.3   Predictors of Internet Usage

Multivariate regression analyses were conducted to test the model, i.e. the association of the background characteristics, psychological factors and unfulfilled information needs with Internet usage. Table 2 shows the results of the whole sample. Younger patients, men, patients with a palliative treatment goal, a more monitoring coping style, more information preferences, and higher fulfilled information and communication needs reported more Internet usage than their counterparts. Contrary to our expectations, education, quality of life, and cancer-related stress reactions were not related to Internet usage.

Table 2. Associations between independent variables and Internet usage ($n = 921$)

	Internet usage		
Background characteristics	**Bèta**	**SE**	**p**
Age	-.120**	.004	.004
Gender (0;1) (1=female)	-.101***	.106	.001
Education (0;1) (1=high) (low=reference cat)	.018	.108	.623
Education (0;1) (1=middle) (low=reference cat)	.021	.107	.562
Quality of Life	-.045	.033	.150
Treatment goal (0;1) (1=curative)	-.098***	.104	.001
Psychological factors	**Bèta**	**SE**	**p**
Cancer-related stress reactions (intrusion)	.052	.035	.102
Monitoring coping style	.365***	.057	.000
Information preferences (0;1) (1= everything)	.086**	.132	.005
Information needs	**Bèta**	**SE**	**p**
Number of unfulfilled information/communication needs	-.078*	.005	.012

*=significant at $p<.05$; **=significant at $p<.01$; ***=significant at $p<.001$.
Final model: $R^2=.204$, $F(23, 910)=10.775$, $p<.001$.

When testing the model separately in the younger (< 65) and the older (≥ 65) group, the results remain the same in the younger group. This means that being male ($\beta = -.083$, $p = .017$), having a palliative treatment goal ($\beta = -.101$, $p = .004$), a more monitoring coping style ($\beta = .395$, $p = .000$), more information preferences ($\beta = .090$, $p = .012$) and higher fulfilled information and communication needs ($\beta = -.106$, $p = .003$) were related to more Internet usage in younger chemotherapy patients. However, in the older group, only a monitoring coping style ($\beta = .295$, $p = .000$) was clearly associated with Internet usage. In addition, highly educated older patients (β = .142, p = .052) tended to use the Internet more often than middle or low educated older patients. The same was found for older men (β = -.133, p = .057) as compared to older women.

4   Conclusion and Discussion

Older cancer patients use the Internet less often than younger ones, but with over 40% of the older chemotherapy patients using the Internet regularly or often, the Internet can be considered an important information source for chemotherapy information for older patients. In the whole sample as well as in the subgroup of younger patients (< 65), men, patients with a palliative treatment goal, a more monitoring coping style, more information preferences and higher fulfilled information and communication needs reported more Internet usage than their counterparts. Education, quality of life, and cancer-related stress reactions were not related to Internet usage. In the older group ($\geq$ 65) only a monitoring coping style, and, to a lesser extent, being male, and having a high education level were related to Internet usage.

The results confirm previous findings that age and a monitoring coping style predict Internet usage for chemotherapy information [13]. Contrary to this previous research, which showed no connection between gender and treatment goal, the present study shows that men and patients with a palliative treatment goal reported more Internet usage than patients without these characteristics. The results indicate that for younger patients, there are many reasons to use the Internet as a source for treatment information, while only older patients with a monitoring coping style use the Internet for this purpose. The previous research also showed that a higher or middle level of education (as opposed to a lower level of education) was related to more Internet use, while the present research finds no such connection, except for the older age group. As the data for the previous study was collected in 2007, this might indicate that the there is still a digital gap in the older generation. Education still seemed to be a dividing characteristic in older patients: higher educated patients used the Internet more often for treatment information about chemotherapy. This is consistent with literature in which an age and education gap in Internet use for information purposes is described [34], [35]. Hence, younger people experience more health benefits from the Internet than older people, while in fact older people have more health information needs [36].

Until now, little was known about the relationship between socio-demographic and medical background characteristics, coping style, information preferences, fulfilled information and communication needs, and Internet usage in younger and older cancer patients. The current study fills this gap and gives more insight in underlying mechanisms. For example, according to the *Elaboration Likelihood Model*, information provision that is tailored to the patients' needs will result in better information processing [37]. Results of this study show that younger patients with more fulfilled information and communication needs report more Internet usage than younger patients with less fulfilled information and communication needs. This indicates that the

Internet can indeed play an important role in needs fulfilment, though this is only found in younger people.

Previous research suggests that medical information is better understood and processed by older people when the information is presented in various ways; for instance by combining interpersonal communication during consultation with the use of media sources [38]. Although older cancer patients in general are found to have a lower monitoring coping style than younger cancer patients [16], results of the current study show that, if older patients have a monitoring coping style, they use the Internet to fulfill their information needs. Cancer patients with a monitoring coping style benefit from receiving a lot of information, as well as emotional support [17]. Thus, the results of this study indicate that the Internet provides opportunities for older patients with a monitoring coping style. This group of older patients is apparently able to find treatment-related information on general Internet websites. This does not mean that older patients with a less monitoring coping style cannot benefit from the Internet. However, they may need more guidance, for instance from their caregivers, in determining which websites are reliable, understandable and applicable to their situation. One of the clearest associations with the use of an information source is it's perceived reliability [13], but it is extremely difficult for older patients to determine whether a website is reliable or not. Moreover, a lot of information on the Internet is written at a higher reading level than the average Internet user has, and many websites are not user-friendly for older people. Although there are existing guidelines to enhance the usability of websites for older people, these are hardly followed. As a result, many websites are twice as hard to use for older than for younger people [39]. It is recommended to pay more attention to the development of websites that are understandable for older people. In addition, the use of patient portals or personal websites, tailored to the individual patient, might add to the usefulness of the Internet for older patients, particularly those with a less monitoring coping style.

To conclude, in line with our assumptions, some factors in the model (i.e., more information preferences and higher fulfilled information and communication needs) are more related to Internet usage in younger patients than in older patients. For cancer-related stress reactions, we assumed that they would play a larger role in the younger group than in the older group, but it was not related to Internet usage in both groups. In the older group only a monitoring coping style, being male and a high education level were associated with Internet usage.

Acknowledgements. This research was carried out in collaboration with the University of Amsterdam, department of Medical Psychology (Dr. Ellen Smets). The study was commissioned by Public Eyes and supported by an unrestricted grant from AMGEN and the Dutch Cancer Society.

References

1. American Cancer Society,
   http://www.cancer.org/acs/groups/content/
   @epidemiologysurv-eilance/documents/
   document/acspc-031941.pdf

2. Statistics Netherlands. Doodsoorzaken; Korte Lijst (Belangrijke Doodsoorzaken), Leeftijd, Geslacht (Causes of Mortality; Short List (Important Causes of Mortality), Age, Gender), http://statline.cbs.nl/StatWeb/publication/ ?VW=T&DM=SLNL&PA=7052_95&LA=NL

3. Signaleringscommissie Kanker van KWF Kankerbestrijding (Signaling Committee Cancer of the Dutch Cancer Society). Kanker in Nederland tot 2020. Trends en Prognoses (Cancer in the Netherlands until 2020. Trends and Prognoses). KWF Kankerbestrijding, Amsterdam (2011)

4. Arora, N.K., Johnson, P., Gustafson, D.H., McTavish, F., Hawkins, R.P., Pingree, S.: Barriers to Information Access, Perceived Health Competence, and Psychological Health Outcomes: Test of a Mediation Model in a Breast Cancer Sample. Patient Education and Counseling 47, 37–46 (2002)

5. Eysenbach, G.: CONSORT-EHEALTH: Improving and Standardizing Evaluation Reports of Web-Based and Mobile Health Interventions. Journal of Medical Internet Research 13 (2011)

6. Statistics Netherlands. ICT Gebruik van Personen naar Persoonskenmerken (ICT Use by Persons Subject to Personal Characteristics), http://statline.cbs.nl/StatWeb/publication/ ?VW=T&DM=SLNL&PA=71098NED&D1=33-133&D2=0,13&D3=a&HD=111219- 1122&HDR=G1,G2&STB=T

7. Lustria, M.L., Cortese, J., Noar, S.M., Glueckauf, R.L.: Computer-Tailored Health Interventions Delivered over the Web: Review and Analysis of Key Components. Patient Education and Counseling 74, 156–173 (2009)

8. KWF Kankerbestrijding (Dutch Cancer Society), http://www.kwf.nl

9. Katz, E., Gurcvitch, M., Haas, H.: On the Usc of thc Mass Media for Important Things. American Sociological Review 38, 164–181 (1973)

10. Perse, E.M., Courtright, J.A.: Normative Images of Communication Media: Mass and Interpersonal Channels in the New Media Environment. Human Communication Research 19, 485–503 (1993)

11. Rubin, A.M.: Uses, Gratifications, and Media Effects Research. In: Bryant, J., Zillman, D. (eds.) Perspectives on Media Effects, pp. 281–301. Lawrence Erlbaum Associates, Hillsdale (1986)

12. Tan, A.S.: Mass Communication Theories and Research, 2nd edn. John Wiley, New York (1985)

13. Muusses, L.D., van Weert, J.C.M., van Dulmen, S., Jansen, J.: Chemotherapy and Information Seeking Behavior: Characteristics of Patients Using Mass-Media Information Sources. Psycho-Oncology 21, 993–1002 (2012)

14. Mor, V., Allen, S., Malin, M.: The Psychosocial Impact of Cancer on Older Versus Younger Patients and Their Families. Cancer 74(S7), 2118–2127 (1994)

15. Jansen, J., Van Weert, J.C.M., Van Dulmen, A.M., Heeren, T.J., Bensing, J.M.: Patient Education about Treatment in Cancer Care. An Overview of the Literature on Older Patients' Needs. Cancer Nursing 30, 251–260 (2007)

16. Ong, L.M.L., Visser, M.R.M., Van Zuuren, F.J., Rietbroek, R.C., Lammes, F.B., De Haes, J.C.J.M.: Cancer Patients' Coping Styles and Doctor-Patient Communication. Psycho-Oncology 8, 155–166 (1999)

17. Miller, S.M.: Monitoring Versus Blunting Styles of Coping With Cancer Influence the Information Patients Want and Need about their Disease. Implications for Cancer Screening and Management. Cancer 76, 167–177 (1995)

18. Van Koerten, C., Feytens, M., Jansen, J., van Dulmen, S., van Weert, J.C.M.: Communicatiebehoeften van Patiënten met Kanker bij Aanvang van een Behandeling met Chemotherapie. Een Onderzoek naar de Rol van Curatief of Palliatief Behandeldoel, Leeftijd en Geslacht (Communication Needs of Cancer Patients Starting with Chemotherapy. A Study into the Role of Curative or Palliative Treatment Goal, Age and Gender). Verpleegkunde. Nederlands-Vlaams Wetenschappelijk Tijdschrift voor Verpleegkundigen 26, 4–12 (2011)
19. Galobardes, B., Shaw, M., Lawlor, D.A., Lych, J., Davey Smith, G.: Indicators of Socioeconomic Position (Part 1). J. of Epidemiology & Community 6, 7–12 (2006)
20. Nederlandse Kankerregistratie beheerd door IKNL (Dutch Cancer Database managed by IKNL)
21. De Vries, M., Van Weert, J.C.M., Jansen, J., Lemmens, V.E.P.P., Maas, H.A.A.M.: Step by Step. The Need to Develop a Clinical Pathway for Older Cancer Patients. European Journal of Cancer 43(15), 2170–2178 (2007)
22. Benjamin, A.E., Matthias, R.E.: Age, Consumer Direction, and Outcomes of Supportive Services at Home. The Gerontologist 5, 632–642 (2001)
23. Silliman, R.A., Troyan, S.L., Guadagnoli, E., Kaplan, S.H., Greenfield, S.: The Impact of Age, Marital Status, and Physician-Patient Interactions on the Care of Older Women with Breast Carcinoma. Cancer 80, 1326–1334 (1997)
24. Bolle, S., Muusses, L.D., Smets, E.M., Loos, E.F., van Weert, J.C.M.: Chemotherapie, Wat Weet u Ervan? Een Onderzoek naar de Publieke Kennis, Perceptie van Bijwerkingen, Informatiebehoeften en het Gebruik van Informatiebronnen met Betrekking tot Chemotherapie (Chemotherapy, What Do You Know About IT? A Study into Public Knowledge, Perception of Side Effects, Information Needs and Information Source Usage). Amsterdam School of Communication Research/ASCoR. Universiteit van Amsterdam, Amsterdam (2012)
25. Aaronson, N.K., Ahmedzai, S., Bergman, B., Bullinger, M., Cull, A., Duez, N.J., et al.: The European Organization for Research and Treatment of Cancer QL-C30: A Quality-of-Life Instrument for Use in International Clinical Trials in Oncology. Journal of the National Cancer Institute 85, 365–376 (1993)
26. Pieterse, A., Van Dulmen, S., Ausems, M., Schoemaker, A., Beemer, F., Bensing, J.M.: QUOTE-Geneca: Development of a Counselee-Centered Instrument to Measure Needs and Preferences in Genetic Counseling for Hereditary Cancer. Psycho-Oncology 14, 361–375 (2005)
27. Van der Ploeg, E., Mooren, T.T.M., Kleber, R.J., Van der Velden, P.G., Brom, D.: Construct Validation of the Dutch Version of the Impact of Event Scale. Psychological Assessment 16, 16–26 (2004)
28. Miller, S.M.: Monitoring and Blunting: Validation of a Questionnaire to Assess Styles of Information under Threat. Journal of Personality and Social Psychology 52, 345–353 (1987)
29. Van Zuren, F.J., De Groot, K.I., Mulder, N.L., Muris, P.: Coping with Medical Threat: an Evaluation of the Threatening Medical Situations Inventory (TMSI). Personality and Individual Differences 21, 16–26 (1996)
30. Thomas, R., Kaminski, E., Stanton, E., Williams, M.: Measuring Information Strategies in Oncology. Developing an Information Satisfaction Questionnaire. European Journal of Cancer Care 13, 65–70 (2004)
31. Van Weert, J.C.M., Jansen, J., De Bruijn, G.J., Noordman, J., Van Dulmen, S., Bensing, J.M.: QUOTEchemo: A Patient-Centered Instrument to Measure Quality of Communication Preceding Chemotherapy Treatment Through the Patients' Eyes. European Journal of Cancer 45(17), 2967–2976 (2009)

32. Rutten, H.J.T., den Dulk, M., Lemmens, V.E.P.P., van de Velde, C.J.H., Marijnen, C.A.M.: Controversies of Total Mesorectal Excision for Rectal Cancer in Elderly Patients. The Lancet Oncology 8, 494–501 (2008)
33. Janssen-Heijnen, M.L.G., Smulders, S., Lemmens, V.E.E.P., Smeenk, F.W.J.M., van Geffen, H.J.A.A., Coebergh, J.W.W.: Effect of Comorbidity on the Treatment and Prognosis of Elderly Patients with Non-Small Cell Lung Cancer. Thorax 59, 602–607 (2004)
34. Bonfadelli, H.: The Internet and Knowledge Gaps A Theoretical and Empirical Investigation. European Journal of Communication 17, 65–84 (2002)
35. Hoffman, D.L., Novak, T.P.: Bridging the digital divide: The impact of race on computer access and Internet use. U.S. Department of Education. Office of Educational Research and Improvement (1998)
36. Oosterveer, D.: Mannen, Jongeren en Hoogopgeleiden Halen Meer Economisch Nut uit Internet (Men, Youngsters and Highly Educated People Get More Economic Benefit from the Internet) (2012),
http://www.marketingfacts.nl/berichten/
mannen-jongeren-en-hoogopgeleiden-halen-meer-economisch-nut-
uit-internet
37. Petty, R.E., Cacioppo, J.T.: The Elaboration Likelihood Model of Persuasion. In: Berkowitz, L. (ed.) Advances in Experimental Social Psychology, pp. 123–205. Academic Press, New York (1986)
38. Sparks, L., Turner, M.M.: The Impact of Cognitive and Emotive Communication Barriers on Older Adult Message Processing of Cancer-Related Health Information: New Directions for Research. In: Sparks, L., O'Hair, H., Kreps, G. (eds.) Cancer, Communication and Aging, pp. 17–47. Hampton Press, Inc., New York (2008)
39. Pernice, K., Nielsen, J.: Web Usability for Senior Citizens: Design Guidelines Based on Usability Studies with People Age 65 and Older. Nielsen Norman Group, Fremont (2002)

Digital Technology to Supercharge Patient-Provider Relationships

Kathryn Joleen VanOsdol

Indiana University Purdue University at Indianapolis, USA
Kathryn_jovan@hotmail.com

Abstract. Recent initiatives promoting the efficiency and effectiveness of the U.S. health care system are grounded in strengthening the relationship between the primary care provider and the patient. Examples of these include Patient Centered Medical Home (PCMH), Medicare Shared Savings Accountable Care Organizations (MSSP ACOs), and Meaningful Use (MU). These incentivized programs re-energize the link between providers and consumers and recognize the use of Health Information Technology (HIT) as key to the success of the models. The objective of this paper is to explore innovative digital processes that supercharge patient-provider relationships by: Health Information Integration; interactive patient surveys, Remote Monitoring Systems (RMS), and the Patient Health Record (PHR); and Data Prioritization through the consolidation and stratification of health information.

Keywords: Accountable Care Organization, Digital, Efficiency, Engagement, Meaningful Use, Medical Home, Patient Centered, Primary Care, Technology.

1 Introduction: The Communication Chasm

In the article entitled "When a Patient Asks, 'Why Won't Anybody Just Talk to Me?'" author Alicair Peltonen recounts her personal experiences with health care communication challenges: "Again and again over the course of months, I felt too intimidated to ask the questions echoing in my mind. Nor did my health care team initiate the conversations I desperately needed."[1] She quotes Harvard School of Public Health professor and former pediatric surgeon, Lucian Leape, as stating that poor patient-doctor communication is "probably the single greatest source of missed information that leads to erroneous treatment, treatment not followed properly, and unnecessary anxiety...an informed patient, who is consulted on their own care, makes different decisions than a passive patient..." Leape, who helped author the 1999 report by the Institute of Medicine that attributed the leading cause of medical mistakes to the fragmented health care system, broadens the scope of accountability with this statement: "Nobody is

---

[1] Peltonen A. (2013) "When A Patient Asks, 'Why Won't Anybody Just Talk To Me?'
   Obtained from:
   http://commonhealth.wbur.org/2013/09/
   patient-doctor-conversation

C. Stephanidis and M. Antona (Eds.): UAHCI/HCII 2014, Part III, LNCS 8515, pp. 415–424, 2014.
© Springer International Publishing Switzerland 2014

responsible for coordinating care...That's the dirty little secret about health care."[2] A 2009 review published in the journal *Medical Care* further demonstrated that "...the odds of patient adherence are 2.16 times higher if a physician communicates effectively."[3] Correspondingly, studies have shown that patient-physician communication barriers are cited in 40% of malpractice suits and "...the dominant theme in these studies' findings was a breakdown in the patient-physician relationship, most often manifested as unsatisfactory patient-physician communication..." [4,5]

Primary care, due to the comprehensive scope it comprises, is frequently a victim of the communication chasm. The American Academy of Family Physicians defines primary care with the following: "Primary care includes health promotion, disease prevention, health maintenance, counseling, patient education, diagnosis and treatment of acute and chronic illnesses in a variety of health care settings (e.g., office, inpatient, critical care, long-term care, home care, day care, etc.)."[6]

Imagine a primary care world where an innovative clinical specialist proposes that their expertise and qualifications will increase patient satisfaction, improve quality of care, and decrease cost. Their aptitude includes assessing patients' support systems, self-care challenges, and tracking patterns of health behaviors. The team member candidate is an expert in motivational interviewing, patient engagement and goal setting, and they perform real-time patient screening and risk assessments that impact clinical decision making at the point of care. The question remains: Are health systems prepared to empower and revitalize patient-provider relationships by employing Technology as the newest member of the primary care team? This presentation examines models and concepts for innovative digital health tools that supercharge the link between providers and patients in the primary care setting.

2   Background: Incentive versus Reality

Initiatives are underway in the U.S. to improve the efficiency and effectiveness of the health care system by promoting the relationship between the primary care provider and the patient. Examples of this include Patient Centered Medical Home (PCMH), Medicare Shared Savings Accountable Care Organizations (MSSP ACOs), and

---

[2] Rabin, R. C. (2013) "Health Care's 'Dirty Little Secret': No One May Be Coordinating Care."
Obtained from: http://www.kaiserhealthnews.org/stories/2013/april/30/coordination-of-care.aspx

[3] Zolnierek, K. B. and M. R. Dimatteo (2009). "Physician communication and patient adherence to treatment: a meta-analysis." Med Care 47(8): 826-834.

[4] Huntington, B. and N. Kuhn (2003). "Communication gaffes: a root cause of malpractice claims." Proc (Bayl Univ Med Cent) 16(2): 157-161; discussion 161.

[5] Moore, P. J., et al. (2000). "Medical malpractice: the effect of doctor-patient relations on medical patient perceptions and malpractice intentions." West J Med 173(4): 244-250.

[6] American Academy of Family Physicians. Policies. Primary Care. Definition #1-Primary Care
Obtained from:
http://www.aafp.org/about/policies/all/primary-care.html

Meaningful Use (MU). These incentivized programs re-energize the link between providers and consumers and recognize the use of Health Information Technology (HIT) as key to the success of these models. PCMH is a comprehensive model of care that promotes the relationship of the patient with their primary care team, recognizing that the coordinated management of care is best achieved by engaging patients with their primary care physicians.[7]   Similarly, the MSSP ACO allows that health systems may share in savings for their successful management of a specified population of patients, with the attribution of the beneficiaries determined by the plurality of primary care services, thus focusing the management of care back to the patient and primary care provider relationship.[8]   Likewise, MU includes incentive payments for the use of electronic health information to: engage patients and families in self-care; promote patient-controlled data; and increase patient access to self-management tools for goal setting and behavior change.[9]   These initiatives have the potential to become innovative translators of care between the provider and the consumer.

Translation of care is needed, as health information communication challenges contribute to poor quality outcomes, preventable high-cost utilization, decreased patient and provider satisfaction, and an increase in medical errors.[10]   These are due to things such as deficient data at the point of care, inefficient electronic health record processes, and lack of interoperability among systems.[11]   On a patient-provider interaction level, these are further complicated by the lack of standardized shared decision making and patient engagement strategies.[12]   Compounding these challenges is the shortage of physicians' time. Yarnall, et al (2009) state the following, "On the basis of recommendations from national clinical care guidelines for preventive services and chronic disease management, and including the time needed for acute concerns, sufficiently addressing the needs of a standard patient panel of 2,500 would require 21.7 hours per day."[13]

---

[7] Ewing, M. (2013). "The patient-centered medical home solution to the cost-quality conuddrum." J Healthc Manag 58(4): 258-266.

[8] McWilliams, J. M., et al. (2013). "Delivery system integration and health care spending and quality for Medicare beneficiaries." JAMA Intern Med 173(15): 1447-1456.

[9] Krist, A. H., et al. (2014). "Electronic health record functionality needed to better support primary care." J Am Med Inform Assoc. doi: 10.1136/amiajnl-2013-002229. [Epub ahead of print]

[10] Carnicero, J. and D. Rojas (2010). "Lessons Learned from Implementation of Information and Communication Technologies in Spain's Healthcare Services: Issues and Opportunities." Appl Clin Inform 1(4): 363-376.

[11] Kortteisto, T., et al. (2012). "Clinical decision support must be useful, functional is not enough: a qualitative study of computer-based clinical decision support in primary care." BMC Health Serv Res 12: 349.

[12] Gordon, J. E., et al. (2014). "Delivering value: provider efforts to improve the quality and reduce the cost of health care." Annu Rev Med 65: 447-458.

[13] Yarnall KSH, Østbye T, Krause KM, Pollak KI, Gradison M, Michener JL. Family physicians as team leaders: "time" to share the care. Prev Chronic Dis 2009;6(2):A59. http://www.cdc.gov/pcd/issues/2009/apr/08_0023.htm. Accessed [January 11, 2014].

Escalating the scope of necessity for linking providers and consumers are two significant events: the exponential increase in the number of expected patients in a physician's practice panel over the course of the next ten years, and an increase in the acuity level of the patients in a physician's panel.[14]   This will be due to a combination of the aging U.S. population, and an imminent increase in the number of insured patients by the expansion provided by the Affordable Care Act (ACA). This will increase the number of patients who are eligible to enroll in Medicaid by approximately 13 million persons by 2023, which is over half of the anticipated 25 million patients to obtain insurance due to the ACA.[15]

The Association of American Medical Colleges (AAMC) states the following: "According to AAMC estimates, the United States faces a shortage of more than 91,500 physicians by 2020- a number that is expected to grow to more than 130,600 by 2025."[16] A recent study published in *Health Affairs* made the following observations related to mitigating the impending provider shortages by the use of Health Information Technology: "We estimate that if health IT were fully implemented in 30 percent of community-based physicians' offices, the demand for physicians would be reduced by about 4–9 percent. Delegation of care to nurse practitioners and physician assistants supported by health IT could reduce the future demand for physicians by 4–7 percent. Similarly, IT-supported delegation from specialist physicians to generalists could reduce the demand for specialists by 2–5 percent. The use of health IT could also help address regional shortages of physicians by potentially enabling 12 percent of care to be delivered remotely or asynchronously. These estimated impacts could more than double if comprehensive health IT systems were adopted by 70 percent of US ambulatory care delivery settings."[17]

3   The Challenge: Organize and Prioritize

What digital applications do health systems, physicians, and patients require to improve efficiency and effectiveness? It is clear that health systems desire to channel patients back to primary care in order to decrease unnecessary high-cost utilization,

---

[14] Petterson, S. M., et al. (2012). "Projecting US primary care physician workforce needs: 2010-2025." Ann Fam Med 10(6): 503-509.

[15] CBO's May 2013 Estimate of the Effects of the Affordable Care Act on Health Insurance Coverage. Obtained from:
http://www.cbo.gov/sites/default/files/cbofiles/attachments/
44190_EffectsAffordableCareActHealthInsuranceCoverage_2.pdf

[16] Association of American Medical Colleges. GME Funding: How to Fix the Doctor Shortage. Projected Supply and Demand, Physicians, 2008-2020. Obtained from:
https://www.aamc.org/advocacy/campaigns_and_coalitions/
fixdocshortage/

[17] The Impact of Health Information Technology and e-Health on the Future Demand for Physician Services. Weiner, Jonathan P., Yeh, Susan, Blumenthal, David.
doi: 10.1377/hlthaff.2013.0680 *Health Aff November 2013 vol. 32 no. 11 1998-2004*

and to improve the quality of preventive and chronic care.[18]   Likewise, primary care providers, in a time-constrained environment, desire to comprehensively address acute, preventive, chronic, and psychosocial care needs through technological processes that do not further contribute to stress and burnout.[19]   In regard to patients, the International Journal of Medical Informatics explored the impact of HIT on patient satisfaction: "Despite being a promising tool to increase patient satisfaction, health information technologies did not show a clear evidence of positive impact on patient satisfaction in this literature review."[20] How then can these seemingly off course trajectories become realigned to obtain mutually beneficial results?

The proposal of this paper is that HIT innovations to link providers and consumers include two complementing areas of focus: Health Information Integration and Data Prioritization.   It is also the premise of this presentation that data integration without prioritization hinders the efficiency and effectiveness of health systems.   Similarly, prioritization for quality improvement is inadequate without comprehensive data integration.   In terms of integration, the following three tools are considered: the use of interactive patient surveys and questionnaires to obtain real-time actionable health information, the incorporation of Remote Monitoring Systems (RMS) to expand the point of care beyond the clinical setting, and leveraging a Patient Health Record (PHR) for patient engagement.   In terms of Prioritization, this includes the two main concepts of: the consolidation of patient health information from across the continuum of care, and the categorization and organization of this health information.   It is proposed that the combined efforts of Health Information Integration and Data Prioritization will have the greatest compounding effects in efficiently linking providers and consumers.

4   Supercharge Step One: Engaged Patients, Efficient Providers

This presentation suggests that an obvious use of patient surveys has traditionally been overlooked; engaging patients to obtain as much relevant and actionable information as possible to inform providers at the point of care.   Many studies have been completed for patients' use of publicly reported data on provider performance, as well as the use of performance reports by providers for quality improvement of technical and health outcomes.[21]   The most common uses of patient survey results include process improvement efforts for appointment wait times, timely triage of phone calls,

---

[18] Basu, J., et al. (2014). "The Small Area Predictors of Ambulatory Care Sensitive Hospitalizations: A Comparison of Changes over Time." Soc Work Public Health 29(2): 176-188.

[19] Babbott, S., et al. (2014). "Electronic medical records and physician stress in primary care: results from the MEMO Study." J Am Med Inform Assoc 21(e1): e100-106.

[20] Rozenblum, R., et al. (2013). "The impact of medical informatics on patient satisfaction: a USA-based literature review." Int J Med Inform 82(3): 141-158.

[21] Safran DG, Karp M, Coltin K, et al. Measuring patients' experiences with individual primary care physicians: results of a statewide demonstration project. J Gen Intern Med. 2006;21(1):13–21.

and customer service.[22]   Research on the use of patient surveys has also found the following: "We identified potentially important correlations between clinical performance and patient reports of clinical interactions and integration of care, reinforcing the need to maintain a focus on patient experiences as part of an overall program to improve chronic disease care."[23]

An innovative digital survey product bridging this gap is Tonic Health, cofounded by Sterling Lanier of Palo Alto, California. In a 2012 interview with *Healthcare IT News*, Mr. Lanier offered the following logical advice in regard to the average ten minute physician visit: "Instead of spending six minutes trying to figure out what's wrong, then four minutes on treatments, why not use the data to spend nine minutes talking about the solution?"[24]   Tonic Health is an interactive and engaging digital patient survey tool, with behind the scenes cloud-based reporting features, and the ability to create and customize surveys that can include intuitive skip logic algorithms based on patient responses and medical history. The survey platform can be deployed on the iPad in the clinic, via a laptop in a patient's home, or via a Smartphone on the go. Tonic's real-time patient screening and on the spot risk scoring capabilities not only optimize care opportunities, but Tonic can also dynamically serve up personalized patient education in the form of videos or articles based on the results of each screening (e.g. patients who screen in as high risk for diabetes may see one type of video, while those who screen in as low risk see another). The result is clear: dramatically higher completion rates of patients willing to offer more information than per traditional paper-based questionnaires, improved accuracy of data collection, labor and workflow efficiencies, significant savings in the form of preventative care, and increased patient satisfaction due to the Disney-like experience provided by the questionnaire platform. Also featured in the February, 2014 edition of *Inc.* magazine in an article entitled "The Startups Saving Healthcare", the author surmises the following: "Tonic provides a partial solution to one of the most vexing challenges in all of the multitrillion-dollar health care industry: How do you get patients to provide the information that health care providers desperately need, and rarely get, in order to improve care while cutting costs?"[25]

5   Supercharge Step Two: Health at Home

An exponentially growing opportunity to link providers and consumers using digital technology is that of Remote Monitoring Systems (RMS). Although more studies

---

[22] Friedberg, M. W., et al. (2011). "Physician groups' use of data from patient experience surveys." J Gen Intern Med 26(5): 498-504.

[23] Sequist, T. D., et al. (2012). "Measuring chronic care delivery: patient experiences and clinical performance." Int J Qual Health Care 24(3): 206-213.

[24] Harris, B. (2012). "3 Ways Tech Can Help Patient Engagement." Healthcare IT News. Obtained from: http://www.healthcareitnews.com/news/ 3-ways-technology-can-facilitate-patient-engagement?page=1

[25] Freedman, D. (2014). "The Startups Saving Health Care." Inc. Obtained from: http://www.inc.com/magazine/201402/david-freedman/ obamacare-health-technology-startups.html

are warranted for this newly emerging technology, recent research has found, "...the use of an RMS is feasible and effective in promoting activation, self-care, and QOL [Quality of Life]."[26]   In their intriguing article in *The American Journal of Medicine* summarizing mobile health in the U.S., the authors of "Telemedicine, Telehealth, and Mobile Health Applications That Work: Opportunities and Barriers" state the following: "Mobile health is currently undergoing explosive growth and could be a disruptive innovation that will change the face of healthcare in the future."[27]   An example of a progressive RMS company is Vivify Health based in Plano, Texas. In a recent mHIMSS article entitled "Mobile Technology; Revolutionizing Healthcare," a Vivify pilot at Christus Health, Texas was featured. Preliminary results showed, "A data review completed for 44 patients who completed the RPMS [Remote Patient Monitoring System] program showed a ROI [Return on Investment] of $2.44" and "In addition to the positive ROI, RPMS patients' utilization of St. Michael Health System decreased – prior to enrollment in the RPMS program, these 44 patients had an average cost of care of $12,937 compared to $1,231 post- RPMS program enrollment."[28] The Vivify Health RPMS is a cloud based application that harnesses evidence based care plans to create customized patient questionnaires that upload patient responses to a care management platform. It also offers an input format for patient recorded biometric data. This supports patient management opportunities such as medication reminders, customizable alerts, and social network integration. Proliferation of RMS is likely to continue, as supported by, "We speculate that implementation of patient-centered medical homes (PCMH) and emergence of accountable care organizations (ACOs) may reduce current barriers to RMT [Remote Monitoring Technology] use in primary care by providing incentives to collaborate and proactively manage patient care."[29]

6   Supercharge Step Three: Stop Boredom, Save Lives

The third link of Health Information Integration is that of Patient Health Records (PHRs). A PHR is "a digital Web-based collection of a patient's medical history in which copies of medical records, reports about diagnosed medical conditions, medications, vital signs, immunizations, laboratory results, and personal characteristics like

---

[26] Evangelista, L. S., et al. (2013). "Examining the Effects of Remote Monitoring Systems on Activation, Self-care, and Quality of Life in Older Patients With Chronic Heart Failure." J Cardiovasc Nurs.

[27] Weinstein, R. S., et al. (2013). "Telemedicine, Telehealth, and Mobile Health Applications That Work: Opportunities and Barriers." Am J Med.

[28] Clifton S, Collins DA, Fanberg H, Ford E, Webster L. (2013) "Mobile Technology; Revolutionizing Healthcare"   Obtained from:
http://himss.files.cms-plus.com/FileDownloads/
2013_Christus%20Health_mHealth%20Readmission%20Pilot%209-13-
13_v6.pdf

[29] Davis, M. M., et al. (2014). "A qualitative study of rural primary care clinician views on remote monitoring technologies." J Rural Health 30(1): 69-78.

age and weight are stored."[30]   The use of PHRs has recently been scrutinized due to the demise of ventures such as Google Health. Although formal research is lacking pertaining to the failure of Google Health, it is speculated that contributing factors were: requiring patients to enter their own data, an inability to inform or entertain users, and a lack of enabling social communication.[31] However, information is emerging to support the use of PHRs, such as Kaiser Permanente's My Health Manager, in which "Use of the system was associated with up to 10 percent fewer visits to the physician and a significant reduction in telephone calls. A survey of members who were actively using this technology showed that most perceived it as useful and easy to use."[32]

One hypothesis for improving the success of PHRs is that broadening the functionality of the PHR by relationships with vendors of health gaming apps and social networking will result in improved patient engagement and behaviour change. An example of this is found with Dossia, a PHR that makes health information actionable by combining it into a single platform that integrates games, social dynamics, incentives, and messaging in a customizable format. As quoted in a recent interview with Forbes magazine, David Goldsmith, Executive Director of the Dossia Consortium states, "We know now that unlocking the real value of PHR's resides in our ability to use data to engage the right patient at the right time."[33]

In the primary care setting, methods need to be further developed to incorporate PHRs into the care continuum. One study shows: "Feedback received from our provider panel included a recommendation to better integrate data from the…central data repository with PHR data to give a more complete view of individual patient records and a dashboard view of their patient panels for use in the provider's clinical workflow."[34] The value of integrating survey, RMS, and PHR data with a centralized data repository is that it minimizes disruptions in clinical workflow and allows for corresponding Data Prioritization.

---

[30] Halamka John D, Mandl Kenneth D, Tang Paul C. Early experiences with personal health records. J Am Med Inform Assoc. 2008;15(1):1–7. doi: 10.1197/jamia.M2562.
http://www.pubmedcentral.nih.gov.proxy.medlib.iupui.edu/
articlerender.fcgi?tool=pubmed&pubmedid=17947615.M2562
[PMC free article] [PubMed] [Cross Ref]

[31] Lohr S. (2011). "Google to End Health Records Service After it Fails to Attract Users." Obtained from: http://www.nytimes.com/2011/06/25/technology/25health.html?_r=0

[32] McDonald K. (2012) "Why Did Google Health Fail?" Obtained from:
http://www.pulseitmagazine.com.au/index.php?option=com_conten
t&view=article&id=954:feature-why-did-google-health-
fail&catid=16:australian-ehealth&Itemid=327

[33] Nosta J. (2013) "For Dossia, Digital Health Isn't Just Personal Anymore." Obtained from: http://www.forbes.com/sites/johnnosta/2013/11/27/for-dossia-digital-health-isnt-just-personal-anymore

[34] Do, N. V., et al. (2011). "The military health system's personal health record pilot with Microsoft HealthVault and Google Health." J Am Med Inform Assoc 18(2): 118-124.

7   Supercharge Step Four: Diagnose the Data

Data Prioritization includes two critical elements: the consolidation of patient health information from across the continuum of care into a dashboard environment that can be categorized and sorted, and the application of risk scoring and prioritization tools. In discussing these two components, the potential exists to accomplish both goals while incurring a small IT footprint.   An example of this is the innovative menu of products of the company Clinigence of Atlanta, Georgia.   Clinigence, a Software as a Service (SAAS) company, found its niche by facilitating the achievement of Physician Quality Reporting System (PQRS) and MU reporting goals. Clinigence expanded these specialized services to ACOs by offering a product that maps data from multiple EMRs and formats the information into a cloud-based dashboard that provides performance outcome measurements for the ACO as an entity, per practice, per physician, and drills down to patient-level health information .[35]   The power of the application is in its ability to link data previously "held captive" in disparate server-based legacy systems to the cloud-based environment, where it creates dashboards that are useful for data analysis by administrators, physicians, case managers, health coaches, and health educators.   The Clinigence platform greatly expands the strategies of patient and population health managers by automating the application of benchmarks to things such as real-time biometric data, medication refill patterns, and overall care plan adherence.   Consider the contrast between the traditional use of claims and demographic data to identify high risk patients, with a dashboard that contains these, as well as actionable information such as referral adherence, utilization patterns, psycho-social needs, patient survey responses, and PHR and RMS summaries.   The result of the combined strength of these digital tools is the prioritization of actionable data that defines the clinician's focus, strengthens the link between providers and consumers, and supercharges patient-provider relationships.

8   Conclusion: The Consumer Connection

The epiphany for U.S. health care systems will be that the standalone EMR will not improve efficiency, decrease costs, and increase provider and patient satisfaction. The integration of adjunct digital platforms has the potential to engage patients, prioritize plans of care, and strengthen the link between patients and providers. In representation of this model, consider the use case of Ms. Smith; a 45-year-old patient of Dr. Wise.   Ms. Smith takes one medication due to a diagnosis of high blood pressure, which is complicated by her obesity.   Her goals include a low salt diet and walking 15 minutes a day, three times a week.   She records her weight, blood pressure, and medication administration schedule using an RMS that automatically

---

[35] "The Importance of Using Data to Improve Care Quality and Lower Costs." (2013). Obtained from: http://www.clinigence.com/news-blog/2014/1/12/the-importance-of-using-data-to-improve-care-quality-and-lower-costs

uploads the readings to a PHR.   Via the PHR, she joined a social network that connected Ms. Smith to others with goals of exercising and making dietary changes, and she downloaded a competitive gaming app that promotes accountability among members of the network. At her 6-month appointment with Dr. Wise, the receptionist who hands her an iPad greets Ms. Smith. Check-in at the doctor's office has been much more enjoyable since the paper survey was replaced with a colorful and interactive digital questionnaire that is based on Ms. Smith's personalized goals and health status.   At the conclusion of the questionnaire an encouraging message congratulates Ms. Smith on achieving her goal of walking three times per week, and that she lost five pounds since her appointment six months ago. The survey tool asks Ms. Smith if she would like to watch a short video on a low salt diet while she is in the waiting room. Ms. Smith watches a two-minute video clip, and at its completion answers a few questions to ascertain her understanding. Behind the scenes, Dr. Wise reviews a dashboard that includes Ms. Smith's RMS values, the progress she is making toward achievement of her goals, any alerts related to the responses Ms. Smith documented on the survey, and a summary of gaps in her chronic or preventive care. A priority of care document is generated for use by the primary care team, which now has nine of the ten minutes of the average primary care appointment remaining to reinforce the most vital link: Ms. Smith.

Accessible Smart
and Assistive Environments

Probabilistic Intentionality Prediction for Target Selection Based on Partial Cursor Tracks

Bashar I. Ahmad[1], Patrick M. Langdon[2], Pete Bunch[1], and Simon J. Godsill[1]

[1] Signal Processing and Communications Laboratory
[2] Engineering Design Centre
Department of Engineering, University of Cambridge, UK
{bia23,pml24,pb404,sjg30}@cam.ac.uk

Abstract. Pointing tasks, for example to select an object in an interface, constitute a significant part of human-computer interactions. This motivated several studies into techniques that facilitate the pointing task and improve its accuracy. In this paper, we introduce a number of intentionality prediction algorithms to determine the intended target *a priori* from partial cursor tracks. They yield notable reductions in the pointing time, aid effective selection assistance routines and enhance the overall pointing accuracy. A number of benchmark prediction models are also restated within a statistical framework and their probabilistic interpretation is utilised to calculate their corresponding outcomes. The relative performance of all considered predictors is assessed for point-click task data sets pertaining to both able-bodied and impaired users. Bayesian adaptive filtering is deployed to smooth highly perturbed mouse cursor tracks that are typically produced by motor impaired users undertaking a pointing task.

Keywords: cursor movement, target assistance, intentionality prediction, Bayesian inference.

1 Introduction

With the proliferation of technological devices and their wide use in work as well as domestic environments, Human-Computer Interaction (HCI) became an integral part of modern life. Pointing at a target is a fundamental task in graphical user interfaces aimed at selecting buttons, menus, etc. Its reliability and accuracy is of a key importance for the design of effective user interfaces. This triggered an immense interest in techniques that facilitate the pointing task by reducing the cursor pointing time and improving its accuracy [1-14]. The problem is particularly challenging given the increasingly diverse population of users, for example motion impaired or able-bodied users, elderly or young users and expert or non-expert users. Accordingly, some users can find the pointing task difficult or even overwhelming at times, especially the motor impaired. In this paper, we introduce probabilistic intentionality predicators to determine in advance the intended target from partial cursor movements in a 2-D set up. The sought objective is to ease and expedite the target selection process on a computer display.

C. Stephanidis and M. Antona (Eds.): UAHCI/HCII 2014, Part III, LNCS 8515, pp. 427–438, 2014.
© Springer International Publishing Switzerland 2014

The characteristics of the cursor movements have been examined in several studies and there is a long history of using Fitts's Law to describe the pointing operation on a computer display and build models of targeting in HCI [1,3,4]. It stipulates that the targeting difficulty is determined by the Index of Difficulty (IoD), which is calculated based on the size of the target and its distance from the starting location. Additionally, the pointing duration can be correlated with the difficulty index. More recently, Kopper *et al* reported that the angular width of a target and the angular amplitude of the movement to the target better model the IoD [5, 6]. An easier and quicker target selection process can be achieved by deploying algorithms that can increase the target size, use larger cursor activation regions, move targets closer to the cursor location, drag cursor to the nearest target [7, 8, 9], etc. However, interactive systems typically display several selectable targets in close proximity. Their layouts have an ever increasing complexity and the targets can have varying sizes and shapes. The inability of the previously mentioned pointing assistive algorithms to determine the intended target in such typical environments was highlighted in [7] as one of their key limitations. It is noted that any erroneous selection can demand additional cognitive as well as movements abilities which can be overwhelming for some users.

As an alternative, researchers have been exploring algorithms that reduce the pointing time and facilitate the selection process by dynamically predicting the intended target on the screen from partial pointing tracks. One of the first target prediction algorithms was proposed by Murata [10], it is dubbed the Bearing Angle (BA) technique. It is based on the premise that the selectable target with the minimum accumulative angle deviation with respect to the partial cursor trajectory is the intended target. It was noted in [11] that BA performs poorly if more than one target is present in the cursor direction of travel, particularly when the cursor is far from the cluster of nominal targets. Previous results on the kinematics of pointing tasks were applied in [11] to show that the cursor movement peak velocity and the distance to the target are linearly related; the destination is accordingly predicted using linear regression. A more complex motion kinematics technique was proposed in [12] assuming a minimum jerk law for pointing motion and fitting a quadratic function to partial trajectory to predict the endpoint(s). However, the cursor tracks for motor impaired users are highly nonlinear since they experience tremor, muscular spasms and weakness [13]. The trajectories exhibit a high level of perturbations with several stops and erratic jumps in rather random directions. This renders the regression-based approaches ineffective for motor impaired users.   In [14], a target predictor that is based on inverse optimal control within a machine learning framework was introduced. It leverages the maximum entropy variant to obtain the probabilities of the selectable target from a partial cursor trajectory via Bayes' rule. The inverse-optimal-control method has a high computational cost compared to the considered methods here. It requires a substantial parameter training routine, e.g. learning the state-action costs, and imposes stringent constraints on the trajectories dynamics.

In this paper, we evaluate a number of probabilistic intentionality prediction algorithms that are characterized by simplicity and low computational complexity. They deliver notable improvements to the pointing process by predicting the correct target from a small number of cursor movement points, for example 20% of the cursor track can suffice to make a correct prediction on the intended target. Bayesian state space filtering, namely Linear Kalman Filtering (LKF), is also deployed to smooth anomalous cursor trajectories. Thus, for users with motor impairments, the substantial achieved reduction in the difficulty level of the pointing task can render an otherwise inaccessible applications accessible. Even small improvements on the efficiency of the target selection process, e.g. saving few milliseconds, can have significant aggregate benefits given the prevalence of interactions through graphical user interfaces.

The rest of the paper is organized as follows. In Section 2, the tackled problem is formulated and the considered probabilistic prediction framework is outlined. In Section 3, a number of prediction models are described and their trade-offs highlighted. They are subsequently tested in Section 4 and conclusions are drawn in Section 5.

2   Problem Formulation and Adopted Approach

The tackled problem is predicting the intended target out of a set of N possible ones $\{B_i: i = 1,2,\dots,N\}$, from a partial cursor movement track $\mathbf{c}_{1:k}$. The latter is defined by $\mathbf{c}_{1:k} \triangleq \{\mathbf{c}_1, \mathbf{c}_2, \dots, \mathbf{c}_k\}$ where $\mathbf{c}_n = [x_{t_n} \quad y_{t_n}]^T$ denotes the recorded cursor coordinates along the x and y axes at time instant t_n; $\mathbf{x}^T$ is the transpose operation. Whereas, t_M is the total time duration it takes the user to select an item on the screen (for example starting at time $t_0 = 0$ for simplicity) and the full cursor track is $\mathbf{c}_{1:M}$. The locations of the selectable targets in the interface are known *a priori* where $\mathbf{b}_i = [b_{x_i} \quad b_{y_i}]^T$ is the position of the "i^{th}" button. We note that the term target and button are used interchangeably in the reminder of the paper.

The intentionality prediction problem is equivalent to calculating the maximum likelihood or Maximum a Posteriori (MAP) for the set of N possible selectable buttons from $\mathbf{c}_{1:k}$. It can be stated as

$$i^*(t_k) = \arg \max_{i=1,2,\dots,N} P(B_i|\mathbf{c}_{1:k}) \tag{1}$$

and $B_{i^*}(t_k)$ is the decided target at time t_k. Let t_C be the time instant at which the intentionality prediction algorithm reaches a correct decision, i.e. $B_{i^*}(t_k)$ is the correct target such that $t_C \leq t_M$.

Following (1) and using Bayes' rule the objective becomes calculating

$$P(B_i|\mathbf{c}_{1:k}) \propto P(B_i)P(\mathbf{c}_{1:k}|B_i) \tag{2}$$

for each of the selectable buttons. Assuming a uniform prior on all buttons, i.e. $P(B_i) = 1/N$ for $i = 1,2,\dots,N$, determining (2) and thereby (1) depends solely on the likelihood probability $P(\mathbf{c}_{1:k}|B_i)$. In a general set up, distinct or weighted probabilities can be allocated to each of the target buttons, e.g. based on the buttons layout or the user profile.

Algorithm 1. Probabilistic MAP Estimator

Input: A partial cursor trajectory at time $\{c_{k-L}, c_{k-L+1}, \ldots, c_k\}$
Output: Intended target $B_{i^*}(t_k)$
  1. Smooth the anomalies in the last logged cursor trajectory; $\hat{c}_k = \mathcal{F}(c_k)$
  2. Calculate the likelihood probability $P(\hat{c}_{k-L:k}|B_i)$ for $i = 1, 2, \ldots, N$ given a chosen prediction model.
  3. Determine the posterior distribution $P(B_i|\hat{c}_{k-L:k})$ of the N selectable targets.
  4. Make a MAP choice using (1).

In a given experiment, it might be desirable to utilise only the last L cursor positions, i.e. $c_{k-L:k} \triangleq \{c_{k-L}, c_{k-L+1}, \ldots, c_k\}$ and $k - L > 0$, to determine $B_{i^*}(t_k)$. A sliding time window is applied to the data and the window width is a design parameter. The adopted prediction approach at time instant t_k is depicted in Algorithm 1. It gives a generic framework encompassing the set of addressed predictors that model $P(c_{1:k}|B_i)$ in Section 3.

It is noted that a practical intentionality predictor should satisfy the following important requirements [14]:

- **Efficiency:** low complexity makes the algorithm amenable to a real-time implementation. This is a critical factor for facilitating the pointing task in graphical user interfaces which are typically completed within a fraction of a second. Off-line computationally intensive algorithms that introduce high delays are not practical.
- **Case independent:** the technique should be independent of the application, selections sequence, target layouts, etc. This is due to the fact that interfaces may significantly vary between different applications and contexts.
- **Adaptability:** the nature of the pointing trajectory is greatly affected by the physical ability of the user, the input device accuracy, level of expertise or experience, etc. An intentionality predictor should be able to take such user capabilities into account.

As it will be apparent in the following sections, the adopted approach and all its associated algorithms fulfil the above requirements. Calculating the posterior probabilities for all the listed algorithms is straightforward and can be case independent. Additionally, the level of performed data smoothing/filtering can be adapted to the user abilities and the level of perturbations in the input data.

Henceforth, various algorithms that allow calculating $P(B_i|c_{1:k})$ are tested on cursor data collected for able and impaired users. The performance of these algorithms is measured in terms of the percentage of time during which the correct button is chosen by the applied predictor; the saving in the pointing time or duration is $t_M - t_C$.

3   Intentionality Prediction Algorithms

Below, a number of algorithms that enable a MAP decision using (1) are described. The objective is achieving performance gains whilst maintaining simplicity and low computational complexity.

3.1   Nearest Neighbour (NN)

This is a simple and intuitive model that relies on selecting the button that is closest to the current cursor position. It relies on measuring the distance between the position of the nominal buttons $\{\mathbf{b}_1, \mathbf{b}_2, \ldots, \mathbf{b}_N\}$ and $\mathbf{c}_k$ at time t_k. It allocates the highest probability to the button with the smallest Euclidian distance $\|\mathbf{b}_i - \mathbf{c}_k\|_2$. In a probabilistic framework, this can be expressed as

$$P(\mathbf{c}_k|B_i) = \mathcal{N}(\mathbf{c}_k|\mathbf{b}_i, \sigma_{NN}^2) \tag{3}$$

where σ_{NN}^2 is the covariance matrix. The observation vector $\mathbf{c}_k$ has a normal distribution with a mean equal to that of the selectable target location in question and a fixed variance whose value is a design parameter. Assuming that the cursor movements at various time instants are independent for simplicity, we reach

$$P(\mathbf{c}_{k-L:k}|B_i) = \prod_{n=k-L}^{k} P(\mathbf{c}_n|B_i). \tag{4}$$

For an equal prior on all the buttons, i.e. $P(B_i) = 1/N$, then (4) suffices to determine the intentionality outcome as per (1) and (2); movements along the x and y axes are reasonably assumed to be independent. It is noted here that the choice of σ_{NN}^2 does not alter the MAP outcome.

3.2   Bearing Angle (BA)

This algorithm is based on the fact that as the cursor is heading towards the target button, the cumulative angle between the direction of travel and the position of the target is minimal [10]. The bearing angle from two consecutive cursor positions with respect to a target can be assumed to be a random variable with zero mean and fixed variance. Hence we can write

$$P(\mathbf{c}_k|\mathbf{c}_{k-1}, B_i) = \mathcal{N}(\theta_{i,k}|0, \sigma_{BA}^2) \tag{5}$$

where $\theta_{i,k} = \angle(\mathbf{v}_k, \mathbf{b}_i - \mathbf{c}_k)$, $\mathbf{v}_k = \mathbf{c}_k - \mathbf{c}_{k-1}$ is the velocity or heading vector. Operator $\angle(\mathbf{a}, \mathbf{b})$ returns the angle between the vectors $\mathbf{a}$ from $\mathbf{b}$ using the dot product definition in a Euclidean space. Equation (5) stipulates that a smaller $\theta_{i,k}$ implies that the "i^{th}" target is more probable; this reflects the rationale behind BA. It follows that

$$P(B_i|\mathbf{c}_{k-L:k}) = \frac{P(B_i)P(\mathbf{c}_{k-L}|B_i)\prod_{n=k-L+1}^{k}P(\mathbf{c}_n|\mathbf{c}_{n-1}, B_i)}{P(\mathbf{c}_{k-L:k})} \tag{6}$$

which incorporates the cumulative sum of the bearing angle depending on the chosen width of the applied time window.

The probabilistic interpretation of BA illustrates that a confidence interval of a width set by σ_{BA}^2 is formed along the direction of travel. It is a wedge-like region and any selectable target that falls within this region is assigned a relatively high probability. With many selectable targets in close proximity from one another, the possibility that the BA model leading to an erroneous prediction is high as noted in [11].

Additionally, as the cursor approaches the true target, the angle $\theta_{i,k}$ can become arbitrarily large leading to small likelihood probabilities and incorrect predictions. Nonetheless, BA tends to make early correct decisions as the users tend to typically head towards the target in the early stages of the pointing task [6, 7].

3.3   Mean Reverting Diffusion (MRD) Model

In a continuous-time, the MAP estimator is based on modeling the cursor movements as a bivariate Ornstein-Uhlenbeck process with a mean-reverting term. It is described by the following stochastic differential equation

$$dc_t = \Lambda(\mu - c_t)dt + \sigma_{MRD}dw_t \tag{7}$$

where Λ is a square matrix that sets the mean reversion rate to steer the evolution of the process, μ is the mean, σ_{MRD} is a square matrix that drives the process dispersion and w_t is a Wiener process [16]. By adopting the above mean reverting diffusion model for the intentionality prediction problem, the mean to which the process should revert to is defined by the location of a selectable target B_i. Hence, $\mu = b_i$ for the "i^{th}" button and the target, which the cursor is drifting towards, is chosen.

Since the cursor positions are available at discrete times, equations (7) should be discretised. Upon integrating (7) over $\mathcal{T} = [t, t + \tau]$ and then discretising the outcome we obtain

$$c_{i,k} = e^{-\Lambda\tau_k}c_{i,k-1} + [I_2 - e^{-\Lambda\tau_k}]b_i + \varepsilon_k \tag{8}$$

where $c_{i,k}$ and $c_{i,k-1}$ are the state vectors with respect to button B_i at the time instants t_k and t_{k-1} respectively. Whereas, $\tau_k = t_k - t_{k-1}$ is the time step and $\varepsilon_k \sim \mathcal{N}(0, \sigma_{MRD}^2)$ is an additive Gaussian noise. Assuming that the cursor movements along the x and y axis are independent, the Λ and σ_{MRD} matrices become diagonal, i.e. $\Lambda = diag(\lambda_x, \lambda_y)$ and $\sigma_{MRD}^2 = diag(\sigma_x^2, \sigma_y^2)$. It follows that the distribution of the conditional state is given by

$$P(c_k|c_{k-1}, B_i) = \mathcal{N}(c_k|\Sigma_{i,k}, \Gamma_k^2) \tag{9}$$

such that

$$\Sigma_{i,k} = e^{-\Lambda\tau}c_{i,k-1} + [I_2 - e^{-\Lambda\tau_k}]b_i \tag{10}$$

and

$$\Gamma_k^2 = \left[\frac{1 - e^{-2\Lambda\tau_k}}{2\Lambda}\right]\sigma_{MRD}^2 . \tag{11}$$

The sought posterior probability is calculated for the MRD model via

$$P(B_i|c_{k-L:k}) = \frac{P(B_i)\mathcal{N}(c_{L-k}|\Sigma_{i,L-k}, \Gamma_{L-k}^2)\prod_{n=k-L+1}^{k}\mathcal{N}(c_n|\Sigma_{i,n}, \Gamma_n^2)}{P(c_{k-L:k})} \tag{12}$$

similar to (6). The reversion rates and the diffusion noise are design parameters that can be tuned to a given data set. It can be noticed that if the pointing cursor is stationary, the MRD MAP reverts to the nearest neighbour model.

3.4   Composite (COM)

The bearing angle model performs poorly when the cursor is moving very slowly since there is no well-defined direction of travel. A composite algorithm uses the BA model whenever the cursor is moving at a velocity that exceeds a certain threshold, i.e. V_T, and switches to the MRD model whenever the cursor speed is below V_T. Selecting the threshold value V_T is a design parameter that requires setting prior to performing the intentionality prediction.

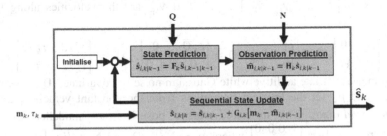

Fig. 1. Simplified block diagram of the LKF; $G_{i,k}$ is Kalman gain

3.5   Weighted Bearing with Distance (WBD)

This model is motivated by the fact that as the cursor approaches the target the bearing angle can take arbitrary values. On the other hand, the direction of travel tends to be a more reliable indication of the destination when the cursor is relatively far from the intended button [1, 5, 13]. Hence, the weighted bearing with distance model fuses the bearing and distance information where the likelihood probability for two consecutive cursor positions is given by

$$P(\mathbf{c}_k|\mathbf{c}_{k-1}, B_i) = \mathcal{N}\left(\theta_{i,k}|0,\ \kappa_{WBD}^2 \Omega_{i,k}^2\right). \qquad (13)$$

Similar to the BA model, the divergence of the bearing from the position of B_i is defined by $\theta_{i,k} = \angle(\mathbf{v}_k, \mathbf{b}_i - \mathbf{c}_k)$; $\Omega_{i,k} = 1/\|\mathbf{b}_i - \mathbf{c}_k\|_2$ is the inverse of the Euclidian norm of distance between the cursor's current position and the "i^{th}" button. Hence, if the cursor is in close proximity to a possible target, bigger $\theta_{i,k}$ values can be tolerated due to the resultant $\Omega_{i,k}$ and vice versa. WBD can seamlessly circumvent the unreliable aspects of BA whilst harnessing its ability to predict the correct target in early stages of the pointing process. Similar to (6) and (12), $P(B_i|\mathbf{c}_{k-L:k})$ of WBD can be calculated.

4   Linear Kalman Filter Based Smoothing

Kalman filter is an adaptive Bayesian filtering approach that is widely used for tracking dynamic signals in real-time due to its robustness and low complexity. It is deployed here to remove involuntary cursor movements typically manifested by large deviations from a direct path between the start point and the target location. Such outliners are caused by motor disorders or situational impairments [13]. Based on several studies on pointing tasks in 2-D environments, e.g. [1, 5, 6, 13], it is reasonable to represent the cursor voluntary movements by the nearly constant velocity model. Accordingly, the discretised state dynamics at the time instant t_k are defined by

$$s_k = F_k s_{k-1} + e_k \tag{14}$$

such that $s_k = \begin{bmatrix} x_{t_n} & \dot{x}_{t_n} & y_{t_n} & \dot{y}_{t_n} \end{bmatrix}^T$; $\dot{x}_{t_n}$ and $\dot{y}_{t_n}$ are the velocities along the x-y axis,

$$F_k = \begin{bmatrix} \hat{F}_k & 0 \\ 0 & \hat{F}_k \end{bmatrix}, \ \hat{F}_k = \begin{bmatrix} 1 & \tau_k \\ 0 & 1 \end{bmatrix}, \ Q = \begin{bmatrix} \rho_x \hat{Q} & 0 \\ 0 & \rho_y \hat{Q} \end{bmatrix}, \ \hat{Q}_x = \begin{bmatrix} \tau_k^3/3 & \tau_k^2/2 \\ \tau_k^2/2 & \tau_k \end{bmatrix} \text{ and } e_k$$

is a zero mean bivariate additive white Gaussian noise of covariance Q. Design parameters ρ_x and ρ_y set the level of deviations from the constant velocity path; their units is $speed^2/time$. The measured cursor positions are modelled as: $m_k = H s_{k-1} + n_k$ and $H = \begin{bmatrix} 1 & 0 & 0 & 0 \\ 0 & 0 & 1 & 0 \end{bmatrix}$ where $n_k \sim \mathcal{N}(0, N)$ and $N = diag\{\sigma_x^2, \sigma_y^2\}$ is the observation noise covariance matrix. Given the Gaussian nature of s_k and m_k, linear Kalman filter depicted in Fig. 1 is the optimal filter in the minimum mean squared error sense [15]; Q and N dictate the level of performed smoothing. The LKF output $\hat{c}_k = \begin{bmatrix} \hat{x}_{t_k} & \hat{y}_{t_k} \end{bmatrix}^T$, which is the smoothed cursor location at time t_k, is used in the adopted Algorithm 1. Additionally, the resulting smoothed velocity vector $\hat{v}_k = \begin{bmatrix} \hat{v}_x & \hat{v}_y \end{bmatrix}^T$ can be used for the BA, COM and WBD models. Fig. 2 shows two cursor tracks for a severely motor impaired user with notable tremor attempting two selections on the interface. The effectiveness of the LKF-based-smoothing is clearly demonstrated in the figure.

5   Experiments

The considered prediction models are tested on two data sets pertaining to: 1) user 1 is able bodied and 2) user 2 is severely motor impaired suffering from notable tremor (see the tracks in Fig. 2). They undertook selection tasks similar to the ISO 9241 with multiple distractors on the screen with a typical layout shown in Fig. 3. Users click the button at the centre of the screen Fig. 3a and then the target button appears with other distractors Fig. 3b. The performance of the adopted model is assessed in terms of the percentage of time the predicator makes a correct decision from a partial cursor track, i.e. the accuracy of the prediction. It is noted that at every observation time, e.g. t_k, the predictive model uses the available track (e.g. $c_{k-L:k}$) and does not assume

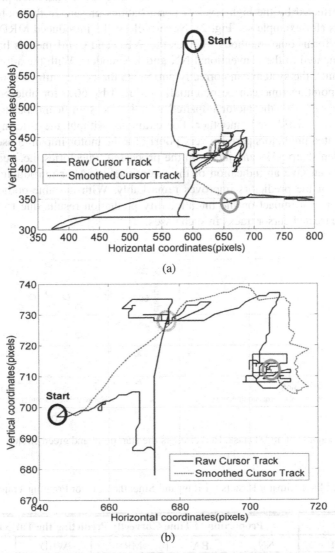

Fig. 2. Two raw and smoothed cursor tracks for a severely impaired user. Start point is the black solid circle, target 1 is the dotted blue circle and target 2 is the solid green circle.

knowledge of how much of the entire trajectory, i.e. $c_{1:M}$, has been completed. Table I exhibits the performance of the considered prediction models with and without the LKF smoother for the two participants. The various design parameters, e.g. L, Λ, σ_{NN}^2, σ_{BA}^2, σ_{MRD}^2 and κ_{WBD} are obtained from Monte Carlo simulations. This is feasible since each model has a maximum of two parameters that alter its MAP outcome. Design parameters that yield the highest percentage of correct predictions are selected.

It can be noticed from Table 1 that the performance of the examined predictors are drastically affected by the high level of perturbations present in the motor impaired cursor tracks (for example see Fig. 2). Nevertheless, the introduced MRD-based predictor outperforms other methods whereas the WBD and COM models bring notable benefits compared to the conventional NN and BA models. With the adopted prediction algorithms, the system can correctly anticipate the target with over 60% accuracy, i.e. the pointing time can be potentially reduced by 60% for able-bodied users. The achieve gains for the motor impaired user is also significant, particularly after introducing the LKF-based smoother. For example, without the filtering operation all the evaluated predictors perform very poorly for the motor-impaired user given the typical sudden sharp jerks and jumps in the processed trajectories, i.e. neither distant nor heading can give an indication of the intentionality. After introducing LKF, the success rate of the predictors improves remarkably. With the able-bodied user, the LKF has marginal impact on the intentionality prediction results due to the smooth nature of the treated cursor tracks in such cases.

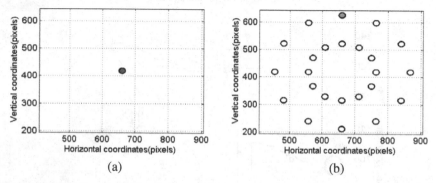

(a)   (b)

Fig. 3. An example of an ISO task. Red circle is the start point and green circle is the target.

Table 1. Map Estimator Results for Raw and Smoothed Cursor Pointing Trajectories

	Proportion of Time Correctly Predicting the Target (%)				
Subject	NN	BA	MRD	WBD	COM
Able-bodied	53.1	31.2	61.8	45.13	56.19
Motor impaired	15.3	4.3	18.6	16.4	14.8
Subject	LKF-NN	LKF-BA	LKF-MRD	LKF-WBD	LKF-COM
Able-bodied	53.3	34.7	62.1	47.3	57.9
Motor impaired	38.4	28.3	44.1	38.8	39.7

6   Conclusions

The adopted probabilistic intentionality prediction approach delivers significant reductions in the pointing durations alleviating difficulties experienced by impaired users. This can be particularly beneficial for assistive interfaces by providing visual feedback, e.g. highlighting predicted target(s) or magnifying them, increasing the movement gain, even making a decision on the user's behalf, etc. The simple Kalman filtering approach is shown to effectively smooth highly perturbed cursor trajectories. This study sets a probabilistic framework and serves as an impetus to further research into more advanced Bayesian filtering algorithms that can better stabilise the pointing movements for irregular position measurements and highly non-linear cursor movement models, e.g. sequential Monte Carlo techniques [17]. Additionally, devising more elaborate models that incorporate the target position (similar to MRD) can be highly beneficial since the filtering operation can produce the sought posterior probabilities, i.e. circumvent the need to separate the smoother from the predictor.

References

1. Oirschot, H.K.-V., Houtsma, A.J.M.: Cursor Trajectory Analysis. In: Brewster, S., Murray-Smith, R. (eds.) Haptic HCI 2000. LNCS, vol. 2058, pp. 127–134. Springer, Heidelberg (2001)
2. Bateman, S., Mandryk, R.L., Xiao, R., Gutwin, C.: Analysis and comparison of target assistance techniques for relative ray-cast pointing. International Journal of Human-Computer Studies, 511–532 (2013)
3. Fitts, P.M., Peterson, J.R.: Information capacity of discrete motor responses. J. Exp. Psych. 67, 103–112 (1964)
4. Mackenzie, I.S.: Fitts' law as a research and design tool in human-computer interaction. Journal of Human Computer Interaction 7, 91–139 (1992)
5. Kopper, R., Bowman, D.A., Silva, M.G., McMahan, R.P.: A human motor behavior model for distal pointing tasks. Int. J. of Human Computer Studies 68, 603–615 (2010)
6. Meyer, D.E., Smith, J.E., Kornblum, S., Abrams, R.A., Wright, C.E.: Optimality in human motor performance: ideal control of rapid aimed movements. Psychological Review 8, 340–370 (1988)
7. McGuffin, M.J., Balakrishnan, R.: Fitts's law and expanding targets: Experimental studies and designs for user interfaces. ACM Transactions Computer-Human Interaction 4, 388–422 (2005)
8. Lane, D.M., Peres, S.C., Sándor, A., Napier, A.H.A.: A Process for Anticipating and Executing Icon Selection in Graphical User Interfaces. International Journal of Human Computer Interaction 2, 243–254 (2005)
9. Wobbrock, J.O., Fogarty, J., Liu, S., Kimuro, S., Harada, S.: The Angle Mouse: Target-Agnostic Dynamic Gain Adjustment Based on Angular Deviation. In: Proc. of the 27th International Conference on Human Factors in Computing Systems, New York, pp. 1401–1410 (2009)
10. Murata, A.: Improvement of pointing time by predicting targets in pointing with a PC mouse. International Journal of Human Computer Studies 10, 23–32 (2005)

11. Asano, T., Sharlin, E., Kitamura, Y., Takashima, K., Kishino, F.: Predictive interaction using the Delphian desktop. In: Proc. of the 186th Annual ACM Smp. on User Interface Software and Technology (UIST 2005), New York, pp. 133–141 (2005)
12. Lank, E., Cheng, Y.N., Ruiz, J.: Endpoint prediction using motion kinematicst. In: Proc. of the SIGCHI Conference on Human Factors in Computing System, NY, pp. 637–646 (2007)
13. Keates, S., Hwang, F., Langdon, P., Clarkson, P.J., Robinson, P.: Cursor measures for motion-impaired computer users. In: Proc. of the Fifth International ACM Conference on Assistive Technologies – ASSETS, New York, pp. 135–142 (2002)
14. Ziebart, B., Dey, A., Bagnell, J.A.: Probabilistic pointing target prediction via inverse optimal control. In: Proc. of the ACM Int. Conf. on Intelligent User Interfaces, pp. 1–10 (2012)
15. Haug, A.: Bayesian Estimation and Tracking: A Practical Guide. John Wiley & Sons (2012)
16. Meucci, A.: Review of Statistical Arbitrage, Cointegration, and Multivariate Ornstein-Uhlenbeck. SSRN Preprint 1404905 (2010)
17. Godsill, S.J., Vermaak, J., Ng, W., Li, J.: Models and algorithms for tracking of maneuvering objects using variable rate particle filters. Proc. of IEEE 95, 925–952 (2007)

Addressing the Users' Diversity in Ubiquitous Environments through a Low Cost Architecture

Tatiana Silva de Alencar[1], Luciano Rodrigues Machado[1],
Luciano de Oliveira Neris[2], and Vânia Paula de Almeida Neris[1]

[1] Flexible and Sustainable Interaction Laboratory - Department of Computing –
UFSCar - São Carlos, SP – Brazil
[2] AGX Technology - São Carlos, SP – Brazil
{tatidealencar,vania}@dc.ufscar.br,
337790@ead.ufscar.br, neroso@msn.com

Abstract. A ubiquitous environment allows the system to infer the users' needs and preferences, making adaptations to the interface. However, the best way to make such adaptations is still under debate by researchers. This paper proposes an architecture that supports the adaptation of user interfaces in ubiquitous environments according to the users' profiles. The proposed architecture is shown simple and low cost, has low implementation complexity and high extension capability. The user profile data are stored on the user's mobile device for privacy. As the profile is defined by the user, it is expected that the interface adaptation occurs more accurately. A prototype is presented as a proof of concept.

Keywords: Ubiquitous Environment, User Profile, Ubiquitous Accessibility, Context-Aware, Adaptive Interface, Raspberry PI.

1 Introduction

The term ubiquitous computing, defined by [22], is used to describe systems which allow their resources to be available everywhere, in an intuitive and transparent way to the user. To achieve transparency of use, [17] computers should anticipate the user's needs and act proactively to provide appropriate assistance. Systems that have this ability are called context-aware [16]. Therefore, in order to sustain the ubiquitous environment existence, the system must proactively oversee and control the context conditions and make the necessary changes by an adaptation process [21].

One of the inputs for the adaptation process should be the users' needs and preferences [15]. In the literature, most of the works which focus on the user interface adaptation is related with the flexibility between different devices [13, 14, 18], but not on the interface adaptation to different types of users. In addition, it is possible to find researches about accessibility in ubiquitous environments that focus on restricted groups of users [1, 12, 20], without considering the interaction needs of different groups in a more universal and inclusive approach.

C. Stephanidis and M. Antona (Eds.): UAHCI/HCII 2014, Part III, LNCS 8515, pp. 439–450, 2014.

Alencar and Neris [3] have demonstrated that known ubiquitous environments partially meet the interaction requirements of visually impaired people, people with low literacy and people with attention deficit and/or memorization problems. These authors argued that ubiquitous environments must be able to adapt themselves to the diverse users' capabilities, related to the physical and cognitive characteristics, and users' interaction preferences.

This paper proposes an architecture that supports the adaptation of user interfaces in ubiquitous environments according to the users' interaction profiles. In this architecture, the users' characteristics and preferences are mapped into an ontology, and are available to ubiquitous applications in an eXtensible Markup Language[1] (XML) file containing the user profile. Aiming to show that it is not necessary many resources[2] to offer adapted interfaces to supply the users' needs and preferences, the proposed architecture is shown simple and low cost by using a Raspberry PI[3] computer. As other advantage of this architecture, we can mention that the user profile data is stored on the user's mobile device (and not in a web server) for privacy. Backup in private storage media is also provided.

In order to prove the concept, a prototype was developed. Considering the emerging context of smart cities, the prototype is set in a bus stop. In this scenario, for instance, a visually impaired person may find it difficult to take the correct bus. The same can happen to an elderly person. The prototype uses a monitor that displays the bus schedules as well as the next bus identification. The system shows the most suitable user interface considering the user's profile.

This paper is organized as follows: Section 2 summarizes the related work on modeling users' profiles for ubiquitous environments. Section 3 shows how the user's profile is mapped, in our proposal, using an ontology. Section 4 presents the proposed architecture for ubiquitous environments that supports adaptive user interfaces, detailing their modules and communication flow. Section 5 presents the prototype build to develop the concept of the proposed architecture and the feasibility study. Finally, we highlight the contributions and limitations of this work and discuss future works in section 6.

2   Related Work

2.1   Architectures for User Diversity in Ubiquitous Environments

In the literature, a few studies on the development of architectures that support the interface adaptation to different users can be found. The architecture proposed by [11] makes use of sensors in the environment to capture contextual information. Data on

---

[1] http://www.w3.org/XML/

[2] Considering that the user may already have a mobile device, the hardware involved in the architecture considers the Raspberry PI (at about US$30.00) and a Bluetooth device (at about US$ 8.00). The software solution is also simple and extensible, making it a low-weight architecture.

[3] http://www.raspberrypi.org/

the user's device are also captured and tests are performed during the interaction with the mobile interface to identify some of the user's characteristics (e.g. disability). This information is sent to a server that queries an ontology to determine the best adaptation to the interface. The changes to be made are sent to the user's device in an XML file.

The Project Aura[4] uses an architecture to adapt the ubiquitous environment according to user location and the tasks he is performing [18]. In this architecture, a Context Observer controls the physical environment and the collected information is sent to a Task Manager. Based on information about the environment and context, and the activity being performed, the Task Manager adapts the interface to the user.

Abascal et al. [2] propose an architecture for adapting interfaces for people with disabilities. In this architecture, the user logs into the interface adaptation system through his mobile device. The system consults an ontology in order to identify the user and determine their needs and preferences. Then the system generates an adapted user interface in eXtensible Hypertext Markup Language (XHTML) and sends to the user's mobile device.

The proposed architectures for [11] and [18] have a medium to high cost due to the use of sensors to identify the user context. Besides the cost, the architecture proposed by [18] has a high complexity in their implementation. In the presented architectures [11, 18, 2], the best interface adaptation is determined by the system, according to the user profile. Although these adaptations are guided by the user needs, the user preferences are not taken into consideration. In [11], the user profile is created during the interaction time. Therefore, in each new interaction, all the identification tasks have to be performed again.

2.2   Modeling Users' Profiles

In this paper, user's profile is defined as a set of characteristics that identifies the users' needs and preferences. These characteristics can be physical (e.g., low vision, visual impairment), cognitive (e.g., attention deficit, memory problems), level of literacy, interests (e.g., news, social networks, books), among others.

In a ubiquitous environment, the details that compound the user's profile may come from various sources, such as sensors, social networking profiles, mobile and semantic web technologies. Each of these sources provides details in different data models. To solve this problem, [10] propose the use of ontologies based on the Simple Knowledge Organization System for the Web[5] (SKOS) in order to model the user's profile with data from these different sources. To provide a standard model, SKOS makes use of Resource Description Framework[6] (RDF), a framework that describes web resources. Using RDF allows the user's profile to be shared among different applications in an interoperable way.

---

[4] http://www.cs.cmu.edu/~aura/

[5] http://www.w3.org/2004/02/skos/

[6] http://www.w3.org/RDF/

Intelligent learning environments also receive data from different sources to provide tailored services and resources to users. To model the user's profile in such environments, [5] propose the use of RDF as a standard model of the user's profile. The proposed architecture combines descriptions and performance requirements from a resource to a particular student in RDF format to make the necessary adjustments. The availability of a standard model allows this profile to be shared with other applications.

Aiming to provide tailored interfaces with focus on the end user, [11] propose an architecture that uses the concepts of Pervasive Computing and a representation of user's profile. The user's profile takes into account their disabilities, preferences, experiences and demographic data. This profile is represented by an ontology expressed in OWL. The ontology is updated through preferences and deficiencies details that are passed by the user application and the data captured by sensors, all made available in an XML file. To perform the necessary adjustments, rules are executed crossing captured data from sensors, user's profile and device profile.

Heckmann et al. [7] propose a General User Model Ontology, an ontology represented in Web Ontology Language (OWL) to uniform interpretation of user models. The GUMO ontology divides the dimensions of the user model in three parts: auxiliary, predicate and range. This ontology makes use of the UbisWorld model [6] to identify the dimensions of the basic user model. The UbisWorld allows the user information representation, such as demographics data, interests, psychological and physiological states, personal characteristics etc.

As can be seen in Table 1, the studies cited do not include all the users' needs and preferences in the user's profile templates. In addition, it is observed that there is a tendency towards the use of XML, either in pure form or as a form of writing in other languages or frameworks such as OWL and RDF.

Table 1. User characteristics present in the user's profile templates: (a) [10], (b) [5], (c) [11], (d) [7]

Paper Users' Characteristics	(a)	(b)	(c)	(d)
Physical	X	X	X	X
Cognitive			X	
Literacy level		X		X
Interests	X	X		X
Interaction preferences			X	X

In our work, the user's profile considers the physical and cognitive characteristics, interests and user's interaction preferences. Furthermore, the proposed architecture makes use of the XML language to describe the user's characteristics and preferences, because of its simplicity and standardization to enable data exchange between applications.

3   Mapping User's Profile Based on an Ontology

Considering that ubiquitous environments must adapt themselves to the different users' characteristics, this paper proposes the use of a more comprehensive user interaction profile that is mapped on an ontology. The GUMO ontology [7] was chosen to model the user profile as it is the most complete among those analyzed (see Table 1).

The classes of the GUMO ontology to be used in modeling or the user profile were chosen based on the application of the UbiCARD technique [4]. The following classes (and their subclasses) were chosen: Basic User Dimensions and Domain Dependent Dimensions. Figure 1 shows the predicates that represent the characteristics, demographics data and user emotional states (Basic User Dimensions).

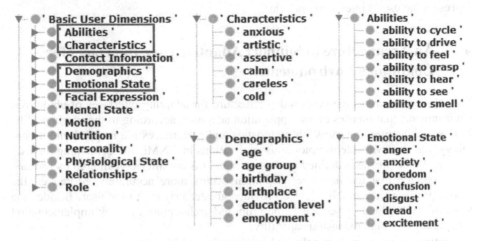

Fig. 1. Predicates that represent the characteristics, demographics data and user emotional states

```
<?xml version="1.0" encoding="UTF-8"?>
<user-profile>
 <statement
  auxiliary = ""
  predicate = ""
  range = ""
  object = ""
  group = ""
 />
</user-profile>
```

Fig. 2. The XML file structure for the user profile representation

The UserML [8] is a markup language for ubiquitous environments divided into two levels: (1) simple XML structure, composed of twenty-five predefined attributes and (2) the ontology that defines the categories. This approach allows applications to use their own ontologies and the UserML language to map them. For this reason, the UserML was chosen as the language to structure XML file that contains the user model profile.

Among the twenty-five attributes of UserML, the following were selected according to the chosen GUMO ontology classes: auxiliary, predicate, range, object, start, end, durability and group (see Figure 2). The attributes start, end and durability are used only for the predicates related to the emotional state.

The next section describes an architecture to support adaptive user interfaces for ubiquitous environments and how an XML file, in the user mobile phone, used to represent the user's interaction profile.

4   An Architecture to Support Adaptive User Interfaces for Ubiquitous Environments

This section describes the proposed architecture for adapting interfaces of ubiquitous environments that focuses on the application adequacy according to the user's profile. In this architecture, the users' characteristics and preferences are mapped into an ontology, and are available to ubiquitous applications in a XML file containing the user profile. As the profile is defined by the user, i.e., it is not inferred/captured by sensors, it is expected that the interface adaptation occurs more accurately. Moreover, the stored profile in the mobile device provides greater privacy to the user. Besides the low cost highlighted in Section 1, the proposed architecture has low implementation complexity and high extension capability.

Aiming to propose a simple and inexpensive architecture, we have adopted a Raspberry PI computer to execute the ubiquitous application. The Raspberry PI is a small computer (as the same size as a credit card) and cheap. It was designed by the Raspberry PI Foundation for children around the world to learn programming. Despite the small size, the Raspberry PI can be used for various tasks and performs as well as a desktop computer.

The proposed architecture is divided into two main areas – user's mobile device and ubiquitous application - as we can see in Figure 3. The user's mobile device contains the XML file describing the profile based on GUMO ontology. The ubiquitous application has the adaptation rules to be applied in the interface according to the user's profile. The data exchange between these devices is controlled by an application in the user's mobile device and in the Raspberry PI. The mobile device application sends the XML file containing the user's profile and the ubiquitous application reads this file and obtains information about the user's needs and preferences.

The communication between the user's mobile device and the ubiquitous application is established via Bluetooth[7]. The data exchange between these devices is

---

[7] http://www.bluetooth.com/Pages/Bluetooth-Home.aspx

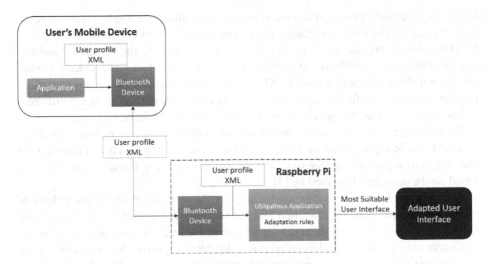

Fig. 3. Proposed architecture for adapting user interfaces in ubiquitous environments

controlled by an application in the user's mobile device and in the Raspberry PI. At first, the mobile device application initializes the Bluetooth and sends a connection request to the application running on the Raspberry PI. After connecting, the mobile device application sends, via Bluetooth, the XML file containing the description of the user's profile. The ubiquitous application reads the XML file and obtains information about the user's needs and preferences.

From the data obtained from the XML file, the ubiquitous application queries that there are adaptations to be performed according to a set of rules defined in the application. As an example, let's consider that the user's profile indicates the user has low vision. In the ubiquitous application there is an adaptation rule which states that when the user has low vision, the application should provide a sound output. If another user indicates in his profile that he prefers textual output and he is elderly, the application must adapt the textual output to the user preference, for instance, increasing the font size of the text. To cope with the concurrency between devices of different users, the ubiquitous application must implement a queue. The requests of each user are met as the progress of the queue. However, if there is no conflict between the requests, the server can attend more than one user at the same time (e.g.: a user needs an audio output and another user needs a visual output from the same information).

5   Proof of the Concept

In order to demonstrate the possibility to provide adaptive interfaces using the proposed architecture, we have been developing a prototype. Considering the emerging context of smart cities, the prototype is set in a bus stop. In this scenario, for instance, a visually impaired person may find it difficult to take the correct bus. The same can happen to an elderly person. The prototype uses a monitor that displays the bus schedules as well as the next bus identification. The system shows the most suitable user interface considering the user's profile, for example, adjusting the font size considering the interaction profile of an elderly person. By identifying the elderly person needs through its interaction profile (XML), the system makes adjustments according to your needs and preferences. As the elderly person indicated in his/her profile that he/she has low vision, the system infers that the font size should be increased.

To test the adaptability of the prototype, we used three different users' profiles. The first profile represents a user with visual impairment, the second an elderly user and the third represents a teenager. The details for creating the users' profiles are based on the personas described by [3].

The visually impaired user is represented by the persona Patricia, the elderly is represented by the persona Francisca and the teenager is represented by the persona Danilo. Their interaction preferences are shown in Table 2. Because not all the information needed for the instantiation of user's interaction profile was available in the description of the personas, some other information was inferred. Based on the information contained in Table 2, the three XML files have been created. Figure 4 shows how the XML file would be instantiated with Francisca's profile.

Table 2. Interaction preferences of the three user's profiles

User / Profile	Patricia persona	Francisca persona	Danilo persona
Input	Keyboard	Voice	Keyboard
Output	Sound	Text	Text
Physical and/or Cognitive characteristics	Visual impairment	Low vision, attention deficit, problems memorizing	-
Interests	Books, Songs, Social Networks	Novels	Games
Literacy level	Higher	Basic	Secondary
Age	20	80	13

A preview of the proposed scenario, considering the three defined profiles and the adjustments to be made are available in Figure 5. The prototype has been implemented in Java language on the Raspberry PI and Java on Android platform in the mobile device. The ubiquitous application runs in a Raspberry PI model B in which an adapter to enable communication via Bluetooth was plugged (see Figure 5). The mobile device application is running on a smartphone with Android operational system in version 2.3.5. The ubiquitous application output is made on a TV via HDMI.

```xml
<?xml version="1.0" encoding="UTF-8"?>
<user-profile>
  <statement
    auxiliary = "has"
    predicate = "AbilityToSee"
    range = "low-medium-high"
    object = "low"
    group = "Abilities"
  />
  <statement
    auxiliary = "has"
    predicate = "Age"
    range = "years"
    object = "80"
    group = "Demographics"
  />
  <statement
    auxiliary = "has"
    predicate = "EducationLevel"
    range = "basic-primary-secondary-higher"
    object = "basic"
    group = "Demographics"
  />
  <statement
    auxiliary = "hasPreference"
    predicate = "Voice"
    range = "primary-secondary"
    object = "primary"
    group = "InterfacePreferences"
    subgroup = "Input"
  />
  <statement
    auxiliary = "hasPreference"
    predicate = "Visual"
    range = "primary-secondary"
    object = "primary"
    group = "InterfacePreferences"
    subgroup = "Output"
  />
</user-profile>
```

Fig. 4. Francisca's profile mapped into XML

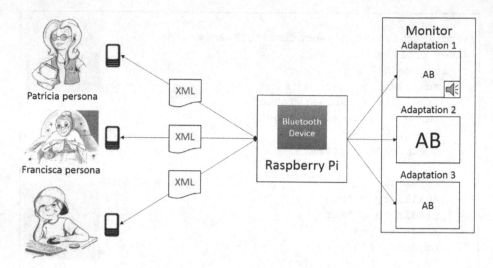

Fig. 5. Proposed scenario

The ubiquitous application has the following modules:

1. Bluetooth Connection Manager;
2. Command Receiver: responsible for receiving the XML file with the user's interaction profile, decoding and making it available to the Command Processor;
3. Command Processor: responsible for performing the adaptation according to the user's profile and the adaptation rules defined in the application.

The mobile device application provides a screen for the user to start or stop the service. When initializing the service, a connection is established between the user's mobile device and the Raspberry PI. The various user requests are placed in a queue and adjustments are performed one by one. In Figure 4 we can see how it is done, for example, adjusting the font size for the interaction profile of Francisca's persona. By identifying the persona Francisca through her interaction profile (XML), the system makes adjustments according to her needs and preferences. In Figure 6, we observe

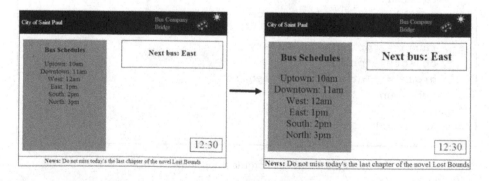

Fig. 6. Adapting the application interface to the persona Francisca

that the font size of the text is increased, since the persona Francisca has indicated that she prefers output as text. However, as the persona has low vision, the system inferred that the font size should be increased.

6   Conclusions and Future Work

This paper presented an architecture for adapting user interfaces of ubiquitous environments considering the user's interaction profile written in an XML specification. As the main contributions of this work, it is possible to highlight:

1. The proposed architecture shows that it is possible to provide adapted user interfaces in a simple, low-cost and extensible approach using a Raspberry PI;
2. Unlike the architectures found in the literature, this allows that the user profile is defined by the user himself, allowing him/er to set his/er needs, preferences and interests;
3. The profile goes with the user (mobility of the profile). As the profile is on the user's mobile device, when the user moves, he/s carries the defined profile. Thus, other applications can easily read it;
4. Furthermore, one of the advantages of this architecture is that the user profile data is stored on the user's mobile device for privacy;
5. This paper contributes to overcoming the challenge indicated by [9]: acquire knowledge of user needs, and provide appropriate solutions for different combinations of users' characteristics and functional limitations.

The prototype developed shows the feasibility of processing different interaction profiles and providing outputs adapted to diverse users. Initially, the treatment of different profiles is done by the simplistic use of a queue. In future work, this issue will be addressed to provide a better solution, for instance considering the user mobile as an output device to deal with the common output device problem. Moreover, future works consider the extension of GUMO ontology to contemplate, for example, information about the user cognitive capabilities. The mobile application for collecting the user profile is in progress.

References

1. Abascal, J., et al.: Automatically Generating Tailored Accessible User Interfaces for Ubiquitous Services. In: Proceedings of ASSETS (2011)
2. Abascal, J., et al.: A modular approach to user interface adaptation for people with disabilities in ubiquitous environments. Internal Technical Report N. EHU-KAT-IK-01-11 (2011)
3. Alencar, T.S., Neris, V.P.A.: Ubiquitous Environments and Brazilian Personas: Can our citizens universally access this technology? In: SEMISH, Curitiba, Brazil (2012)
4. Alencar, T.S., Neris, V.P.A.: Sistemas Ubíquos para Todos: conhecendo e mapeando os diferentes perfis de interação. In: IHC, Manaus, Brazil (2013)

5. Dolog, P., Nejdl, W.: Challenges and benefits of the semantic web for user modelling. In: AH 2003 Workshop at WWW 2003 (2003)
6. Heckmann, D.: Introducing situational statements as an integrating data structure for user modeling, context-awareness and resource-adaptive computing. In: ABIS (2003)
7. Heckmann, D., Schwartz, T., Brandherm, B., Schmitz, M., von Wilamowitz-Moellendorff, M.: Gumo – The General User Model Ontology. In: Ardissono, L., Brna, P., Mitrović, A. (eds.) UM 2005. LNCS (LNAI), vol. 3538, pp. 428–432. Springer, Heidelberg (2005)
8. Heckmann, D., Krueger, A.: A User Modeling Markup Language (UserML) for Ubiquitous Computing. In: Brusilovsky, P., Corbett, A.T., de Rosis, F. (eds.) UM 2003. LNCS, vol. 2702, pp. 393–397. Springer, Heidelberg (2003)
9. Margetis, G., Antona, M., Ntoa, S., Stephanidis, C.: Towards Accessibility in Ambient Intelligence Environments. In: Paternò, F., de Ruyter, B., Markopoulos, P., Santoro, C., van Loenen, E., Luyten, K. (eds.) AmI 2012. LNCS, vol. 7683, pp. 328–337. Springer, Heidelberg (2012)
10. Martinez-Villaseñor, L.M., Gonzalez-Mendoza, M., Hernandez-Gress, N.: Towards a Ubiquitous User Model for Profile Sharing and Reuse. In: Sensors (2012)
11. Martini, R.G., Librelotto, G.R.: Uma abordagem para a personalização automática de interfaces de usuário para dispositivos móveis em Ambientes Pervasivos. In: SEMISH, Curitiba, Brazil (2012)
12. Miñón, R., Abascal, J., Aizpurua, A., Cearreta, I., Gamecho, B., Garay, N.: Model-Based Accessible User Interface Generation in Ubiquitous Environments. In: Campos, P., Graham, N., Jorge, J., Nunes, N., Palanque, P., Winckler, M. (eds.) INTERACT 2011, Part IV. LNCS, vol. 6949, pp. 572–575. Springer, Heidelberg (2011)
13. Nakajima, T., et al.: Middleware design issues for ubiquitous computing. In: MUM 2004, pp. 55–62. ACM, New York (2004)
14. Newman, M., et al.: Designing for Serendipity: Supporting End-User Configuration of Ubiquitous Computing Environments. In: Proceedings of ACM DIS 2002 (2002)
15. Saha, D., Mukherjee, A.: Pervasive computing: a paradigm for the 21st century, pp. 25–31. IEEE Computer Society, New York (2003)
16. Schilit, B.N., Theimer, M.M.: Disseminating active map information to mobile hosts. IEEE Network, 22–32 (1994)
17. Schmidt, A.: Context-Aware Computing: Context-Awareness, Context-Aware User Interfaces, and Implicit Interaction. The Encyclopedia of Human-Computer Interaction (2013)
18. Sousa, J.P., Garlan, D.: Aura: an Architectural Framework for User Mobility in Ubiquitous Computing Environments. In: Proceeding of the 3rd Working IEEE/IFIP Conference on Software Architecture, Montreal (2002)
19. Tandler, P.: Software Infrastructure for Ubiquitous Computing Environments: Supporting Synchronous Collaboration with Heterogeneous Devices. In: Abowd, G.D., Brumitt, B., Shafer, S. (eds.) UbiComp 2001. LNCS, vol. 2201, p. 96. Springer, Heidelberg (2001)
20. Vanderheiden, G.: Anywhere, Anytime (+Anyone) Access to the Next-generation WWW. In: Computer Networks and ISDN Systems, pp. 1439–1446 (1997)
21. Yamin, A.C.: Arquitetura para um Ambiente de Grade Computacional Direcionado às Aplicações Distribuídas, Móveis e Conscientes do Contexto da Computação Pervasiva. Thesis (Ph.D. In: Computer Science) - Institute of Informatics, UFRGS, Brazil (2004)
22. Weiser, M.: The Computer for the 21st Century, pp. 94–104. Scientific American (1991)

A Comparative Study to Evaluate the Usability of Context-Based Wi-Fi Access Mechanisms

Matthias Budde, Till Riedel, Marcel Köpke,
Matthias Berning, and Michael Beigl

TECO, Karlsruhe Institute of Technology (KIT), Karlsruhe, Germany
budde@teco.edu
http://www.teco.edu/~budde

Abstract. This paper presents a comparative study of six different tag and context based authentication schemes for open Wi-Fi access. All of the implemented methods require only a smartphone and an *HTML5* capable webbrowser, making them interchangeable and easy to incorporate into existing infrastructure. We recruited 22 participants for the study and used two standardized questionnaires as well as additional metrics to assess whether further investment in a systematic usability analysis seems prudent. The evaluation shows that suitable alternatives for Wi-Fi authentication exist and points out their limitations and opportunities.

Keywords: Universal Access, Practical Security, Usability, User Experience, User Study, Interfaces, Device Association, Authentication, Wi-Fi, Smart Environments, Context.

1 Introduction

Future computing environments – as driven by the notions of ubiquitous computing and ambient intelligence – are expected to give rise to information technology that is embedded in everyday life and is spontaneously formed from ubiquitous devices, objects, and services that we can easily access. While humans understand how to access physical resources at their disposal, it is often harder in a digital world. Accessible digital resources are a key factor to assistance and inclusion, especially in public spaces. Open Wi-Fi access, e.g. through hotspots, creates many issues (access control, liability and legal issues) on the user and institutional side, as malicious parties cannot be kept out of the network. This is why today, usually username and password, entered into a web interface (a.k.a. *captive portal*), are required to access wireless infrastructure.

Providing seamless wireless network service is not only about network quality but also about user experience and ease of access has become an important factor for quality of life. Adding an extra burden on users – particularly technically non-literate users or ones with special needs – actually excludes many people from access, especially when using complicated *username:password* schemes with media breaks. As a step towards the proliferation of accessible networks, this work evaluates the usability of ways for associating handheld devices to Wi-Fi networks, while also regarding implementation and practical feasibility.

C. Stephanidis and M. Antona (Eds.): UAHCI/HCII 2014, Part III, LNCS 8515, pp. 451–462, 2014.
© Springer International Publishing Switzerland 2014

2   Related Work

A great variety of schemes have been proposed in the past to pair mobile devices for spontaneous interaction, many of which could also be applied for the use case of authenticating to a Wi-Fi hotspot. One solution proposed is the use of Out-of-Band (OOB) information to establish a shared secret. Holmquist et al. [6] as well as Mayrhofer et al. [12] proposed to couple devices using their accelerometers by shaking them simultaneously. This, however, is not easily applicable to systems involving static infrastructure. A method to generate a shared secret from ambient audio was investigated by Sigg et al. [16]. These technical publications do not take human factors into account, which we targeted in this work. Several other authors conducted comparative user studies on the usability of device pairing or Wi-Fi setup. Kostiainen et. al. [9] used formative interviews to assess user needs in home network access control and proposed a conceptual system for setup and management. Both Uzun et. al. [18] and Kainda et al. [8] analyzed device pairing by different textual interfaces. Kumar et. al. [10] included variants of eight device pairing methods in a large study implemented on a common platform. The usability assessment is mostly based on automatically logged user actions with no qualitative feedback. Ion et al. [7] used mock-ups to investigate the usability of device pairing methods with regard to perceived security needs in different real-life situation. Their findings indicate that the usability as well as user preference depend on the context of the pairing situation.

3   Methodology

In this work, we conducted a user study to explore six different methods suitable to replace classic *username:password* authentication for public Wi-Fi. In addition to token based methods we adapted we adapted two relevant OOB techniques and included a recent approach using surface-confined Wi-Fi [3] as context based methods. The methods were selected to fulfill the following constraints:

- *Non-mediated*: The user can perform the login at any time by himself.
- *Intuitive*: Wi-Fi hotspots are broadly used by ordinary non-expert users.
- *Platform-independent*: Mobile devices and OSs are diverse and volatile.
- *Explicit*: The system can record consent of the user when connecting.

The last constraint distinguishes the evaluated methods from access control based on *Geofencing* [14] or overprovisioning [4], which both allow confining Wi-Fi networks to certain physical boundaries, enabling location based access. Although it can be argued that *implicit* access is generally preferable, additional to fulfilling legal contstraints, the proposed explicit methods do not require overprovisioning in the infrastructure and are therefore also deployable in an light-weight and interchangable fashion.

For platform-independence, we selected methods that can solely be implemented using web technology, thus easily be adapted to user needs and incorporated into *captive portals*. For this paper we implemented all on top of *HTML5* features like `GetUserMedia()` and `GetDeviceMotion()`. This has the aditional benefit that the schemes are interchangeable and a set of different methods can be offered to respect user preferences or hardware constraints. The source code of the implementations will be released as part of the *Global Public Inclusive Infrastructure* (GPII) component repository and are freely available[1].

Username:password. This authentication scheme is well-known and standard today. A user enters his credentials into a form and presses a login-button to gain access. We included it as a base line and to back the obvious hypothesis that this scheme is not well suited for handheld devices.

QR Codes. By encoding a URL containing the login credentials into a QR code it can be scanned with any camera phone. We accessed the camera image through *HTML5* and decoded it using a *JavaScript* library (*jsqrcode*).

NFC. Login information can also be stored as URL in a *Near Field Communication* (NFC) tag and accessed remotely with many modern phones. An alternative would have been NFC-based *Wi-Fi Protected Setup*, which we refrained from using due to known vulnerabilities [19] and lacking personalizability.

2DST Sheet. A detailed description of the *Two-Dimensional Signal Transmission* (2DST) waveguide sheet was published in previous work [3]. To log on, users connect to the open Wi-Fi and the *captive portal* page prompts them to place the device on the sheet (see Figure 1) and acknowledge the coupling. The device can subsequently be removed from the sheet and access is granted.

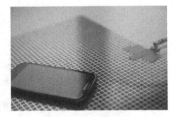

Fig. 1. Phone on 2DST sheet

Kinect. We adapted the *Point&Control* system [2] that uses the *Microsoft Kinect* (first generation) for user-device association based on the user context. The *captive portal* page prompts the user to press a button and raise an arm to connect. If the gesture is matched by the Kinect, access is granted. For this usability test we used this very simple scheme, that does not match the accelerometer pattern of the phone with the *Kinect* model for added contextual prove, which is possible on most modern devices also using *HTML5* [5].

Audio Context. The last context-based method employs ambient audio as OOB channel, as used in *Pintext* paring [16]. The entropy of generated fingerprints generally makes them suitable to be used as a shared secret [15]. To log in, a user presses a button on the *captive portal* and both phone and server record for eight seconds. A server synchronizes[2] both recordings, calculates fingerprints and compares them. If they are sufficiently similar, access is granted.

---

[1] https://github.com/teco-kit
[2] In our tests synchronization significantly slowed down this scheme, as acurate time sync could not be realized in *HTML*.

3.1   Task and Session Structure

Participants were asked to connect to an open Wi-Fi, authenticate their device using the given mechanism and open a browser to access a web page. For this, they were given a *Samsumg Galaxy SIII* smartphone, which supported all of the six methods. The test sessions were conducted in an office at our lab – in German or English, depending on the subject's preference. Participants were welcomed and guided to the test room one at a time (1-on-1 moderated sessions, see Figure 2). The test's setup and intention were introduced and subjects read and signed a privacy statement. Subsequently, the moderator collected demographic data (age, gender, etc.) and some information on the subject's habits regarding technology use (frequency of handheld Wi-Fi access, usage of public Wi-Fi hotspots, etc.) by means of a pre-test questionnaire. After that, the main phase of the test commenced: Subjects, in turn, completed the task – i.e. log on to the Wi-Fi and open a website – for each method and fill in a questionnaire. The order of the six methods was shuffled to avoid biases from practice or fatigue. Each method was explained beforehand and written descriptions of how to proceed were available throughout the test. After repeating the three steps for each method, the participant was asked to fill in the post-test questionnaire. Sessions took between 52 and 100 minutes, with an average of 69 minutes.

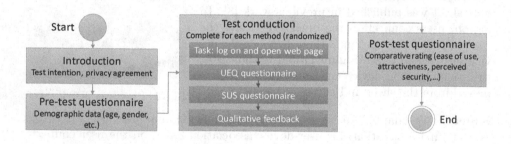

Fig. 2. Session structure each participant ran through during the user study

3.2   Participants

We recruited 22 participants aged between 20 and 48, eight of them female. All of them attended voluntarily without being offered a reward. Figure 3 shows the data on demographics and participants' habits collected using the pre-test questionnaire. The subjects composed a well-educated group, accustomed to the use of mobile devices and working in different fields, the majority pursuing technical professions. None were security experts. All participants reported accessing the Internet once or more per day. Most (14) also daily used handheld mobile devices to connect to Wi-Fi networks, some weekly (3). Three participants said that they rarely accessed Wi-Fi with a handheld device and two never at all. Most subjects often used public Wi-Fi hotspots, only one never did, and two rarely. All others

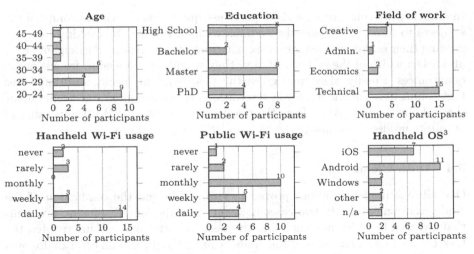

Fig. 3. (Top) Participants by age, completed level of education and field of work or studies. (Bottom) Frequency of Wi-Fi network access with a handheld device respectively using open Wi-Fi hotspots, as well OS's installed on subjects' personal devices[3].

accessed public Wi-Fis at least monthly, four even daily. Overall, the subject group is suitable for an initial assessment of the selected methods, as they are digitally literate and familiar with the presented task.

3.3   Questionnaire Design

The study we conducted is mostly summative, with additional formative aspects. We were looking to find out whether the proposed solutions could in principle satisfy user needs. To quickly assess both usability and user experience of the tested schemes, we considered different standardized questionnaires. The *System Usability Scale (SUS)* [1] has been applied to a wide range of systems in the past 20 years, from printers over phones to desktop and web applications. Subjects express their level of agreement to ten simple statements using a five-point Likert. It is slim, short term viable and yields a single score as result, which is already generalizable at relatively small sample sizes [17]. As alternative, we looked at the *User Experience Questionnaire (UEQ)* [11]. It consists of 26 pairs of opposing attributes (e.g. *annoying* and *enjoyable*). Users express their agreement with them on a seven-point Likert. The UEQ yields six different scores for the categories *attractiveness, perspicuity, dependability, efficiency, stimulation,* and *novelty.* We decided to use both UEQ and SUS, as they can be filled in quickly and we were interested to see if they yielded consistent results, since the SUS focuses on usability while the UEQ aims at assessing the whole user experience.

Aside from summative data from the two questionnaires, we also collected three to five qualitative statements about what the subjects liked and disliked about each system. All of this was done separately for each of the methods.

---

[3] Three participants chose multiple options.

In addition, we constructed a short post-test questionnaire which prompted the subjects to directly compare the systems with each other, by ranking them regarding their ease of use, perceived security and attractiveness. Participants were also asked which of the systems (if any) they would recommend to friends or acquaintances. Finally, they were given the possibility to specify additional free text comments. The moderator also recorded any unprompted statements made throughout the test. Aside from the questionnaires, we recorded the number of attempts needed to complete the task and the time to do so.

3.4 Data Cleansing

Overall, our implementations proved to run stably and the conduction of the study went smoothly. In two cases however, we experienced software problems that led to difficulties in completing the task: A software crash interrupted the task completion in six cases of the *Audio Context* login and an error dialog was shown. In these cases, the task was repeated and participants were instructed to disregard the first failed attempt. Failed tries were not included in the results for task times or number of attempts. In two instances involving the 2DST sheet, a software bug prevented the correct recognition of the device by the sheet, leading to an unusually high number of tries (12 respectively 8 attempts). To avoid skewed results, the data from these two runs was removed from the set.

Regarding the final three ranking questions, subjects explicitly were given the option to rank two systems equally by assigning the same ordinal number. However this lead to some participants using *competition ranking* (i.e. leaving a gap in the ranking when several systems tied) and others using *dense ranking* (no gaps). To reach a realistic ranking when averaging over all participants, we transformed the data to *fractional ranking* scores, as those have the property that the ranking numbers' sum is the same as under strict ordinal ranking.

4 Results

This section presents the results of our analyses. First, we show the quantitative metrics (attempts, task time), followed by the SUS and UEQ scores. Finally, comparative statements and qualitative feedback ratings are presented.

4.1 Quantitative Performance Metrics

Table 1 shows the number of attempts and the time needed to perform the login task (both overall and averaged per attempt). NFC was the only scheme which took all subjects only one attempt, all others had to be repeated at least once by at least one participant. While this was seldomly necessary for *username:password* (2, mistyping) and *Audio Context* (4, fingerprints too different), it happened more often with the 2DST sheet (6, device removed from sheet to early). More than a third of the subjects had to repeat their attempt using QR codes (8, recognition failed) or the *Kinect* (9, tracking failed). Regarding task

Table 1. Automatically collected metrics (sorted by median time per attempt)

Meth.	# Attempts					Task time (overall)					Task time (per attempt)				
	min	max	med.	mean	conf.[4]	min	max	med.	mean	conf.	min	max	med.	mean	conf.
NFC	1	1	1	1.00	n/a	2s	15s	6s	6.5s	1.36	2s	15s	6s	6.5s	1.36
Kinect	1	4	1	1.64	0.38	7s	57s	11s	19.3s	5.66	7s	17s	10s	10.5s	1.16
2DST	1	3	1	1.45	0.33	7s	56s	14s	19.3s	5.81	7s	34s	11s	13.2s	2.65
QR	1	3	1	1.55	0.33	10s	91s	33s	44.9s	11.90	6s	81s	26s	30.4s	7.51
Pwd	1	2	1	1.09	0.42	34s	153s	51s	60.3s	1.67	34s	111s	51s	54.4s	1.25
Audio	1	2	1	1.18	0.17	77s	381s	126s	157.3s	33.43	77s	215s	119s	130.3s	16.25

times, all methods except *Audio Context* performed significantly faster than entering passwords. Again, NFC stood out, closely followed by *Kinect* and 2DST sheet. The use of QR codes still took only half the time of entering text credentials, while the audio login took much longer due to the long processing times.

4.2 SUS and UEQ Scores

Figure 4 and Table 2 show the UEQ category results, the overall UEQ score as well as the SUS score over all participants. When looking at SUS scores, a percentile rank of below 60.0 is considered poor and an indicator for severe usability problems, while values over 80.0 are generally good [17], 100.0 being the maximum possible. Regarding the UEQ score, values below -0.8 indicate a negative rating, over 0.8 a positive one, and in between neutral. However, Schrepp et al. [13] point out that the actual interpretation of the ratings depends on the weight of the categories in the concrete application and intended user group. For normal end users, they regard *attractiveness* as most important, followed by *perspicuity* and *dependability*, and thirdly *efficiency*. The authors also provide a benchmark which is based on 163 studies with a total of 4818 participants and sets the score boundary between above-average and below-average different for the individual categories (*attractiveness*: 1.09, *perspicuity*: 0.9, *dependability*: 1.06, *efficiency*: 0.84 , *stimulation*: 1.0, and *novelty*: 0.63).

Basing our interpretations on these preliminary considerations, the ratings show a slightly different picture than the performance metrics before: Judging from the SUS scores, for *Kinect* and QR, no compelling conclusion can be drawn from the SUS score. Both NFC and the 2DST sheet login can be considered good systems with no apparent usability problems, while *Audio Context* seems to have severe issues. *Username:password* barely scores better than ambient audio, only just exceeding 60.0 points.

When looking at the UEQ, we see a difference between the overall UEQ and the SUS score: The overall UEQ rating for the *Kinect* based system is better than that of QR codes, and *Audio Context* scores higher than *username:password*.

Regarding the most relevant UEQ categories, the use of passwords scores high in the categories *perspicuity* and *dependability*, while receiving low ratings for *attractiveness* and *efficiency*. This illustrates the additional information that can be drawn from the UEQ scores. Similar observations can be made for the

---

[4] All confidence intervals (±) in this work are constructed at a 95% confidence level.

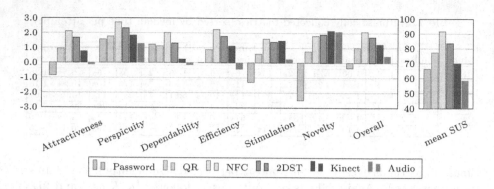

Meth.	UEQ category scores						SUS score		
	attrac.	perspic.	depend.	effic.	stimul.	novel.	median	mean conf.	
	mean conf.	mean conf.	mean conf.	mean conf.	mean conf.	mean conf.			
Pwd	**-0.85** 0.45	1.56 0.50	1.22 0.31	0.00 0.51	-1.30 0.41	-2.50 0.32	63.8	66.3 6.02	
QR	0.94 0.48	1.76 0.33	1.11 0.41	0.88 0.46	0.59 0.41	0.76 0.44	73.8	77.7 5.56	
NFC	**2.11** 0.36	**2.72** 0.21	**2.02** 0.40	2.24 0.39	1.60 0.37	1.81 0.40	**95.0**	**91.6** 4.45	
2DST	**1.67** 0.38	**2.31** 0.34	1.30 0.45	1.78 0.35	1.39 0.45	1.90 0.45	**86.3**	**83.5** 4.72	
Kinect	0.75 0.60	1.83 0.43	**0.22** 0.50	1.13 0.38	1.48 0.40	2.16 0.29	72.5	69.9 7.67	
Audio	-0.12 0.60	**1.27** 0.48	-0.15 0.32	-0.42 0.39	0.24 0.42	2.10 0.41	55.0	58.5 8.70	

Fig. 4. and Table 2. Mean UEQ scores and confidence per category (left) and mean and median SUS scores (right) for each Wi-Fi access method.

other systems: While the QR method scores more or less average in all remaining categories, it performs well regarding *perspicuity*. Both NFC and the 2DST sheet login clearly score high in all categories. According to the UEQ scores, the main shortcoming of the *Kinect* scheme is *dependability*, which is in line with the observations made from the performance metric *number of attempts* while the *efficiency* score adequately reflects the short completion times of the scheme. *Audio context* scores badly across the board, with the exception of the categories *perspicuity* and *novelty*. An aspect clearly differing from the performance metrics are the non-task related hedonic quality aspects, that express how *novel* and *stimulating* users percieve a system to be [11]. Not surprising, the password scheme has a very low rating here, while the context-based methods score high.

4.3   Comparison and Preferences

The last section of the post-test questionnaire specifically prompted the users to rank the six methods compared to each other. The resulting ranking (see Figure 5) is consistent for the two aspects *usability* and *attractiveness*: NFC clearly spearheads, followed by the 2DST sheet, QR codes, *Kinect* and then *Audio Context*. The classic *username:password* scheme came out last. The rankings so far are in agreement with the UEQ *attractiveness* rating.

Interestingly, the *perceived security* ranking paints a different picture: Generally, participants felt that the token based methods were more secure than the context-based schemes (see Figure 5).

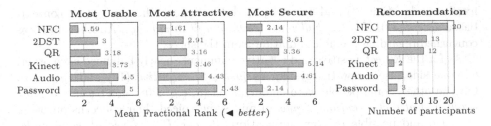

Fig. 5. Subjective ranking of the methods regarding usability, perceived security and attractiveness (left) and which schemes participants would recommend (right)

Altogether, almost all (20) participants stated that they would recommend NFC as Wi-Fi access method to friends or acquaintances. More than half would recommend using QR codes (12) or the 2DST sheet for contextual access (13). Notably, despite the otherwise rather poor ratings of the audio based scheme, still five participants would recommend the system, more than the classic password (3) or the *Kinect* based scheme (2).

4.4   Qualitative Statements and User Feedback

As expected, the study confirmed that *username:password* credentials are not suitable for Wi-Fi authentication on mobile devices. While users rate the method as *intuitive* (8) and secure (10), almost all users said that *smartphones are inadequate for entering random strings* (18). As unique property, subjects saw that *text is memorizable* (*P06*), providing an abstract token. Regarding QR codes, we observed that opinions were divided: Participants both describe the method to be *intuitive* (15) and *complicated* (9) as well as *fast* and *slow* (9 each). Some (6) also stated that they either experienced or anticipated problems in bad lighting. (*P07: the shadows of hand and phone interfered*). Regarding the necessary permission for the browser to access the camera, *P22* reported: *giving deep system access without exactly knowing what is going on makes me uneasy.*

Concerning NFC, participants predominantly gave positive comments (see Table 3): Most subjects characterized it as *intuitive* (18) and *fast* (17). However, a few users (5) also voiced technical concerns, ranging from fear of high energy consumption (*P14: NFC always on?*) or losing the tag to security concerns, as the phone did not ask permission before opening the webpage. Participant *P01* also specifically disapproved that *one has to use both hands.* Some users (4) also pointed out that not every device features NFC (e.g. *P15: my iPhone doesn't have an RFID reader*).

Table 3. Amount of positive and negative comments (both prompted and unprompted)

Method	Pos.	Neg.	Ratio
NFC	82	25	3.28
2DST	73	37	1.97
QR	57	48	1.19
Kinect	70	62	1.13
Passwd	46	47	0.98
Audio	48	78	0.62

Regarding the 2DST sheet, users reported that it was *innovative/cool* (6) as well as *fast* (13) and *easy* (21) – emphasizing that they needed to do very little (*P06: that's it?*). Some users perceived the system as limited in terms of being fixed to a location (3) and one subject did not grasp the concept of context-based access (*P01: big and bulky and would not fit in my bag*). Another user was concerned regarding possible radiation from the sheet.

As for the *Kinect*, positive and negative comments nearly balanced each other: On one side, users saw the system as *fast* (13), *intuitive* (14) and *cool* (13). On the other, some people were embarrassed (8, e.g. *P08: don't want to jump about and attract attention in public*) and some voiced their concerns on being recorded and possible privacy implications (2, e.g. *P05: sense of being under surveillance*). Others again liked the aspect of performing an activity in order to log on (8). Regarding the *Ambient Audio* login, the users' main issue was the *long wait* (21), followed by technical concerns, such as interference from *handling noises* or unreliability in *silent ambiences* (2, e.g. *P11: especially problematic for mutes*). Four users expressed disbelief that the method would work at all (*P13: I have the feeling that this will often fail*). Regarding the security, the method felt both *insecure* (5, e.g. *P18: I guess that many false positives occur*) and *very secure* (4) to the users. As with the *Kinect*, privacy concerns were also expressed (2). On the other hand, participants characterized the system as *innovative* (8) and *intuitive/magic* (12, e.g. *P07: great, I don't have to do anything*).

General comments mostly concerned lack of understanding regarding context-based access applicability (e.g. *P18: I don't see use cases, except maybe in trains*).

5   Discussion

We implemented six *HTML5*-based techniques for associating handheld devices to Wi-Fi networks and evaluated them regarding their usability. As expected, it backed that *username:password* credentials are unsuitable for handheld Wi-Fi access, and that the other five schemes may – to a varying degree – present viable alternatives.

Our study yielded some interesting results: A general observation is that purely summative studies may not reflect the full range of relevant aspects. Although both SUS and UEQ seem suitable to determine if severe issues exist, caution should be exercised when using them to rank systems. While we can see that they generally show similar tendencies, the UEQ addresses the whole user experience and its categories can provide helpful additional insights regarding the area possible problems may reside in. This is especially true for systems whose SUS score lies in the "gray area" between 60.0 and 80.0 percent. Placing too much emphasis on mere speed or completion rates as a factor may be misleading as well, especially in the context of usable security. In this area, it is important to augment standard usability testing with some metric that specifically addresses aspects like perceived security, trust, etc.

The multitude of different user statements revealing interesting issues – both actual and perceived – underlines the importance of also collecting qualitative feedback. While for the two best performing schemes (NFC and 2DST) most metrics are in agreement with each other, singular issues are revealed by other metrics, such as qualitative feedback for NFC or the number of attempts with the sheet. For some methods, only the full range of metrics paints an adequate picture for the assessment of the system, especially those on which opinions are divided: The *Kinect* achieved average to high summative ratings and the second to best completion times, but subjects perceived it as insecure and least recommended it. As for the *Audio Context* scheme, despite mostly bad ratings and performance, more than half of the subjects regarded it as intuitive and almost a quarter would recommend it. This illustrates that multiple metrics also allow discerning between fundamental issues and specific problems that can e.g. be attributed to the implementation and may be remedied in the future.

An important realization regarding methods involving cameras or microphones was that many participants voiced their concerns on being recorded and possible privacy implications, as well as a sense of being under surveillance. We conclude that systems involving video or audio recording should probably be avoided, and if such methods are considered, it is important to convey to the users that their privacy is protected. Furthermore, deep system access by web apps (e.g. camera or sensor access or automatically opening scanned URLs) should be transparent and only occur with user consent. When considering methods involving visible activity, embarrassment is an important factor, even if the *Kinect* based scheme caused both positive and negative feedback regarding the activity. We conclude that the applicability of such a system depends strongly on the situation, user group and maybe also cultural aspects. As a design guideline for systems that involve little interaction (*Ambient Audio*) and/or losing focus of the screen (as sometimes seen with *Kinect* or *2DST*), non-visual feedback such as an auditory signal is advisable to indicate success of the association process.

6   Conclusion and Future Work

We believe that good integration of classic usability studies and metric based analyses, as well as an analysis of other requirements on the user side (hardware features, OS, etc.) and the operators side (infrastructure, maintenance cost, etc.) needs to be conducted in order to come to a meaningful assessment of the viability of a method. As we collected very different statements regarding concerns and the acceptance of systems from technically versed and unseasoned users, we conclude that usable security systems should ideally be evaluated in a real-world context to assess which methods users would actually choose and keep using.

In future work we plan to study the most suitable methods addressing especially technically non-literate users and users with special needs. We also plan to further evaluate the barriers that hinder including novel, multimodal *HTML*-based context and user sensing methods – such as the alternative login methods presented in this work – in real applications. This includes further assessment of the potential of basing such systems on web technology, as this makes systems easy to interchange or include into existing applications in a modular fashion.

Acknowledgements. This work was partially funded by the European Union under project *Prosperity4All*, grant *610510*. We thank Daniel Karl for his implementation support as well as all study participants, especially Klaus Rümmele and his staff.

References

1. Brooke, J.: SUS - A quick and dirty usability scale. Usability Evaluation in Industry 189 (1996)
2. Budde, M., Berning, M., Baumgärtner, C., Kinn, F., Kopf, T., Ochs, S., Reiche, F., Riedel, T., Beigl, M.: Point & Control – Interaction in Smart Environments: You Only Click Twice. In: UbiComp 2013 Adjunct., pp. 303–306. ACM (2013)
3. Budde, M., Köpke, M., Berning, M., Riedel, T., Beigl, M.: Using a 2DST waveguide for usable, physically constrained out-of-band Wi-Fi authentication. In: 2013 ACM Conference on Pervasive and Ubiquitous Computing, pp. 221–224. ACM (2013)
4. Faria, D.B., Cheriton, D.R.: No long-term secrets: Location-based security in over-provisioned wireless lans. In: Hot Topics in Networks (HotNets-III) (2004)
5. Hauber, M., Bachmann, A., Budde, M., Beigl, M.: jActivity: Supporting Mobile Web Developers with HTML5/JavaScript Based Human Activity Recognition. In: 12th International Conference on Mobile and Ubiquitous Multimedia. ACM (2013)
6. Holmquist, L., Mattern, F., Schiele, B., Alahuhta, P., Beigl, M., Gellersen, H.: Smart-Its Friends: A Technique for Users to Easily Establish Connections between Smart Artefacts. In: Abowd, G.D., Brumitt, B., Shafer, S. (eds.) UbiComp 2001. LNCS, vol. Ubicomp, p. 116. Springer, Heidelberg (2001)
7. Ion, I., Langheinrich, M., Kumaraguru, P., Čapkun, S.: Influence of User Perception, Security Needs, and Social Factors on Device Pairing Method Choices. In: SOUPS 2010. ACM (2010)
8. Kainda, R., Flechais, I., Roscoe, A.W.: Usability and security of out-of-band channels in secure device pairing protocols. In: SOUPS 2009 (2009)
9. Kostiainen, K., Rantapuska, O., Moloney, S., Roto, V., Holmstrom, U., Karvonen, K.: Usable access control inside home networks. In: WOWMOM, pp. 1–6 (2007)
10. Kumar, A., Saxena, N., Tsudik, G., Uzun, E.: A comparative study of secure device pairing methods. Pervasive and Mobile Computing 5(6), 734–749 (2009)
11. Laugwitz, B., Held, T., Schrepp, M.: Construction and evaluation of a user experience questionnaire. In: Holzinger, A. (ed.) USAB 2008. LNCS, vol. 5298, pp. 63–76. Springer, Heidelberg (2008)
12. Mayrhofer, R., Gellersen, H.-W.: Shake well before use: Authentication based on accelerometer data. In: LaMarca, A., Langheinrich, M., Truong, K.N. (eds.) Pervasive 2007. LNCS, vol. 4480, pp. 144–161. Springer, Heidelberg (2007)
13. Schrepp, M., Olschner, S., Schubert, U.: User Experience Questionnaire Benchmark Praxiserfahrungen zum Einsatz im Business-Umfeld. In: Usability Professionals 2013 (2013)
14. Sheth, A., Seshan, S., Wetherall, D.: Geo-fencing: Confining Wi-Fi coverage to physical boundaries. In: Tokuda, H., Beigl, M., Friday, A., Brush, A.J.B., Tobe, Y. (eds.) Pervasive 2009. LNCS, vol. 5538, pp. 274–290. Springer, Heidelberg (2009)
15. Sigg, S., Budde, M., Ji, Y., Beigl, M.: Entropy of Audio Fingerprints for Unobtrusive Device Authentication. In: Beigl, M., Christiansen, H., Roth-Berghofer, T.R., Kofod-Petersen, A., Coventry, K.R., Schmidtke, H.R. (eds.) CONTEXT 2011. LNCS, vol. 6967, pp. 296–299. Springer, Heidelberg (2011)
16. Sigg, S., Schuermann, D., Ji, Y.: PINtext: A Framework for Secure Communication Based on Context. In: Puiatti, A., Gu, T. (eds.) MobiQuitous 2011. LNICST, vol. 104, pp. 314–325. Springer, Heidelberg (2012)
17. Tullis, T., Albert, W.: Measuring the User Experience: Collecting, Analyzing, and Presenting Usability Metrics. Elsevier Science (2010)
18. Uzun, E., Karvonen, K., Asokan, N.: Usability analysis of secure pairing methods. In: Dietrich, S., Dhamija, R. (eds.) FC 2007 and USEC 2007. LNCS, vol. 4886, pp. 307–324. Springer, Heidelberg (2007)
19. Viehböck, S.: Brute forcing Wi-Fi Protected Setup. Wi-Fi Protected Setup (2011)

The FOOD Project: Interacting with Distributed Intelligence in the Kitchen Environment[*]

Laura Burzagli[1], Lorenzo Di Fonzo[1], Pier Luigi Emiliani[1], Laura Boffi[2], Jakob Bak[2], Caroline Arvidsson[2], Dominic Kristaly[3], Leonardo Arteconi[4], Guido Matrella[5], Ilaria De Munari[5], and Paolo Ciampolini[5]

[1] CNR-IFAC, via Madonna del Piano, 10 50019 Sesto Fiorentino (FI), Italy
[2] Copenhagen Institute of Interaction Design, Toldbodgade 37b, 1253, Copenhagen, Denmark
[3] Vision Systems SRL, Str. Aurel Vlaicu 61bis, 500188 Brasov, Romania
[4] Indesit Company SpA, via Lamberto Corsi 55, 60044 Fabriano (AN), Italy
[5] Università degli Studi di Parma, Parco Area delle Scienze 181/a, 43124 Parma, Italy
{l.burzagli,l.difonzo,p.l.emiliani}@ifac.cnr.it,
{l.boffi,j.bak,c.arvidsson}@ciid.dk,
kdominic@vision-systems.ro, Leonardo.Arteconi@indesit.com,
{guido.matrella,ilaria.demunari,paolo.ciampolini}@unipr.it

Abstract. Kitchen activities involve complex and articulate interactions with heterogeneous technologies and devices. In this paper, outcomes of the FOOD AAL-JP project are presented, related to the development of a kitchen environment implementing ambient-assisted-living features, aimed at increasing safety, autonomy, engagement and reward in dealing with food-related activities.

Keywords: ambient assisted living, smart kitchen, user-centered design.

1 Introduction

Many among daily living activities, are related to food: grocery shopping, food preparation, cooking, eating and kitchen washing-up are indeed a relevant share of the daily tasks. Besides its obvious link with health, food is important as a mean for social engagement as well: from time immemorial, having food together is a way for keeping and strengthening good relationships with family, friends or in more formal contexts. Also, food is a prominent cultural media, it is strongly connected to local cultural heritage, and is currently gaining more and more popularity in TV shows, books and magazines. Food impacts on daily life, therefore, well beyond its mere sustenance aspects. Notably also, food activities are among most complex daily living activities, very often requiring to the user considerable knowledge and mastering of a number of techniques, tools, appliances. Moreover, kitchen work implies several safety concerns (related to fire, flood, sharp tools, food preservation…). The altogether makes the management of kitchen activities a challenging and multi-faceted component of daily living, essential to support independent life and useful in fostering social participation.

---

[*] On behalf of the FOOD AAL-JP consortium.

C. Stephanidis and M. Antona (Eds.): UAHCI/HCII 2014, Part III, LNCS 8515, pp. 463–474, 2014.
© Springer International Publishing Switzerland 2014

Due to this, great effervescence is showing up in the market of kitchen appliance (so-called white goods). A growing number of ICT-enabled devices is coming out from research labs, and is approaching the user's market. Most innovative functions are related to appliance connectivity, remote operation and alternative user's interfaces (based on smartphones, tablet, or touch panels). Kitchen appliances, however, differ from most widespread consumer electronics with many respects. When considering a kitchen oven, for instance, interaction requirements are quite apart from those, e.g., of a personal portable audio device:

- The intended audience is much wider, including family members having different cooking and technology skills, different ages, feeding habits and preferences, and possibly dealing with disabilities and age-related impairments. This calls for the adoption of design-for-all principles, caring for usability and accessibility.
- The aimed lifetime of a kitchen appliance is usually much longer than most consumer electronic devices, possibly overpassing the lifespan of a given technology generation. Flexibility and re-configurability are needed to ensure consistent longevity to the on-board ICT components.
- Severe environmental conditions are to be accounted for. Due to heat, moist and dirt, rugged hardware is needed, and suitable interaction modes (e.g., hands free) have to be taken into account.
- Finally, kitchen daily routine usually implies interaction with more than one device: the adoption of a separate, independent (and possibly not uniform) interfaces schemes for each appliance is expensive, unpractical and unfriendly to the users. A more uniform and general approach needs to be implemented, this however requiring some standardization and interoperability efforts to designers and manufacturers.

The FOOD project, funded in the framework of the third call of Ambient Assisted Living Joint Program (AAL-JP), starts from the considerations above and aims at developing specific AAL services, dedicated to the kitchen environment, to support elderly people in carrying out food-related daily living activities and interacting with home appliances in a much simpler, safer and rewarding way. The project started in September, 2011and will last until February 2015. It involves 9 partners, coming from 5 European countries Denmark, (Italy, Romania, Sweden, The Netherlands).

A year-long pilot phase is just started, involving 30 households located in Italy, Romania and The Netherlands, in order to account for a wide variety of customs, cultural, social and economical features. The project is led by Indesit, a large company manufacturing white goods and ranking among lead positions in the European kitchen appliance market. Due to this, solutions devised within the project are being deployed in a truly market-oriented view, inherently accounting for sustainability and practicality.

2   FOOD Technology

The FOOD technical vision [1] is based on the seamless integration of sensors and "intelligent" appliances, aimed at offering innovative functionalities in the house, as well as Internet- based services and applications. Among them, specific emphasis is placed on enabling access, through a natural interface, to information and communication in different social environments.

The FOOD infrastructure includes first a field, peripheral layer of connected devices: environmental sensors and appliances communicate through a wireless network architecture, exploiting the IEEE 802.15.4/ZigBee protocol. The adoption of a wireless, standardized protocol reduces system intrusivity and allows for better interoperability, reconfigurability and flexibility. The main technical challenge, to this regard, was that of incorporating connectivity features within white goods, coping with tight cost constraints of a highly competitive market and with inherent safety needs. Two alternative approaches were followed: with reference to high-end, electronic-intensive machines, such as ovens, washing and dish-washing machines, connectivity is obtained by deploying a networking node within the on-board control electronics of the appliance. This enables bi-directional user interaction, i.e., status monitoring as well as active control are made possible. Within the FOOD project, a "smart oven" has been designed and introduced, based on such an approach.

Simpler devices, involving little or no active control needs (e.g. a fridge) have been monitored through external "add-ons", i.e., sensor boxes providing information about the appliance status without actually being part of the appliance itself. For instance, a small box placed inside the refrigerator allow for inferring opening of the door, internal temperature and humidity; in case of fridge replacement, the box can be easily moved to the new appliance, thus not adding to the appliance cost itself. Similarly, a sensor box is placed close to the hob plate, allowing for monitoring its status. Other environmental sensors account for safety monitoring (flood, fire/smoke, gas leak) and for tracking user interaction (presence sensors, door/drawer opening sensors).

Through the ZigBee network, data coming from the field are gathered at a central unit: here, data are abstracted, i.e., meaningful information is made independent of the actual physical sensor details. To this purpose, a suitable data structure has been devised, based on a basic ontology of the kitchen scenario. Data are stored in a database, which in turn enables supervision of the system and feeds a service-oriented architecture, providing local and remote services with web services for interacting with the system. User interfaces, therefore, access the system knowledge base in a standardized way, possibly allowing for multi modal interaction and for interoperability. Mostly important, through abstraction, kitchen related information converge within a unique interface scheme, almost independent of the actual control panels of each appliance, thus making it possible to control a variety of devices in a uniform, homogeneous fashion.

3   FOOD Services

Based on the infrastructure described so far, the FOOD project envisages a number of services related to feeding activities: besides more straightforward tasks (such as shopping list compilation, recipes management, etc.) the project aim at providing the users with innovative functions, preserving independence in daily life and eliciting inclusive potentials of food-related matters. A first service classification was made, based on the involved networking level and of the interface features; four main levels of services were identified:

Table 1.

Level	Short description	Interface	Example
0 **Basic**	Stand-alone services provided by sensors or basic functionalities of household appliances.	Sound alert/appliance display	Oven lock door Flood alarm
1 **Intermediate**	Services based on data provided by household appliances and processed locally by the gateway	Appliances displays or external display	Energy consumption monitoring, appliance status check, reminders, shopping list compilation
2 **External**	Services with external providers	External display, Internet connection	e-commerce, social network
3 **Advanced**	Services combining appliance data and external providers	Tablet, PC, mobile, TV	See examples below

To design such services, a user-centered approach was exploited: however, a simple assessment of "user's needs", to be translated into system requirements, was felt to be ineffective in guiding the design process, since the project was not meant to just identify and improve actual weaknesses in the elderly daily life or current kitchen technology dedicated to them. A holistic approach was pursued instead, looking at kitchen activities in the more general framework of lifestyle and daily tasks, and investigating their links to physical and mental wellbeing.

At the beginning of FOOD project an extensive field work in Italy, The Netherlands and Romania was carried out, aiming at meeting elderly in their own context (their home, neighborhood, and city) and at gaining insights on the process of ageing through direct observation and interaction. More specifically, their perspectives on food, food preparation, eating, shopping, cooking and social aspects of food were investigated: *what motivates elderly to cook and eat? What role does food play in relation to their health and physical and mental activities?*
Insights were gathered and organized, clustering them in categories (planning food, getting grocery, cooking, eating, storing food) and enabling the partnership to identify a set of emerging "opportunity areas":

- **Proactive behavior against ageing watersheds:** elderly challenges their brain and body with activities that are undermined by the aging, from filling crosswords to refresh their cognitive capability to going out to the day care to keep a social life.
- **Keeping elderly involved in their context as active characters:** being aware of services and possibilities offered in their neighborhood works as a motivation to make advantage and take part to their local community.

- **Freedom to find their own custom solution:** in order to suit their needs and overcome their limits, elderly evolve new behaviors and adapt their environment and equipment to them.
- **Food as a touch point of elderly social life:** around food, elderly enact their active role in the family and may rediscover a social life in seniority.
- **Support network as a scaffolding for elderly:** elderly reorganize their social network according to the help and support they need, often making neighbors and shop keepers become more crucial than relatives.

Based on this, a number of scenarios were described, suitable for evaluating potential services to be implemented and their impact on users' daily lives. A number of actions involving the FOOD system are highlighted in the following:

Scenario 1: *Maria Rossi is 75 years old. She does not have any permanent disability, but a normal decrease of visual acuity and hearing. Sometimes, she forgets what she is supposed to do. In the morning, when she is waiting for the milk to warm, the fridge tells her: "Maria, did you forget that you invited your granddaughter and her husband for dinner tonight?" Maria does not want to admit it with the fridge and she replies that obviously she did not forget. However, can the fridge suggest a menu for the dinner? The fridge proposes a list of dishes, according to the tastes and dietary habits of the guests, who often have dinner with the grandparent. Maria replies that the menu is OK, but fish is too expensive due to the economic crisis. Can the fridge suggest a less expensive alternative? She agrees with the new proposal, but she asks the fridge to look for a new recipe, different from the one used some months ago. The fridge navigates trough the Web and selects some recipes that, according to its knowledge, the guests could like. After the selection made by Mrs. Rossi, the fridge, on the basis of the RFIDs on the available products, finds out what is lacking for the execution of the recipe. After the authorization by Mrs. Rossi, it connects with the supermarket, asks for the necessary goods and arranges a delivery time compatible with the preparation of the dinner. Finally, it programs itself for helping Mrs. Rossi in cooking at the right time and for activating the kitchen appliances (for example, for switching on the oven). In the meantime the gas is switched off before the milk can spill. The kitchen tells Mrs. Rossi that the milk is warm enough.*

Scenario 2: *Guido Bianchi's wife died some time ago. He is not expert with the housework and particularly with cooking. He is not seriously disabled, but he is slightly depressed and this reduces his attention about elementary actions, as switching off the gas or closing the door of the fridge. It happened yesterday evening and the fridge made him aware of the problem with a sound signal. Today at 1 p.m. he has not yet moved from the sofa to prepare lunch. The sensors that monitor activity near the stove inform the FOOD system, which in turn emits a speech signal to make Guido aware that it is lunch time. Then Guido stands up. His tablet, suitably programmed, suggests a recipe compatible with the diet suggested by his doctor for a person who is diabetic. The tablet on which Guido takes note of what food he bought and has eaten, confirms that he has at home all necessary ingredients. He starts to cook according to the single steps suggested by the tablet, but midway he has some doubts. He calls his daughter using Skype. He gets help for cooking and is also very* *happy to hear his daughter's voice. The food is ready. The gas is switched off. No alarm signal is audible. He sit down to eat, but before he calls the daughter to tell her that he was able to cook the food. Since the recipe is simple and the dish is tasty, he decide to* **share it on the network** *and asks other people's comments. The "network" friends are happy to be contacted, because it means that Guido is less depressed than yesterday.*

Scenario 3: *Giovanni and Vanda are old married people. Giovanni is becoming not self-sufficient, due to mild dementia. Therefore, Vanda, even if she suffers of cardiac and visual problems, is able to cope with the situation with the help of the children, who do not live with them. Moreover, Giovanni and Vanda are living in a small village and the neighbours are willing to help, for example taking care of the shopping or sharing time with Giovanni when Vanda has some urgent need outside home. The children are also able to help her remotely using the Skype videoconferencing system.*

At home, they have installed an intelligent control and communication systems, based on the computers in the appliances and an external service provider. The modern home appliances help Vanda in her everyday activities. The **interaction with them is simple**, *both using their panels or the tablet coming with them. With the tablet, she can also control them when she is not at home.*

They are also able to take care of the **power consumption**. *Giovanni was taking care of it, but now he not able any more. Moreover, the data* **are accessible also by the children**, *who can help if the parents spend more than their income allows. Moreover, security is not a problem as well. Water, gas and the running of the appliances are under control and the alarm signals are active.*

Every week the children, who have trained Vanda to use the home system, bring up to date the list of the activities to be carried out. They are shown at the right time on the tablet or on the display of the oven. The tablet allows her to enlarge the text on the screen and this is very useful due to her reduced visual ability.

She likes the home system. For example, she is not afraid any more to forget some medicament for the husband. **The home system takes care of reminding it.**

At the beginning, Vanda had some problems to accept the tablet, but now she is comfortable with it. It contains the **list of the shops**, *the list of what the family needs every week and with some effort from her side the list of what is really available at home. Shopping is easier. From the tablet she can* **call the shops** *or send a message. She has a set of standard messages, prepared by the children. They are able deal with her everyday needs. She is now accustomed to this virtual butler able to help in many tasks. Vanda leads a secluded life at home with the husband. She lacks the contact with her friends and she discusses this problem with the service provider. She likes to cook in general, but now there is the additional problem that she and the husband must follow specific regimens due to their illnesses. A* **service for the exchange of recipes** *is set up, based on video-telephony. She can discuss of food and recipes with friends,* **get the recipes from a common database**, *see what* **they are cooking in their kitchens**, *and show what she is doing thus giving the possibility to correct errors. She is in a community of people with the same interests and can be helped with her diet.*

Within the project, only a subset of functionalities suggested by the scenarios above have been implemented, due to time, costs and effort constraints: a number of possible services enabled by the FOOD environment were devised, classified according to the schemes above and to the involved system components, and eventually mapped onto the opportunity areas. A sample, non-exhaustive list of services may include:

Environmental Control: deals with safety and energy managements. Provides the user with safety warnings and alarms, and monitors current energy consumption of kitchen appliances, manages load balancing to prevent black-outs (due to excessive power request), task scheduling, e.g., according to hourly energy tariffs.

Food Management: includes management of databases related to available food and recipes, allowing the user to plan her/his meal according to what's actually available in the food storage, to dietary prescriptions and habits, and looking for suitable recipes.

Shopping: helps the user in compiling a shopping list and keeping track of the food inventory. Also, it may enable, depending on local conditions, access to e-commerce facility or connection to local grocery shops.

Cooking Companion: enable users (possibly suffering from mild cognitive impairments) to carry out cooking tasks by providing them with step by step guidance. Selected video recipes may be available in a video format, guiding the user though all subsequent steps. A suitable user interface is needed, and the system should be capable of getting feedback from appliances and sensors (just to check if the oven has been set at the appropriate temperature, for instance), in order to issue context-aware messages and automatically manage the video flow.

Wellness Monitor: information gathered from appliances and sensors are exploited to infer behavioral patterns, to be correlated with wellness and health conditions [2]. Simple checks can be carried out on the frequency of using main appliances: for instance, if the fridge has not been opened for two days, this may indicate lack of appropriate feeding. Not using stove/oven for a period may suggest loss of motivation/interest in eating/preparing food, etc. In a more general sense, an overall "kitchen activity" evaluation can be carried out, allowing for early identification of problems inducing functional and psychological decline. From repetitive/disordered activity patterns, also hints about possible cognitive issues can be worked out.

Senior Chef: is a social networking application for physical   neighborhood, aimed to create opportunities of engagement with local seniors in planning meals, shopping and eating together. FOOD technology is exploited for supporting networking activity.

Cooking Academy: is a cooking tutoring network run by elderly in favor of their peers, in order to   share their recipes, e.g.,   with foreign caregivers of   elderly, chef of elderly homes and single elderly who need/want to learn cooking in their late age.

Ready Steady Cook: oriented toward food education, exploits networking system facility to connect user's kitchen with professional chefs and nutritionists, sharing the cooking time and interactively guiding users toward rewarding experiences in preparing tasty and healthy foods.

Not all of the above service has been implemented yet, while all of them went through a subsequent development design step known as "service blueprinting" [3], whose aim is to map all the interested actors, touchpoints and technologies involved in a service onto an user journey.

4   Designing and Iterating the FOOD Services and Interfaces

4.1   The Process of Service Blueprinting

As IDEO service designer Fran Samalionis frames [3] when designing a service with a focus on whatever driver (may it be business, technology or customer), we need to bring along the whole process all the other dimensions that the user experience consists of. Failures happens as soon as we ignore or consciously leave out from the process actors, stakeholders, technologies, artifacts and interfaces that the service is constituted of. When designing a service, you are actually taking care of an ecology that needs to be nurtured, and not just survive, through every design decisions and implementations that is taken and carried out and through every interactions that happens at different levels among the components of the service.

In order to describe the service ecology, the tool known as "service blueprint" comes to help to map the various actors and components of the service and the interactions among them along time.

The service blueprint tool has been adopted by the FOOD consortium and partners teamed up in groups to address the services listed in section 3, working together and iterating the blueprints. A template to facilitate the blueprinting process has been developed and distributed to partners, with brief instructions on how to use it especially meant for those ones which were dealing with such a process for the first time.

The service blueprint starts with laying down an user journey in its timeline, step after step, revealing the hidden and less obvious ones we do not use to think of when we describing a service. For the FOOD project we envisioned that more than one user could be involved in a particular user journey, such as of course the elderly person, his/her caregiver, the shopkeeper, etc. depending on the service and the particular scenario we were considering (Fig. 1).

Soon after the user journey, we mapped the touchpoints, which are all the different tangibles through which an user accesses the service along its timeline and subsequent steps. For the FOOD services, the touchpoints cover a big range of possibilities: from the computer, the phone, the tablet and any kind of FOOD paper leaflet, to the kitchen appliances or alarms interfaces, such as the oven display (Fig.2).

It is essential to think of all the touchpoints in totality when we start describing a service in order to come up with a coherent system that fits the steps of the user journey and its logical sequence. Regarding what an user is aware of while using a service, the user journey and the touchpoints are known to him/her, that is why in the blueprint map they are placed above the so called "line of visibility", laying onto the "on stage" area of the map.

Below the line of visibility instead, laying in the "back-stage" area, all those actors and components of the service which are not immediately interacting and visible to the users stand, such as the FOOD system component (the oven, the sensors, etc), the medical doctor, the national health service, the FOOD nutritionist, just to give some few examples (Fig.3).

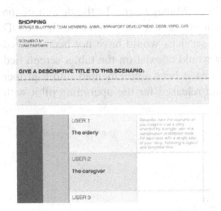

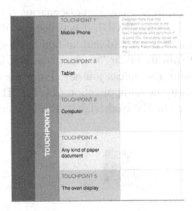

Fig. 1. A detail from the blueprint template showing the prospective multiple users in a FOOD Shopping service user journey and the instruction to fill it in

Fig. 2. A detail from the blueprint template showing some of the possible touchpoints

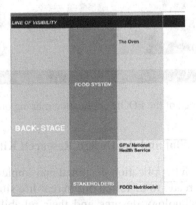

Fig. 3. A detail from the blueprint template showing some of the back-stage components blow the visibility line

The collective activity of blueprinting in groups allowed drafting different user journeys per each service, each journey describing a particular scenario of use. Moreover, the process helped out revealing misunderstandings among partners about their preconceived ideas of the services and allowed to agree on a shared vision of them to be implemented into working prototypes.

In the pipeline of the prototype implementation, the service blueprints were also preparatory to the wireframe process of the FOOD service application, running on tablet. The blueprints were then handled to the partner in charge of developing the wireframes and GUI for the FOOD app.

Mock ups of the screens have been developed (Fig.4) for some of the services mapped out in the blueprints, such as the Shopping, a basic version of Cooking Companion, Safety and some scenarios from the Food Management. In the design of the wireframes and GUI, it was decided that in order to let the users perceive the FOOD app as a consistent and unified experience, the services would have not been labeled and split into their "working" names, but they would coexist on the tablet screen tied up into a seamless journey. Later the services have been implemented into a proper working tablet application (the FOOD app) and released for the upcoming pilot with seniors in The Netherlands, Romania and Italy.

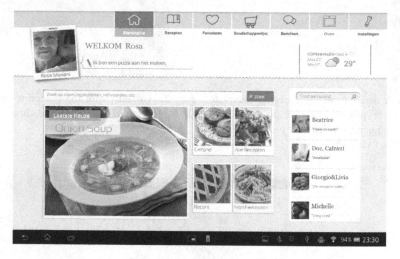

Fig. 4. A mock-up screen of the FOOD application running on tablet, dutch version

4.2   The Kick-Off the Pilot and the Design Research Kit

With the initial FOOD tablet application designed and implemented, the Pilots of the FOOD project are finally ready to be tested out in real-life situations. Pilots purpose is twofold: *i)* testing the technology designs and their reliability under the stress and unforeseen circumstances that arise during in-situ use and, *ii),* understanding the uptake and appropriation of the technological innovations by the elderly participants – and whether this incurs actual changes in their dietary and social habits.

These two agendas are being dealt with through the pilot in two overarching Pilot research tracks. There is an evaluation of the developed service and technological innovations, in both qualitative and quantitative terms, to assess the functionality, usability and feasibility of such socio-technical service systems through actual implementations. The second track is concerned with further developing the developed systems based on the real-life feedback from the Pilot implementations.

The project has planned and executed the initial steps of the Pilot deployment of the services at the time of writing. The pilot planning has taken the above aspects into consideration through testing the systems developed as iterative prototypes deployed in a live use-context, rich with socio-technical inter-weavings of extra-system-specific dependencies and contingencies. This is done through enlisting the collaboration of the project consortium's user-group partners, who can closely follow and support the daily use of the services by the Pilot participants.

The Pilots consist of three very different European locations, each with their own set of cultural values and traditions, namely Brasov, Romania; Fabriano, Italy and Eindhoven in the Netherlands.

The elderly participants of these locations speak three different languages, have three different cuisines and differ in various ways in their social make-up. The Pilot planning, therefore, is focused around the user-group partners deploying specific site teams that engage with the elderly participants in their local language and with a cultural understanding that can facilitate the introduction of the developed service systems.

The deployment has been split into two parts: introduction of the participants to the hardware and services, and a following data gathering phase, where quantitative data from the implemented systems as well as qualitative data gathered directly from the participants. The gathering of quantitative data will be described elsewhere, but for the qualitative data gathering we would like to describe in more detail the process involved in the collection and its intent, as it is a crucial part of testing and further developing the systems through the holistic approach mentioned in section 3.

Initially the system introductions to the elderly participants has to be preceded by instructions to the site teams in each Pilot location, to train the involved staff how to instruct the participants in using the services and related technical devices. Detailed manuals of the software have been developed, in collaboration with the user groups partners. Manuals serves as a physical support object in both the training of site teams and participants and as boundary objects between the different cultural and technological life-worlds of participants and developers.

The training process involves introducing the site teams to the software interface, the manual;, how to instruct the elderly participants and how to collect qualitative data on subsequent visits.

To enable qualitative feedback from the participants, a design research tool kit is given to the elderly, to help them remember specific experiences with the services and to ease sharing at the subsequent visits of the site teams. The design research tool (Fig.5) consists of two equally important share-back parts: a physical diary where the participant writes, on a regular basis, negative and positive feedback about the interaction with the hardware, and about their habitual patterns in everyday life, since installation, in terms of physical and mental well-being as well as social interaction enabled by technological services. The second part of the design research kit consists of a photo gallery together with a physical description document, both tightly connected to the written journal. This encourages the elderly participant to interact with the tablet and take photographs of important situations connected to their experiences.

The diary and the photo gallery work as two parts of the same feedback collection, with the intention of providing the elderly with the chance to share feedback in different media. After the initial Pilot kick-off in Brasov it has already become clear that providing both a physical and a digital feedback possibility is crucial, since the participants have very different levels in terms of usage experience of digital device.

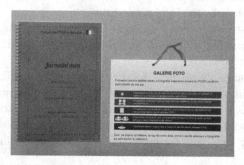

Fig. 5. The Design Research Kit, Romanian version: diary and photo gallery

In the months following the Pilot kick-off Pilot locations will be visited by research team on a 2-6 months basis, to gather and analyse data collected by the site team members. Such data, together with diary entries and pictures, will provide interesting insights for the actual use and further development of the FOOD technologies.

After the one-year period of the Pilot, the qualitative data from the participant sites will get synthesised into a qualitative evaluation of the Pilot phase in terms of usability and impact on the daily life of the participants, as well as recommendations for developing the services into more market-ready solutions, based on meaningful and contextualised interactions for the elderly users.

Acknowledgements. This work was carried out in the framework of AAL-JP project (project code AAL-2009-3-66), jointly funded by EU and national agencies of participating members.

References

1. Allen, J., Boffi, L., Burzagli, L., Ciampolini, P., De Munari, I., Emiliani, P.L.: FOOD: Discovering Techno-Social Scenarios for Networked Kitchen Systems. In: Encarnação, P., Azevedo, L., Gelderblom, G.J. (eds.) Assistive Technology: From Research to Practice, AAATE 2013, vol. 33, pp. 1143–1148. IOS Press (2013)
2. Losardo, A., Grossi, F., Matrella, G., De Munari, I., Ciampolini, P.: Exploiting AAL Environment for Behavioral Analysis. In: Encarnação, P., Azevedo, L., Gelderblom, G.J. (eds.) Assistive Technology: From Research to Practice, AAATE 2013, vol. 33, pp. 1121–1125. IOS Press (2013)
3. Moggrdge, B.: Designing Interaction. Cambridge. The Mit Press (2007)

Services and Applications in an Ambient Assisted Living (AAL) Environment

Laura Burzagli, Lorenzo Di Fonzo, and Pier Luigi Emiliani

Institute of Applied Physics (IFAC), National Research Council (CNR), Florence, Italy
{l.burzagli,l.difonzo,p.l.emiliani}@ifac.cnr.it

Abstract. As part of the AAL programme, the FOOD project is developing a smart kitchen and is setting up local and remote ICT applications to support feeding in a secure and comfortable environment. The implementation of an application to help people with diabetes in choosing a correct diet is used as an example of the emerging complexity of ICT applications in an Ambient Intelligence environment. Suggestions for possible future approaches to the development of Ambient Intelligence environments and complex applications are offered.

Keywords: AAL, e-Inclusion, services.

1 Introduction

Recently, interest has grown in the emergence of an Information Society as an Ambient Intelligence (AmI) environment and in the study of how it is possible to avoid exclusion of people, with main reference to people with activity limitations and elderly people. As a part of the AAL (Ambient Assisted Living) European programme dealing with elderly people, the FOOD[1] Project (Framework for Optimizing the prOcess of FeeDing), under the responsibility of the Italian Company Indesit[2], is developing a smart kitchen. It contains interconnected sensors and kitchen appliances and allows access to local and remote (Internet) applications dealing with all aspects of feeding (e.g. from accessing databases of recipes and getting ingredients for cooking to socialising around food topics with friends). The FOOD system (networked appliances and a selection of services/applications) are now in a pilot phase in apartments of older people in Italy, The Netherlands and Rumania [1].

In smart housing, up to now most emphasis has been on problems related to safety and health care, because, as prerequisites to an independent life, people need to live in a safe environment and be in good health. A lot of technology has been developed for these applications (e.g. sensors, remote control services, e-Health services), often as an answer to a specific problem and not integrated in a comprehensive living ecosystem. It is now time to take also care of well-being of people in their living environments, aiming to grant them comfort, entertainment, possibilities of social contacts,

---

[1] http://www.food-aal.eu
[2] http://www.indesitcompany.com/inst/en/index.jsp

C. Stephanidis and M. Antona (Eds.): UAHCI/HCII 2014, Part III, LNCS 8515, pp. 475–482, 2014.
© Springer International Publishing Switzerland 2014

etc. This is the aspect of the FOOD activity in the focus of the present paper. As an example, the problems relevant to set up an application to support people with diabetes in choosing a correct and pleasant diet is outlined.

However, as all successful activities, the FOOD project has contributed to point out limitations of the present approach to the development of intelligent environments and support applications, particularly for groups of people with activity limitations (sometimes partial and/or potential as in the case of older people). The diet application, for example, implies a level of complexity asking for a more general approach to the implementation of the entire home system. Therefore, a possible structured approach to its development is proposed and briefly described.

2   Design of Smart Environments: The Present Situation

One of the main features of research and development in smart housing is to be technology driven. A new technology is available and attempts are made not only to avoid new forms of exclusion, but also, hopefully, to use it to support specific user groups. Normally, the problems of a group or several groups of people with activity limitations are the starting point of development. They are expressed in questions as, for example, the following: how can people, who are blind or have (minor) decreases of ability to see as many elderly people, live independently in a smart house? How can they use the available technology? How can they be supported by this technology?

Another common feature is that, in many cases, accessibility to ICT and human machine interaction aspects are the focus of activity. Obviously, they represent a basic element, but the concern about them may have a limiting effect on the functionalities[3] to be considered as components of the applications to be implemented. Only functionalities that can easily be made available through the planned interface are considered, without an analysis of other different interaction options, often available, for a more appropriate implementation of the applications.

As an example, in the FOOD project two interaction options have been considered from the very beginning. The first is distributed and based on the interfaces of the single appliances. The second is aimed to allow the control of the entire kitchen and the connection with the outside world. It is based on a tablet using the Android operating system. In this case, interaction with the environment is taken back to the normal model of interaction with a computer (windows, menus, etc.), using the accessibility supports offered by the operating system itself or available in the Google Play market (for example a screen reader for blind persons).

A more general and abstract approach should be adopted. The starting point should be the identification of activities that people must carry out to live an independent and satisfactory life (for example in the case of FOOD: acquisition of food, access to recipes, cooking and so on). On the basis of the identified activities the environment (networked appliances, sensors, and services/applications) should be designed and implemented, considering all user groups that can be reasonably served (Design for

---

[3] In this paper, functionality and service are used as synonyms.

All) in planning its layout, number and type of appliances, number and type of interactions. Then, when necessary i.e. when difficulties are present for the completion of necessary tasks, suitable technological supports should be examined, also considering possible clashes of interest among different user groups and choosing the solution that maximises advantages (e.g. reduction of cost, number of people who can use it). Finally, if the chosen technological solutions are not suitable for some user groups, special adaptations could be looked for (Assistive Technology).

The lack of a structured approach and the limitations of the interaction technology available in the FOOD environment led to a partially unsatisfactory situation. While the analysis of the needed applications and of its component functionalities was made at a general and abstract level, the implementation had to take into account the technological limitation related to industrial constraints (availability of standard appliances with limited possibility of modifications and a pre-defined tablet interface).

3   Identification of the Necessary Functionalities

The design and implementation of a kitchen, where people can take care of feeding independently and comfortably, can be structured in the following steps:

- Identification of activities necessary for feeding;
- Identification of applications necessary to allow people to carry out the activities and/or to support them, when necessary. They can be based on technology (both local and remote) and on the support by people (e.g. cooperative networks);
- Splitting up of the applications into functionalities contributing to their implementation. This is necessary, because the same functionality can be re-used in many applications (for example, a database facility can be used in applications dealing with recipes, food availability, diet and so on);
- Identification of interactions relevant for accessing available functionalities. This is the level where accessibility concerns should be considered. Ideally, applications and their functionalities should only be chosen on the basis of the foreseen benefit for all users. Then, if some users have interaction problems, the effort of offering an accessible version should be made;
- Choice of technology for the implementation of the environment and relevant applications;
- Implementation of the AmI environment;
- Evaluation.

Presently, the identification of activities and functionalities to support them is often made on an ad hoc way, for example with interviews with end users, often in an inadequate number. This can be useful when different options are available and it is necessary to investigate what is more convenient for a person or a group of people. However, general knowledge about activities to be carried out for feeding and their connection with necessary abilities have been widely investigated and made available in a structured form in the WHO ICF document [2] and its developments. WHO ICF is a widely accepted document, produced through the agreement of people around the world. It is well structured and, therefore, usable in mechanised procedures. Moreover, the ICF classification can be used as it is or expanded if necessary. In ICF, activities relevant for feeding are classified, including difficulties that people with activity limitations could encounter in carrying them out. Moreover, the classification has been extended to consider the impact of food on health, e.g. on the diabetes disease [3].

After the definition of activities and sub activities, the identification of functionalities, necessary to support these activities (feeding, in the FOOD project), is necessary. They include technological functionalities available in the kitchen and/or remotely and human support. Examples are: control of the single appliances, access to recipes documentation in electronic format, access to social networks to get information and to discuss about food topics, etc. This identification must be done (Design for All [4] [5]) taking into account the abilities of all people who are supposed to use the kitchen. So far, no interaction aspect needs to be taken into account, but only functional ones: for example, the use of complex descriptions of recipes can create difficulties to older people with decreased cognitive capabilities, independently from the form of interaction. In the case study, the identification of additional functionalities for taking care of the diet for people with diabetes was necessary, as shown in the following section.

4   Emergence of Complexity – Diet for People with Diabetes

Even if a correct and balanced diet is beneficial for all people, some of them have diseases that need avoidance of a specific food or a careful balance of the entire diet.

The diet for people with diabetes is considered here as a case study to show that taking care of it leads to a level of complexity that is incompatible with the intelligence available in the smart kitchens presently proposed. It is maintained that new structured procedures for assembling the environment, setting up applications and controlling the entire system are needed.

If the person in the kitchen has an allergy or a disorder as the coeliac disease or a high cholesterol level, it easy to advise her about possible problems with food. They are binary (yes/no) situations. It is easy to go through the recipes or the shopping list and send warnings as shown in Fig. 1, where the output of an application set up in FOOD is shown.

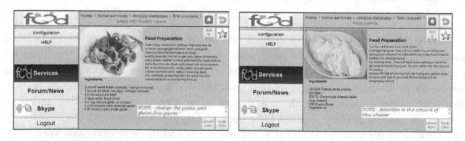

Fig. 1. Warnings for people with coeliac disease or high cholesterol level

With people with diabetes, the situation is much more complex. Given a food, it is not possible to tell them that it is not advisable to eat it. It suitability depends on:

- The food eaten in the previous days;
- The food possibly available in the near future (if information is accessible);
- The average health situation of the single person;
- The present situation (real time measurements).

A lot of knowledge is necessary:

- About the disease (different forms of diabetes);
- About foods and their calorie content;
- About possible interactions among food items;
- The medical history of the patient;
- Its diet history;
- The real-time situation.

Therefore, the possibility of reasoning on this knowledge must be available.

A lot of knowledge is indeed available about different aspects of the problem, which has been already formalised in ontologies [6], for example on food and the different aspects of the diabetes disease [7]. Expert systems [8] exist able to reason about different aspects of the disease and support health care professionals and patients. This means that the environment cannot only be augmented with sensors and networked appliances, able to give simple warnings and/or offer adapted interactions for people who have sensorial or cognitive lacks of abilities. It must be able to reason on formalised information to take care of all aspects relevant for a secure and comfortable life.

5   A Possible Future

Even if it is obviously difficult to influence the development of basic technology, it is in principle possible to control its integration in environments, able to cope with complex problems as the one briefly outlined in the previous section.

Fig. 2 is a simplified sketch of the procedure that designers and implementers should use in setting up intelligent environments. At the same time, it describes the way the system itself should be able to run and evolve to take care of the complex tasks needed to grant people a comfortable and independent life at home and of the evolution of the technological environment. The main feature of the procedure is that it must be based on formalised knowledge of all aspects relevant for design and implementation of the environment, using which designers and/or the system itself can reason in order to optimise its behaviour.

Once necessary activities of people and system functionalities to support them have been identified, developers must decide and implement the right assembly of the building blocks (home appliances and sensors), the way functionalities are made available, and the type(s) of suitable interactions.

This implies knowledge about:

- The environment under study (in this case, the kitchen and all activities related to feeding in general and to people with diabetes in particular);
- The applications of interest (e.g. ontologies about food and different aspects of diabetes);
- The different functionalities that it is necessary to make available;
- User abilities, considered from the perspective of contents (e.g. complexity of the language to be used in connection with the cognitive abilities of the potential users);
- Characteristics of technology and its interface protocols;
- Users' interactions capabilities and possible accessibility supports.

User information is particularly critical. At the design and development stage, this is supposed to be used to plan the necessary functionalities and interactions. Everything that is crucial to allow the control reasoning system to adapt the environment and functionalities to the single user must be made available.

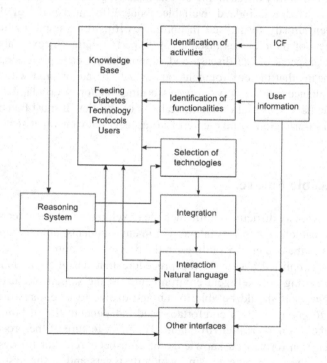

Fig. 2. A structured design and implementation procedure

If one looks at Fig. 2 from the perspective of the implemented system, the knowledge base becomes a mechanised (ontology-based) database and the reasoning system is not any more the designer, but an artificial intelligence inference machine. The reasoning system must be able to interconnect the (normally heterogeneous) technological building blocks of the environment and to adapt the entire system to the identified needs of the users, considering the behaviour of the individual building blocks and the complete resulting environment, the information contents of the services/applications, and the foreseen interactions. More in detail, it must be able:

- To monitor possible changes in the definitions of activities to be carried out (e.g. evolution of ICF);
- To acquire user behaviour and formalise it in the ontologies;
- To evolve the functionalities of the environment and applications, as a result of changes in the knowledge about activities, evolution of technology, and changes in needs and preferences of users;
- To get information about evolution of technology and its functionalities, integrating, when necessary, the required changes in the system;
- To get information about possible evolution of interaction features of the emerging environment and integrate it in the system.

Moreover, it must be able to monitor usage of the entire environment in real time, acquiring and formalising possibly varying usage patterns in order to adapt continuously its behaviour to user requirements.

From the interaction perspective, it is important to observe that in complex situations as the ones emerging in ambient intelligence environments, interaction cannot only be analysed from the perspective of giving the user access to the available interface. A real exchange of information between people and the system, which must be able to assist them, learn from their behaviour, test the validity of its assumptions and react to explicit requests, must be established.

People are normally used to exchange information through face-to-face conversation in "natural language". Speech is the "natural" interface among them. Therefore, the interaction between environments and people living in them should be mainly based on a dialogue in natural language. Interfaces based on windows, menus, command lines are only a poor way out of the real problem, due to limitations of present technology. However, trends of developments in information technology and artificial intelligence (see, for example, the SIRI applications by Apple [http://www.apple.com/ios/siri/] and the Watson project by IBM [http://www-03.ibm.com/innovation/us/watson/]) show real possibilities of a successful evolution in this direction.

Obviously, also a communication in natural language may create interaction problems to some groups of people with activity limitations. They must be identified and formalised, and the reasoning system is supposed to introduce the necessary adaptations as a function of the user and activity the carried out. Apparently, natural language interaction is considered a promising and viable possibility, where industry is heavily investing. In the meantime, it will be necessary to work with suboptimal solutions, as the ones considered in the FOOD project. Problems potentially caused by these interactions must be carefully analysed and formalised to allow the control of the corresponding interfaces by the reasoning system.

6   Conclusions

Ambient intelligence is offering interesting new possibilities to allow a comfortable life for all citizens and to support independent life of people with activity limitations. A prerequisite is that information about the environment itself, the available technology and users must be carefully collected and represented in a formalised form, to be used by the designer or an artificial intelligence reasoning system to adapt the environment to the individual users.

An application dealing with the suggestion of a diet for people with diabetes has been   used as a case study to show that the smart home system must evolve to exhibit a real intelligent behaviour, not only from the perspective of adapting interaction to users but also in producing relevant information.

A similar conclusion can be reached discussing problems of safety in the house, which must be able to infer needs of intervention not only from physical sensors (e.g. gas switched on, leaking taps), but also from the behaviour of its inhabitants.

References

1. Allen, J., Boffi, L., Burzagli, L., Ciampolini, P., De Munari, I., Emiliani, P.L.: FOOD: Discovering Techno-Social Scenarios for Networked Kitchen Systems. In: Encarnação, P., Azevedo, L., Gelderblom, G.J., Newell, A., Mathiassen, N.E. (eds.) Assistive Technology: From Research to Practice. Assistive Technology Research Series, vol. 33, pp. 1143–1148. IOS Press (2013)
2. WHO International Classification of Functioning, Disability and Health (ICF). World Health Organization, Geneve (2001)
3. Ruof, J., Cieza, A., Wolff, B., Angst, F., Ergeletzis, D., Zaliha, O., Kostanjsek, N., Stucki, G.: ICF Core Sets for Diabetes Mellitus. J. Rehabil. Med. (suppl. 44), 100–106 (2004)
4. Emiliani, P.L., Burzagli, L., Billi, M., Gabbanini, F., Palchetti, E.: Report on the impact of technological developments on eAccessibility. DfA@eInclusion Project D2.1 (2008), http://www.dfaei.org
5. Emiliani, P.L., Aalykke, S., Antona, M., Burzagli, L., Gabbanini, F., Klironomos, I.: Document on necessary research activities related to DfA. DfA@eInclusion Project D2.6 (2009), http://www.dfaei.org
6. Kehagias, D., Kontotasiou, D., Mouratidis, G., Nikolaou, T., Papadimitriou, I.: Ontologies, typologies, models and management tools. OASIS Project D1.1.1 (2008), http://www.oasis-project.eu
7. Cantais, J., Dominguez, D., Gigante, V., Laera, L., Tamma, V.: An example of food ontology for diabetes control. In: Proceedings of the International Semantic Web Conference 2005, Galway, Ireland (2005)
8. Snae, C., Brückner, M.: A Food-Oriented Ontology-Driven System. In: Second IEEE Conference on Digital Ecosystems and Technologies, pp. 168–176 (2008)

Energy@home: Energy Monitoring in Everyday Life

Stefano Corgnati[1], Elena Guercio[2], and Simona D'Oca[1]

[1] TEBE Research Group, Department of Energetics,
Politecnico di Torino Corso Duca degli Abruzzi 24, 10129 Torino, Italy
{stefano.corgnati,simona.doca}@polito.it
[2] Telecom Italia, Research & Prototyping via G. Reiss Romoli 247, 10100 Torino, Italy
elena.guercio@telecomitalia.it

Abstract. Goal of the research is to assess evaluations of the innovative smart monitoring system Energy@home for domestic electricity consumption. Aim of the Energy@home system is to provide householders with a persuasive tool that allows to manage energy consumption more efficiently. A combination of persuasive communication strategies such as graphical real-time and historical feedbacks to encourage competitiveness against "similar" households are provided to users through domestic user-friendly interfaces and combined with personalized energy saving prompts sent via newsletters. The Energy@home system was tested on 52 users selected all over Italy. From the qualitative standpoint, the system was evaluated easy to use and useful from 95% of trial users. The average system evaluation on a 1-to-10 scale was 7.8. From the quantitative standpoint, the Energy@home system motivated domestic consumer to save more than 9% in the electricity bill and emerged as an effective tool in reducing stand-by consumption on average above 15%.

Keywords: Energy, User Experience, Persuasive Stimuli, User Interface, Changing behavior.

1 Introduction

Moving towards a model to understand household behaviour, the human decision to behave in a certain way is driven by a wide range of internal and external factors [1]. Specifically, in the area of domestic energy consumption, there is a need to take into account the physical, social and cultural factors that influence and/or constrain a user's choices and behaviours, such as age, gender, social class, income, geographical position and political differences, aside from information provision and economic incentives [2]. Achieving energy conservation is a double challenge, partly technical and partly human. Thus, disciplines such as sociology, social psychology, anthropology and building physics are increasingly relevant to understand findings into behavioural patterns of energy consumption in households.

To address the human side of energy efficiency, theories of persuasive communication and attitude change must be coupled together with available home automation technologies displaying energy information, with the aim of educating, motivating, incentivizing and persuading domestic user towards energy saving behaviours.

C. Stephanidis and M. Antona (Eds.): UAHCI/HCII 2014, Part III, LNCS 8515, pp. 483–492, 2014.
© Springer International Publishing Switzerland 2014

The goal of this study is to assess and provide evaluations of the innovative smart monitoring system Energy@home for domestic electricity consumption. The aim of the Energy@home system is to provide householders with a persuasive tool that improves awareness of energy behaviour in their homes and allows them to manage their energy consumption more efficiently. A combination of persuasive communication strategies such as graphical real-time and historical feedbacks and comparison tools to encourage competitiveness against "similar" households are provided to users through domestic user-friendly interfaces and combined with personalized energy saving prompts sent via web-newsletters.Besides, qualitative techniques to collect data from users during the Energy@home trial are applied, such as questionnaires and focus groups, with the aim to gather information on occupant behaviour related to electricity energy use in homes.

2   Problem Statement

Although significant improvements in energy efficiency have been achieved in home appliances and lighting, this alone is not enough: the electricity consumption in the average EU-25 household has been increasing by about 2% per year during the last 10 years [3]. Moreover, occupant behaviour at home can enormously vary on the base of different energy related behavioral patterns: accordingly, Andersen in 2012 [4] demonstrated that energy consumption in almost identical dwelling might increase up to three times. Interestingly, results of several studies [5, 6, 7, 8, 9, 10, 11] underlined that the energy saving potential by improving occupant behaviour is on the average about 15%.

The concept of displaying energy consumption to domestic consumers in order to promote energy saving behaviours has been suggested since the 1980s [12, 13, 14]. Existing real-time energy monitoring tools allow users to visualize and to manage more efficiently their electric energy loads at home.

Field studies on environmental behaviour [15, 16, 17, 18] conceptualized persuasive strategies, pointing out that energy consumer may be influenced by antecedent (general) and consequence (feedback) information. Antecedent strategies announce the availability of positive or negative consequences through information, prompts, demonstration and commitments. Consequence strategies provide rewards and feedback, following particular energy behavior that has been observed and monitored.

From the literature concerning feedback information, there is still little clarity on how best to achieve energy-saving potential in dwellings. A study conducted by Harkins and Lowe [19] gave evidence to the fact that if users are given a goal to reach, they feel a sense of satisfaction of achievement from reaching that goal. Moreover, it is believed that there is a social driver at work in the presentation of energy use in comparative fashion. Van Houwelingen and Van Raaij [20] stated that if users are shown how much energy they are using compared to others, they may well get satisfaction from knowing they are doing better than others. If households learn they use more energy than other similar households, it is assumed they will be motivated to reduce consumption and possibly more so than those other households.

Regarding the feedback display's form, it is important to examine how the type of unit of power used to convey energy consumption influences the consumer. Hayes and Cone [21] emphasized that using the kWh as display unit would be the most obvious choice among technicians for identifying electricity energy use. Moreover, people may not understand the relevance of the amount of energy they are using to the effect it has on environment or economy. For this reason, home energy saving potential must be communicate to end users also in terms of economic and environmental impacts.

3   Energy@home System

The Energy@home project envisions a communication web platform that provides users with information on their household consumption by means the direct visualization of the energy loads on smart appliances displays, smart phones or personal computers. The system is based upon graphical user/friendly interface, information exchange and persuasive feedback information related to energy usage, energy consumption and energy tariffs in the home area network. The system's general architecture of the Energy@home system is reported in figure 1.

Two parallel energy efficiency strategies are tested with the aim of reducing domestic electric loads. The "human-sided" strategy focuses on potentialities in influencing the occupants' use of domestic equipment through information and feedbacks (web based graphical user interface). The "machine-sided" strategy focuses on the automatic management and shifting of domestic energy loads.

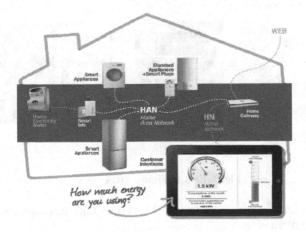

Fig. 1. Energy@home system

4   Energy@home Trial

In 2013 Telecom Italia managed a trial with 52 households to test the Energy@home system both from a technological (system efficiency) and user-experience (system usability) point of view. Among the selected trial sample, 20 households installed a photovoltaic meter, 9 households have 4.5 and 6 kW contractual power meters and 23 households have 3 kW contractual power meter. Trial users were dislocated in different Italian regions and differed for house typology (condo vs. detached house) and family members (from two to six households). They were also different for the propensity to save energy.

Telecom Italia managed the trial in collaboration with Enel Distribuzione and Indesit Company, all founding members of the Energy@home Association (Energy@home: http://www.energy-home.it/). Every participant of the Energy@home trial installed (by himself or through a specialized technician) the Energy@home kit including: a smart gateway, 5 smart plugs, a smart info (turning into "smart" the traditional electrical meter) and a zigbee washing machine (see fig. 2). A web based app allowed every user to access his/her energy data directly at home or remotely (office, another home, mobility...) and to see household breakdown consumption as a function of Watt (stand-by power), kWh (appliances' consumption details, historical consumption data, overload warnings, etc.) or Euros (spending forecast). Trial users had also access to a web-platform community connecting people involved in the trial. Scope of the web-community was to allow users to compare peer consumption data or to ask for suggestions or technical support.

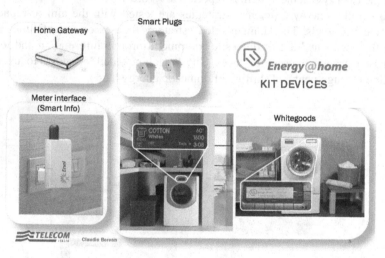

Fig. 2. Energy@home kit devices

The trial was managed in order to test the system both from a technical and user experience point of view.

During the trial we collected both qualitative and quantitative data. Quantitative data are related to log files that indicate the "click number" on different visualization options of the system like energy cost, energy consumption, appliance details, number of access to the system, and data sent from every device in terms of watt and watt/hour. Quantitative data are also related to statistical data about changes in user behaviour after specific "persuasive stimuli" we sent them through 8 newsletters every 15 days of system use.

Fig. 3 shows the 8 the persuasive stimuli sent through newsletters to the participants. The participants were grouped in 10-12 people and newsletters were sent in different periods to different groups of users.

8 newsletters: everyone was sent with test and "graphical position" of user in comparison with others							
Prompts on energy consumption with reference to family type	Prompts on stand-by energy consumption	Suggestion of actions to reduce stand-by energy consumption	Prompts on refrigerator energy consumption	Which is the most energy consuming appliance?	Prompts on smart washing machine energy consumption (Part I)	Prompts on smart washing machine energy consumption (Part II)	Visualization of changes in energy consumption load

Fig. 3. Persuasive stimuli in newsletters

Qualitative data concerns a direct daily communication channel settled with trial users. Trial users communicate with the experimenter team (comments, problems, questions, suggestions…) through email. Persuasive stimuli were sent by email and qualitative users' responses were collected and associated to direct observation of behavior changes. These information were analyzed to highlight social and contextual drivers in home energy uses as well as correlations with statistical quantitative data to explain behavioral changes. Furthermore, users information were collected through an online forum (directly accessible from graphical user interface), focus groups and online questionnaires. Two questionnaires were distributed. The first one gathered detailed information about the sample of trail users in order to correlate household typology to their consumption data. The second one was sent after about one year of Energy@home system usage. It collected data related to system usage, habits, satisfied needs and unsatisfactory experiences related to the Energy@home system and it took about 20 minutes to be filled in. Most of the items had multiple-choice answers, moreover some open questions were inserted in order to better identify user opinions on perceived system benefits and possible optimizations of system usage in the real context of use.

Two focus groups were settled in order to gather information related to the users' satisfaction, to find confirmation to the evidences of the questionnaire as well as to evaluate new concepts about energy management, evolution and business model. Finally strengthens and weaknesses of the system were highlighted and the voice of the users were used as a guide to next improvements.

5   Main Results

5.1   Qualitative Analysis: Focus Groups, Questionnaires and Spontaneous Feedback

Data were collected through emails, newsletters' feedbacks, forum, focus group and questionnaires. Data from different sources are consistent and complement each other:

more than 70% of the sample responded to the questionnaire (39 users among 56) and about 75% of the sample sent at least one feedback or suggestion during the trial. Besides, a first focus group (8 trial users with 3kw meter) was managed to test the satisfactory level of the system usage as well as to deepen the questionnaire findings.

Main qualitative results of the trial are summarized, selected from the questionnaire's results.

In a scale from 1 to 10, the average respondents' vote of the system is 7.8. Trial users considered the system "innovative" and "effective" in its energy saving potential. 56% of the users interacted with the system every day; 77% of the users looked at graphical interface at least one day/week (33% 2-3 times/week; 13% everyday).

The system is considered easy to use and useful from 95% of interviewed people. Moreover, trial users would be pleased to keep system at home after the trial (88%) and they would suggest the system usage to their friends (74%). Above 34% of the sample would pay the system about 2 euros/month or a corresponding percentage between 10-25% of the economical saving obtained by the system usage (31%); just 13% of the interviewed wouldn't pay for the system usage.

Three main perceived strengths of the Energy@home system are:

- Consumer awareness regarding stand-by consumption.
- Reduction of wasteful behavior.
- Ease of use

Some weaknesses have emerged too:

- Smart plugs are too bulky
- Inadequate number of smart plugs
- Technical problems of various types (reported by individuals, not always significant for the entire group).

Focus groups were useful to confirm questionnaires data and overall to deepen knowledge related to users' motivations, drivers in energy saving behaviors, customers' needs and suggestions about the system.

5.2   Persuasive Stimuli

Results of the research demonstrate that:

- The Energy@home system motivates users to change their behavior and generated a savings of more than 9% [Fig. 4].

Results in figure 4 show the amount of energy saving after 8 months of system usage where each month is compared with the same month of the previous year: about 77% of the users (10 over 13) achieved energy savings after installing the Energy@home system in their homes, on average 9% of savings were measured corresponding to 5.6 TWh[1]. Significantly, the "best case" user managed to lower its electricity energy consumption up to -40%.

---

[1] Analysis performed for a basis of 61.3 TWh of annual domestic electricity consumption in Italy (AEEG, 2013).

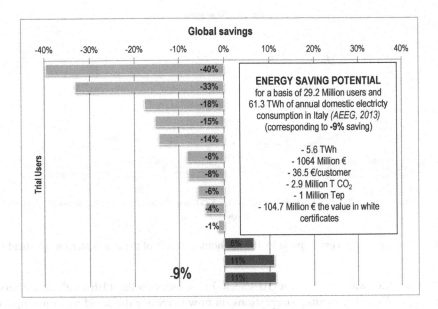

Fig. 4. Global energy saving achieved during the trial testing phase of the Energy@home system

In the Italian context, assuming that energy saving would be achieved by 29.2 million Italian electricity domestic consumers,[2] in one year a total amount of 1064 Million € can be saved, equivalent to 35.6 € saved in the electricity bill from every Italian family. This saving corresponds to avoiding the emission of 2.9 Million tons of CO_2 and a value of the corresponding white certificates of 104.7 Million Euro, i.e. 3.6 €/customer.

- The Energy@home system is an effective tool to reduce the contractual power.

Analysis of the energy loads of trail users having contractual powers of more than 3 kW were performed in order to understand the percentage of time of effective need of 4.5 kW or 6 kW. This study highlights that only one over 8 trail users exploited the potentiality of the contractual power they paid for. All these users can lower their contractual power and go back to the 3 kW contract with an economic saving in their energy bill of more than 180 €/year.

The Energy@home system is an effective tool to motivate users to reduce the stand-by consumption on average above 15% [Fig. 5].

Analysis of the standby power was performed on data related to 10 trail users of the Energy@home system. The stand-by consumption of each trial home was assumed as the minimum electrical consumption recorded over the 24 hours with a 2 minutes acquisition step. These values were then aggregated into a daily mean of stand-by consumption, for each of the 10 trail users. Results highlight that the standby was on the average above 66 W.

---

[2] (AEEG, 2013).

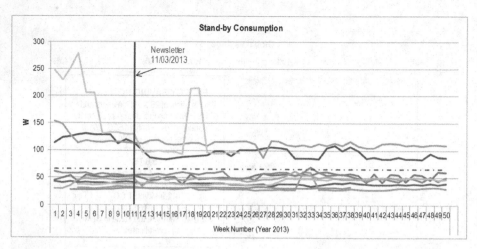

Fig. 5. Standby energy consumption in 10 trial homes. Effect of the newsletter on the stand-by consumption

- A newsletter was sent to these 10 selected trail users on the 11th week of monitoring (11/3/2013), providing suggestions on how to reduce the stand-by consumption in their homes. Significantly, it emerged that educating users in reducing the stand-by power of their appliances results in the greatest energy savings at home. The effectiveness of this communication is summarized here:
  - 6 over 10 trial users reduced the home stand-by consumption, after receiving the newsletter.
  - Trial users reduced on average their stand-by power of -15% (11.5 W).
  - The "best practice" user managed to reduce the stand-by power of -40% (80 W) corresponding to an annual energy saving of above 125 €.
  - Thanks to the decrease in stand-by power, the "best practice" user managed to reduce up to 23% of his/her domestic electricity consumption.
- The Energy@home system is an effective tool to motivate users in shifting their consumption in the off-peak time ranges on the average of 5%. Based on national regulation, economic tariff of domestic electricity energy varies based on three hourly categories:
  - F1: from Monday to Friday 8 – 19 (peak hours)
  - F2: from Monday to Friday 9 – 8 (off-peak hours)
  - F3: Weekends and Holidays (off-peak hours)

Energy consumption for 18 selected trail users was organized into three hourly categories, corresponding to the two-hour tariff applied by Enel Servizio Elettrico (electricity supplier). For each trail user, the consumption recorded during peak hours (F1 tariff) was compared to the consumption recorded during off-peak hours (F2 ad F3).

Results show that electricity consumption of trail users using the Energy@home kit moved from peak to off-peak tariff consumption on average of 5% with respect to the same months of 2012.

6   Conclusions and Next Steps

The Energy@home system is an effective tool in reducing electricity energy consumption at home on the average among 9%. Results demonstrate that more than 77% of the testing-users achieved energy savings, after installing the Energy@home system in their homes. "Best-case" trial user managed to lower his/her electricity energy consumption up to -40%. Significantly, whether this energy saving would be achieved by 29.2 million Italian electrical domestic consumers, in one year a total amount of 1064 Million € can be saved, equivalent to 35.6 € saved in the electricity bill from every Italian family. This saving corresponds to avoiding the emission of 2.9 Million tons of CO_2 and a value of the corresponding white certificates of 104.7 Million Euro, i.e. 3.6 €/customer. Qualitative responses from users indicate that the system is effective and easy to use and "helps" users to reduce consumptions and electrical costs in everyday life. Most important, people perceived their changes in consumption behavior.

Further improvements are needed to enhance system reliability and effectiveness. A goal for future control devices in dwelling is to became a cost-effective tool able to raise user awareness regarding energy uses in homes and hence to guide users towards more energy savings behaviors.

References

1. Fabi, V., Andersen, R.V., Corgnati, S.P., Bjarne, W.O., Filippi, M.: Description of occupant behaviour in building energy simulation: state-of-art and concepts for their improvement. In: Fabi, V., Andersen, R.V., Corgnati, S.P., Bjarne, W.O., Filippi, M. (eds.) Proceeding of Building Simulation 2011: 12th Conference of International Performance Simulation Association, Sydney, November 14-16,
2. Shove, E.: Converging Conventions of Comfort, Cleanliness and Convenience. Journal of Consumer Policy 26, 395–418 (2003)
3. European Commission, EU energy trends to 2030. Publications Office of the European Union, Luxembourg (2009) ISBN 978-92-79-16191-9
4. Andersen, R.: The influence of occupants' behaviour on energy consumption investigated in 290 identical dwellings and in 35 apartments. In: Proceedings of Healthy Buildings 2012, Brisbane, Australia (2012)
5. Wood, G., Newborough, M.: Dynamic energy-consumption indicators for domestic appliances: environment, nehaviour and design. Energy and Buildings 35, 821–841 (2003)
6. Wood, G., Newborough, M.: Design and Functionality of Prospective of Energy Consumption Displays. In: Proceeding of the 3rd International Conference on Energy Efficiency in Domestic Appliances and Lighting (EEDAL 2003) (2003)
7. Ueno, T., Sano, F., Saeki, O., Tsuji, K.: Effectiveness of an energy-consumption information system on energy savings in residential houses based on monitored data. Applied Energy 83, 166–183 (2006)
8. Ueno, T., Sano, F., Saeki, O., Tsuji, K.: Effectiveness of displaying energy consumption data in residential houses. Analysis on how the residents respond. In: Proceeding of 2006 American Council for an Energy Efficient Economy (ACEEE) Summer Study on Energy Efficiency in Buildings (2006)

9. Ouyang, J., Hokao, K.: Energy-saving potential by improving occupants' behavior in urban residential sector in Hangzhou City, China. Energy and Building 41, 711–720 (2009)
10. Faiers, A., Cook, M., Neame, C.: Towards a contemporary approach for understanding consumer behaviour in the context of domestic use. Energy Policy 35, 4381–4390 (2007)
11. Hokao, J.O.K.: Energy-saving potential by improving occupants' behavior in urban residential sector in Hangzhou City, China. Energy and Building 41, 711–720 (2009)
12. Miller, S.: New Essential Psychology: Experimental Design and Statistics. Routledge, London (1984)
13. Stern, P.: What psychology knows about energy conservation. American Psychologist 47, 1224–1231 (1992)
14. Wilhite, H., Ling, R.: Measured energy savings from a more informative energy bill. Energy and Buildings 22(2), 145–155 (1995)
15. Dennis, M.L., Soderstrom, E.J., Koncinski, W.S., Cavanaugh, B.: Effective dissemination of energy related information. American Psychologist 45(10), 1109–1117 (1990)
16. Winnett, R.A., Leckliter, I.N., Chinn, D.E., Stahl, B.: Reducing energy consumption: the long-term effects of a single TV program. Journal of Communication 34(3), 37–51 (1984)
17. Seligman, C., Darley, J.M.: Feedback as a means of decreasing residential energy-consumption. Journal of Applied Psychology 62, 363–368 (1977)
18. Darby, S.: The effectiveness of feedback on energy consumption. A review of the literature on metering, billing and direct displays. In: Proceedings of ACEEE Summer Study on Energy Efficiency in Buildings (2008)
19. Harkins, S.G., Lowe, M.D.: The Effects of Self-Set Goals on Task Performance. Journal of Applied Social Psychology 30(1), 1–40 (2000)
20. Van Houwelingen, J.T., Van Raaij, W.F.: The effect of goal setting and daily electronic feedback on in-home energy use. Journal of Consumer Research 16, 98–105 (1989)
21. Hayes, S.C., Cone, J.D.: Reducing residential electricity energy use: payments, information, and feedback. Journal of Applied Behavior Analysis 10, 425–435 (1977)

Integrating Computer Vision Object Recognition with Location Based Services for the Blind

Hugo Fernandes[1], Paulo Costa[2], Hugo Paredes[1], Vítor Filipe[1], and João Barroso[1]

[1] INESC-TEC and UTAD – University of Trás-os-Montes e Alto Douro, Vila Real, Portugal
{hugof,hparedes,vfilipe,jbarroso}@utad.pt
[2] School of Technology and Management, Polytechnic Institute of Leiria, Leiria, Portugal
paulo.costa@ipleiria.pt

Abstract. The task of moving from one place to another is a difficult challenge that involves obstacle avoidance, staying on street walks, finding doors, knowing the current location and keeping on track through the desired path. Nowadays, navigation systems are widely used to find the correct path, or the quickest, between two places. While assistive technology has contributed to the improvement of the quality of life of people with disabilities, people with visual impairment still face enormous limitations in terms of their mobility. In recent years, several approaches have been made to create systems that allow seamless tracking and navigation both in indoor and outdoor environments. However there is still an enormous lack of availability of information that can be used to assist the navigation of users with visual impairments as well as a lack of sufficient precision in terms of the estimation of the user's location. Blavigator is a navigation system designed to help users with visual impairments. In a known location, the use of object recognition algorithms can provide contextual feedback to the user and even serve as a validator to the positioning module and geographic information system of a navigation system for the visually impaired. This paper proposes a method where the use of computer vision algorithms validate the outputs of the positioning system of the Blavigator prototype.

Keywords: location-based, services, blind, navigation, computer vision, object recognition.

1 Introduction

Moving from one place to another is a difficult challenge that involves obstacle avoidance, staying on street walks, finding doors, knowing the current location and keeping on track through the desired path, until the destination is reached. While assistive technology has contributed to the improvement of the quality of life of people with disabilities, with major advances in recent years, people with visual impairment still face enormous limitations in terms of their mobility. Nowadays, navigation systems are widely used to find the correct path, or the quickest, between two places. In recent years, several approaches have been made to create systems that allow seamless tracking and navigation both in indoor and outdoor environments. However there

C. Stephanidis and M. Antona (Eds.): UAHCI/HCII 2014, Part III, LNCS 8515, pp. 493–500, 2014.
© Springer International Publishing Switzerland 2014

is still an enormous lack of availability of information that can be used to assist the navigation of users with visual impairments (or other kinds of impairment), as well as a lack of sufficient precision in terms of the estimation of the user's location. All these factors combined, maintain a situation of large disparity between the availability of such technology among users who suffer from physical limitations and those who do not suffer such limitations. To address the task of finding the user location in indoor environments several techniques and technologies have been used such as sonar, radio signal triangulation, radio signal (beacon) emitters, or signal fingerprinting. All these technologies can be, and have been, used to develop systems that help enhancing the personal space range of blind or visually impaired users. In the case of outdoor environments, some hybrid systems have been proposed that use GPS as the main information source and use radiofrequency for correction and minimization of the location error. Another hybrid approach may be the use of computer vision algorithms to work together with global positioning. In a known location, the use of object recognition algorithms can provide contextual feedback to the user and even serve as a validator to the positioning and information system modules of a navigation system for the visually impaired. This paper proposes a method where the use of computer vision algorithms validate the outputs of the positioning system.

Section 2 presents related work in the field of navigation systems and the determination of the user's location, whether indoor or outdoor. Specifically some works are presented which focus on user's with visual impairment. Section 3 describes how the prototype addresses the problem of creating a navigation system for the blind. Section 4 presents some final considerations regarding the techniques used in object recognition.

2   Related Work

Location and navigation systems have become very important and widely available in recent years as a tool for finding the quickest or optimal route to a specific destination or simply to retrieve contextual information about the environment and nearby points-of-interest (POI). To determine the user's location most of these systems use the Global Positioning System (GPS), but since GPS signals are greatly degraded inside of buildings they only work well in outdoor environment.

To address the task of finding the user location in indoor environments several techniques and technologies have been used such as sonar, radio signal triangulation, radio signal (beacon) emitters, or signal fingerprinting. All these technologies can be, and have been, used to develop systems that help enhancing the personal space range of blind or visually impaired users [1]. Another technology widely used in this context is Radio-Frequency Identification (RFID). RFID tags are built-in with electronic components that store an identification code that can be read by an RFID tag reader. In recent years some research teams [2][3][4] have developed navigation systems based on this technology. In the case of outdoor environments, some hybrid systems have been proposed that use GPS as the main information source and use RFID for correction and minimization of the location error. The research team at the University of Trás-os-Montes e Alto Douro (UTAD) has an extensive work in terms of accessibility and rehabilitation. In the last few years, the team has given major focus to visual impairment and on how existing technology may help in everyday life applications. From an extensive review of the state of the art and its best practices, three main projects have been developed: the SmartVision [5][6], Nav4B [7] and Blavigator [8] projects.

The main goal of the SmartVision project was to develop and integrate technology for aiding blind users and those with severe visual impairments into a small portable device that is cheap and easy to assemble using off-the-shelf components. This device should be extremely easy to carry and use, yet providing all necessary help for autonomous navigation. It should be stressed out that the device was designed to be an extension of the white cane, not a replacement, and to be "non-invasive", issuing warning signals when approaching a possible obstacle, a point-of-interest or when the footpath in front is curved and the heading direction should be adapted.

In this sense, the SmartVision prototype addressed three main applications: (1) local navigation for centering on footpaths etc. and obstacle avoidance, in the immediate surroundings, but just beyond the reach of the white cane; (2) global navigation for finding one's way; and (3) object/obstacle recognition, not only on the shelves in a pantry or supermarket, but also outdoor: bus stops, taxi stands, cash machines (ATM) and telephone booths. The Nav4B project aimed to be an extension of the work done in the SmartVision project.

The new prototype, developed by the Blavigator project is built with the same modular structure as the SmartVision project. The Blavigator project aimed at creating a small, cheap and portable device that included all the features of the SmartVision prototype, with added performance optimization.

3   Blavigator Prototype

3.1   Modular Structure of the Prototype

The prototype is composed by the same modules that compose the SmartVision prototype: Interface, Geographic Information System (GIS), Navigation, Location, Computer Vision/Object Recognition and the central Decision Module (Fig. 1).

The Interface Module is responsible for the user interface. The system outputs information through vibration (haptic actuator present in the electronic white cane) and through text-to-speech technology (per user request or in the presence of relevant contextual information).

The Geographic Information System keeps a local representation of the data stored in a dedicated remote server supported and maintained by the Blavigator project. The Geographic Information System (GIS) in the remote server stores data about all the points-of-interest, layers, etc., in a MySQL database. All the required CRUD (create, read, update and delete) operations are available through a web application interface (Fig. 2).

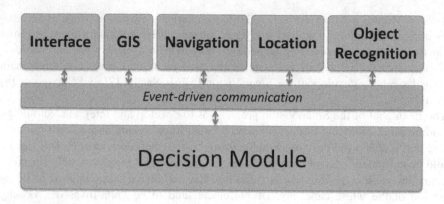

Fig. 1. Modules of the Blavigator prototype

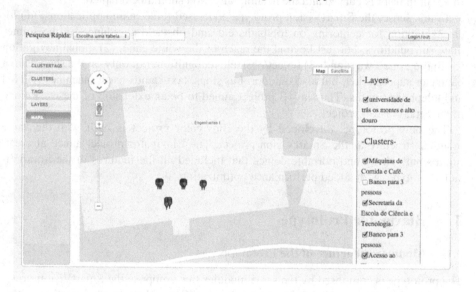

Fig. 2. Points of Interest (POI)/Objects/Layers stored in the Geographic Information System

The Navigation Module, by request of the Decision Module (and user input), uses data from both the Location Module and the GIS to calculate the optimal route to a specific destination (point-of-interest), to guide the user through the calculated route and to provide contextual information about the user's surroundings.

The Computer Vision/Object Recognition Module is used to validate the information retrieved by the Location Module in combination with the GIS Module. In other words, when the Location Module informs the system about a new coordinate, the central Decision Module queries the GIS about which objects are expected to be found in the user's surroundings. Then, knowing which nearby objects may be found, object recognition algorithms and the device's built-in camera are used to search for these objects. Once an object is found, this information is used to validate the outputs from the Location Module and, at the same time, feed the user with contextual information, extending the reach of the traditional white cane.

3.2   Navigation Software, User Setup and System Interface

When a new geographic coordinate in sensed by the Location Module, the mobile application (software) can handle this input in one of two ways (or modes) according to the user's requirements: Navigating or Touring. If the user wants to navigate to a specific point-of-interest, the system uses the current coordinate and the destination coordinate to calculate a route between the two points. Then, each input from the Location Module triggers the Navigation Module to keep the user on his track. On the other hand, if the user wants to stroll around, as if sightseeing, the system uses the current coordinate to query the GIS Module about relevant features (points-of-interest) in the user's surroundings. There is an 'alert' level within the software that can be modified by the user to filter the types of alerts he wants to be warned about. This is a support system that must not be intrusive neither an obstacle by itself, overriding the will of the user.

The interface between the user and the mobile software application is bidirectional (Fig. 3).

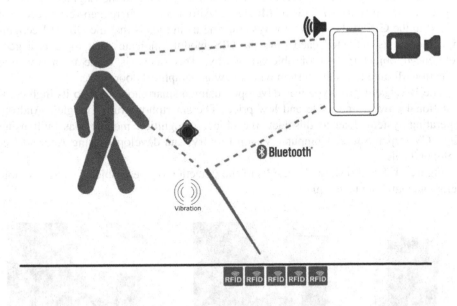

Fig. 3. User setup and system interface

The user interfaces the software using a small joystick placed conveniently in the white cane. The joystick works in four directions and has a press button as well (a total of five switches). This joystick is used to navigate the software application and the inputs are sent via Bluetooth. When the software needs to provide feedback to the blind user, text-to-speech technology is used. This type of audio cues is used only at specific locations (such as dangerous areas or important points-of-interest) or by user request, if he feels the need to know with more detail the contents of his surroundings.

No interface is made with the mobile device itself, directly. The mobile application is designed to be interfaced exclusively using text-to-speech and the joystick.

3.3   Computer Vision Object Recognition

Regarding the Computer Vision module, which is the focus of the proposed work, its function is to extract information about the surrounding environment so as to enhance the navigation of a blind person. This paper proposes the use of algorithms for recognizing certain elements often found in the environment and which contribute significantly to a secure mobility of the user. These algorithms are used to create a library of routines able to individually recognize the elements in the surrounding environment and are activated according to the elements expect to be found in the place where the user is located, at every moment. In addition, object recognition is often a computationally demanding task which gets more and more demanding as the number of elements to be detected the image gets larger. This module must be able to provide indications in real time.

To test this idea, three different objects commonly found in the Engineering building of the University of Trás-os-Montes e Alto Douro where geo-referenced and stored in the GIS of the Blavigator system. The main idea is that the Object Recognition module is activated each time the GIS module indicates that there is a geo-referenced object (or set of objects) nearby. This query is made each time the Location Module feeds the system with a new geographical coordinate.

The Blavigator prototype was developed using a smartphone, due to its high computational power, small size and low price. The smartphone runs Google's Android operating system. Due to this fact, the object recognition module was built using OpenCV (Open Source Computer Vision Library) and developed using Android Developer Tools.

Figures 4, 5 and 6 show the results of the detection of these objects using a simple template matching technique.

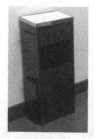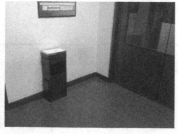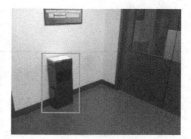

Fig. 4. Detection of trash can in the corridor (case #1)

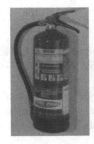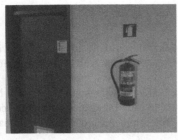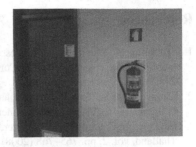

Fig. 5. Detection of fire extinguisher in the corridor (case #2)

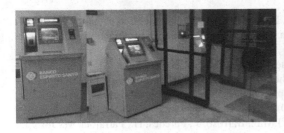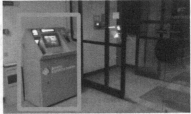

Fig. 6. Detection of ATM in the main hall (case #3)

It is important for the recognition of picture elements to be activated according to the type of elements known to be close to the blind person at each specific moment.

4   Final Remarks

As there are often several important elements in the environment simultaneously is very important that algorithms are simultaneously very robust and very fast. The elements in the examples shown in Figures 4, 5 and 6 were detected using a simple template matching technique. This technique was used for its simplicity in these initial tests and to prove the concept presented in this paper. However this technique is also known to be extremely time consuming and also known to fail the detection when there is a big mismatch between the template's size and pose when compared to the actual size and of the object in the image.

To overcome this issue the extraction of this information in the image can be made using "Machine Learning" techniques, in particular through the use of Artificial Neural Networks (ANN), "Support Vector Machines" (SVM) for pattern recognition, or through the use the "Wavelet Transform." The robustness of the detection of features in the image can be increased using techniques invariant to scale, using methods such as SIFT ("Scale-invariant feature transform") or SURF ("speeded Up Robust Features").

References

1. Strumillo, P.: Electronic interfaces aiding the visually impaired in environmental access, mobility and navigation. In: 3rd Conference on Human System Interactions (HSI), pp. 17–24 (2010)
2. Chumkamon, S., Tuvaphanthaphiphat, P., Keeratiwintakorn, P.: A Blind Navigation System Using RFID for Indoor Environments. In: 5th International Conference on In Electrical Engineering/Electronics, Computer, Telecommunications and Information Technology, Thailand, vol. 2, pp. 765–768 (2008)
3. Willis, S., Helal, S.: RFID Information Grid for Blind Navigational and Wayfinding. In: Proceedings of the 9th IEEE International Symposium on Wearable Computers, Osaka, pp. 34–37 (2005)
4. D"Atri, E., Medaglia, C., Panizzi, E., D"Atri, A.: A system to aid blind people in the mobility: A usability test and its results. In: Proceedings of the Second International Conference on Systems, Martinique, p. 35 (2007)
5. du Buf, J.M.H., Barroso, J., Rodrigues, J.M.F., Paredes, H., Farrajota, M., Fernandes, H., José, J., Teixiera, V., Saleiro, M.: The SmartVision navigation prototype for the blind. In: Proc. Int. Conf. on Software Development for Enhancing Accessibility and Fighting Info-exclusion (DSAI), pp. 167–174 (2010)
6. Fernandes, H., du Buf, J., Rodrigues, J.M.F., Barroso, J., Paredes, H., Farrajota, M., José, J.: The SmartVision Navigation Prototype for Blind Users. Journal of Digital Content Technology and its Applications 5(5), 351–361 (2011)
7. Fernandes, H., Faria, J., Paredes, H., Barroso, J.: An integrated system for blind day-to-day life autonomy. In: The Proceedings of the 13th International ACM SIGACCESS Conference on Computers and Accessibility, Dundee, Scotland, UK (2011)
8. Fernandes, H., Adão, T., Magalhães, L., Paredes, H., Barroso, J.: Navigation Module of Blavigator Prototype. In: Proceedings of the World Automation Congress, World Automation Congress 2012, Puerto Vallarta (2012)

Home Control via Mobile Devices: State of the Art and HCI Challenges under the Perspective of Diversity

Sarah Gomes Sakamoto[1], Leonardo Cunha de Miranda[1], and Heiko Hornung[2]

[1] Department of Informatics and Applied Mathematics,
Federal University of Rio Grande do Norte (UFRN), Natal, Brazil
sarahsakamoto@ppgsc.ufrn.br, leonardo@dimap.ufrn.br
[2] Institute of Computing, University of Campinas (UNICAMP), Campinas, Brazil
heix@gmx.com

Abstract. With technological advancements in recent decades, home environments incorporate several electronic appliances in order to facilitate activities and improve users' quality of life. The increasing complexity of household appliances makes their management a nontrivial task. Mobile devices emerge as excellent platforms to enable control over such a range of appliances, providing convenience, flexibility and several interaction possibilities. However, home control via mobile devices also present some challenges, among others regarding the diversity of users. This paper presents the state of the art in home control via mobile devices. Based on an analysis of these solutions, we identify and discuss Human-Computer Interaction (HCI) challenges under the perspective of diversity. In addition, we propose a set of guidelines in order to minimize or overcome these challenges. This work may support design process of new solutions and future research focusing on domestic environment.

Keywords: diversity, domotics, smart home, home automation, mobile application.

1 Introduction

Home is a physical space which comprises social and human aspects, referring to propriety or state of mind, and reflects the lifestyles of the inhabitants [1,2]. The interplay of individual and cultural values make home a complex space. With technological advancements in recent decades, a home environment may incorporate several electronic appliances in order to facilitate activities and improve users' quality of life. These household electrical appliances increased in complexity and functionality, and present different interfaces and controls. With increasing complexity of appliances, it can be expected that interaction becomes more complex as well. With increasingly complex systems, it is necessary to make these functionalities available to all users, in an easier and more effective way.

Mobile devices – e.g. mobile phones, tablets and smartphones – emerge as possible platforms to enable control over such a range of appliances. They have already been adopted by users from different economic and social backgrounds, are equipped with

C. Stephanidis and M. Antona (Eds.): UAHCI/HCII 2014, Part III, LNCS 8515, pp. 501–512, 2014.
© Springer International Publishing Switzerland 2014

several features, provide integration through a single interface are convenient to carry, and make home control possible even when not at home (e.g. in the case of the smartphone). This scenario fits the needs of users in modern societies and enables several interaction possibilities.

Much work focused on the development of solutions in this domain, especially on technical issues (cf. Section 2). However, it is important to consider Human-Computer Interaction (HCI) aspects in development of new solutions. According to Saizmaa and Kim [3], HCI studies have focused mostly on the interaction between humans and technology, not considering the importance of home aspects. Nonetheless, it is essential to consider the relation between users, technology and the domestic environment. There are some challenges of home control via mobile devices related to the diversity of users. Interface and interaction design for this context must consider these differences.

This paper presents the state of the art in home control via mobile devices. Based on analysis of these solutions, we identify and discuss HCI challenges under the perspective of diversity. In addition, we propose a set of guidelines in order to minimize or overcome these challenges. We argue that this work might support design process of new solutions and future research focusing on domestic space.

The paper is organized as follows: Section 2 presents the literature solutions composing the state of the art; Section 3 introduces HCI challenges for this context under the perspective of diversity; Section 5 discusses research issues and additionally presents the proposed guidelines; Section 6 concludes.

2   State of the Art

This section presents the state of the art of mobile devices for controlling elements of domestic environment, in the contexts of smart homes as well as home automation. The literature solutions are organized according to the kind of interface/interaction they present via mobile devices.

2.1   Textual Command Interface

Some solutions do not provide graphical interfaces to support user's interaction. They enable users to control their home through text commands, which are interpreted by home systems. These solutions use mobile telephony services to enable communication, and commands are sent via SMS (Short Messaging Service), using mobile phone.

Alheraish et al. [4], El-Medany and El-Sabry [5], Ahmad et al. [6], Khandare and Mahajan [7], Zhai and Cheng [8], Li et al. [9] and Felix and Raglend [10] propose monitoring and control systems which enable users to control household appliances, sending a message to switch appliances on or off, and check statuses. These solutions are implemented in circuit and use several sensors (e.g. fire, motion and temperature). These works focus on illumination control or home security, for example, intrusion detection, door locking or monitoring. Solutions [7,8] also use cameras. An example of a control command [7] is "STARTDEVICE 1; STOPDEVICE 4", to turn an appliance on and turn another appliance off. Al-Ali et al. [11] focus on energy management, providing functions to users and utility companies. Users may send commands such as "Turn ON AC, Turn OFF WM" to turn air-conditioning on and washing machine off.

2.2 Textual Interface with Visual Layout

Although different interfaces may be designed for appliance control through mobile devices, several works still provide simple graphical interfaces, with textual information through forms and menus. Each appliance is represented by a name, which may be the appliance's category or an identifier, such as "device 1". Users change an appliance's status using elements such as text fields, check boxes and radio buttons. It provides an enhanced interaction in comparison to textual command interfaces mentioned in the previous Section 2.1.

Some works [12,13,14,15] demonstrate this improvement and provide a dual-approach, i.e. communication occurs via SMS or an application. Both forms may be used, but the application acts as an abstraction layer for interaction since users interact with visual interface elements instead of typing commands. These applications were implemented in Java (J2ME). In the same way as interfaces, home management evolves and some systems provide other functions in addition to on/off switches, such as ventilation level [13] and lighting intensity control [14]. In [16], users may check power consumption of plugged appliances and control home via PDA applications with Bluetooth or via mobile phones with SMS. Other solutions only provide application interfaces. The solution proposed in [17] also enables users to change an appliances voltage level. HouseAway [18] provides a HTML page, the solutions in [19,20,21] provide applications with textual menus, implemented in mobile C and GVM platform, Java and Python for Symbian platforms. Systems in this section use microcontrollers, except [15], which uses an X10 controller with power line communication. Moreover, all works focus on development of a system architecture, not on HCI aspects.

2.3 Graphical Interface

With the improvement of processing power and the growth of available resources in mobile devices, several works introduced graphical elements to promote user interaction. These interface designs use colors, icons, charts, images and videos in order to provide a better user experience. Some solutions focus on development of applications and others on complete systems, but they show a particular concern regarding user interface, unlike works of the previous sections.

Yeoh et al. [22] present the e2Home system, which enables switching home appliances on or off and controlling a mobile robot. Users interact with a PDA application or sending textual commands via e-mail. It follows the dual-approach, in which application is an abstraction layer. Its interface shows icons for each appliance along with its name and a select list with its status, and a 2D home map for robot control.

Oh and Kim [23] present a similar work, which proposes to control a mobile robot through an Android smartphone for home monitoring. The application interface only displays the captured images at the center of smartphone screen and direction buttons.

In [24], a local security system is proposed for Android devices. Users can lock, unlock and check a door status from a short distance. The application displays the door status and four buttons, the system uses Arduino and Bluetooth. Solutions [25,26] provide control over appliances, image capture and alerts for security breach. HASec [25] provides an iOS application with visual elements following the iPhone Human Interface Guidelines. SmartEye [26] has a Java application which shows a home plan in 2D view, with appliances in their respective home space and color scheme to help users identifying appliances status. Rahman and Saddik [27] present a mobile client to control real home objects through 3D avatar interaction, using Second Life virtual interface. Since mobile devices lack processing power to render such 3D graphics, it uses a virtual display technique based on remote rendering graphics at a desktop computer. The implemented prototype supports touch events, such as swipe and tap, and provides illumination control, using X10 controllers.

Other systems present functionalities that are more complex. Home-in-Palm [28] provides an Android smartphone application to configure automatic changes based on time or a user's location. In [29], users may define rules, schedule tasks and set priorities, interacting with an iPhone application, an iPad client and a web client. Homer [30] provides two different applications, for iPad and iPhone, and enables users to define rules using a language based on triggers, conditions and actions, with clauses like "when", "do" and "if". The system uses a framework based on OSGi, HTTP and JSON. Dickey et al. [31] provide a cloud service-based system with an iPad application, which uses touchscreen interaction. Its interface uses several visual elements, such as touch buttons similar to on/off switches, and regulators to control light intensity with simple finger dragging. System also displays charts and uses Arduino with X10 and ZigBee communication. Solutions [32,33] generate user interfaces automatically. uniKNX [32], an iPhone application, uses configuration files, provided in system deployment, to aid systems integration with mobile device. Based on these files, it generates interface elements at runtime and provides local control. The mobile phone application presented in [33], has been implemented in ASP .NET and Java-Script, and enables users to for example open/close doors, turn lights on or off, and change color and intensity.

2.4   Multi-modal Interface and Direct Manipulation

Current mobile devices are equipped with specialized technologies and features. Accelerometers, camera, and NFC (Near Field Communication) are common examples. There are different forms of interaction beyond textual or graphical user interface, and some solutions already explore these technologies in interface and interaction design. The following solutions focus on home appliances control addressing some possibilities.

Suo et al. [34] present HouseGenie, a solution for touchscreen smartphones. It provides multi-modal interaction, integrating recognition engines of speech and handwriting, and enables to "fusion" multiple modes of interaction, e.g. when selecting an object with a click or touch and performing and action on this object by voice. It supports click, hold and drag-and-drop gestures, its interface uses several visual elements and displays a 2D home map. It uses an OSGi-based infrastructure to interconnect home appliances. Costa et al. [35] focus on interface design and also provide multi-modal interaction on their accessible interface design proposal to home control. This work provides voice and touchscreen interaction, and the design is based on icons and quadrants, targeting people with visual, hearing, motor and cognitive disabilities. The proposal was implemented over a tablet with Bluetooth communication. Kühnel et al. [36] propose using three-dimensional gestures with a smartphone for home control. The prototype was implemented for the iPhone, using accelerometer data for gesture recognition, and combining touchscreen GUI interaction for more complex actions.

Chueh and Fanjiang [37] propose a context-aware application with automatic interface generation and direct manipulation. Appliances are discovered using NFC of a smartphone, and their descriptions are downloaded through Bluetooth. The application then generates the interface based on user context. It enables local control and uses Arduino. The prototype provides TV control. Solution [38] proposes combining computer vision and ubiquitous computing. In this approach, users point a smartphone camera towards a target appliance in order to recognize it, and then select a function. It requires every appliance to have a visual fingerprint, which can be a photo or visual descriptions. Chen et al. [39] propose a touch-driven interaction system to control household appliances. Users touch target devices with a smartphone, which then captures appliance data and combines it with context information. That way, touch actions are translated into control actions. As a demonstration, three applications were implemented, to control a stereo system, media activities on TV, and to connect a smartphone to a Wi-Fi network.

Based on an analysis of these works, we identified some HCI challenges under the perspective of diversity, which we present in the next section.

3   HCI Challenges under the Perspective of Diversity

When referring to diversity, we consider users with different characteristics, including culture, age, education, gender, technical skills, knowledge, cognitive skills or use conditions. The domestic environment, due to its heterogeneous nature, always aggregates a heterogeneous set of users and diverse use situations. According to Huang [40], a key HCI challenge in mobile application design is how to make such devices usable and affordable to a heterogeneous set of users. To overcome this issue, it is necessary to consider social and contextual factors [41] in order to comprehend users' needs in their context of use, i.e. home control. The literature presented in the previous section outlines the state of the art in home control via mobile devices. Based on an analysis of these works, we identify and discuss HCI challenges under the perspective of diversity for this specific domain, which are presented below.

Home View: In order to control their homes, users must manage functions provided by household appliances, which are located in the domestic space. However, how to (re)present this space to all dwellers? Many solutions represent home as an appliances list, with no reference to the corresponding home space the appliances belong to [12,13,14,17,20,21,22,25,31]. Other solutions separate them according to location, based on room selection, such as [33]. Other approaches are to represent home as an architectural plan in a 2D-view with appliances in their respective real positions, such as in [26], or as 3D environment with virtual objects, as proposed in [27]. The 3D approach might enhance immersion and aid in elements assimilation. However, some people might have difficulties to navigate in these virtual environments. According to [34], devices identification and monitoring is faster and clearer in 2D-panoramic view than in 3D-view. Even so, 2D map representation might impose difficulties to interpretation, and changes in appliances arrangement might require map restructuring. Moreover, there is also the barrier of displaying spatial representations, 2D or 3D, in restricted screen-size devices, such as the smartphone. On the other hand, appliances lists may aid users to find the target appliance with symbolic recognition, with no spatial processing. However, it may not be as immersive as spatial representations. How to (re)present this space in order to assist diverse users with different characteristics to identify appliances through mobile devices constitutes a relevant challenge in this context.

Control Complexity: Solutions for home control involve management of a wide range of appliances, with different functions. Appliances with increasing functions make their control a very complex task. Their control via mobile devices is even more difficult, given the intrinsic characteristics of these platforms. Higher complexity functions, such as rule definition like in [29,30], bring even more challenges. According Manternaghan apud Manternaghan and Turner [30], users would like to control their home in a way that does not resemble programming. But policy definition usually uses conditional statements and commands, which requires a programming-like interaction. Nylander et al. apud Suo et al. [34] claim that users prefer using a smartphone instead of a computer to control appliances, since it is more convenient. Since smartphones have screens with limited size, a challenge for interaction design is to enable this wider range of appliance management through these devices. Providing solutions which enables users with different characteristics and usage situations to manage their home amidst this complexity constitutes another challenge.

Interface and Interaction Flexibility: Regarding interface flexibility, the configuration of appliances in a home might change over time, e.g. new appliances might be added, removed or changed in position. The application interface must reflect these changes, including the customization of automatically assigned identifiers may require customization. Some applications [13,16,32] reference household appliances and rooms as identifiers. These identifiers might be application or manufacturer defaults, might not represent the respective object/place efficiently or logically from a user's point of view. However, in many cases, graphical interface and system are tightly coupled, which makes modifications more difficult. Regarding interaction flexibility, many solutions provide only one form to interact with system. Among 36 solutions presented in the state of the art, only 3 provide multi-modal interaction [34,35,36]. Although some solutions [37,38,39] explore other forms of interaction, they do not enable users to use other interaction modes. This excludes people who cannot use a particular interaction form [42], for example, in the case of a disability or a temporal limitation due to a specific context of use. For example, a person doing a household chore, such as washing the dishes, might temporarily not be able to interact with a touchscreen interface. This challenge has not been addressed/solved in most of the work presented in the previous section.

Individuality and Multi-person Interaction: People share space and appliances with other residents at domestic environment. Several people can control several appliances, simultaneously or at different times. These appliances usually provide a single interface, common for all users. Despite home being a shared environment, each individual has a personal relationship with the space. Even if interface modification is enabled, if it remains common to all users, issues regarding individuality and diversity still persist. For example, users may accomplish routine tasks in specific way according preference (e.g. configure light intensity at a specific value). This characteristic is individual and user interface must reflect it. Another example is regarding names of home spaces. Even if application provide modifying names, for example, from "Room 1" to "John's Room", each user should define a particular name, such as "My Room", which reflects the own vision of home space. It is therefore necessary to provide solutions to equitably attend all users, but also reflect the users' individuality in each interaction, and it imposes a challenge to this context.

Privacy: Since home is a space that entails individual and personal values, we must consider privacy in solution design for domestic spaces. Solutions for home control involve appliances and environment monitoring, which bring to light the challenge of preserving people's privacy. Several works presented in the previous section provide home security systems [4,5,6,7,8,25,26]. In order to detect intrusion, these systems monitor the environment extracting private data from cameras or sensors. The camera usage to capture image and videos in several works [7,8,14,23,25,26] aims to provide better visualization, greater reliability and feedback, but it may impact user privacy. The privacy issue must also be considered in solutions that use context information or sensor data captured from mobile device, as in [39]. Data from user profiles, such as used in [28], also highlights privacy issues, since it contains user preferences and several personal information regarding domestic routine. Home is a sacred environment in diverse cultures and the privacy concept might vary among individuals as well as among cultures. Thus information regarding domestic space requires great attention and imposes a challenge for new solutions design under this context.

Internationalization and Localization: With globalization, potential users of software are not restricted to a country or region. Home environment is a concept presented in different cultures across the world, it is thus important that home control applications may be used by users from different nations and cultural backgrounds. However, these applications are often developed to support a single language, imposing a challenge for diversity. None of the solutions presented in the previous section mention multi-language support.

3.1   Guidelines

Considering the challenges presented in the previous section, we propose a set of guidelines in order to minimize or overcome them. In this paper we consider the concept of guideline as addressed by Stephanidis et al. [43,44], as a general statement that applies in a particular context, typically subject to further interpretation so as to reflect the requirements of a particular organization or design case. Below we present our guidelines for the context of home control via mobile devices.

Consider the Dwellers' Perspective: Interface and interaction design of solutions must consider each dweller's perspective to (re)present this space, such as space division, references, rooms and names.

When adopting a spatial representation, offer an alternative non-spatial representation: Spatial representations, such as maps or virtual environment simulations require human spatial reasoning skills, which may hinder access by all users.

Abstract Low-Level Information of Home Control: Application interfaces must abstract low-level details, highlighting information and simplifying home management and control. It must provide high-level interaction, e.g. users must interact with elements that group information and specific resources.

Provide Policy Management in "Natural" Approach: If a solution provides policy management, provide user interaction in the most "natural" way possible, in a way that does not seem like programming software. Practical alternatives to aid in this process may include graphical elements usage, such as figures, natural language and gestures.

Enable Simple and Complex Tasks Accomplishment: The solution design must account for people with different goals and levels of "mastery", i.e. for both beginners and advanced users, to access basic or complex functions, through mobile interface. Some possible alternatives include configuration features and interface levels (e.g. beginner, intermediate and advanced) based on users usage and knowledge.

Provide Several Forms of Interaction: Thus, people with no ability to interact through a certain form of interaction might use another one to accomplish tasks. Mobile devices provide several features, such as audio, voice and sensors, which enables designers to go beyond the GUI.

Provide a Dynamic Interface, Decoupled from System Functionalities: Provide a dynamic interface, which reflects changes, such as new appliances and floor layout. New appliances might bring new functionalities. Different vendors might implement functionalities differently. Decoupling would hide these details from users and provide them with a unified interface that adapts to changes. This interface should allow users to modify interface elements, such as identifiers and icons, as well as to insert new images (e.g. regarding new appliances inserted into the system).

Promote Individuality on Interface/Interaction: Provide features to enable users to personalize some interface elements and interaction with system. Thus, solution matches the user's interests, reflecting their individual characteristics and personal relation with the environment, attempting specific and personal needs. Saving user preferences, routine actions and setup values may contribute to personalize interface/interaction and reduce manual repetition in mobile devices.

Consider Privacy on Environment, Device and User Context: The solution design must consider privacy regarding domestic space, the context data captured from both, environment and mobile device, as well as personal information provided by users. Some alternatives include consent and setup features, and all information under this context regarding personal values must be considered.

Provide Internationalization and Localization: The mobile application for home control must provide internationalization and localization, supporting translation of interface elements to another idiom.

4   Discussion

Differently from other works (e.g., [40,41,45,46]), this paper focuses on HCI challenges for the specific domain of home control via mobile devices. Some works expose HCI challenges for mobile devices [40,41,45]. However, these challenges only cover issues related to device characteristics and do not take into account the use context of such devices, e.g. home control. Likewise, works presenting challenges for home automation [46] only address challenges regarding the domestic context and do not consider restrictions relevant to mobile devices. This work addresses both concerns under the perspective of diversity, presenting identified challenges and relating them with literature solutions.

The set of guidelines presented in this paper requires substantial interpretation by designers, which might be considered a drawback. Furthermore, the guidelines were not experimentally validated, and only reflect knowledge and intuition on the specific subject. However, we chose this format because our goal was to provide a high level support to designers in this specific domain, supporting them to consider and reflect upon relevant points which might minimize or overcome the challenges identified in this work. As our literature review has shown, interaction design of domotic environments is a relatively new area. Once we gathered more empirical data of designing and evaluating systems in this domain, the guidelines might be refined and made more operable defining more concrete recommendations or success criteria.

Although the problem domain of home control includes terms such as smart home, most of the found literature focused on home automation. Therefore, it is important to stress that this paper do not focus on specific issues regarding ubiquitous computing [47]. Furthermore, despite recent advances concerning mobile devices, many solutions still lack usage of new forms of interaction. Most of the state of the art solutions still provide interaction through traditional GUI and several works do not consider HCI aspects. Nowadays mobile devices present a huge impact in users' everyday lives, thus new mobile interfaces and interactions are expected to improve users' experiences. Identifying challenges in this context is the first step to tackle them and provide a better interaction.

5   Conclusion

This paper has presented the state of the art and HCI challenges in solutions for home control via mobile devices. The contribution of this paper is to summarize current literature solutions considering HCI aspects and identify challenges under the perspective of diversity, contextualized to this specific domain. In addition, we propose a set of guidelines, which may guide the design process of new mobile applications focusing home control. Our goal is to support designers to consider relevant points highlighted by the challenges and to minimize or overcome them.

Future work will involve a design, implementation and evaluation of app to control household appliances following the proposed guidelines. Furthermore, research about other forms of interaction with mobile devices for this context is required in order to extend the usage possibilities and attend user and situation diversity.

Acknowledgments. This work was partially supported by the Brazilian Federal Agency for Support and Evaluation of Graduate Education (CAPES), by the Institute of Computing at University of Campinas (IC/UNICAMP), and by the Physical Artifacts of Interaction Research Group (PAIRG) at Federal University of Rio Grande do Norte (UFRN), Brazil.

References

1. Mallett, S.: Understanding Home: A Critical Review of the Literature. The Sociological Review 52, 62–89 (2004)
2. Frolich, D., Kraut, R.: The Social Context of Home Computing. In: Harper, R. (ed.) Inside the Smart Home, pp. 127–162. Springer (2003)
3. Saizmaa, T., Kim, H.-C.: A Holistic Understanding of HCI Perspectives on Smart Home. In: 4th Int. Conf. on Networked Computing and Advanced Information Management, pp. 59–65. IEEE (2008)
4. Alheraish, A., Alomar, W., Abu-Al-Ela, M.: Programmable Logic Controller System for Controlling and Monitoring Home Application Using Mobile Network. In: IEEE Instrumentation and Measurement Technology Conference, pp. 24–27. IEEE (2006)
5. El-Medany, W.M., El-Sabry, M.R.: GSM-based Remote Sensing and Control System Using FPGA. In: Int. Conf. on Computer and Communication Engineering, pp. 1093–1097. IEEE (2008)
6. Ahmad, A.W., Jan, N., Iqbal, S., Lee, C.: Implementation of ZigBee-GSM based Home Security Monitoring and Remote Control System. In: 54th International Midwest Symposium on Circuits and Systems, pp. 1–4. IEEE (2011)
7. Khandare, M.S., Mahajan, A.: Mobile Monitoring System for Smart Home. In: 3rd Int. Conf. on Emerging Trends in Engineering and Technology, pp. 848–852. IEEE (2010)
8. Zhai, Y., Cheng, X.: Design of Smart Home Remote Monitoring System based on Embedded System. In: IEEE 2nd Int. Conf. on Computing, Control and Industrial Engineering, pp. 41–44. IEEE (2011)
9. Li, X., Yuan, Q., Wu, W., Peng, X., Hou, L.: Implementation of GSM SMS Remote Control System based on FPGA. In: Int. Conf. on Information Science and Engineering, pp. 4–6. IEEE (2010)

10. Felix, C., Raglend, I.J.: Home Automation Using GSM. In: Int. Conf. Signal Processing, Communication, Computing and Networking Technologies, pp. 15–19. IEEE (2011)
11. Al-Ali, A.R., El-Hag, A.H., Dhaouadi, R., Zainaldain, A.: Smart Home Gateway for Smart Grid. In: Int. Conf. on Innovations in Information Technology, pp. 90–93. IEEE (2011)
12. Van Der Werff, M., Gui, X., Xu, W.L.: A Mobile-based Home Automation System. In: 2nd Int. Conf. on Mobile Technology, Applications and Systems, pp. 1–5. IEEE (2005)
13. Al Mehairi, S.O., Barada, H., Al Qutayri, M.: Integration of Technologies for Smart Home Application. In: IEEE/ACS Int. Conf. on Computer Systems and Applications, pp. 241–246. IEEE (2007)
14. Yuksekkaya, B., Kayalar, A.A., Tosun, M.B., Ozcan, M.K., Alkar, A.Z.: A GSM, Internet and Speech Controlled Wireless Interactive Home Automation System. IEEE Transactions on Consumer Electronics 52, 837–843 (2006)
15. Shahriyar, R., Hoque, E., Naim, I., Sohan, S.M., Akbar, M.: Controlling Remote System Using Mobile Telephony. In: 1st Int. Conf. on Mobile Wireless Middleware, Operating Systems, and Applications, pp. 1–7. ICST (2008)
16. Lien, C.-H., Bai, Y.-W., Lin, M.-B.: Remote-Controllable Power Outlet System for Home Power Management. IEEE Trans. Cons. Electr. 53, 1634–1641 (2007)
17. Ali, U., Nawaz, S.J., Jawad, N.: A Real-time Control System for Home/Office Appliances Automation, from Mobile Device through GPRS Network. In: 13th IEEE Int. Conf. on Electronics, Circuits and Systems, pp. 854–857. IEEE (2006)
18. Mandurano, J., Haber, N.: House Away: A Home Management System. In: IEEE Long Island Systems, Applications and Technology Conference, pp. 1–4. IEEE (2012)
19. Yoon, D.-H., Bae, D.-J., Kim, H.S.: Implementation of Home Electric Appliances Control System based on the Mobile and the Internet. In: International Joint Conference, pp. 3730–3733. IEEE (2006)
20. Debono, C.J., Abela, K.: Implementation of a Home Automation System through a Central FPGA Controller. In: IEEE Mediterranean Electrotechnical Conf., pp. 641–644. IEEE (2012)
21. Piyare, R., Tazil, M.: Bluetooth based Home Automation System Using Cell Phone. In: IEEE 15th International Symposium on Consumer Electronics, pp. 14–17. IEEE (2011)
22. Yeoh, C.-M., Tan, H.-Y., Kok, C.-K., Lee, H.-J., Lim, H.: e2Home: A Lightweight Smart Home Management System. In: 3rd Int. Conf. on Convergence and Hybrid Information Technology, pp. 11–13. IEEE (2008)
23. Oh, H.-K., Kim, I.-C.: Hybrid Control Architecture of the Robotic Surveillance System Using Smartphones. In: Int. Conf. on Ubiquitous Robots and Ambient Intelligence, pp. 782–785. IEEE (2011)
24. Potts, J., Sukittanon, S.: Exploiting Bluetooth on Android Mobile Devices for Home Security Application. In: IEEE Southeastcon, pp. 1–4. IEEE (2012)
25. Das, S.R., Chita, S., Peterson, N., Shirazi, B.A., Bhadkamkar, M.: Home Automation and Security for Mobile Devices. In: IEEE Int. Conf. on Pervasive Computing and Communications Workshops, pp. 141–146. IEEE (2011)
26. Atukorala, K., Wijekoon, D., Tharugasini, M., Perera, I., Silva, C.: SmartEye Integrated Solution to Home Automation, Security and Monitoring through Mobile Phones. In: 3rd Int. Conf. on Next Generation Mobile Applications, Services and Technologies, pp. 64–69. IEEE (2009)
27. Rahman, A.S.M.M., Saddik, A.E.: Remote Rendering based Second Life Mobile Client System to Control Smart Home Appliances. In: IEEE Int. Conf. on Virtual Environments Human-Computer Interfaces and Measurement Systems, pp. 1–4. IEEE (2011)

28. Marusic, L., Skocir, P., Petric, A., Jezic, G.: Home-in-Palm - A Mobile Service for Remote Control of Household Energy Consumption. In: 11th Int. Conf. on Telecommunications, pp. 109–116. IEEE (2011)
29. Kugler, M., Reinhart, F., Schlieper, K., Masoodian, M., Rogers, B., André, E., Rist, T.: Architecture of a Ubiquitous Smart Energy Management System for Residential Homes. In: 12th Annual Conference of the New Zealand Chapter of the ACM Special Interest Group on Computer-Human Interaction, pp. 101–104. ACM (2011)
30. Maternaghan, C., Turner, K.J.: A Configurable Telecare System. In: 4th Int. Conf. on Pervasive Technologies Related to Assistive Environments, pp. 1–8. ACM (2011)
31. Dickey, N., Banks, D., Sukittanon, S.: Home Automation using Cloud Network and Mobile Devices. In: IEEE Southeastcon, pp. 1–4. IEEE (2012)
32. Bittins, B., Sieck, J., Herzog, M.: Supervision and Regulation of Home Automation Systems with Smartphones. In: 4th UKSim European Symposium on Computer Modeling and Simulation, pp. 444–448. IEEE (2010)
33. Kartakis, S., Antona, M., Stephanidis, C.: Control Smart Homes Easily with Simple Touch. In: Int. ACM Workshop on Ubiquitous Meta User Interfaces, pp. 1–6. ACM (2011)
34. Suo, Y., Wu, C., Qin, Y., Yu, C., Zhong, Y., Shi, Y.: HouseGenie: Universal Monitor and Controller of Networked Devices on Touchscreen Phone in Smart Home. In: Symposia Workshops on Ubiquitous, Autonomic and Trusted Computing, pp. 487–489. IEEE (2010)
35. Costa, L.C.P., Almeida, N.S., Correa, A.G.D., Lopes, R.D., Zuffo, M.K.: Accessible Display Design to Control Home Area Networks. IEEE Transactions on Consumer Electronics 59, 422–427 (2013)
36. Kühnel, C., Westermann, T., Hemmert, F., Kratz, S., Müller, A., Möller, S.: I'm Home: Defining and Evaluating a Gesture Set for Smart-Home Control. Int. J. Hum.-Comput. Stud. 69, 693–704 (2011)
37. Chueh, T.-F., Fanjiang, Y.-Y.: Universal Remote Control on Smartphone. In: International Symposium on Computer, Consumer and Control, pp. 658–661. IEEE (2012)
38. Belimpasakis, P., Walsh, R.: Fusing Mixed Reality and Networked Home Techniques to Improve User Control of Consumer Electronics. In: IEEE Int. Conf. on Consumer Electronics, pp. 107–108. IEEE (2011)
39. Chen, L., Pan, G., Li, S.: Touch-Driven Interaction via an NFC-Enabled Smartphone. In: IEEE Int. Conf. Pervasive Comp., pp. 504–506. IEEE (2012)
40. Huang, K.-Y.: Challenges in Human-Computer Interaction Design for Mobile Devices. In: World Congress on Engineering and Computer Science, pp. 236–241 (2009)
41. Wobbrock, J.O.: The Future of Mobile Device Research in HCI. In: CHI Workshop What is the Next Generation of Human-Computer Interaction?, pp. 131–134 (2006)
42. Sainz de Salces, F.J., England, D., Llewellyn-Jones, D.: Designing for All in the House. In: Latin American Conference on Human-Computer Interaction, pp. 283–288. ACM (2005)
43. Stephanidis, C., Akoumianakis, D., Sfyrakis, M., Paramythis, A.: Universal Accessibility in HCI: Process-Oriented Design Guidelines and Tool Requirements. In: 4th ERCIM Workshop on User Interfaces for All, pp. 1–15 (1998)
44. Akoumianakis, D., Stephanidis, C.: Propagating Experience-based Accessibility Guidelines to User-Interface Development. Ergonomics 42, 1283–1310 (1999)
45. Dunlop, M., Brewster, S.: The Challenge of Mobile Devices for Human Computer Interaction. Personal Ubiquitous Comput. 6, 235–236 (2002)
46. Brush, A.J.B., Lee, B., Mahajan, R., Agarwal, S., Saroiu, S., Dixon, C.: Home Automation in the Wild: Challenges and Opportunities. In: Annual Conference on Human Factors in Computing Systems, pp. 2115–2124. ACM (2011)
47. Weiser, M.: The Computer for the 21st Century. Scientific American 265, 94–104 (1991)

Novel Consumer-to-Product Interactions with Context-Aware Embedded Platforms

Sönke Knoch, Matthieu Deru, Simon Bergweiler, and Jens Haupert

German Research Center for Artificial Intelligence
Research Department Intelligent User Interfaces
Saarbrücken, Germany
{firstname.familyname}@dfki.de

Abstract. In this work we suggest a new device to instrument everyday objects in the end-user life cycle phase that makes everyday life easier for the elderly. The instrumentation of products, such as food, transforms them into smarter and more intelligent products. The equipped product notifies the user when food is spoiled and—interconnected with other smart products—advises against side effects that occur when food is consumed while a certain medication is ingested. We describe the considerations that were made towards a first prototype from a technical perspective. An interaction model was developed, a requirements analysis performed and several design and development considerations made. An architecture shows the information flow between sensors, actuators, and the Internet of Things. In the end, the prototype of a product sleeve is presented that is easy to handle and intuitive to operate. A feedback study is planned in the near future.

Keywords: Internet of Things, smart/intelligent products, prototyping.

1 Introduction

The proportion of elderly in the population has increased. According to the German Federal Office of Statistics [1], about one person out of seven was younger than the age of 15 years in Germany in 2010. Worldwide, only Japan had a lower rate of young people in the same year. This increasing number of old persons leads to an increasing demand in care services. New technologies can allow these growing populations of elderly to live in better conditions at home for a longer time. Sensing capabilities of old people that are fading away can be absorbed by smart devices with sensors and specific features in the smart home [2] of the future. In contrast to systems which try to detect critical situations by monitoring a person's vital parameters [3] or by interpreting movement patterns [4], we seek to make life easier by instrumenting the living environment. Following the ideas of the Internet of Things [5] and Ubiquitous Computing [6], future environments will become more intelligent when a net of intelligent, smart objects is present on a larger scale.

C. Stephanidis and M. Antona (Eds.): UAHCI/HCII 2014, Part III, LNCS 8515, pp. 513–524, 2014.
© Springer International Publishing Switzerland 2014

The input modalities of an intelligent, smart product collect a huge amount of data during its life cycle, so called "Big Data" [7], that can be stored in digital product memories as demonstrated by Brandherm and Kröner [8]. Context-aware computing [9] adds value to raw sensor data as it helps to understand it [10]. The object memory model (OMM) as discussed in the W3C OMM Incubator Group [11] provides a format to structure data on these "smart labels". Associated data is stored on the physical artifact's label or in the digital cloud, depending on the storage capabilities of the label and the amount of data to store. A framework and a set of tools to handle OMMs is suggested by Haupert [12]. It allows the creation of new applications to digital object memories. We will apply the OMM to the product sleeve, because it allows us to store information in a structured and easy to access manner and at the same time it supports the upload of code snippets [13]. Code snippets define a logical rule, to perform an action (e.g., alert the user) when a certain threshold (e.g., freezing temperature) is reached.

As in many cases, objects and products today are not instrumented on grounds of costs, we suggest an intelligent product sleeve—the Ring—that makes products kinetic, tangible, smarter, and more intelligent when it is slipped on a product. While products in the future will be endued with radio frequency identification (RFID) chips [14], the product informs the sleeve smoothly about its identity and origin over near field communication (NFC). Products with barcodes are scanned with an inbuilt optical sensor or another device in the Internet of Things, e.g., a smartphone. In comparison to systems that are integrated into an object, the concept behind the product sleeve improves the cost-benefit ratio of instrumentation as it is reusable and adaptive. Therefore, we follow the concept of "Incycling" as suggested by Brandherm, Kröner, and Haupert [15].

In the following section, we will summarize related work. In Section 3 the underlying scenario for the application of the suggested prototype is described. Then, in Section 4 the instrumentation of an object, the interaction between objects and between humans and objects is modeled. In Section 5 we define the requirements based on the scenario and the interaction model from a hardware perspective. Design and software engineering decisions are depicted in the Sections 6 and 7. Finally, we summarize the results and give an outlook on future work in Section 8.

2   Related Work

Milky [16] is an anthropomorphic milk carton that presents a new way of emotional interaction with products. The instrumented milk carton has a touch screen and sensors as input modalities and WLAN and ZigBee to communicate with other devices. The milk carton shows emotions via a face on the screen. If a customer comes closer to Milky, it blinks with its eyes and plays acoustic sounds to catch the customer's attention. As the instrumentation of such a milk carton might be too expensive, the product sleeve presented in this work depicts a cheap alternative way of product instrumentation, which is reusable and follows the idea of "Incycling" [15]. The product sleeve was developed for home scenarios, while Milky unlocks its full potential primarily in shopping scenarios.

Mother and its Motion Cookies [17] were presented at the CES 2014 and represent one central node (Mother) with power plug and several sensor nodes (Motion Cookies) that send data to the central node. The basic package comes with one movement sensor, one thermometer, one range sensor, and one adaptive sensor node supplied by battery. These sensor nodes can be attached to objects, such as bottles, in the user's household to allow them to communicate their status to the mother following the idea of the Internet of Things. In comparison to the Mother network, the product sleeve is independent and needs no central entity as it forms the network in an ad-hoc manner.

Smart Products as described by Mülhäuser [18] can interact with the user in all life cycle phases. The product sleeve makes a product smart and is meant to be a home application. Thus, the human-to-product interaction model was developed for the end user life cycle phase. Capabilities, such as sensors, LEDs, and communication interfaces, support a natural and intuitive interaction with the equipped product. The interaction modalities are able to analyze the environment and to derive conclusions based on this knowledge. The results of this process are communicated to the user in form of guidance. A guidance is a recommendation what the user can do with the equipped product that has been in a certain environment for a while (since the moment of equipping). A minimalistic design supports natural and intuitive interaction. The product sleeve also allows the integration of the product into smart environments, such as a smart kitchen [2].

Towards smart products Meyer, Främling, and Holmström [19] suggest the term *Intelligent Product*. According to Gershenfeld [20], the barrier between things and the digital world has to melt in the near future and it already has looking at the last decade. The complete connection of both, the physical and the digital world remains a challenge for the future. In industrial settings, intelligent products already experienced a change through the introduction of Auto-ID technologies, where the MIT Auto-ID Center played and now the Auto-ID Labs play a crucial role. Auto-ID technologies allow products to communicate their current state to the machines that handle the product. For example, Kröner et al. [21] demonstrate the interaction with digital product memories by showing how a robot handles fragile and non-fragile objects in different ways, throwing them into the basket or placing them carefully on the table. All these changes and new opportunities resulting from the rise of new technologies trigger a shift from centralized to distributed computing in production. These changes may end up in the Fourth Industrial Revolution, Industry 4.0 [22], a research strategy exclaimed by the German Federal Ministry of Education and Research. In this context, the Internet of Things, Cloud Computing, and Big Data are the most influential factors.

According to the classification for intelligent products by Meyer et al. [19], the suggested product sleeve has a level of intelligence that is called *problem notification*. Because of its ability to detect problems and communicate them to the user its intelligence is above simple information handling. Still, it has not reached the level of decision making which is up to the user. Its nature could be better described as a decision support system. The location of intelligence is an *intelligence at object* and partly an *intelligence through network*. On the one hand, the object instrumented with the sleeve has all computational power, storing capacities, and connectivity that is necessary and, thus can be called a big smart device or embedded platform. On the other hand, knowledge about objects in the vicinity may influence notifications and decision support. Finally, regarding the aggregation level of intelligence the product sleeve is an *intelligent container*, as it is aware of an object that might be intelligent by itself. It registers if an object is removed or attached, adapts and processes the object's knowledge, and is not an intelligent item that only manages information and notifications about itself.

3   Scenario

John is an old person who has difficulties to manage the challenges of everyday life. He suffers from mild cognitive impairments and forgetfulness. Nevertheless, John would rather not move to a retirement home. A care service supports him and passes by every day to undertake a few basic tasks, e.g., shopping, cleaning, and looking after the patient's condition. The time for these tasks is limited, such that the service only has half an hour for each visit. In the time left, John is on his own. Because his senses are fading away while getting older, it has become more difficult for him, e.g., to deal with the groceries in the household. The information on the packages is printed in very small letters and is hard to read. It has also become harder for John to smell or see if a product is spoiled. The product sleeve that is attached to food by the employee of the care service when she brings the groceries and places them into the fridge, visualizes product information in such a way that John can recognize it easier and detects spoiled food by the product's date of expiry. As the product sleeve follows the idea of "Incycling", it can be reused on similar products in the future. An inbuilt accelerometer recognizes movement when the product is grabbed by John and alerts him if the product has expired. A red light and an acoustic alert hint at the potentially spoiled food. If the food is okay and the storage of the food was all right—appropriate temperature and brightness—then the light shines green.

4   Interaction Model

4.1   Object Instrumentation

The sleeve device is charged in a charging cradle and can be applied to a variety of products. Our prototype was made to carry bottles and other drinking vessels, such as beverage cartons commonly utilized to carry milk or juice. To instrument the object with the sleeve device, the RFID interface has to be placed very close to the product's RFID chip to allow the device to read the data on the chip. If no

RFID chip is available at the product, the barcode is scanned with the camera of the device or of a smartphone. Once the data is transmitted, the device can fetch additional information over its Wi-Fi connection. Related snippets are downloaded to build the basis for notifications on status changes of the product. Now, the newly instrumented product has become a smart, intelligent product and can be used as usual with its additional, newly won features.

4.2 Human-to-Object Interaction

Human-to-object interaction is triggered in two ways indirectly and directly. An indirect interaction is given when the sensors detect that the user is paying attention to the object. Movement detection, brightness, and distance measurements register when the object is grabbed. If a notification is waiting in the queue to get communicated, it is now released. The output modality depends on the priority of the notification. High priority notifications are released automatically. The object vibrates, shows red light over the LED, and plays the message over the audio speaker. An example for such a high priority notification would be that the milk has expired. Low priority notifications are visualized over an orange light. If the user wants to hear the notification he or she can push the button to hear the notification. An example for a low priority notification would be that the milk is almost finished. If there are no notifications in the queue the LED shows green light. To rate the notification, the user has to press the one touch button interface that provides a feedback function.

4.3 Object-to-Object Interaction

Multiple instrumented objects that use the OMM to store data can also interact with each other. Over Web service discovery the objects know about the existence of each other and can generate notifications based on code snippets [13] they have automatically downloaded. One example is the suggestion of receipts. For example, the milk can suggest to make pancakes if it registered a carton of eggs in the same fridge. This would be a low priority notification. An example for high priority notifications are side effects that occur when a certain kind of food is consumed while the patient is ingesting a certain medication. For instance, drinking grapefruit juice can increase the level of medicine in the blood, which can increase the risk of side effects. Calcium channel blockers, a medication to decrease blood pressure in patients with hypertension, can interact with grapefruit juice and increase the level of medicine in the patient's blood. The system prevents the consumption of both and requests the user to seek advice from the pharmacist or doctor. As the product sleeve in its current, prototypic state is not suitable to be attached to pills, the interconnected object would be an intelligent medicament blister, as suggested by Nesselrath et al. [2].

5 Requirements

To support the interaction model presented in Section 4, a set of requirements for the device can be derived.

5.1 Input Modalities

An accelerometer is necessary to detect movements of the device. A distance measurement module allows to detect if a person or object is close to the Ring. A light sensor will detect the brightness around the object. This function is necessary to check for example, if the fridge is open or not and to monitor the storage conditions. To supervise storage conditions, a temperature and humidity sensor will provide an additional sense.

5.2 Output Modalities

To answer the question about the visualization, it is important to discuss the target group of users and the planned shape of the product. The users will be elderly who experience a fading away of their senses through normal aging up to mild cognitive impairments. An easy-to-use and self-explaining user interface has to be developed to support such users. Touchscreens might provide a lot of capabilities, but are difficult to fit in a round shaped device that fits around a bottle. For that reason, we will use LEDs to visualize the state of the product (in good condition, in bad condition, there might be an issue) that illuminate the product sleeve in green, red, or orange light. To communicate the content of the notification to the user, an easy to recognize output modality has to be chosen. As displays are difficult to integrate and hard to read, especially for the elderly, natural language output in form of spoken words seems to be most appropriate. From a hardware point of view, this requires the integration of a speaker. For people suffering of deafness, the visualization is submitted to a screen device in the vicinity, e.g., the television or the tablet. If not understood at the first time, the playback of the natural reader can be played back again by pressing the button.

5.3 Communication

A camera is on-board to provide an interface to read visual tags, such as bar-codes. NFC allows to read and write information that is stored on RFID chips. Over Wi-Fi the connection to the Internet can be established to fetch additional information that might be necessary to generate product related notifications. ZigBee is a communication protocol that allows wireless communication between devices consuming low energy. To allow communication between objects in the vicinity in an energy saving way, a ZigBee module is integrated.

5.4 Power Supply

To run the required functionality, an appropriate power supply is necessary. The intended hardware to realize all input and output modalities is consuming little power. Main consuming components are the CPU and the communication module. So it is an advantage if some of the main consumers known from the smartphone domain (cf. [23], [24]), such as LCD and GPS, are not inbuilt. To

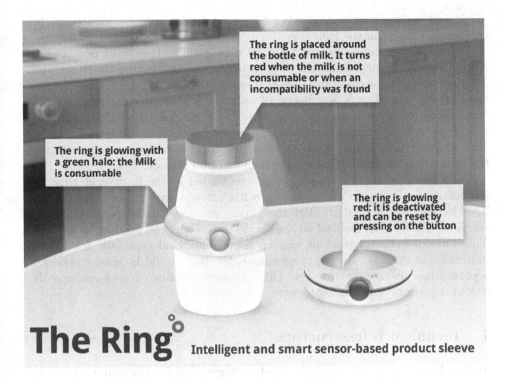

Fig. 1. Shape of the Ring

load the mobile power supply, the product sleeve is placed in a charging cradle that loads the device wireless. This way of charging is easy to handle for the care service and the elderly, as no cable has to be plugged in and out.

6   Design

The design of the Ring follows the philosophy of creating a minimalistic device. The object instrumentation as described in Section 4.1 has to be very easy. Additionally, there should be only one intuitive "interface" between device and user. We realize this idea with a one button interaction. The button is integrated in an elastic band. It changes its color according to the tracked sensor information, which trigger low or high priority notifications. When, for example, the milk is in good condition and no compatibility problems with medicines or the metabolism of the consumer were found, it will turn green. On the other hand, if there is a potential problem with the milk, the button will turn red. When recommendations and suggestions—low priority notifications—are generated the button will turn orange. In order to amplify this visual signal and to provide a direct, clearly visible feedback to the user, a small flexible LED stripe is placed around the elastic band. This stripe will glow accordingly red, green, or orange. These colors are amplified by sequences of light impulse. The batteries and the sensors are placed in the elastic band making it completely autonomous. Figure 1 shows the design concept of the Ring.

The one button concept plays a central role. It allows the caring personnel to easily reset the status of the ring by pressing the central button for 10 seconds. This action resynchronizes the parameters and the sensors, for example, when the ring was placed on a new bottle of milk. To parametrize the ring, wireless communication is used: over an app and a Wi-Fi module, the caring personnel can set up several parameters depending on the patient's health or metabolism. This configuration defines when the ring has to glow and what parameters of the milk are taken into account over the integrated sensors.

The consumption of the patient is also registered by the Ring: each time the patient takes the bottle and opens it, a log entry is written into the storage. This information is used to alert the caring personnel if the patient has not correctly followed the medical advices and "consumed" the product as advised. This kind of behavior tracking can be useful and vital especially for elderly patients. For example, during the summer, the Ring could be used to check if a person has drunk enough water. This prevents a feeling of weakness and the risk of dehydration during heat waves.

7   Technical Infrastructure

To develop a first prototype of the product sleeve that fits the requirements described in Section 5, we decided to use the Microsoft .NET Gadgeteer platform. Microsoft .NET Gadgeteer provides a platform that is easy to learn and represents a good basis for quick prototyping networked devices for the Internet of Things [25].

The core component of the prototype that was developed in this approach based on a GHI Electronics Spider Board running the .NET Micro Framework. There are different types of sensors that can be connected to this Gadgeteer platform. The sensor interpretation layer that can be seen in Figure 2 gathers information of the current environment to set situational parameters. These parameters are necessary in order to make an evaluative statement and establish the basis for estimations and forecasts. In the implemented prototype, we use a moisture and temperature/barometer sensor combined with an accelerometer and gyroscope module. A barometer module analyzes the current weather situation and will check if, for instance, milk is beginning to turn sour in the following hours. Additionally, a mobile accumulator provides the power supply for the modules and the Gadgeteer board.

On the software side, the framework for estimation and forecasting based on sensor knowledge is written in C#, the standard programming language for the .NET framework. The evaluation and case analysis will be based on defined rules. Once a rule matches, an action is triggered and sent to the Presentation Manager. This module initiates the appropriate form of visualization, supported by pre-defined acoustic alerts. Not every use case allows the use of a touchscreen, but a touchscreen has the advantage that information can be displayed directly.

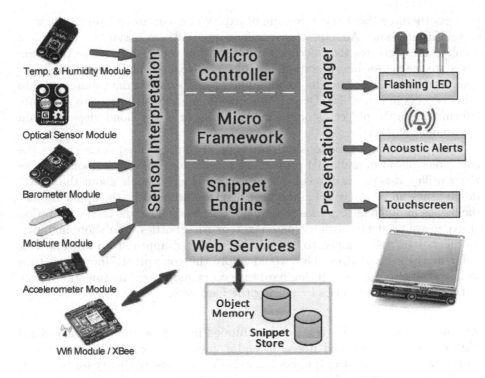

Fig. 2. Technical Architecture and a Set of Selected Sensors

It encourages the user to interact directly via gesture. In this way, for example, a conscious acknowledgement is obtained and given that a warning has been read. In its minimal lightweight variant that can be seen in Figure 1, the system can also be assembled just with LEDs that show the relevant states and illuminate the Ring. In this case, the status varies from red to green, from inedible to edible. A network layer enables the access to Web services over a Wi-Fi connection. Conditions and information can be sent to the server that hosts all object memories and receives updates from the snippet store.

8   Conclusion and Future Work

In this work, we presented the Ring that instruments everyday objects and transforms them into smart, intelligent objects. Its context-awareness allows the communication of notifications about the state of the attached object to the user. The realization showed that the system supports both, the interaction between humans and objects as well as between interconnected objects, follwing the idea of the Internet of Things. As an application, we suggested the household of an elderly person. The Ring can be used to reinforce the person's decreasing senses.

It alerts the user about the exceeding of expiry dates or about side effects with certain medications. An interaction model supports these scenarios. A technical architecture regulates the information flow within the device, where the main parts are the Sensor Interpretation, the Web service, and the Presentation Manager. The Web service provides a communication interface to data sources and to other objects in range. The Object Memory Model (OMM) is used to structure information in the object's storage, in the device or in the cloud, depending on the amount of data.

We are building a good-looking prototype of the presented device using the Gadgeteer platform and a 3D printer. To receive some feedback about the device's utility, it is planned to consult a group of elderly people about the operational fitness in everyday life in the near future. Additionally, the application of the device in different scenarios is planned. One example is the instrumentation of expensive products, such as champagne or wine bottles, in a shopping environment. It is also planned to extend the suggested approach to objects with different shapes and sizes. This would apply the concept of "Incycling" to a wider range of products reducing hardware costs and the environmental impact in future shopping scenarios by reusing the hardware.

Acknowledgment. This research was funded in part by the German Federal Ministry of Education and Research under grant number 01IA11001 (project RES-COM) and 01IS13015 (project SmartF-IT). The responsibility for this publication lies with the authors.

References

1. Statistisches Bundesamt (Destatis): Just released - statistical yearbook (October 2012),
   www.destatis.de/EN/PressServices/Press/pr/2012/10/PE12_351_p001.html
   (accessed at January 29, 2014)
2. Nesselrath, R., Haupert, J., Frey, J., Brandherm, B.: Supporting persons with special needs in their daily life in a smart home. In: 2011 7th International Conference on Intelligent Environments (IE), pp. 370–373 (2011)
3. P, G.: HOPE- eectronic gadget for home bound patients and elders: Create the future design contest (June 2012),
   http://contest.techbriefs.com/2012/entries/medical/2659
   (accessed at January 29, 2014)
4. Dovgan, E., Lutrek, M., Pogorelc, B., Gradiek, A., Bruger, H., Gams, M.: Intelligent elderly-care prototype for fall and disease detection. Slovenian Medical Journal 80(11) (January 2011)
5. Ashton, K.: That 'internet of things' thing (June 2009),
   www.rfidjournal.com/articles/view?4986 (accessed at January 29, 2014)
6. Weiser, M.: Some computer science issues in ubiquitous computing. Commun. ACM 36(7), 75–84 (1993)

7. Zaslavsky, A., Perera, C., Georgakopoulos, D.: Sensing as a service and big data. arXiv:1301.0159 [cs] (January 2013), Proceedings of the International Conference on Advances in Cloud Computing (ACC), Bangalore, India (July 2012)
8. Brandherm, B., Kröner, A.: Digital product memories and product life cycle. In: 2011 7th International Conference on Intelligent Environments (IE), pp. 374–377 (2011)
9. Dey, A.K.: Understanding and using context. Personal Ubiquitous Comput. 5(1), 4–7 (2001)
10. Perera, C., Zaslavsky, A.B., Christen, P., Georgakopoulos, D.: Context aware computing for the internet of things: A survey. IEEE Communications Surveys & Tutorials Journal abs/1305.0982 (2013)
11. Kröner, A., Haupert, J., Seiler, M., Kiesel, B., Schennerlein, B., Horn, S., Schreiber, D., Barthel, R.: Object memory modeling (September 2011), www.w3.org/2005/Incubator/omm/XGR-omm-20111026/ (accessed at January 29, 2014)
12. Haupert, J.: Domeman: A framework for representation, management, and utilization of digital object memories. In: Augusto, J.C., Bourdakis, V., Braga, D., Egerton, S., Fujinami, K., Hunter, G., Kawsar, F., Lotfi, A., Preuveneers, D., Binabdulrahman, A.W., Zamudio, V. (eds.) 9th International Conference on Intelligent Environments (IE 2013), July 18-19, pp. 84–91. IEEE, Athen (2013)
13. Kröner, A., Haupert, J., Hauck, C., Deru, M., Bergweiler, S.: Fostering access to data collections in the internet of things. In: Narzt, W., Gordon-Ross, A. (eds.) UBICOMM 2013, The Seventh International Conference on Mobile Ubiquitous Computing, Systems, Services and Technologies, pp. 65–68. IARIA (September 2013) (Best Paper Award)
14. Resatsch, F., Sandner, U., Leimeister, J.M., Krcmar, H.: Do point of sale RFID-Based information services make a difference? analyzing consumer perceptions for designing smart product information services in retail business. Electronic Markets 18(3), 216–231 (2008)
15. Brandherm, B., Kröner, A., Haupert, J.: Incycling: Sustainable concept for instrumenting everyday commodities. In: Proceedings of the 2011 International Workshop on Networking and Object Memories for the Internet of Things, NoME-IoT 2011, pp. 27–28. ACM, New York (2011)
16. Deru, M., Bergweiler, S.: Milky: On-product app for emotional product to human interactions. In: Proceedings of the 15th International Conference on Human-Computer Interaction with Mobile Devices and Services, MobileHCI 2013, pp. 552–557. ACM, New York (2013)
17. Sen.se: Mother (January 2014), http://sen.se/store/mother (accessed at January 29, 2014)
18. Mühlhäuser, M.: Smart products: An introduction. In: Mühlhäuser, M., Ferscha, A., Aitenbichler, E. (eds.) Constructing Ambient Intelligence. CCIS, vol. 11, pp. 158–164. Springer, Heidelberg (2008)
19. Meyer, G.G., Främling, K., Holmström, J.: Intelligent products: A survey. Computers in Industry 60(3), 137–148 (2009)
20. Gershenfeld, N.A.: When things start to think. Henry Holt, New York (1999)
21. Kröner, A., Haupert, J., GeaFernndez, J., Steffen, R., Kleegrewe, C., Schneider, M.: Supporting interaction with digital product memories. In: Wahlster, W. (ed.) SemProM. Cognitive Technologies, pp. 223–242. Springer, Heidelberg (2013)

22. German Federal Ministry of Education and Research and German Federal Ministry of Economics and Technology: Project of the future: Industry 4.0 (March 2013), www.bmbf.de/en/19955.php (accessed at January 29, 2014)
23. Carroll, A., Heiser, G.: An analysis of power consumption in a smartphone. In: Proceedings of the 2010 USENIX Conference on USENIX Annual Technical Conference, USENIXATC 2010, p. 21. USENIX Association, Berkeley (2010)
24. Niskanen, I., Kantorovitch, J.: Towards the future smart products systems design. In: 2011 IEEE International Conference on Pervasive Computing and Communications Workshops (PERCOM Workshops), pp. 313–315 (2011)
25. Hodges, S., Taylor, S., Villar, N., Scott, J., Bial, D., Fischer, P.T.: Prototyping connected devices for the internet of things. Computer 46(2), 26–34 (2013)

Activity Recognition in Assistive Environments: The STHENOS Approach

Ilias Maglogiannis[1], Kostas Delibasis[2], Dimitrios Kosmopoulos[3],
Theodosios Goudas[1], and Charalampos Doukas[4]

[1] Dept. of Digital Systems, University of Piraeus, 18534, Greece
{imaglo,goudas}@unipi.gr
[2] Dept. of Computer Science and Biomedical Informatics, 35100, Greece
kdelib@dib.uth.gr
[3] TEI of Crete, Dept. of Informatics Engineering, 71004, Greece
dkosmo@ie.teicrete.gr
[4] Dept. of Information and Communication Systems Engineering, 83200, Greece
doukas@aegean.gr

Abstract. The paper presents the research conducted within the framework of the STHENOS project (www.sthenos.gr), which aims at the development of methodologies and systems for assistive environments. The proposed systems and applications are capable of recognizing the human activities and assist disabled or elder persons in performing every day activities and detect abnormal situations such as a fall or long periods of inactivity. The paper includes the technical details of the proposed activity recognition methodology using fisheye video cameras and wearable sensors. Initial results have proven the feasibility of the adopted approaches and the efficiency of the implemented system.

Keywords: Assistive Environments, Pervasive Healthcare, Activity Recognition, Fisheye video, Wearable sensors.

1 Introduction and Related Work

The aging of the global population obviates the need for systems able to monitor people in need in their personal or hospital environment. The isolated processing of data coming from visual or other sensors has reached it limits; however, the incorporation of multimodal information may lead to more robust recognition of human behavior. In this paper we present our research within the framework of the STHENOS project (www.sthenos.gr). STHENOS aims at the development of methodologies and tools to develop pervasive human-centered systems and applications, to recognize the human state (identity, emotions and behavior) in assistive environments using audiovisual and biological signals. STHENOS is envisaged to offer services such as support for the aged and disabled persons, measurement of their activity level and detection of critical situations from audiovisual content and signal collections.

A major concern in an assistive environment is how to transform the low-level signals to semantic knowledge and use it to identify security and safety events [1], [2].

C. Stephanidis and M. Antona (Eds.): UAHCI/HCII 2014, Part III, LNCS 8515, pp. 525–536, 2014.
© Springer International Publishing Switzerland 2014

Special sensor nodes with networking capabilities are required for collecting and transmitting activity related data (i.e., accelerometer and audio-visual data). These sensors can be attached on several locations on the subject's body or in the surrounding environment. A monitoring node is required for collecting the aforementioned data and performing required processing in order to enable an estimation of the human status. Recorded video frames can provide feed to a video tracker that tracks the movement of the patient's body and generates body shape features (i.e., coordinates of a bounding box containing the subject's body). Recorded sounds can be further utilized in order to detect emergency events like distress speech expressions or body fall sounds. Additionally, in the cases where the human is the sound source, the localization of the latter in conjunction with visual trajectory information can provide more robust estimation of the actual incident and avoid false alarms generated by other sound sources. The data are properly transformed in a suitable format for the classifier and the classification phase begins. Based on a predefined classification model (i.e., train model), the patient status is detected (i.e., emergency status when an emergency event is detected, normal status otherwise). Apart from the indication of an emergency incident (e.g., a patient fall), an estimation of the severity of the incident can be provided based on the patient's behaviour after the fall as recorded by visual sensors; visual inactivity or soft activity combined with distress sounds originating from patient's location suggest that patient has not lost consciousness and is trying to recover from the fall. In case that no visual or sound activity is recorded after the detected fall, the incident can be classified as serious. In previous works by us [9] several channels have been used for detecting behaviour.

In the visual channel there are several challenges that need to be addressed, e.g., illumination changes and occlusions concerning the visual input from cameras. The illumination is easier to control in home environments; to mitigate occlusions a network of cameras is often used. Robust methods for visual monitoring (tracking) of humans in adverse conditions have been presented in [3], [4], or by using holistic features [5]. The tracking methods, which typically use particle filters, have to be adapted and extended for the specific environment and target requirements. Specifically, the appropriate features to track have to be defined, as well as the appropriate object model. As already mentioned tracking may be performed using also non visual sensors such as audio. Microphone arrays can be used for target monitoring in two levels: firstly at low level using features extracted from the signal and secondly at higher level using sequences of extracted 3D positions. Apart from that, neurophysiological data can be employed to provide an overall context of the human state. The automated behavior modeling, using vision or other sensors is highly desired, given the complexity of the executed everyday tasks. A deviation from the model might signify a health problem of the monitored person. The general treatment is still an open issue, however machine-learning offer flexible frameworks such as Hidden Markov Models, Conditional Random Fields etc. The behavior recognition problem will be treated as a time series classification task, separately in the bio-signals and video modalities. To this end the main methodologies are the ones that use a statistical model (generative) and the ones that calculate a similarity between different time series models (discriminative). In the past we have used such techniques to model normal and abnormal actions like walking, running, abrupt motion in [6] using a camera network.

The adopted approach in the STHENOS project involves the utilization of visual and non-visual sensors. The main problems of using visual sensors (cameras) are the occlusions and the illumination changes. Thus we have experimented with fisheye cameras possible to resolve occlusions. In addition we have extracted holistic image representations after background subtraction and utilized human models to find human silhouette and pose. For the non-visual channel the acquisition of healthcare data (like heartbeat, body temperature, oxygen saturation and related biosignals) and patient context (like location, and activity status measured by accelerometers) can be utilized. In order to properly identify various events of interest, such as falls using the different sensor and information channels described previously, specific fusion and classification techniques have been utilized concerning mainly the visual modality so far, i.e., RGB and depth images [2]. Motion and audio data will be similarly preprocessed and will be fused and classified using a number of different classification methods (e.g., neural networks, support vector machines, etc.). The overall architecture of the envisaged STHENOS system is illustrated in Figure 1. Since the project is still in progress, we present here the modules that are already implemented focusing on activity recognition using fisheye video cameras and wearable sensors.

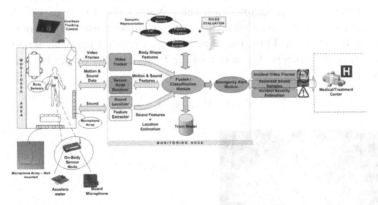

Fig. 1. The STHENOS system architecture illustrating basic modules: motion, sound, visual perceptual components and respective equipment and the aggregation node

2   The Visual Module Enabling Silhouette Detection and Human Pose Recognition

One of the most important system modules is the visual one. It is based on a) a novel model of the fisheye camera that enables the extraction of the direction of view of each pixel of the video frame, b) a 3D parametric model of a human and c) an evolutionary algorithm that recovers the parameters of the 3D human model, based on an objective function that compares the proposed to the currently observed one. The module components and their interconnections are illustrated in Fig. 2.

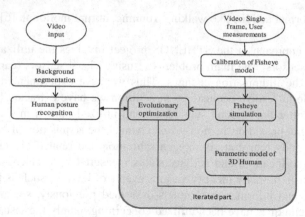

Fig. 2. The camera module components

2.1   Fisheye Camera Model

The main objective of the work described in this section is to establish a one-to-one relation between the image pixel and the direction of view that is recorded in this pixel, defined in spherical coordinates by its azimuth and elevation angles. The characteristic of the fisheye camera is that it can cover a field of view of 180 degrees. In this work we use a model to simulate the image formation using the fisheye camera, so that given the real-world position of an object (x,y,z), we may calculate the image coordinates (j,i) of its pixels. The action of the fisheye model M can be written in the general form

$$(j,i) = M\ (x, y, z) \tag{1}$$

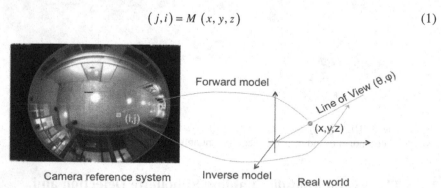

Fig. 3. The forward and inverse fisheye model

The details of the proposed model, which is illustrated in Figure 3, are presented in [7]. The process of the camera model calibration defines the values of the unknown parameters. The fisheye camera was permanently installed on the roof of the university laboratory. Therefore, the parameters of the fisheye camera model need to be determined only once and they will be utilized in processing of every subsequent captured video sequence. For this reason the user provided the position of several landmark points on a single video frame. The real world coordinates of these landmark points were also measured, with respect to the reference system. Let

$$\left(x_{im}^{i}, y_{im}^{i}\right) = M\left(x_{real}^{i}, y_{real}^{i}, z_{real}^{i}; p, x_{sph}, y_{sph}\right) \tag{2}$$

denote the position of the i-th landmark points on the video frame, according to the parameters of the current model M (note that superscripts are not powers). x_{real}^{i}, y_{real}^{i} z_{real}^{i}, are the coordinates of the world point i which is projected to the camera. p is the ratio z_{sph}/z_{plane} x_{sph}, y_{sph} are .... The values of the model parameters are obtained by minimizing the error between the expected and the observed frame coordinates $\{(X_{im}^{i}, Y_{im}^{i})\}, i = 1,...,N$ of the landmark points, as following:

$$\left(p, x_{sph}, y_{sph}\right) = \arg\min_{p, x_{sph}, y_{sph}}\left(\sum_{i=1}^{N_{p}}\left(\left(X_{im}^{i} - x_{im}^{i}\right)^{2} + \left(Y_{im}^{i} - y_{im}^{i}\right)^{2}\right)\right) \tag{3}$$

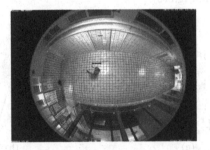

Fig. 4. Visualization of the resulting fisheye model calibration

This minimization is performed using brute force exhaustive search. We would like to emphasize that this operation is only performed once after the initial installation of the fisheye camera and does not need to be executed in real time. The resulting calibration of the fisheye model is shown in Fig. 4, where a virtual grid is laid on the floor and on the two walls of the imaged room. The grid is then rendered on the captured frame, using the fisheye model, in order to assess the accuracy of the fisheye model calibration. The user defined landmark points are shown as 'o', whereas their projected location on the video frame, using the calibrated model are shown as '*'.

2.2 The Human Shillouette Model

For modeling the human body a number of approaches use simple geometric primitives such as cylinders. For the preliminary results presented in this work, we utilized a free triangulated model of a standing human [http://www.3dmodelfree.com/models/20966-0.htm], consisting of approx. 27.000 vertices. Since we are interested in projecting the human model through the fisheye camera in real time, we discard the triangle information of the model and we treat it as a cloud of points. We also applied a vertex decimation process to reduce the number of vertices by a factor of 8.

The vertices of the model were labeled manually using logical spatial relations, into 5 classes: right and left arm (RA, LA), right and left leg (RL, LL) and the rest of the body (torso and head). The pose of the human is modified by changing the position of the hands and legs independently, using the following controlling parameters:

Legs are allowed to rotate round the Y axis with respect to the hips (thus they remain on the sagital - YZ plane). Arms are allowed to rotate round the shoulders. In Fig 5(a) the arms are shown along the coronal plane, whereas in Fig. 5(b) the left arm (black vertices) is shown at a rotated position around the Y axis (thus on the sagital plane). Thus, one angle is required to describe the motion of each leg, whereas two parameters are required to describe the position of each arm. The rotation of the hands involves rotations around the X and Y axis. The human model is used to produce a simulated (rendered) segmented video frame that is compared to the actually segmented one. Figure 6 illustrates this concept, where a model of a standing man is shown in Figure 6(a). The model is scaled to height=1.8m and is placed at several locations in the imaged room, touching the floor (b). The rendered frame using the fisheye model is shown in Fig.6(c).

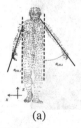
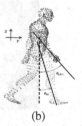

(a)   (b)

Fig. 5. The model of the human (anterior view and right view), with labels as color. The axis of the limbs and their angles with the vertical human axis, that define the parameters of the 3D human model, are also shown.

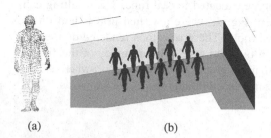
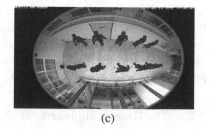

(a)   (b)   (c)

Fig. 6. (a) The 3D model of a standing man, (b) scaling the model to height=1.8 m, touching the floor and reproducing the model at several locations of the imaged room and (c) rendering the 3D human models through the calibrated fisheye lens

2.3   Matching the Human Model with the Segmented Frame

The human pose can be extracted by recovering the values of the parameters of the human model. Let us denote I_M the binary image of the parametric model generated by the fisheye model and I_S the segmented image of the corresponding video frame. The objective function is defined as following:

$$f(\mathbf{p_m}) = \sum_{\substack{image \\ domain}} I_M \cap I_S - \sum \overline{I}_M \cap I_S - \sum I_M \cap \overline{I}_S \qquad (4)$$

where, $\overline{I}$ denotes the boolean negative of I, $\cap$ denotes the boolean AND operator and the summation is done over the whole image domain. Thus, the objective function is defined as the number of non-zero pixels of I_M on non-zero pixels of I_S minus the number of non-zero pixels of I_M on zero pixels of I_S minus the number of zero pixels of I_M on non-zero pixels of I_S. It is evident that for the ideal set of model parameters, the value of the objective function should be maximized. Due to the large number of parameters and the complexity of the objective function, which cannot be written in closed form and its derivatives cannot be analytically computed, we employed a Genetic-based optimization approach as described in [8]. For these initial results, the step of evolutionary optimization is not performed in real time.

3   The Non-visual Module Enabling Activity Classification

The non-visual module is based on signals acquired by wearable and environmental sensors and consists of three components: a wearable/textile part that has been designed for maximum user convenient, a mobile part that adds additional patient context awareness and a repository / data analysis component that provides all the essential interfaces for collecting the data and tools for managing the latter.

3.1   The Wearable Devices Component

For the wearable part we have used textile accelerometers and a heartbeat chest strap by Polar (www.polar.com). The latter sensors are connected to a textile version of the Arduino open hardware microcontroller platform, called LilyPad (http://arduino.cc/en/Main/ArduinoBoardLilyPad). Arduino is an open-source single-board microcontroller. The hardware consists of a simple open hardware design for the Arduino board with an Atmel AVR processor and on-board I/O support. The software consists of a standard programming language compiler and the boot loader that runs on the board. The LilyPad Arduino is a microcontroller board designed for wearable and e-textiles. It can be sewn to fabric and similarly mounted power supplies, sensors and actuators with conductive thread. For the connection between the Polar monitor and the microcontroller, the Polar HeartRate Module has been utilized. Lilypad collects data through the appropriate embedded software and transmits them on an Android-based mobile phone through a Bluetooth interface. An appropriate application has been developed for the Android that collects the data and forwards them to the data repository. The application stores also the acquired data on the mobile's memory card for future usage of retransmission in case of communication problems.

3.2   The Mobile Component

The mobile component has also been developed using the Arduino platform. It consists of additional sensors like an air quality sensor and wireless networking modules that provide direct connectivity to the Internet. The modules can be either a WiFi or a 3G/GPRS modem depending on whether indoor and/or outdoor functionality is provided. The purpose of developing and using an additional mobile sensor unit is twofold: a) to demonstrate the feasibility of existing microcontroller platforms in communicating directly with the Internet and the presented system and b) more sensors can be added ad-hoc on the system since both the hardware (the Arduino platform) and the developed software provide such features.

3.3   The Repository and Data Analysis Component

The specific component is essential for collecting the sensor data and enabling further analysis. A Cloud infrastructure would serve the tasks of on line storage and processing in the best way for such an application, thus we have initially utilized the Okeanos Cloud Infrastructure (https://okeanos.grnet.gr/home/), which is available for the Greek Universities. Sensor data are transmitted using a lightweight REST API that enables direct communication from the Arduino Lilypad microcontroller when direct wireless connectivity is available. The Weka core library has also incorporated into the system allowing the deployment of the motion analysis platform and context awareness platform.

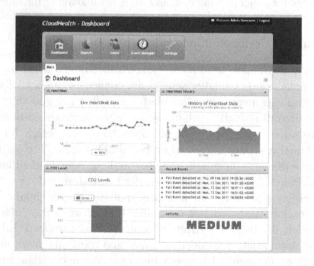

Fig. 7. The graphical interface of the web management application on the Cloud

The system is able to acquire motion, heartbeat and air quality data and display them in real time on the appropriate graphical interface (see Figure 7). It also performs real time classification of the motion data and provides an estimation of the user's activity and alerts in case of an emergency indication (e.g., a fall incident estimation).

4   Initial Experimental Results

4.1   Results from the Camera Module

The camera module has been tested using number of indoor videos, acquired by the fisheye Mobotix Q24 hemispheric camera, which was installed on the ceiling of the imaged room. Results from a number of frames are shown in Figure 8. The segmented frames are shown in green, the fisheye rendered 3D human is shown in red and their intersection in yellow. It becomes evident that the proposed system is able to extract the human pose from the fisheye video frames, although the original segmentation is incomplete, contains holes, or non-human background, as it can be seen the last frame, where parts of the moving door are segmented as video foreground.

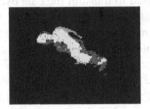
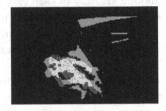

Fig. 8. The resulting pose recognition from 2 random frames of the acquired fisheye videos

Fig. 9(a) shows an exemplar frame of one of the video sequences acquired. The resulting 3D human model, after fitting the fisheye-rendered parametric 3D human model to the segmented frame is shown in (b), using real world Cartesian coordinate system. The actual fisheye-rendered 3D human model is shown in (c). It can be observed that the proposed algorithm was able to detect the specific human pose.

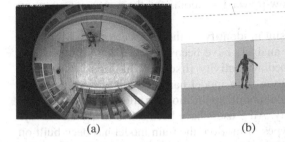
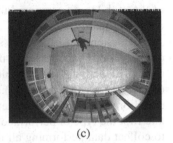

(a)   (b)   (c)

Fig. 9. (a) An original video frame showing a human, (b) the 3D model with its parameters fitted to the segmented original frame and (c) the fisheye-rendered 3D model in a simulated frame

The generation of the 3D parametric human model is performed very fast, with approximately 1 msec including the required geometric transformations. The rendering of a 3D human model with 2.500 vertices through the modeled fisheye camera is also performed very fast (i.e in 1.5msec in an average PC). The calculation of the objective function (Eq. 4) requires approximately 8 msec for a 3D model with 2.500 vertices and a frame of 480x640 pixels, although the number of pixels in the frame does not drastically affect the execution time. All timing was performed using an Intel(R) Core i5-2430 CPU @ 2.40 GHz Laptop with 4 GB Ram, under Windows 7 Home Premium.

4.2   Results from the Non-visual Module

In the context of the initial module evaluation 5 users have been equipped with the sensors described in Section 3. All of them (average height males aged between 25 - 35) have used both the wearable and mobile monitoring units while performing every day activities. The sampling rate for the accelerometer values has been at 10 samples per second (indicated as an acceptable rate for identified falls by previous works as in [9], for heartbeat data once per heartbeat detected and for air quality data every 1 minute. The mobile gateway in each case is used to transmit the data over a commercial 3G network to the Okeanos cloud infrastructure. The differences between two sequential acceleration values have been transmitted at the same rate whereas the average heartbeats per minute have been calculated and transmitted every second respectively.

During the initial experimentation with the system, a drop packet rate of 20-30% has been detected. This fact is either due to the Arduino low resources for high rate sampling of sensors and transmitting the data at the same time, or due to network congestion because of the repetitive REST calls at such a high sampling rate (i.e. 10 acceleration samples per second). In order to address this issue, a memory buffer has been introduced on the Arduino side that collects motion data during a 10 second time frame and then transmits the latter to the Cloud. This way the drop rate has been minimized between 2-5%, which is quite acceptable for the application. Regarding power consumption, the wearable part (powered by one AAA battery) was able to last for at least 18 hours while the mobile part could not last more than 6 hours. This difference can be explained by the more energy-intensive communication mechanism (3G) of the mobile unit compared to the low-power Bluetooth, and the power consumption of the air quality sensor.

The system has been quite successful in identifying the user's activities. More specifically, activities based on motion analysis have been classified into three categories: high activity (like running), medium activity (like walking) and low activity (e.g., lying on bed or sitting). Initially a train model has been built using the Weka core library and modifying the Android mobile application for allowing users to annotate first the type of performed activity. All 5 users have been asked to use the sensors to collect data performing all three types of motion: the train model has been built on 20 minutes of jogging and fast walking, 30 minutes of walking and 60 minutes of performing low activity. The mobile application has transmitted the data and the corresponding motion type as selected by the user. After collecting the data the training model has been built on the Cloud. A number of different classifies have been evaluated using the initial motion and heartbeat data. The features utilized for building the classification models are the acceleration changes in the X, Y and Z axis, the input from the gyroscope (tilt) sensors (a tilt value for each axis) and the average heartbeat rate (beats per minute). Four classes were examined, namely jogging, fast walking, walking and sitting/low activity). We achieved an accuracy of 86% by using the Naive-Bayes [10].

5   Discussion and Conclusions

The presented research within the STHENOS project aims at the development of a reliable system of environment awareness for the monitoring, the recognition of activities and the detection of the Patients' and Elders' state. For the development of the above system we have presented the technical details of the two basic modules that gather information from the visual and the non-visual channels. The implementation so far has illustrated the proof of concept of the methodologies proposed by the STHENOS project. Regarding the visual channel further work will include, the adoption of a more robust statistical 3D model for the human and the refinement of the fisheye model, using more parameters to increase its accuracy. Finally more efficient implementation of the evolutionary algorithm based optimization will be explored for the determination of the 3D model parameters. These approaches include exploiting the converged population from the previous frames to initialize the search for the current frame and/or restricting the parameter range according to their optimal values from the previous frames. The fact that the evolutionary algorithm is highly parallelizable may also be exploited. This will allow near real time execution of the final pose and activity determination step.

The non-visual module on the other hand may not provide accurate identification of the pose or a specific action, however the estimation of activity levels and the detection of emergency events such as falls is feasible. An important aspect of the proposed system that needs to be further examined is the creation of generic classification rules for various motion types using the training set obtained by various users. Such a feature would increase the acceptance of the proposed system by a higher number of users, since it would not require the initial training phase. Key issues arising also from such a system include social issues about acceptance and training with the technology. Other open issues that need to be addressed are the security of privacy of data and the energy efficiency of the textile sensors and microcontroller platform, in order to extend the system autonomy.

Acknowledgment. The authors would like to thank the European Union (European Social Fund ESF) and Greek national funds through the Operational Program "Education and Lifelong Learning" of the National Strategic Reference Framework (NSRF) - Research Funding Program: \Thalis \ Interdisciplinary Research in Affective Computing for Biological Activity Recognition in Assistive Environments for financially supporting this work.

References

1. Maglogiannis, I., Vouyioukas, D., Aggelopoulos, C.: Face Detection and Recognition of Human Emotion Using Markov Random Fields. Personal and Ubiquitous Computing 13(1), 95–101 (2009), doi:10.1007/s00779-007-0165-0
2. Makedon, F., Le, Z., Huang, H., Becker, E., Kosmopoulos, D.: An Event Driven Framework for Assistive CPS Environments. In: ACM SIGBED Review - Special Issue on the 2nd Joint Workshop on High Confidence Medical Devices, Software, and Systems (HCMDSS) and Medical Device Plug-and-Play (MD PnP) Interoperability, vol. 6(2), pp. 28–36 (2009)
3. Makris, A., Kosmopoulos, D., Perantonis, S., Theodoridism, S.: A Hierarchical Feature Fusion Framework for Adaptive Visual Tracking. Image and Vision Computing 29(9), 594–606 (2011)
4. Kosmopoulos, D., Doulamis, A., Makris, A., Doulamis, N., Chatzis, S., Middleton, S.: Vision-based production of personalised video. Signal Processing: Image Communication 24(3), 158–176 (2009)
5. Kosmopoulos, D., Chatzis, S.: Robust Visual Behavior Recognition. IEEE Signal Processing Magazine 27(5), 34–45 (2010)
6. Antonakaki, P., Kosmopoulos, D., Perantonis, S.: Detecting Abnormal Human Behavior using Multiple Cameras. Signal Processing 89(9), 1723–1738 (2009)
7. Delibasis, K., Goudas, T., Plagianakos, V., Maglogiannis, I.: Fisheye Camera Modeling for Human Segmentation Refinement in Indoor Videos. In: Proc. of 6th ACM International Conference on Pervasive Technologies Related to Assistive Environments (PETRA 2013). ACM, Rhodes (2013), doi:10.1145/2504335.2504375
8. Goldberg, D.: Genetic Algorithms in Search, Optimization, and Machine Learning. Addison Wesley (1989) ISBN:0201157675
9. Doukas, C., Maglogiannis, I.: Emergency Fall Incidents Detection in Assisted Living Environments Utilizing Motion, Sound and Visual Perceptual Component. IEEE Transactions on Information Technology in Biomedicine 15(2), 277–289 (2011)
10. Kohavi, R.: Scaling Up the Accuracy of Naive-Bayes Classifiers: A Decision-Tree Hybrid. In: Second International Conference on Knowledge Discovery and Data Mining, pp. 202–207 (1996)
11. Kosmopoulos, D.I., Doliotis, P., Athitsos, V., Maglogiannis, I.: Fusion of color and depth video for human behavior recognition in an assistive environment. In: Streitz, N., Stephanidis, C. (eds.) DAPI 2013. LNCS, vol. 8028, pp. 42–51. Springer, Heidelberg (2013)

Evaluation of the Human Factor in the Scheduling of Smart Appliances in Smart Grids

Jânio Monteiro[1,2], Pedro J.S. Cardoso[1], Rita Serra[1], and Licínia Fernandes[1]

[1] ISE, University of Algarve, Portugal
[2] INOV, Lisbon, Portugal
jmmontei@ualg.pt

Abstract. Recently there has been an increase of interest in implementing a new set of home appliances, known as Smart Appliances that integrate Information Technologies, the Internet of Things and the ability of communicating with other devices. While Smart Appliances are characterized as an important milestone on the path to the Smart Grid, by being able to automatically schedule their loads according to a tariff or reflecting the power that is generated using renewable sources, there is not a clear understanding on the impact that the behavior of such devices will have in the comfort levels of users, when they shift their working periods to earlier, or later than, a preset time. Given these considerations, in this work we analyse the results of an assessment survey carried out to a group of Home Appliance users regarding their habits when dealing with these machines and the subjective impact in quality caused by either finishing its programs before or after the time limit set by the user. The results of this work are expected to be used as input for the evaluation of load scheduling algorithms running in energy management systems.

Keywords: Smart Grids, Home Grids, Human Factor, Comfort Level, Smart Appliances, Mean Opinion Score.

1 Introduction

Currently we are witnessing an increase in the energy produced by renewable sources, either motivated by the increase in the cost of oil exploitation or by an increment in environmental concerns, with its higher expression in the energy obtained from wind and photovoltaic sources. In this context, the traditional view of a distribution grid that uses centralized generators to provide power to consumers is being replaced by a "smart grid" solution where energy production is based in a Distributed Generation (DG) [1]. The power generated by these energy sources however varies according to environmental conditions which are not controllable. In this scenario the traditional role of consumers is being replaced by a more proactive one, not only in the sense that they should be able to produce energy locally, for self-consumption and/or feed it into the electrical grid, but also in the sense that they are expected to adjust their demand according to the power that is being produced.

C. Stephanidis and M. Antona (Eds.): UAHCI/HCII 2014, Part III, LNCS 8515, pp. 537–548, 2014.
© Springer International Publishing Switzerland 2014

In this context, several scientific works [2][3][4] have analyzed the importance of an efficient management of home grids by consumers, or by an Energy Consumption Scheduling device (ECS). The role of an ECS is to optimally schedule loads in order to better harness the energy produced locally or shift them to work at the periods of time when the rate is lowest, while reflecting user preferences. This also requires that loads, like HVAC (heating, ventilation and air conditioning) and Home Appliances, should be able to communicate with the ECS device and shift their working periods, or adjust the power they consume, according to the power generated locally from renewable sources, or according to a supplier's tariff, which in turn may change dynamically.

By creating a new range of appliances that integrate Information Technologies, the Internet of Things (IoT) [5], with the ability of communicating and respond dynamically to the varying tariffs, a reduction on CO_2 emissions to the atmosphere is possible [6], while ensuring at the same time higher returns on investments made in renewable energy sources. Due to this, as described in [7], Smart Appliances are characterized as an important milestone on the path to the Smart Grid.

In this scenario, one important feature associated with the ECN is to prevent electrical overloads that may happen when several appliances are scheduled to work in the same period of time in the search for a lower cost or tariff. In this case the ECN should decide which appliance is expected to work first and which ones should be scheduled to work later, reflecting a level of priority that should be commensurate with the user preferences. In fact, while overloads may prevent the user from using the ECN, the quality of the scheduling algorithm from a user perspective will also determine how it will be used.

While the shifting of the working periods of some of equipment do not have a clear correlation with the comfort levels of users, like for instance a swimming pool pump, the changing of the working periods of other appliances - like clothes washing machines, clothes dryer and dish washer - have a direct impact in people's routines and therefore affect the perception of the quality of the ECS algorithm. In fact, while the efficiency of a demand side management (DSM) algorithm that runs in an ECS is proportional to the level of flexibility that users impose to their appliances, we believe that that flexibility will depend on the correct assessment of user preferences made by the ECS.

Since an optimum or nearly optimum solution in terms of cost may imply changing the work period of the machine to several hours before the limit, or make it finish some minutes after the pre-set time limit, the Objective or Multi-objective Function of the scheduling algorithm should include an assessment of user preferences.

While the human factor in the scheduling of residential loads has been included in some algorithms [8][9], as far as we know there isn't any study that clearly defines the comfort level curves of the major appliances according to their time variation.

Given these considerations, in this work we analyze the results of an assessment survey carried out to a group of 44 users, concerning their habits and the subjective impact in quality that the clothes washers, clothes dryer and dish washer appliances have, when they finish their programs before and after a pre-set time limit. The results of this work are expected to be used in the evaluation of load scheduling algorithms running in ECS devices.

The rest of this paper is organized as follows. Section 2 describes the methodology used in the subjective assessment of user preferences. Section 3 presents the obtained results comprising the frequency and time-of-use of the appliances, distribution of type of tariffs, value given to an ECS device and assessment of the impact in quality caused by changing the moment when appliances finish their programs. Section 4 concludes the paper, pointing out future developments of this work.

2   Methodology Used in the Subjective Assessment Survey

In order to evaluate the user habits and its preferences when managing of home appliances, an online based survey was created covering the following issues: the assessor's frequency in using home appliances, time of use of such appliances, type of electrical tariff contracted with the electricity provider, the level of importance given to a device that controls home appliances and the subjective impact in quality caused by changing the moment when appliances finish their programs.

For the evaluation of the subjective impact caused by changing the moment when a clothes washer, clothes dryer or dish washer finishes its program a five-grade scale was used with each level mapping to a certain quality, as follows: 1- Bad Quality; 2- Poor Quality; 3- Fair Quality; 4- Good Quality and 5- Excellent Quality. As users are expected to have different levels of tolerance to delay according to their daily routines, different conditions were evaluated comparing usage at week versus weekend days and at distinct times of the day.

The results of these tests were afterwards analyzed by obtaining the Mean Opinion Score (MOS) for each appliance and condition, using equation (1):

$$\bar{u}_{mct} = \frac{1}{N} \sum_{1}^{N} u_{imct} \tag{1}$$

In equation (1), Nm represents the number of observers that use appliance m, and uimct represents the score of observer i, for appliance m, in condition c and delta time t. We have considered the values of delta time t to be negative (i.e., t<0) when the appliance finishes its program before the time limit set by the user, positive when it finishes after the limit set by the user, or zero when it finishes the program at the limit set by the user.

The MOS results obtained from equation (1) were afterwards used to obtain a regression function. The function used for regression was:

$$f(t) = \alpha + e^{\beta + \chi t} \tag{2}$$

The values of α, β and χ were obtained minimizing the distance between equation (2) and the set of umct points. For each appliance m and condition c, two regression functions were considered, one for t≤0 and another for t≥0.

In the following section we present the results obtained from the assessment survey.

3   Results and Analysis

The assessment panel which answered the survey was selected by invitation among retired persons, middle age individuals and college students, all of them in Portugal. The majority of questionnaires were answered online, resulting in a total of 44 answers.

3.1   Frequency and Time-of-Use of the Appliances

In the first question we have evaluated the frequency of usage of the clothes washers, clothes dryer and dish washer appliances by each individual. The results of these answers are shown in Table I.

Table 1. Frequency of usage of the clothes washers, clothes dryer and dish washer appliances

Assessor:	Clothes washer	Dish Washer	Clothes Dryer
Does not use it	0,0%	**25,0%**	**61,4%**
Use it rarely	2,3%	2,3%	**25,0%**
On average use it once per month	4,5%	2,3%	6,8%
On average use it once per week	11,4%	6,8%	4,5%
On average use it two or three times per week	**29,5%**	20,5%	0,0%
On average I use it more than three times per week	**52,3%**	**43,2%**	2,3%

As it can be verified, among the three appliances covered in this study, the clothes washing machine is the most commonly used one, with nearly 82% of the subjects using it more than twice per week. Regarding the clothes dryer on contrary only 2,3% of the subjects use it more than twice per week, while it is not used at all by 61,4% of the persons that answered the survey.

Table 2. Time-of-use frequency of the appliances in weekdays (DW) and weekend (WE)

Time of Day	Clothes washer		Dish Washer		Clothes Dryer	
	WD	WE	WD	WE	WD	WE
From 7am to 10 am	11,5%	6,1%	0,0%	2,3%	0,0%	4,8%
From 10am to 12am	11,5%	**37,9%**	5,7%	4,5%	8,3%	14,3%
From 12am to 6 pm	11,5%	**30,3%**	5,7%	27,3%	8,3%	**28,6%**
From 6 pm to 12 pm	**46,2%**	15,2%	**62,9%**	**50,0%**	41,7%	**42,9%**
From 12pm to 10am	**19,2%**	10,6%	**25,7%**	15,9%	**41,7%**	9,5%

In the following question we asked for the time-of-use frequency of these appliances, differentiating weekdays from weekends. Table 2 presents these results.

As it can be verified, while during weekdays these appliances tend to be used between 6 pm and 7 am (of the following day), at the weekend they tend to be used earlier. This is more clearly verified in the case of the clothes washing machine, which at weekends is mostly used between 10 am and 6 pm, while the other two appliances are predominantly used between midday and midnight.

3.2   Type of Tariffs Distribution and Recognized Importance of an ECS Device

As the results in the previous section may reflect the type of tariff that users have, we asked assessors to specify it. These results are presented in Figure 1. As verified, half of the assessors had a time of use type of tariff, either comprising two or three time periods.

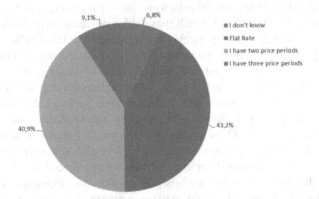

Fig. 1. Distribution of the electrical tariffs contracts among the assessment panel

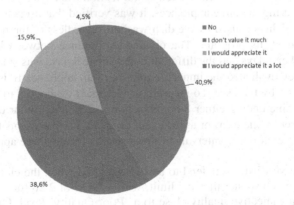

Fig. 2. Importance given to a device capable of managing appliances automatically

When correlating the type of tariff with the time of use of the appliances, we verified that all of the assessors that use their appliances between midnight and 7 am had a time of use contract, driving them to change their routines.

When we asked users to state the level of importance that they recognize in having a device capable of scheduling their appliances automatically, around 45% of assessors didn't consider it relevant, as shown in Figure 2.However, among those users that have a time of use type of tariff (corresponding to nearly 50% of the survey universe), 95% of them considered it relevant. Among them 45% stated that they would appreciate it and 50% stated that they would appreciate it a lot.

3.3   Assessment of the Impact in Quality Caused by Changing the Moment When Appliances Finish Their Programs

In this section we evaluate the impact in quality (or comfort) that a scheduling device would have when changing the work period of appliances to end before or after the limit set by the user.

Before being asked to answer the following part of the survey, users were first instructed to consider a scenario in which they had a device in their homes capable of managing their appliances, so they would save money in electrical bills.

In the first group of questions we started by evaluating the impact in quality that a delay of either 7, 15, 30 or 60 minutes would cause in a user, considering that the appliance was set to finish at a certain hour. As those impacts may depend on the type of appliance and on the time frame where the machine is expected to work, we asked assessors to consider different situations comprising: weekend days and either 7 am, 7 pm or 11pm in weekdays. These results are shown in Figures 3, 4 and 5, which represent the MOS results and the associated 95% confidence intervals respectively for the clothes washers, clothes dryer and dish washer appliances.

In terms of the clothes washing machine, the results show that users tend to be less tolerant to delays at 7 am and 11 pm, when compared to 7 pm and weekend days. Regarding the clothes dryer appliance the tolerance to delays tends to increase between 7 am, 7 pm and 11 pm in weekdays and from those days to the weekend.

When comparing the three appliances, it was verified that users tend to be more tolerant with the delays caused by the dish washer, regardless of the moment when it is supposed to finish its program. The obtained difference between MOS of the dish washer at weekend days and the different hours of weekdays was small.

We have then evaluated the impact in quality of an appliance finishing sooner than the time limit set by the user. To measure it, we asked evaluators to grade the quality level of a machine ending either 8 hours, 4 hours, 2 hours, 1 hour or 30 minutes before the limit set by the user, or at the exact hour. Figure 6 presents the MOS and the associated 95% confidence intervals of these results for the three appliances analyzed in this study.

As it can be verified, users tend to be less satisfied when the clothes washing machine finishes much sooner than the limit, with a MOS of 2.26 for a 8 hours advance, translating to a subjective quality close to a 'Poor Quality' level. One of the reasons causing this dissatisfaction could be the fact that people don't like to leave clothes wet inside the washing machine for long periods of time.

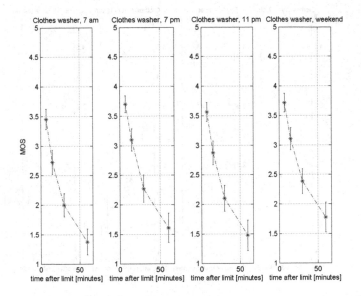

Fig. 3. MOS and associated 95% confidence intervals for the assessment of a clothes washing appliance finishing 7, 15, 30 and 60 minutes later than expected, at different hours and days of the week

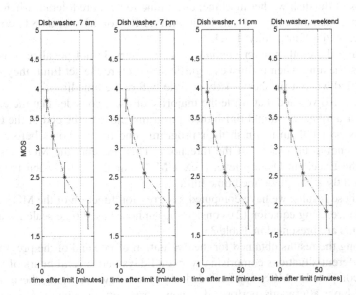

Fig. 4. MOS and associated 95% confidence intervals for the assessment of a dish washer appliance finishing 7, 15, 30 and 60 minutes later than expected, at different hours and days of the week

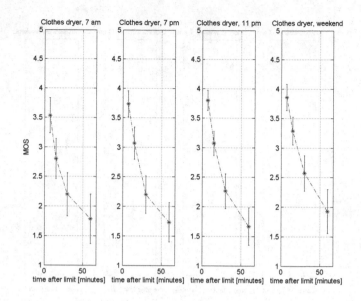

Fig. 5. MOS and associated 95% confidence intervals for the assessment of a clothes dryer appliance finishing 7, 15, 30 and 60 minutes later than expected, at different hours and days of the week

In terms of the dish washer machine, users tend to be more tolerant when it finishes much sooner than the expected time limit with a MOS of 2.75 for an 8 hours advance, slightly below the 'fair quality' level.

Regarding the clothes dryer appliance, while users do not penalize it as much as the clothes washing when it finishes significantly before the set limit, they tend to be more satisfied when it finishes exactly or little before the time limit.

We have also verified that while the majority of users consider that the clothes and dish washer appliances should finish their programs close to the end of the time limit, some users prefer them to finish their programs one or two hours before the limit, instead of ending up exactly at the threshold. This prevents the MOS results from reaching the Excellent Quality level (i.e., a MOS equal to 5.0), when the appliance finishes exactly at the predefined time limit.

Given these results, we have computed a regression function of the MOS values for each appliance using equation (2), considering an hour based time scale for all curves. These results are presented in Table 3.

Regarding the results obtained for the evaluation of late end of the programs, since we had different situations comprising weekend days and several hours of weekdays, we have computed a MOS that included all these answers. Using these new MOS points we have afterwards performed a new curve fitting. Figure 7 presents these MOS points, together with the curve fitting curves using equation (2) for the three types of appliances. Table 4 presents the regression results of these MOS points.

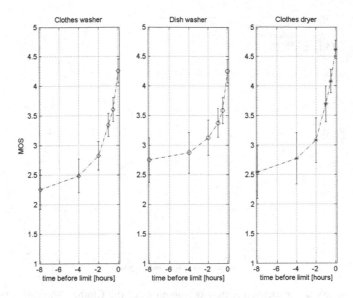

Fig. 6. MOS and associated 95% confidence intervals for the assessment of a clothes dryer, dish washer and clothes dryer appliances finishing sooner than the time limits set by the user

Table 3. Statistical parameters resulting from the regression of MOS points when the appliances finish their programs later than the set limit, in different time frames

Fitting Results	Weekdays			Weekend
	7 am	7 pm	Midnight	
Clothes Washer				
α	1.1655	1.1389	1.1828	1.4077
β	1.1296	1.1480	1.1293	1.0575
χ	-2.6680	-1.9437	-2.3894	-2.0964
Standard Deviation	0.0278	0.0616	0.0356	0.05136
Correlation Coefficients	0.99985	0.99916	0.99974	0.99934
Dish Washer				
α	1.4082	1.5535	1.4546	1.2878
β	1.0585	1.0051	1.0550	1.1109
χ	-1.8726	-1.8610	-1.7796	-1.6507
Standard Deviation	0.0677	0.0674	0.1286	0.1230
Correlation Coefficients	0.99876	0.99863	0.99535	0.99596
Clothes Dryer				
α	1.7558	1.5505	1.4366	1.6690
β	1.0465	1.1234	1.1602	1.0756
χ	-3.9491	-2.9447	-2.6600	-2.3944
Standard Deviation	0.0435	0.0527	0.2226	0.0268
Correlation Coefficients	0.99962	0.99948	0.99991	0.99984

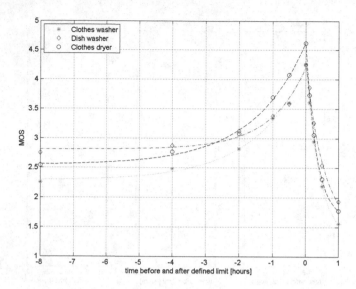

Fig. 7. MOS points and associated regression functions of the Clothes Washing, Dish Washer and Clothes Dryer appliances

The combined analysis of Figure 7 and Table 2, shows that these curves represent a good aproximation to the MOS points, with correlation coeficients higher than 0.99.

Table 4. Statistical parameters resulting from the regression of the MOS when the appliances finish Before the set Limit (BL) and After the set Limit (AL)

Fitting Results	Clothes washer		Dish Washer		Clothes Dryer	
	BL	AL	BL	AL	BL	AL
α	2.28360	1.2361	2.81172	1.4296	2.54453	1.6253
β	0.65824	1.1122	0.32819	1.0568	0.73273	1.0940
χ	0.63582	-2.2738	0.91504	-1.7900	0.62390	-2.9560
Standard Deviation	0.07081	0.03578	0.09419	0.0938	0.05393	0.0084
Correlation Coefficients	0.99732	0.99972	0.99111	0.99754	0.99865	0.9999

Table 5. Priority levels of the three appliances to be considered in scheduling algorithms

Priority	Condition - Selecting Appliance to finish:		
	Much sooner	Near the pre-set time	Later than time limit
High	Dish Washer	Clothes Dryer	Dish Washer
Medium	Clothes Dryer	Dish Washer and	Clothes Dryer
Low	Clothes Washer	Clothes Washer	Clothes Washer

Given these results, we have categorized the importance given to the appliances in three levels of priority (High, Medium and Low). These prioritization results are shown in Table 5 and may be considered by scheduling algorithms.

4   Conclusions

The main contribution of this paper include the results of the frequency, time-of-use distribution and the regression functions that measure the impact in quality caused by changing the moment when appliances finish their programs.

The high percentage of users with a time-of-use type of tariff that consider it relevant to have an ECS device capable of scheduling appliances automatically is a good indicator of the importance of such devices in the near future.

Regarding the tolerance to delays of the three appliances in this study, it was verified that users tend to be more tolerant with the delays of the dish washer, regardless of the moment when it is supposed to finish its program.

On the other hand, users tend to be less satisfied when the clothes washing machine finishes much sooner than the limit, with a MOS that is close to the Poor Quality level. Regarding the clothes dryer appliance, while users do not penalize quality as much as the clothes washer when it finishes significantly before the set limit, they tend to be more satisfied when it finishes exactly or little before the time limit.

Finally, the regression results of the MOS points using equation (2), show that the obtained functions and parameters have achieved a good approximation to the MOS points and thus can be considered a good representation of the human assessment of quality, in the scheduling of these appliances.

Acknowledgments. This work was supported by the Portuguese QREN R&TD Project Number 30260, "Managing The Intelligence" (MTI).

References

1. Shen, S.: Empowering the Smart Grid with Wireless Technologies, Editor's Note. IEEE Network Magazine (May/June 2012)
2. Erol-Kantarci, M., Mouftah, H.T.: Wireless Sensor Networks for Cost-Efficient Residential Energy Management in the Smart Grid. IEEE Transactions on Smart Grid 2(2) (June 2011)
3. Infield, D.G., Short, J., Horne, C., Freris, L.L.: Potential for domestic dynamic demand-side management in the UK. Presented at the IEEE Power Eng. Soc. Gen. Meet., Tampa, FL (June 2007)
4. Stamminger, R.: Synergy potential of smart appliances Univ. Bonn, Bonn, Germany (March 2009), http://www.smart-a.org, Deliverable 2.3 of work package 2 from the Smart-A project
5. What the Internet-of-things Will Mean for the Smart-grid. IEEE Smart Grid (June 2011), http://smartgrid.ieee.org/june-2011/
95-what-the-internet-of-things-will-mean-for-the-smart-grid

6. The Impact of Smart Grid Residential Energy Management Schemes on the Carbon Footprint of the Household Electricity Consumption. In: Erol-Kantarci, M., Mouftah, H.T. (eds.) 2010 IEEE Electrical Power & Energy Conference (2010)
7. Arrival of Smart Appliances is a milestone on the path to the Smart Grid. IEEE Smart Grid (October 2011),
   http://smartgrid.ieee.org/newsletter/october-2011/
   415-arrival-of-smart-appliances-is-a-milestone-on-the-path-
   to-the-smart-grid
8. Esser, A., Kamper, A., Franke, M., Most, D., Rentz, O.: Scheduling of electrical household appliances with price signals. In: Operations Research Proceedings, pp. 253–258. Springer (2006)
9. Bozchalui, M., Hashmi, S., Hassen, H., Canizares, C., Bhattacharya, K.: Optimal Operation of Residential Energy Hubs in Smart Grids. To appear in IEEE Transactions on Smart Grid (July 2012) (accepted)

Technical Progress in Housing Environment and Its Influence on Performing Household Chores

Przemyslaw Nowakowski

Wroclaw University of Technology, Faculty of Architecture
Prusa st. 53/55, 50-317 Wroclaw, Poland
przemyslaw.nowakowski@pwr.wroc.pl

Abstract. Technological conveniences became permanent elements of people's lives. Various appliances help out with daily chores and shape the standards of our lives. They are accessible thanks to well-developed and efficient manufacturing. The basic role of those diverse technological products is to reduce both physical and mental effort involved in people's work and, consequently improve the comfort of life. Using those numerous appliances requires, among others, special knowledge and training, which may cause various stressful situations.

The presentation focuses on the following problems: comparison of the technological advancements in former and contemporary households, the role of the appliances in performing household chores, changes in the routine activities (disappearance of some chores and appearance of new ones), the influence of a higher standard of living on labour and time input, elimination of various appliances as a result of changes in commodity market, reduction in the ability of using modern appliances (especially among the elderly and the disabled) and the consequences of using new technologies and information technology in households.

Keywords: household, technological progress, ergonomics, household chores.

1 Introduction

Nowadays, almost all activities are performed using various technological appliances. The majority of societies living in industrialized countries would not be able to perform everyday activities without numerous appliances. This dependency is visible both on macro economical scale and among individual households.

The tools with help out with everyday chores have accompanied people since the prehistoric times. Together with the specialization of labour and distinction of various professions, the concentration of technological utensils took place mainly in the work environment. The industrialization of production and spreading of various "consumption goods" led to a bigger supply of numerous appliances also in households. The technological advancements were created to simplify the household chores and to improve the comfort and efficiency of leisure time. Although the appliances improving human labour were being brought into general use, the scope of household chores

C. Stephanidis and M. Antona (Eds.): UAHCI/HCII 2014, Part III, LNCS 8515, pp. 549–557, 2014.
© Springer International Publishing Switzerland 2014

did not quite diminish. The use of the appliances often requires additional loads of work. Moreover, using the complicated utensils sometimes leads to various stressful situations.

In many regions of the world there is a centuries-old tradition of organized labour and, connected with it, production of technological developments. Even urban areas where most of the population live can be called a "technological development". Also individual people are constantly surrounded with technological utensils at their homes and in their work environment. Having various technological equipment in households has always been a synonym of high social status and wealth. Moreover, often enough it was also an attribute of power. Many of the technological appliances had a significant influence on people's lifestyles and various social changes. Among them we can distinguish: communication media (print, computer, Internet), transportation (horse carriage, car, plane), machines enabling production (machines powered by animals, water etc., steam engine, internal combustion engine, electrical machine and production robot).

2   Labour and Technology in Former and Contemporary Households

Throughout the centuries the households were miserly equipped, if we look at it from today's perspective. It was not until the second half of 19th century, thanks to the development of industrial production, when the households were started to be equipped more intensively with various appliances. The modern technological standard of housing became common after the second World War. Therefore, it can be stated that this previously unknown level of technological advancement of everyday life has lasted for about 50 years. Two full generations became accustomed to this particular style and standard of living, and, as a result, handling technology has become a routine. Performing everyday activities resulted in disappearance of conscious perception of some abiding technological systems. Using water supply network, electrical grid (power) and telecommunication network (telephone) is so common that no one anymore takes notice of those conveniences, which did not exist in former times. Together with gradually more and more advanced technology appears a dissonance between the potential possibilities of usage of modern appliances and their actual use in everyday life. In case of more advanced technologies (e.g.: computer systems, electronic devices), their functions are very rarely used in full scope, especially outside the work environment, e.g. in a household.

The degree to which the modern households are equipped with electric appliances does not influence the differentiation of measurable labour input (e.g.: shopping, preparing of meals, doing the washing up, doing the washing, ironing, cleaning etc.). This variable is influenced by the number of members of family and their life cycles (single person, couples with and without children, etc.). The highest intensity of the abovementioned chores falls mainly on women during the period when they take care of small children and on the householders who take care of people of special needs, such as the severely ill and elderly relatives. The aforementioned findings come from the research of labour input conducted in the American households from the end of 1930s till the end of 1980s. Paradoxically, in spite of the technological advance and common use of modern appliances, which help people out with various laborious chores, the input of labour does not decrease, but remains the same. On the other hand, the German research indicates that there are considerable saves in time thanks to use of such appliances as: washing machine, dishwasher, vacuum cleaner or microwave. However, the time which is saved is spent on new chores, which were not performed in former households, and which are related to a higher demand in providing the feeling of comfort to household members [4]. Also the following contrary tendencies can be visible:

- disappearance or minimizing of some laborious chores typical of former households, nowadays almost not encountered;
- the increase in input and frequency of chores which formerly were performed relatively rarely;
- occurrence of chores which were not known before.

Thanks to the modern heating systems and ovens it is not any more necessary to fire up and maintain fire, to provide firewood, to clean furnace and to dispose of ash. Other chores that are almost nonexistent in modern households are: sewing and darning etc. Because of the industrialization of production and food manufacturing, and creation of a dense network of shops, members of households ceased to stock up and make preparations of fruit and vegetables. Nowadays, independent food preparation is considered as a hobby, which is notably limited because of necessary inputs of work. Also baking and preparing noodles and pasta is substituted with ready-made products.

On the other hand, many of the house chores were significantly intensified during the last few decades. In modern households people stock considerably more clothing, linen and dishes. Considering the increase in hygienic demands this situation results is a need to wash and iron more clothes and to do more washing up. In addition to those continually more common chores there are other activities, such as: sorting, folding, drying, putting the items in various places in the house. Also the cleaning chores were extended which was a result of a considerable increase in the equipment of modern households.

Nowadays householders spent more time on preparing meals that they used to. A couple of dozen years ago mainly simple dishes (such as: soups and one-ingredient dishes) were prepared, often for two days. Prepared meals were just heated up on the next day. Thanks to the modern prosperity and a wide offer of food products and ready-made dishes people are encouraged to prepare diverse and fresh meals every day. However, preparation of exotic or dietary meals often requires additional loads of work and special equipment or seasonings.

A distinct issue is a considerable increase in the time spent on grocery shopping. People used to buy their supplies in the closest grocery stores, because the retail prices were similar and cars were a rare commodity. In those days, because of big competition between numerous supermarkets, people prefer to commute to shops in order to get the best value for their money. However, searching for bargains, sales and deals is time-consuming, and going to a remote shop requires to have an own car. Commuting to shops inclines householders to prepare a detailed shopping list, which is also time-consuming. The fact that the shops are open longer than they used to, also during weekends and bank holidays, encourages to do the shopping in more diverse times [4]. This convenience relieved people of the duty of going shopping regularly in specified periods of time and in fact prolonged performing of house chores even to late night hours and Sundays.

Over dozen of years a stabilized and leveled rhythm of work and relaxation was predominant. Both men and women used to come back from work at the same time, which favoured preparing warm meals together, as a family. Preparing dinner often coincided with coming home of children from school. However, the last twenty-year period can be characterized by a more elastic work time, a need to work overtime and sometimes a need of working two jobs. Therefore the household members come back home in different times and they pass each other by during the meal times. The diversification of the work rhythm requires coordination of spending time together as a family. Also having to stay at work late sometimes requires changing plans for spending an evening together. What helps with such a coordination is popularization of a telephone (especially mobile phones). However, talking on the phone with other household members is time-consuming and it often requires a beforehand change of plans [4].

Simple technological devices do not require special qualifications and preparation to operate them. Moreover they are not that susceptible to failures. If they are used in a correct way they operate for a long time, sometimes even exceeding their moral wear. More complicated equipment, such as mechanical devices (powered with engines) and electronic devices more often require a special training and precautions when using them, in order to avoid their failure or causing an accident.

In modern conditions of high supply for household appliances and a decline in their prices, the producers take various actions in order to save money by changing the technological process which results in a quicker wear of products. At the same time, their special construction excludes a simple and cheap repair and exchanging of a broken component. The repairs are connected with a pricy exchange of bigger modules or an exchange of a considerably new module for a brand new one.

A big competition in the market also caused some considerable changes in the grocery offer and in the usage of some kitchen appliances. Numerous appliances were transformed or even removed from the modern households because of the industrial transformation of food and selling it in various forms. Among them we can distinguish:

- food processors (portioned and shredded vegetables and freshly squeezed fruit and vegetable juices);
- slicers (loaves of bread and cold-cuts already sliced in shops);
- meat grinders, hatchets and mallets (meat portioned in shops by grinding, slicing, selling of steak and stew meat, and pieces of chicken etc.);
- coffee grinders, mortars and pestles (availability of grained packed coffee and packaged herbs and spices);

- rolling pins, breadboards, makitras, dough pestles etc. (different types of dumplings, noodles and other semi-prepared foods, various types of pasta, pizza, pies and cakes sold in packages or on its own).

The current offer of semi-processed and ready-made products is widely diverse in case of culinary types, quality and price range, which enables to meet diversified needs. Many of the ingredients contained in ready-made meals does not differ from traditional home-made dishes. Thanks to it, numerous household chores connected with preparing and processing the ingredients, as well as, cleaning after those processes are not performed any more while preparing complex meals. Also using various equipment which was invented in order to aid with the aforementioned kitchen chores became obsolete. Resignation from those "old-fashioned" conveniences enabled people to attain measurable advantages, such as avoiding expenses connected with purchasing some kitchen appliances and saving some additional storage space in kitchen.

The main goal of using technical appliances is improving the quality of life through, among others:

- gaining free time;
- reducing the labour;
- removing the barriers (e.g. architectural and social), development of feeling of independence;
- improving of labour productivity and efficiency;
- gaining the feeling of safety and eliminating of risks.
- However, technology also has some drawbacks. It causes the occurrence of new chores and various stressful situations. That results in a decrease in the feeling of comfort of living because of:
- the increase in the labour input and intensity;
- the increase in dependency from technical appliances and loss of independence;
- unequal possibilities of using the appliances resulting from, for instance: age and experience;
- additional chores connected with preparing and cleaning after using the equipment;
- exceeding expectations concerning the equipment leading to discomfort and even frustration;
- an increase in payments (costs of the appliances and maintenance costs);
- strains on the microclimate (noise, vibrations, overheating of air, electromagnetic radiation, etc.);
- negative influence on the environment (excessive consumption leading to shrinking of the natural resources and producing of waste) [2].

3   Technology and Interpersonal Relations in Households

Technological conveniences influence not only performing of everyday chores, but also some social relations. In household environment this focuses mainly on the relationships between the members of households. Modern multimedia (TV, computer games, etc.) cause loosening of family ties. Numerous chores connected with taking care of children and the elderly require a personal involvement without using technological equipment [3].

Modern technology plays a special role in bringing up children. In the kitchen space there have been considerable amendments concerning feeding little children. Nowadays there is a wide range of ready-made foods for infants and young children which enables caretakers to reduce laborious work connected with daily preparation of balanced meals. It is also possible to meet growing culinary demands of children and adults. The separate assortment of ready-made products is aimed at people suffering from various food allergies and gluten intolerance.

Technicization of everyday life and almost all spheres of human activity leads to creating urban areas and household environment which is hostile to children. Children's play areas are constantly shrinking and the technological devices used by adults become threats to them. Reconciliation of career and bringing up children is becoming more and more difficult. Moreover, it is also difficult to take care of children while performing household chores, because a child is exposed to numerous dangers (burns, cuts, etc.). Modern technological security systems enable to raise the safety standards, nevertheless, adults should still keep their constant attention on their children. On the other hand the possibility of playing outside independently is nowadays becoming limited because of various threats and possibilities of injuries. Moreover, new city facilities are built on areas previously allocated to children, such as playgrounds [5]. Playing outside home is no longer a popular activity and children spend their spare time in flats which sometimes disturbs adults with performing daily household chores.

Formerly, performing various household chores demanded also involvement of children, who sometimes worked as much as the adults. Especially seasonal works (preparing fruit and vegetable preserves and making stock), routine cleaning chores and taking care of cattle required help from children. Participation in household chores was a form of preparing children to their adult lives and integrating the generations within a family. Nowadays, as previously mentioned, the majority of seasonal chores connected with making food supplies does not take part in modern flats anymore and a lot of routine chores require using complicated equipment. As a result, children are basically excluded from participation in household chores (and integration with their parents through work) and their duties are usually limited to maintaining the order in their rooms. Also the complicated usage of kitchen appliances, sharp tools or fear of expensive table settings being destroyed results in isolating children from preparing and serving meals together with adults.

The development of information technology aims at enabling communication with the outside world for those workers who are telecommuting. Thanks to an easy transfer of information the comfort of life can be easily raised. Modern media are targeted not only towards adults but also children. All age groups live in this "media chaos" which leads to social disintegration and atrophy of inter-generational bonds within particular families (because of: TV, Internet, computer games). As a result, participation of all members of family in housekeeping becomes even harder to organize. Those tendencies are noticed by adults who try to engage their children in performing household chores. However, parents do it because of pedagogical, rather than, practical reasons, as children are not able to really help them with performing the chores [4].

4   Household Technology and Ecology

In the light of "sustainable development" tendencies and attempts to preserve the natural resources it seems that the western civilization reached its peak in the saturation with consumption goods, especially various appliances aiming at helping with everyday activities. However, recently slow changes can be observed. Consumers become more interested in the quality of goods they purchase therefore a more advanced technology is applied in order to meet customers' high demands while using less resources and materials. Also, nowadays, more popularity is gained by immaterial values, such as information and feeling of comfort connected with limitation of consumption (literal – eating less food, and figurative – producing more and consuming less).

The functioning of households has changed considerably over the last couples of dozen of years. The members of households became more prosperous and acquired various properties and household appliances which need spending additional time on maintenance. The civilizational development also caused an increase in hygienic standards of living. Therefore maintaining the house nowadays requires intensified work in the areas of doing the laundry, ironing and cleaning. Also the kitchen chores have become more extended in time due to the diversification of menu and changing of the times of meals. The consumption becomes gradually more based on highly processed products.

Current high hygienic standards require using technologically advanced products of personal hygiene and cleaning supplies. Using some of those supplies causes skin exhaustion and immunodeficiency. Moreover numerous detergents have a negative impact on the natural environment, especially on the water supplies.

Food products undergo considerable transformations using chemical substances (in order to, for instance: gain mass, reduce the time of ripening or prolong their shelf life). Food designed and produced in a laboratory is usually flavorsome and nutritious and stays fresh longer. However, it is also harmful for people's health causing, e.g.: obesity, cardiovascular diseases and allergies. The intensified agriculture production is also unfavourable for the natural environment as it leads to: deforestation, soil contamination and disturbances in the natural water cycle.

5   Technical Conveniences and Subjective Feeling of Comfort of Living

In mechanization process human labour is replaced by machines. Its shift aims at reducing the most difficult, toilsome and monotonous chores. Together with mechanization the share of human labour both in physical (using muscles) and psychic (using mind) sense decreases significantly [1]. On the other hand, technicization of household environment led to, among others: disappearance of many stimuli which used to be representatives of the special role of the household. One example can be open fire, which was used for heating and cooking. Its colouring and beaming warmth fostered creating an enjoyable atmosphere and provided pleasant stimuli for people's senses. Fire also encouraged family members to bond and gather around it. However, making a fire, maintaining it and cleaning the hearth was a laborious and time-consuming task. Also the fire usually did not give enough energy. Because of those inconveniences, currently people ceased to use open fire in their households. Nevertheless, many people still remember about the advantages of an open fire that is why they try to compensate for its loss. It has become popular to light candles, burn wood in a fireplace or coal in a barbecue. Also using such appliances as: washing machine, fridge, halogen oven or cooker hood resulted in disappearance of various smells. In former households the smells changed depending on the performed chores, for instance: the smell of soap during doing the laundry, the smell of roasted meat and baked pies. The natural smells of fruit or flowers are replaced by artificial air fresheners. In spite of all those subjective inconveniences, nowadays, it seems impossible to resign from household appliances which objectively provide high quality of work and enable users to relax.

Despite their functional usefulness, traditional appliances, for some users, are also sources of many nostalgic feelings. Former appliances become exhibits in various museums and in private collections. Very often they have a sentimental meaning to their owners. On the other hand, modern appliances are often bought because of their esthetic qualities. They are also regarded as a symbol of wealth and particular lifestyle.

6   Summary

Using numerous appliances and technical devices resulted in reducing human labour in household chores. However, along the technicization of everyday life comes an increase in psychic burdens. Factors like: flexibility of work, increase in hygienic standards, growth in products supplies, competition on the job, service and goods market demand adjusting the household chores to changing social conditions. Running a modern household requires detailed organization, division of duties and performing a lot of additional chores. Among those additional duties we can distinguish: various preliminary and cleaning chores, which often are not visible in the day balance. That is why despite numerous technological improvements, a notable gain in "free time" is not visible. One of the recompensations is actual or apparent freedom in organizing free time into house and work-related duties, which then leads to further dependency from other organizational chores [4].

Many of the aforementioned chores could not be performed without modern conveniences found in modern households. A certain dependency can be seen between civilizational development (technology in house and work environment) and cultural changes in everyday life (extension of working time and appearance of new chores).

Despite appreciable improvement in household chores thanks to using various devices (e.g. household appliances), the traditional household model did not change significantly. Still the bigger share of housework and bringing up children is delegated to women, who are still perceived as guardians of hearth, though only figuratively. Potential users believe that applying new technologies will make the chores more efficient, shorter and less laborious [4]. However, basing on previous experience it appears that the technological progress needs to be accompanied with social stabilization of living conditions and protection of households from various dangers in the working environment (being overloaded with work, fear of losing one's job etc.).

Applying of technological conveniences did not bring "a relief from household chores", as exchanging human labour with machines is still limited. Technological progress enables reducing various activities and elimination of numerous old, routine chores. Nevertheless, together with social changes it discredited the traditional order and division of roles in household, as well as the authority of women as housewives [3]. Although running a house nowadays is a job with a "manager-like" status it seems to be even less appreciated in modern societies living in industrialized countries.

References

1. Giedion, S.: Die Herrschaft der Mechanisierung. Ein Beitrag zur anonymen Geschichte, p. 557. Europäische Verlagsanstalt, Hamburg (1994)
2. Heßler, M.: Mrs. Modern Women. Zur Sozial-und Kulturgeschichte der Haushaltstechnisierung, p. 28. Campus Verlag GmbH, Frankfurt/Main (2001)
3. Hoepfner, W.: Geschichte des Wohnens.Von 1945 bis heute. Aufbau – Neubau – Umbau, pp. 768, 771–772. Deutsche Verlags-Anstalt, Stuttgart (1999)
4. Meyer, S., Schulze, E.: Technisiertes Familienleben. Blick zurück und nach vorn, Berlin. Edition Sigma, p. 25, 29, 34, 181, 194, 201 (1993)
5. Nowakowski, P., Charytonowicz, J.: Ergonomic Design of Children's Play Spaces in the Urban Environment. In: Stephanidis, C. (ed.) UAHCI 2007 (Part II). LNCS, vol. 4555, pp. 517–526. Springer, Heidelberg (2007)

Shadow Cooking: Situated Guidance
for a Fluid Cooking Experience

Ayaka Sato[1], Keita Watanabe[2], and Jun Rekimoto[1,3]

[1] The University of Tokyo, 7-3-1 Hongo, Bunkyo-ku, Tokyo 113-0033, Japan
[2] Meiji University, 4-21-1 Nakano, Nakano-ku, Tokyo 164-8525, Japan
[3] Sony Computer Science Laboratories, 3-14-13 Higashigotanda,
Shinagawa-ku, Tokyo 141-0022, Japan
{ayakasato,rekimoto}@acm.org,
watanabe@fms.meiji.ac.jp

Abstract. Cooking is one of the most popular activities at home; however, preparing a new dish by reading a recipe is not a trivial task. People might lose their current position in the recipe, misunderstand the required amount of ingredients, and generally become confused by the step that should be followed next. Shadow Cooking guides users with situated, step-by-step information projected on a kitchen counter. It consists of a depth camera and a projector, which are installed above the kitchen counter. Shadow Cooking instructs the user on the steps to follow by projecting information directly onto the utensils and ingredients. The system also integrates a digital kitchen scale with the recipe such that the user is automatically prompted with the required weight based on the ingredient currently being measured. In addition, we have connected the system with remote locations in order to enable a user to communicate with other cooks easily.

Keywords: Accessibility of Smart Environments, cooking, AR, kitchen, measuring.

1 Introduction

Cooking is a staple domestic activity around the world. Such activity provides a feeling of sufficiency; therefore, cooking is important beyond just providing nourishment. However, there are many steps involved in cooking and it requires some knowledge, which makes cooking difficult, especially for beginners. Even people with experience are likely to make mistakes when preparing a recipe for the first time.

Cooking by following a recipe is not a trivial task. A cook has to be aware of the steps that have been completed, and be equally aware of the steps that follow next. However, different cooking books will frequently list several steps within one sentence or one block of text, such that the cook can sometimes lose their place in the recipe. Meanwhile, the cook might attempt to simultaneously focus on their current activity and try to understand what to do next. This type of balancing can cause mistakes, such as missing steps or inadvertently using the wrong amount of an ingredient.

C. Stephanidis and M. Antona (Eds.): UAHCI/HCII 2014, Part III, LNCS 8515, pp. 558–566, 2014.
© Springer International Publishing Switzerland 2014

Given that cooking is a real-time task, excessive efforts to understand the recipe can interrupt the cooking activity itself, which could result in an improperly cooked dish.

The other problem with current recipes is measurement. If the weight of an available ingredient (for example, meat) is different from the weight specified on a recipe, the amount of all the other ingredients must be recalculated accordingly. However, recalculating ingredients is an extremely cumbersome task that can cause mistakes when done incorrectly.

We conducted a pilot study to observe the mistakes that are most likely to occur with common written recipes. We used a muffin recipe, and both beginners and experienced cooks participated. We found that beginners were not familiar with measuring units, such as grams, cups, spoons, and milliliters, and as a result, they often made mistakes by using the wrong measuring tools. Beginners were also confused as to which utensil to use when the recipe only indicated to "mix" and used a spatula when a whisk was more appropriate. Both beginners and experienced cooks became confused with units such as "tablespoon" and "teaspoon," or inadvertently missed steps, such as forgetting to use flour where the recipe indicated to "...mix sugar, flour, baking powder and oil..." These results illustrated to us that the current style of recipes commonly used at homes can easily cause users to make mistakes.

In this paper, we propose a system that guides cooks by displaying a single step directly onto the cooking environment; the step displayed varies according to the user's progress. This enables users to recognize immediately the step to follow, thus helping the user to avoid mistakes and cook smoothly.

2   Related Work

Recently, several experimental systems have been developed to enhance the kitchen.

The method of integrating a recipe with a real kitchen is used in several systems [1, 2, 3, 4, 5]. CounterActive [1] projects a recipe to a kitchen counter that the user can operate by touching the counter. Panavi [4] is a sensor-embedded frying pan that manages user by recognizing the temperature of the frying pan. However, with these systems, users are still required to read instructions and be aware of their current step in the recipe and the following step. Kitchen of the Future [6] installed several monitors, cameras, and foot switches in an entire kitchen such that users were not required to see a recipe from a distance location. However, Kitchen of the Future does not recognize user's action. Cooking Navi [7] and Video CooKing [8] synthesize multimedia such as videos and photographs in order to make text-based recipes more understandable. These systems help users know detailed information. Some systems specialize in recognizing user's activities and objects within the kitchen [10, 11, 12]. Adding depth images to normal images enables such systems to recognize fine-grain kitchen activities, such as mixing and the number of spoonful ingredients that have been poured into a cooking implement [11].

In contrast to these systems, our system is more focused on supporting the entire cooking process according to the context of cooking, rather than merely recognizing cooking activities.

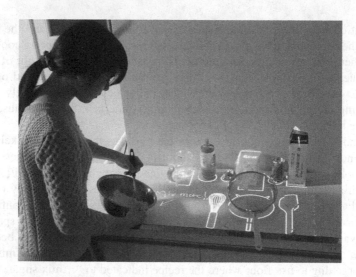

Fig. 1. An operation scene from the Shadow Cooking system. Cooking instructions are directly projected onto the kitchen counter and cooking objects. The instructions move forward according to the user's progress.

3   Shadow Cooking

As explained in the previous sections, the problem with written recipes lies in the separation of the real cooking workspace and the recipe itself. Previous works that merged the kitchen with recipes did not attempt to solve this problem, and a cook is still required to read the recipe, or the user must decide when to proceed to the next step; therefore, it is still possible for the cook to commit mistakes. Our research supports a merged kitchen and recipes, and it guides users according to their situation. Our system aims to decrease the possible mistakes and confusion in cooking in order to facilitate a fluid cooking experience.

Our proposed system, called Shadow Cooking, is a system that projects a guide directly onto the work surface, in accordance with a real-time situation (Fig. 1). The system recognizes the user's current progress in the recipe and guides the next action step-by-step. The real environment and the recipe are integrated in two ways. One is spatial (i.e., information is projected onto the position of actual ingredients) and the other is chronological (i.e., instruction information is projected according to the current progress of actual cooking). Thus, we expect the cooking activity to proceed uninterrupted, without the necessity to read a recipe. Our system aims to allow users to place their full attention on the cooking activity.

3.1   System Configuration

Shadow Cooking consists of a computer, a depth camera, a projector, and a digital kitchen scale (Fig. 2). The depth camera and the projector are installed above the kitchen counter to detect objects and project a visual guide directly onto the ingredients and utensils. A kitchen scale is installed with a Bluetooth chip that sends weight information to the computer in real time. After a recipe is selected, a step-by-step guide is projected onto the objects according to the user's current status in the recipe.

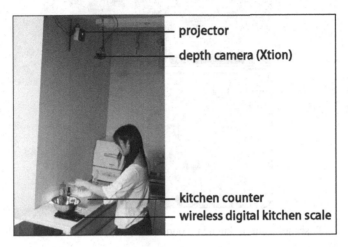

Fig. 2. Configuration of the system. The wireless digital kitchen scale tracks the quantity of an ingredient that the user has poured into the scale.

3.2   Recognition of the User's Cooking Context

The depth camera recognizes the existence of objects at specific locations on the kitchen counter in order to determine whether the user is following the instructions. The recognition is based on depth; therefore, once the user has placed an object on the specified place and the depth has been recorded, the system would not fail to recognize objects because of hands moving over them. To distinguish objects, we set the lower and higher height of each object; the system then recognizes the existence of the objects when the depth value is within these two thresholds at the designated position on the kitchen counter. This is an extremely simple method, but it can effectively detect typical incorrect situations, such as incorrectly placing a milk carton instead of butter.

Fig. 3-(2) shows the recognition screen from the depth camera. The blue lines indicate that an object exists in its designated position. Further, the digital kitchen scale is used to recognize the currently used amount of ingredients. Steps move forward by tracking the movement of objects and the currently used weight. For steps that cannot be determined through these two actions, the user can simply place a hand over the hand outline in order to move to the next step (Fig. 4-(2)).

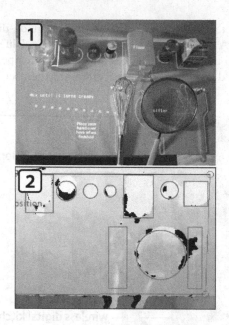

Fig. 3. (1) A real scene from a kitchen counter, (2) a corresponding depth image for recognition

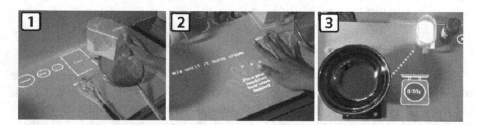

Fig. 4. Operation steps. (1) The user sets all the ingredients and utensils onto the projection. (2) The steps move forward by detecting the movement of objects and the scale amount, or by placing hands over an image as shown. (3) The user follows the instructions visualized with lines and some words. In this figure, the system is instructing the user to place 50 grams of sugar into a bowl.

3.3   System Usage

The system follows the steps indicated in this section to guide the user.

Step 1: Preparation. After selecting a recipe, the user sets all the ingredients and utensils onto the shadows as shown in Fig. 4-(1). After placing all the ingredients, the system will automatically proceed to the next step in the recipe.

Step 2: Adjustment (Optional). Optionally, the user can adjust the quantity of the recipe according to the specific weight of an ingredient. To adjust, the user would pick up the ingredient from the counter and place it on the scale; the amounts for the remaining ingredients are adjusted automatically.

Step 3: Cooking Along with Shadow Cooking. After step 2, the user can place a hand over the hand outline to start cooking. The user cooks based on arrows, numbers, and short instructions to progress. Steps proceed according to the movements of objects. For example, if the step is to "Put 50 grams of flour into a bowl," an arrow is directed from the flour to the bowl and a circle image shows the remaining amount that needs to be added and the amount that has been added already, as shown in Fig. 4-(3). When the user picks up the wrong ingredient or adds too much, an alert is displayed. When an ingredient is not needed anymore, its shadow disappears from the counter, or the user is guided to wash the utensil to use it again.

3.4   Trial

We conducted a trial to observe the performance of the system and to verify whether the user interface is appropriate. Two subjects (a male and a female) used the system to cook muffins. The male subject did not have any experience in cooking pastries; the female subject cooks several times a year. We explained only the usage of a standard digital kitchen scale: it has two buttons, one is to power the apparatus on and off; the other is to reset to zero grams any object on the scale. We did not explain how to use the system. Moreover, we recorded videos from a camera above the kitchen counter and to the side in order to observe the participants' handling of the utensils. Additionally, we interviewed the subjects after the test.

Consequently, both subjects did not make any mistakes and both answered that there was no difficulty understanding the instructions. However, the female participant responded that when the instructions indicated to "Mix well," she felt unsure as to how well to mix. In addition, both subjects had an inclination to pour more liquid, such as milk, than was necessary.

4   Remote Instruction

Novice cooks have a poor knowledge regarding cooking, and the information provided in recipes is frequently inadequate to guide beginners; for example, generally, recipes have no indication as to the proper heat level at which to cook certain dishes, or how to cut ingredients. Further, beginners might be unaware of how to manage unexpected circumstances, such as overheating, or a mixture not appearing as expected. On the other hand, experienced cooks, who cook daily, have sufficient knowledge such that they can arrange recipes in their own way, and adjust the heat level and taste according to their experience. Novice cooks cannot perform such changes without experience, and experienced cooks lack the opportunity to share their knowledge and sense of cooking.

With Shadow Cooking, we present another feature: experienced cooks can advise other cooks who are cooking in real time and from remote locations. A USB camera is attached to the ceiling of a cook's kitchen, and the adviser can observe the actions of the cook through video displayed from a touchscreen tablet (Fig. 5). The adviser can then guide the cook in two ways: (1) through voice chat, and (2) through annotation of hand-written messages using a conductive pen. For (1), users can simply chat about cooking; for (2), when the adviser writes a message directly on the video using the tablet, the written contents are projected immediately onto the same position on the cook's kitchen counter. This annotation enables users to communicate directly, and even demonstrate instructions that might be difficult to express using words only. Moreover, the adviser can ensure that the cook is following instructions correctly. We expect this feature to help novice cooks in acquiring more cooking knowledge than their present experience. We also expect this feature to aid users in inheriting home cooking skills; for example, a mother can teach a child who lives away from home.

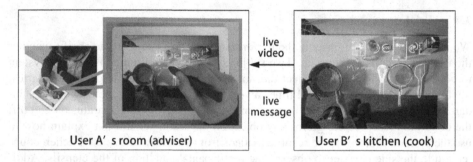

Fig. 5. An adviser from a remote location advises a cook using live video from the camera placed at the ceiling of the cook's kitchen. The adviser can then speak and write instructions; the written messages are then projected directly onto the kitchen counter.

5   Discussions

In this section, we discuss present problems and future work.

5.1   Supporting Other Cooking Processes

Our work assists the complete flow of cooking using weights and depth changes. For the trial, we used a recipe for muffins, which mainly consisted of measuring and mixing ingredients. There are several other processes involved in cooking, such as frying, steaming, and cutting. The processes that necessitate heat require temperature management; however, it is difficult to determine the appropriate temperature, and the process cannot be reversed once a given dish has been overcooked. We consider that previous studies, which visualize heat temperature by numerical methods [4] or heat maps [14], are valid and users can evaluate visually whether they are applying the correct temperature. The process of cutting is also difficult, especially for novice cooks, because there are several methods for cutting ingredients, for example, chopping, slicing, and mincing; moreover, cutting requires practice. We consider that it is effective to combine a video database, similar to the database that VideoCooking [8] incorporates into its system, or videos recorded by other cooks, such as CookTab [15].

5.2   Combination of Other Measuring Tools

In the trial, we observed that the subjects poured too much liquid because pouring speed is fast and it is difficult to control small amounts, compared with flour. The authors of this work have previously developed a system called "smoon" [13], a measuring spoon that automatically adjusts its capacity according to recipe data (Fig. 6). We consider that this type of measuring tool is more suitable for liquids.

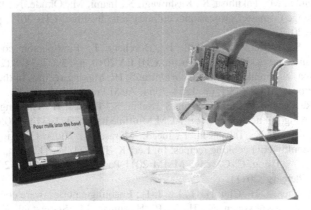

Fig. 6. Our previous work developed a utensil called "smoon," which is a measuring spoon that automatically adjusts its capacity according to recipe data

5.3   Miniaturizing the System and Applying to Other Activities

The current system requires the installation of several devices in the kitchen. Recently, USB cameras, projectors, and depth cameras can be miniaturized and can be connected to a tablet. If the entire system is miniaturized and becomes portable, it can be used for other situations, for example, to perform other activities on a table, such as knitting, sewing, and soldering circuits.

6   Conclusion

In this paper, we proposed a cooking support system called "Shadow Cooking" that aims to integrate recipes with real-time cooking. Because the recipe steps are progressively shown, and the position of ingredients and utensils spatially correspond to real ingredients and utensils placed on a kitchen counter, a user can concentrate on the activity of cooking, instead of diverting their attention on attempting to understand the recipe. Our user evaluation confirmed that this system helps users, and both beginner as well as experienced cooks can prepare a dish equally correctly, without any prior knowledge of the recipe.

References

1. Ju, W., Hurwitz, R., Judd, T., Lee, B.: Counteractive: An Interactive Cookbook for the Kitchen Counter. In: Proc. CHI EA 2001, pp. 269–270 (2011)
2. Suzuki, Y., Morioka, S., Ueda, H.: Cooking Support with Information Projection onto Ingredient. In: Proc. APCHI 2012, pp. 193–198. ACM Press (2012)
3. Ikeda, S., Asghar, Z., Hyry, J., Pulli, P., Pitkanen, A., Kato, H.: Remote assistance using visual prompts for demented elderly in cooking. In: In Proc. ISABEL 2011, pp. 1–5. ACM Press (2011)
4. Uriu, D., Namai, M., Tokuhisa, S., Kashiwagi, S., Inami, M., Okude, N.: Experience "panavi": challenge to master professional culinary arts. In: Proc. CHI 2012, pp. 1445–1446. ACM Press (2012)
5. Mennicken, S., Karrer, T., Russell, P., Borchers, J.: First-person cooking: a dual-perspective interactive kitchen counter. In: CHI EA 2010, pp. 3403–3408 (2010)
6. Siio, I., Mima, N., Frank, I., Ono, T., Weintraub, H.: Making recipes in the kitchen of the future. In: Proc. CHI EA 2001, pp. 1554–1554. ACM Press (2004)
7. Hamaoka, R., Okabe, J., Ide, I., Satoh, S., Sakai, S., Tanaka, H.: Cooking navi: assistant for daily cooking in kitchen. In: Proc. ACM Multimedia, pp. 371–374 (2005)
8. Doman, K., Kuai, C.Y., Takahashi, T., Ide, I., Murase, H.: Video CooKing: Towards the synthesis of multimedia cooking recipes. In: Lee, K.-T., Tsai, W.-H., Liao, H.-Y.M., Chen, T., Hsieh, J.-W., Tseng, C.-C. (eds.) MMM 2011 Part II. LNCS, vol. 6524, pp. 135–145. Springer, Heidelberg (2011)
9. Chi, P.-Y.P., Chen, J.-H., Chu, H.-H., Lo, J.-L.: Enabling calorie-aware cooking in a smart kitchen. In: Oinas-Kukkonen, H., Hasle, P., Harjumaa, M., Segerståhl, K., Øhrstrøm, P. (eds.) PERSUASIVE 2008. LNCS, vol. 5033, pp. 116–127. Springer, Heidelberg (2008)
10. Hooper, C.J., Preston, A., Balaam, M., Seedhouse, P., Jackson, D., Pham, C., Ladha, C., Ladha, K., Plötz, T., Olivier, P.: The French Kitchen: Task-Based Learning in an Instrumented Kitchen. In: Proc. UbiComp 2012, pp. 193–202. ACM Press (2012)
11. Lei, J., Ren, X., Fox, D.: Fine-grained kitchen activity recognition using RGB-D. In: Proc. UbiComp 2012, pp. 208–211. AMC Press (2012)
12. Ziola, R., Grampurohit, S., Nate, L., Fogarty, J., Harrison, B.: OASIS: Creating Smart Objects with Dynamic Digital Behavior. In: Interacting with Smart Objects, Workshop at ACM IUI (2011)
13. Watanabe, K., Sato, A., Matsuda, S., Inami, M., Igarashi, T.: Smoon: A Spoon with Automatic Capacity Adjustment. In: VRIC 2012 Proceedings, Laval Virtual 2012 France (2012)
14. Kita, Y., Rekimoto, J.: Thermal Visualization on Cooking. In: Proceedings of the 23rd International Conference on Artificial Reality and Telexistence (2013)
15. Sato, A., Tsukada, K., Siio, I.: CookTab: smart cutting board for creating recipe with real-time feedback. In: Proc. of UbiComp 2012, pp. 543–544. ACM Press (2012)

Smart Houses in Cloud4all: From Simulation to Reality

Boyan Sheytanov[1], Christophe Strobbe[2], and Silvia de los Ríos[3]

[1] Astea Solutions, Sofia, Bulgaria
bsheytanov@asteasolutions.com
[2] Hochschule der Medien, Stuttgart, Germany
strobbe@hdm-stuttgart.de
[3] Life Supporting Technologies, Universidad Politécnica de Madrid, Madrid, Spain
srios@lst.tfo.upm.es

Abstract. The Global Public Inclusive Infrastructure (GPII), which is being developed by the Cloud4all project and several other R&D projects, is a framework to ensure that everyone who faces accessibility barriers due to disability, ageing, etc. can use computers, mobile devices, the Internet and all the information and services available through these media. One of the goals of the Cloud4all project is to investigate this "auto-personalisation from preference sets" (APfP) in a domestic environment. To this end, the project is developing an online simulation of a smart house containing several devices with adaptive user interfaces such as a multimedia system and a washing machine with a display. For demonstration purposes, the simulation allows visitors to select the preference sets of seven personas with a variety of disabilities, i.e. visual, auditory, cognitive and motor impairments.

The Smart House Living Lab is a real accessible house equipped with the usual services of a conventional house where different ICT technologies (sensors and actuators) are distributed extensively in the living lab technical areas such as ceilings and walls, remaining invisible to users. It is managed by the Life Supporting Technologies Group of the Universidad Politécnica de Madrid; and it is also a member of the European Network of Living Labs [4].

This paper shows the Smart Houses online simulation developed within Cloud4all and its integration with the Smart House Living Lab at UPM.

1   Auto-personalisation from Preference Sets in Cloud4all

Cloud4all uses "preference sets" (known as profiles in some other contexts) to identify the needs and preferences of its user. These preference sets might be generic or specific to the context of a given application, device, platform, or environment. Based on the preference set, the Cloud4all system determines the best assistive technologies and user interfaces that will make IT systems and content accessible. In the case of the Smart House online simulation, we want to demonstrate how various user needs can be accommodated by typical home appliances.

We have targeted a wide variety of disability groups to show the capabilities a Smart Home can achieve with the help of Cloud4all. Re-using personas defined in the AEGIS [2] and ACCESSIBLE [1] projects, we have determined the needs and

C. Stephanidis and M. Antona (Eds.): UAHCI/HCII 2014, Part III, LNCS 8515, pp. 567–574, 2014.
© Springer International Publishing Switzerland 2014

preferences for various user types. Some excerpts from Cloud4all's preference sets for these personas are shown below.

Paulina Reyes

```
{
    "http://registry.gpii.org/common/adaptationType": [{"value": ["audio
description", "audio representation", "tactile representation"]}]
    "http://registry.gpii.org/common/language": [{"value": "es"}],
    "http://registry.gpii.org/applications/uk.co.jads.android.speechRate":
[{"value": 5}]
}
```

Maurice Nalobaka

```
{
    "http://registry.gpii.org/common/genericFontName": [{"value": "sans-
serif"}],
    "http://registry.gpii.org/common/fontSize": [{"value": 18}],
    "http://registry.gpii.org/common/foregroundColor": [{"value":
"#FFFFFF"}],
    "http://registry.gpii.org/common/backgroundColor": [{"value":
"#000000"}]
}
```

Nitesh Sarin

```
{
    "http://registry.gpii.org/common/language": [{ "value": "en-GB"}],
    "http://registry.gpii.org/common/magnification": [{ "value": 2.0 }],
    "http://registry.gpii.org/common/invertImages": [{ "value": false }],
    "http://registry.gpii.org/common/tracking": [{ "value": "mouse" }],
    "http://registry.gpii.org/applications/com.aisquared.zoomtext.application
Priority": [{ "value": 0 }],
    "http://registry.gpii.org/applications/com.microsoft.windows7.themes": [{
"value": "Windows 7 Basic" }],
    "http://registry.gpii.org/applications/com.microsoft.windowsphone7.backgr
oundColour": [{ "value": "#FFFFFF" }],
    "http://registry.gpii.org/applications/com.microsoft.windowsphone7.foregr
oundColour": [{ "value": "#000000" }],
}
```

Edward Hodgins

```
{
    "http://registry.gpii.org/common/language": [{ "value": "en-GB"}],
    "http://registry.gpii.org/common/visualAlert.usage": [{ "value": "pre-
ferred" }],
    "http://registry.gpii.org/common/visualAlert.systemSounds": [{ "value":
"window" }],
    "http://registry.gpii.org/common/voiceRecognition.microphoneGain": [{
"value": 1.0 }],
    "http://registry.gpii.org/common/voiceRecognition.volume": [{ "value":
1.0 }],
    "http://registry.gpii.org/common/voiceRecognition.dictation": [{ "value":
true }],
    "http://registry.gpii.org/common/voiceRecognition.commandAndControl.vocab
ulary": [{ "value": "Natural" }],
    "http://registry.gpii.org/common/adaptationPreference.adaptationType": [{
"value": "visual representation" }],
    "http://registry.gpii.org/common/adaptationPreference.language": [{ "val-
ue": "en" }]
}
```

Mikel Vargas

```
{
    "http://registry.gpii.org/common/onscreenKeyboard": [{ "value": true }],
    "http://registry.gpii.org/common/-provisional-initDelay": [{ "value":
0.120 }],
    "http://registry.gpii.org/common/cursorSpeed": [{ "value": 0.850 }],
    "http://registry.gpii.org/common/cursorAcceleration": [{ "value": 0.800
}],
    "http://registry.gpii.org/common/-provisional-mouseEmulationEnabled": [{
"value": true }],
    "http://registry.gpii.org/common/stickyKeys": [{ "value": true }],
    "http://registry.gpii.org/common/-provisional-slowKeysEnable": [{ "val-
ue": true }],
    "http://registry.gpii.org/common/slowKeysInterval": [{ "value": 0.4 }],
    "http://registry.gpii.org/common/-provisional-debounceEnable": [{ "val-
ue": true }],
    "http://registry.gpii.org/common/debounceInterval": [{ "value": 0.20 }],
```

```
    "http://registry.gpii.org/common/language": [{ "value": "es-ES"}],
    "http://registry.gpii.org/common/-provisional-speechRecognitionOn": [{
"value": true }],
    "http://registry.gpii.org/common/controllerWindow": [{ "value": "show"
}],
    "http://registry.gpii.org/common/microphoneGain": [{ "value": 1.0 }],
    "http://registry.gpii.org/common/dictation": [{ "value": false }],
    "http://registry.gpii.org/common/mouseControl": [{ "value": false }],
    "http://registry.gpii.org/common/automaticDelay": [{ "value": 0.0 }],
    "http://registry.gpii.org/common/automaticScanRepeat": [{ "value": 3 }],
    "http://registry.gpii.org/common/scanSpeed": [{ "value": 0.5 }],
    "http://registry.gpii.org/common/keyHeightRelative": [{ "value": 5 }],
    "http://registry.gpii.org/common/keyWidthRelative": [{ "value": 3 }],
    "http://registry.gpii.org/common/keySpacingRelative": [{ "value": 1 }],
    "http://registry.gpii.org/common/doubleClickSpeed": [{ "value": 0.4 }],
    "http://registry.gpii.org/common/absolutePointing": [{ "value": true }],
}
```

Peter Vandezande

```
{
    "http://registry.gpii.org/common/language": [{ "value": "en-GB"}],
    "http://registry.gpii.org/common/screenEnhancement.magnification": [{
"value": 2.0 }],
    "http://registry.gpii.org/common/screenEnhancement.invertImages": [{
"value": false }],
    "http://registry.gpii.org/common/screenEnhancement.screenMagnification":
[{ "value": "ZoomText" }],
    "http://registry.gpii.org/application/ZoomText.priority": [{ "value": 0
}],
    "http://registry.gpii.org/common/mouseEmulation": [{ "value": "Keyboard"
}],
    "http://registry.gpii.org/common/voiceRecognition.microphoneGain": [{
"value": 0.5 }],
    "http://registry.gpii.org/common/voiceRecognition.dictation": [{ "value":
true }],
    "http://registry.gpii.org/common/voiceRecognition.commandAndControl.vocab
ulary": [{ "value": "Natural" }]
}
```

The purpose of these preference sets for the chosen personas is to cover a wide range of user needs – so that we can see how they apply in a domestic environment. To this end, we have also carefully selected a range of appliances and devices that appear in almost every home. When defining the adaptations for each appliance, we have tried to be as realistic as possible – e.g. washing machines don't usually have a big display, but it is not uncommon for it to be touch screen. Similarly, we have tried to make the interfaces presented as close as possible to real products on the market – while still allowing a certain level of customization that might not be currently available. Table 1 below shows the personas chosen, the devices chosen, and a mapping of appliances that support adaptations for the needs of a given persona.

Table 1. Target groups and device adaptations

Target group/device	Blindness	Night blindness	Low vision	Hearing impairments	Motor problems	Cognitive limitation
Persona	Paulina Reyes	Maurice Nalobaka	Nitesh Sarin	Edward Hodgins	Mikel Vargas	Peter Vande-zande
Multimedia system	X	X	X	X	X	X
Smart phone	X	X	X	X	X	X
Air conditioning remote	X	X				
Kitchen appliances	X	X	X	X		X
House sensors		X		X	X	X

It is easily seen that the simulation covers a wide range of needs, even for devices with small displays, such as AC remotes. Thus its users are able to get a better idea of how Cloud4all's auto-personalisation from preferences applies to a domestic environment.

2   Smart Houses Online Simulation

The Smart Houses online simulation provides a graphics interface depicting a typical house (Fig. 1). A user is able to choose a room, which is followed by an animation that slowly transitions to that room. The devices and appliances in the room are highlighted and the user can pick any of them to be transferred to the device interface.

Each device shows a default user interface that can later be adapted to the user needs (Fig. 2) – such as increasing the font size, applying high contrast theme, changing the volume, etc.

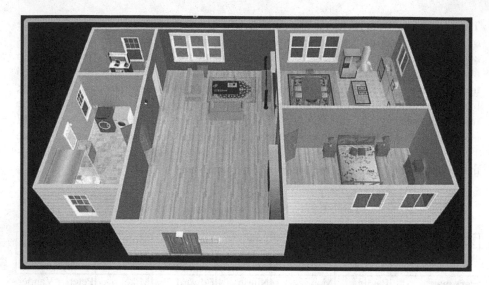

Fig. 1. The home page of the Smart Houses online simulation

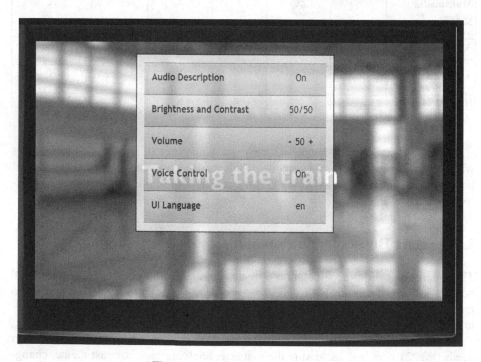

Fig. 2. The multimedia system menu

There are two ways to explore the simulation – you can either type your Cloud4all token to determine the best setting for you on each of the devices, or choose one of seven predefined personas. They allow visitors to easily get an impression of the adaptive interfaces in the simulation without going through the process of creating their own preference set. The simulation will not only be of value to the Cloud4all project but also to other smart home projects that may take advantage of the open-source simulation to explore and show different smart home features and functions. Beyond that, the online simulation is connected to the Smart House Living Lab of the Universidad Politécnica de Madrid (UPM), one of the Cloud4all partners.

3   Smart House Living Lab at UPM

The Smart House Living Lab at UPM serves as a research and development environ-ment in the Ambient Intelligence context of technology and services to prevent, care and promote the health and welfare of people, support for social inclusion and the independent living of fragile and dependent groups, in all stages of the value chain: training, experimental research, technological development and technology transfer.

With an area of over 150 m², it features modern control technology, monitoring and regulation of the environment. It consists of 3 distinct areas:

- User area: approximately 100 m² where currently a house is simulated (with kitch-en, bathroom, bedroom and living room), but it is an open space where any scena-rio required can be simulated.
- The Control room: which has a unique view of the user through a one-way mirror and holds the communication and monitoring systems and server technologies.
- Area of Interaction in Virtual Reality: used for studying both, the user interaction with devices prior to prototyping in reality and for training them in their use. It serves for rapid prototyping of new services.

The Smart House Living Lab appliances are controlled through KNX [3]. Different technologies are used and can be applied to develop new applications and services. The Smart House Living Lab provides infrastructure for interaction with ICT technol-ogies in the fields of communication, interaction, security, control and comfort.

The Cloud4all Smart House online simulation provides an innovative accessible user interaction model, taking advantage of Cloud4all accessibility features, to access and control the smart house appliances of the Smart House Living Lab.

Conclusion

The Smart House online simulation developed within the Cloud4all project and its integration with the Smart House Living Lab at UPM provide a glimpse into the fu-ture, when technology will be accessible to everyone everywhere – starting from their own home. They also show the power of Cloud4all to make accessibility easier for everyone – with no need for repeated complex configurations on every device.

Acknowledgements. Work presented in this paper has been researched within the Cloud4all project. Cloud4all is a R&D project that receives funding from the European Commission under the Seventh Framework Program (FP7/2007-2013) under grant agreement n° 289016. The opinions expressed are those of the authors and not necessarily those of the funding agency.

Additional acknowledgements to CIAMI project (PAV-100000-2007-397) for the Smart House Living Lab at UPM, which was partially funded by Plan Avanza (Information Society, Ministry of Industry, Tourism and Trade of Spain).

References

1. ACCESSIBLE project, http://www.accessible-eu.org/ (March 2014) (retrieved)
2. AEGIS project – Open Accessibility Everywhere, http://www.aegis-project.eu/ (March 2014) (retrieved)
3. KNX – the Worldwide STANDARD for Home and Building Control, http://www.knx.org/ (November 2013) (retrieved)
4. The European Network of Living Labs, http://www.openlivinglabs.eu/ (November 2013) (retrieved)

Building a Recognition Process of Cooking Actions for Smart Kitchen System

Fong-Gong Wu and Tsung-Han Tsai

Department of Industrial Design, National Cheng Kung University, Tainan, Taiwan
fonggong@mail.ncku.edu.tw, scott0510@hotmail.com

Abstract. Smart kitchen should be focusing its development on the actual interaction with users and the environmental objects rather than emphasizing on complicated instructions and feedback. Unfortunately, the current techniques can only be designed to identify motions and basic actions. The main purpose of this paper is to analyze and research user motions and actions involved in the process of cooking, including ingredient preparation, and to discover multiple action identification characteristics for the user and cooking utensils. By using the video analysis, ultimately, the project will use these characteristics to establish a reliable cooking-action database. Our study can distinguish between similar actions. The model is primarily used to identify, understand and differentiate the extent of the intellectuality of user motions. This model may be used in the future in the application to cooking support systems or other smart kitchen developments.

Keywords: Smart Kitchen, Human Behavior Taxonomies, Motion analysis, Video analysis, Decision Tree Learning.

1 Introduction

Nowadays, people's daily lives are closely related to technologies. Particularly our family lives with the accelerating pace of technological innovation, which has always been the focus of life. Also, many activities have been created within the family environment. If the environment can be made to reciprocate this behavior and respond to human behavior, it will lead to several advantages [1]. To provide useful devices which are most closely related to daily life, an intelligent family lifestyle has comprehensively seen the direction of future development worldwide.

Combined with various sensing technologies, the smart home system is also used to monitor and analyze the daily routine behaviors of residents. When unusual behaviors are sensed which are different to those being established in the system database, then residents might have some potential problems which needed to be further understood, like physiological or physical disease problems. Different systems may choose different sensing technologies based on its purpose. In general, technologies most commonly used by existing smart home systems are mainly divided into two main categories—Direct Environmental Sensing and Infrastructure Mediated Systems [2]. Direct Environmental Sensing takes advantage of certain facilities like camera or

C. Stephanidis and M. Antona (Eds.): UAHCI/HCII 2014, Part III, LNCS 8515, pp. 575–586, 2014.
© Springer International Publishing Switzerland 2014

RFID to offer considerably useful information for identification of actual activities of human beings, yet the installation and maintenance costs are relatively higher. Infrastructure Mediated Systems, however, merely need to install sensors on certain existing facilities. Compared to the Direct Environmental Sensing which has to use a large number of simple binary sensors in an area, the Infrastructure Mediated Systems can relatively lower the complexity of installation and maintenance costs.

In order for the system to be able to correctly guide the user on cooking steps, it is necessary to first think about how to let the system know when the user has completed an action [3]. Three ways which can be used are as follows: (1) User notification; (2) Use of an IC tag; and (3) System recognition. The first way allows the user to directly notify the system by pressing a button so that the system knows that a certain action has been completed. The user then follows the directions for the next step.

The User centric Smart Kitchen System was created based on this design in which the system directly identifies the movements of the user and then gives support and feedback to the user if necessary. In general, the system is designed to identify hand locations, postures or cooking utensils. Food ingredients are not identified, as too many characteristics, such as colors, shapes, grains and textures make identification very difficult. There are several pieces of equipment which can be used for identification; besides the RFID identification system motioned above, an identification technique based on image identification is also available. The latter does not add any electronic tag on objects or the user, but directly turns a screenshot into pictures or images by using cameras or thermal imaging detection. Images or pictures used to take a screenshot could be a set of logistic, systematic totem. Not adding an image on the kitchenware or cooking tools for simple identification by the appearance is also workable. Many of the recent dining and auxiliary systems employ this type of identification technique to identify and recognize hand gestures and basic movements.

Smart kitchen should focus its development on the actual interaction with the user and the environmental objects, rather than emphasizing on complicated instructions and feedbacks. Those extra and unwanted motions do nothing but easily distract the user [4]. If the operation of smart equipment and the feedback approaches are inconsistent with the behaviors that the users are familiar with, or even force the user to have to re-learn and adapt to new ways of interaction, then such a design may contrast with the original idea for better quality or even causes more inconvenience. Nevertheless, as mentioned in the prior section, the development of existing smart kitchen systems focus relatively on the systematic application and the integration of the system and environment, like the cooking support system, for example, which emphasizes on the integral process planning of the cooking guide.

Cooking usually involves many complex actions, rather than merely simple ones like picking up or cutting. It is not enough for a smart system to identify hand movements [5]. Thus, in order to allow the system to better understand which movements and actions are being carried out by the user, it should first build an integrated action data set as references for the system to map user actions and movements.

The main purpose of this paper is to analyze and research user motions and actions involved in the process of cooking, including ingredient preparation, and to discover multiple action identification characteristics for the user and cooking utensils.

Ultimately, the project will use these characteristics to establish reliable Human Action Recognition Process. The model is primarily used to identify, understand and differentiate the extent of the intellectuality of user motions. This model may be used in the future and applied to the cooking support system or other smart kitchen developments, such as the auxiliary system of recipe amplification. In addition, because our study investigates the kitchen of smart home, our target environment is focused on home kitchen not commercial kitchen, which may be different not only in spatial allocation but also in cooking actions.

Miyawaki and Sano [6] developed a cooking navigation system utilizing the virtual agent, which is made by augmented reality tech to assist user to accomplish all cooking actions.

The scope of the research, which involves Human Behavior Analysis (HBA), widely ranges into applications from several fields, such as motion detection, background extraction and high-leveled abstraction behavior models [7]. Prior to conducting the behavior analysis, however, it is necessary to first define the relationship of layered behavior. There is plenty of literature related to HBA taxonomies [8] defined three layers of taxonomy. This first layer is called "action primitive" or "motor primitive", an action layer which is made up of a series of different or repeated action primitives. If the layer is involved in a wider range, including objects or interaction between the user and the environment, then it is called an "action layer". Let's take the action of making coffee as an example. A single arm or hand motion is called "action primitive", putting the teapot on the stove or picking up a cup from a table is called "action", and the whole process of making coffee is so-called an "activity".

Chaaraoui et al. [7] categorized HBA as being divided into four layers: motion, action, activity and behavior according to semantics and time frame. The layer of "motion" is mainly used to detect the "movement" or something like the measurement of eye position or head posture. At the "action" layer, it has not been merely used to differentiate human motions; rather, it includes the interaction between humans and objects. "Second" is used as a measurement unit; an "activity" is made up of all types of "actions", which are measured anywhere from several seconds to several minutes, such as cooking or taking a shower. As a result, to better understand a user's activity, it is necessary to identify and classify a series of actions. The final layer is called "behavior", in which the time unit ranges from a single day to several weeks. It is used to detect the subject's abnormal behaviors in advance, such as discovering whether the subject suffers from some symptoms of a disease, like Alzheimer's disease (AD), for example, through observing and analyzing lifestyle, habits, and routine behaviors.

The method of defining behavior based on different layers is very helpful for doing relevant research, as the researchers can effectively identify the preferred layers they are going to identify, and avoid unwanted ones. To summarize the above classifications, this study focuses on the exploration of the "action" layer, including the operational interactions between humans and utensils. The "activity" of "cooking" is made up of these series of "actions".

2   Methods

2.1   Content Analysis

Frequent cooking actions must be listed first before being recognized and understood by the system. The research for this study is set in the home kitchen, and the target user is set to be those who frequently use the kitchen, regardless of gender. It is believed to be more appropriate to collect the cooking actions from general commercial recipe books. Later, the ideal target data can be analyzed and induced based on the Content Analysis. Content Analysis is a methodology of quantitative analysis which is based on the contents of the literature. It converts non-quantitative texts into quantitative data for the purpose of establishing meaningful classification items to analyze specific characteristics, features, or trends.

According to the definition, the research scope of this study is defined at the very beginning. A Western cuisine recipe book, which ranked number 1 in the current market, was selected. This recipe book provides 119 dishes. Any verb used to describe the cooking procedure of each recipe will be extracted and recorded into a form of Microsoft Excel. Because the difference between "Action" and "Motion" has been clearly defined previously in this study, this study will record and extract from the texts of the selected recipe book those actions which have an interactive relationship with the objects, such as shredding or stirring. As a result, some motions like stretching out or raising a hand or certain cooking activities such as boiling or roasting, will not be counted and included in this research.

2.2   Expert Interview

Those actions, which are extracted from the texts of the selected recipe book, may partially differ from those performed in real life, or actually are the same ones but merely with a different description in the text. Therefore, before determining the final target actions, this study will conduct an expert interview to evaluate and correct those action items listed previously.

This study constructed an open-ended interview with two professors who have professional backgrounds in cooking. Through these two professors' expertise, the interview aims at determining which actions are suitable for the research scope of this study.

2.3   Recording Cooking Action Videos

When the action items are decided, video recordings will be conducted to record these actions. The first step for video recording is to set the environment as well as the recording equipment. The filming environment is set in a home kitchen, rather than in a laboratory. From this picture it is clear that the work area of the kitchen is divided into three parts: stove, countertop, and sink. Then the action demonstration and video recording will be conducted based on the work areas which correspond to different action items. This study chose subjects with cooking experience for this action demonstration because, first, the research scope is set in a home kitchen, and second, the action items are selected and established from the texts of recipe books.

Concerning the kitchenware, according to the action list we presented, a general kitchen knife is selected for the cut action, and other utensils are rod and turning shovel. The knife tip and shank are respectively tagged with a round green sticker (with a 16 mm), that makes it clearly stand out from the background of the environment. This round green sticker is used as a feature point for image analysis (As Figure 1). Moreover, the distance of two dots between the utensil tips and shank is different. This is used as a reference for determining the displacement of the z-axis (in an orthogonal relation with the image screen). The distance between the camera and the kitchenware is 90 cm.

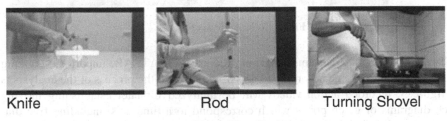

Knife   Rod   Turning Shovel

Fig. 1. Utensils

Concerning the video recording equipment, a camera with a resolution of 1920*1080 pixels at 30fps is selected, the distance of utensil and camera is 90 cm. When the recording environment and video equipment are all set, it's time for recording the cooking actions. At the beginning of the recording, a pure action, which simply operates the kitchenware without food, will be recorded. Later, the main purpose for the operators to hold the knife and repeat the chopping actions on the same side is to calculate errors in the video analysis, which is used to define the green color coordinate, followed by the implementation and recording of all kinds of actions. Every single action is operated by a single operator, with a single action lasting for 15 seconds. While filming, operators will be asked to hold the utensil vertically toward the countertop, and start the action after the recording has started for one second. When all of these files are saved, set and well organized, the next step will be to make the video set for the analysis of the action parameters.

2.4   Video Analysis

After completing the recording work, videos will be converted to Avi format which will be imported to the MATLAB for image analysis. First, according to the different environment, the green points on the utensils will undergo an RBG Coordinates Analysis, which will find the parameter threshold of the green points among red, blue and green colors. The purpose of doing so is to adjust parameter threshold of two green points captured by each video (Figure 2).

The steps of analysis are as follows: First, execute the file named RGB_ROI_ColorAnalysis_ReadVideo after turning on MATLAB. Second, type the file path which you want to analyze and then circle the green dots on the utensils by cross cursor tool, and the analysis results of RGB color spaces will be obtained after clicking. Then definite the color spaces of green dots according to the results.

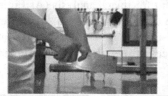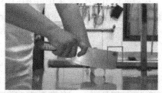

Fig. 2. Color Analysis Process

Then, execute the file named Motion_Record by MATLAB, import the cooking action videos one by one according to classification, and the process of the analysis is as figure 3, recorded action videos will be analyzed for later establishing moving track diagrams of green points which correspond to a time axis, including five diagrams of analyzed results— Amplitude and Frequency on the X-axis Y-axis and Z-axis and variations of two-point distances. Also it will make a video output of the analysis process.

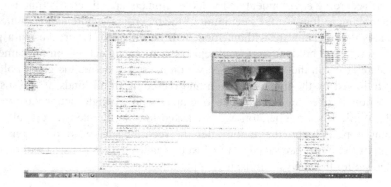

Fig. 3. Video Analysis Process

2.5   Data Analysis

After completing the analysis of all videos, each action group, such as cooking action groups for slicing or dicing, will be undergo a data analysis to identify the parameter difference of sub-actions in each group, define each parameter's threshold, and finally analyze and organize each action group as diagrams to establish a database of action parameters.

Attribute Analysis. There are several steps after analyzing action videos: First, we organize the peak data of the diagram into Microsoft Office Excel. Second, classify the data that might be Key attribute from the action videos into a table, columns are action classes and rows are attribute classes. And then, save the file as Comma separated Value (CSV) after completing the table for machine learning to proceed researching.

Decision Tree Learning. After building data table, we start to precede Decision Tree Learning by Weka. Weka is free software for data analysis and predictive modeling which is written by java and the developer is University of Waikato in New Zealand. There are many standard data mining tasks and operator methods to choose, and the operating interface is very easy for users. Plus, it is able to be operated in almost every system, including Linux, Windows, OS X and etc.

First, open the Weka, click "Explorer" and choose the database table which is csv file from the "Preprocess" label, and we can see some numerical value of table classes and data. And then move the cursor to "Classify" label, click the "Choose" button, choose the Decision Tree Learning methods. This research is completed by representative operator method called SimpleCart. At last, choose the "Start" button to start analyzing, and the results will be presented in the "Classifier Output" column.

The analysis results are the classification results of SimpleCART Decision Tree, different attribute data thresholds, total Correctly Classified Instances and Precision, and detailed accuracy by class, including Precision and Recall. At last, proceed Confusion Matrix by the analysis result and then present the final matrix.

3   Analysis and Results

3.1   Cooking Actions Taxonomies

The first half of this study mainly organizes general actions for cooking by first analyzing a Western cuisine recipe book through Content Analysis. Later, a preliminary action list is established and then given to cooking professionals for revision and to solicit suggestions for completing a final list of cooking action items.

In the first phase of conducting the Content Analysis, a total of 119 dishes will be recorded with 1,607 verbs. 45 different action items will be obtained after organization.

Table 1. The sub-actions list (Recipe)

Action	Sub-action					
	Cut	Slice	Cut into two	Cut into stick	Julienne	Chop
Cut	Mince	Dice	Cube	Gash	Cut into angularity	Cut into segments
	Cut into rods					
Press	Mush	Crash				
Frying	Frying	Shallow-Fry	Stir-Fry			

Then, these 45 action items will be grouped based on operational attributes. For example, those actions, such as Slicing, Cubing or Julienning, are all associated with a knife; therefore, all of them will be categorized under the general classification of cutting. Finally, a total of 27 action items will be organized in order to conduct a simple descriptive statistical analysis for calculating the total percentage of each item. Table1 showed sub-actions list of some actions. The Above results will later be given to two professors who are cooking experts for correction.

Based on the ideas and feedback given by cooking experts and the observation of some cooking videos, partial items with similar actions will be revised. Finally, a final list of actions will be completed as shown in Table 2.

Table 2. The sub-actions list (Final)

Action	Sub-action					
Cut	Cut	Slice	Cube	Dice	Julienne	Mince
Press	Mush	Crash				
Frying	Frying	Shallow-Fry	Stir-Fry			

3.2   Cooking Actions Video Set

After analyzing the color space, we will get three figures which show the color distribution of RGB individually. We definite the green dots spaces as Index_NonSelect=find(Normal_R>0.133 | Normal_G<0.602 | Normal_G>0.684 | Normal_B<0.275) according to the results data, red value for <0.133, green value for <0.602 and >0.684, blue value for 0.275 which is not detected, the location of green dots on the moving utensils is able to be identified precisely through this method. Because there is no certain testing place for this experience, the color space of green dots will be dissimilar under different circumstances in the video. To precisely catch the moving green dots, we will do color space analysis to adjust data before analyzing the videos recorded under different circumstances.

Fig. 4 showed the image of reference video which is purposed to analysis the chromaticity coordinates of green point and calculate the error of video analysis. The following is the video images of similar action groups.

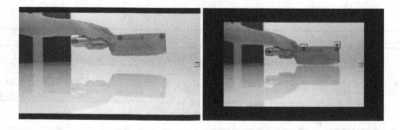

Fig. 4. Image of reference video

3.3 Video Analysis Results

Base on the correspondence of green point's locus and timeline in reference video, we can export four diagram and data of Amplitude on X Y and Z-axis, Frequency on X Y and Z-axis and variation of two-point distances. At first, we analyzed the reference video, try to correct the accuracy and calculate the error, and then analyzed the action video sets we recorded before.

According to the variation of two-point distance, divide the differences between maximum and minimum variation by two-point distance, then we can get the error of our video analysis, which is approximately 1.9%.

The following are the video analysis results of Cut action(cube slice shred dice and mince), which contained three figures, including the displacements of X-axis, displacements of Y-axis and variation of two-point distances. X-axis represented the vertical axis on the image perpendicular to countertop; Y-axis represented the horizontal axis on the image, as to Z-axis it's orthogonal to the image. We can see the amplitude differences from the first two figures. If the variations of two-point distances decrease, it means that the utensils are moving away from the camera, so we can see it represents the displacements of the Z-axis. Then it used the Fourier transformation to calculate each action's movement frequency on each of the three axis and find out the representative number of frequency. We can see the peak frequency of each action, the three axis number of peak frequency is its movement frequency.

3.4 Motion Elements Database

After video analysis, we will get the data of cooking movements. In addition to organizing amplitude and frequency of the data, we also observe the possible key differences from the action videos, and classify the representative data into tables, then precede the Decision Tree Learning analysis to get the result path.

In addition to calculating the general value of video analysis results such as amplitude and frequency; meanwhile, we also observe cooking movements to figure out the key attributes to separate two similar movements and then put them into the chart. From the analysis result of chart, we figure out that there are some observable differences in the frequency part; therefore, we use the frequency of all movements as presetting attribute in this research.

In the cutting classifications, we figure out that the displacement on the Z-axle of stripping is bigger than slicing in the same time observably. The displacement will be increasing because that the chunk-shaped ingredients are bigger than flake-shaped ones. The observed differences also reflect on the result chart of video analysis, which is the slope of amplitude on the Z-axle of the two movements. The greater the slope the more displacement per unit time, on the contrary, the smaller. At last, organizing the key data into charts and then built motion element database.

There is no significant difference in other movement classifications except for frequency; therefore, we use it on the three axles as attribute of the movement.

4   Discussion

It is important for smart kitchen systems to accurately identify the actions performed by users. It's also the core of cooking support systems. We started by analyzing the verbs occurring frequently in recipes and made classifications. A total of 119 dishes were recorded with 1,607 verbs. 46 different action items were obtained after organization. Actions that are performed by the same utensils were grouped together. We had classified 27 items, of which four items have sub-actions. Then we asked experts to refine this list, combining and modifying some action items, and finally getting a total of 26 action items, including four actions with sub-actions. These action items represent the most commonly used actions in cooking behavior. The second stage is to record the cooking action video set. Although there are already many available action video sets, since we have sorted out a list of actions in this study, we recorded them ourselves. This cooking action video set can also supply other studies with a resource for other image analysis methods.

The most important part was that our study has achieved significant results on the identification of the various actions. Based on the results, we analyzed the action's amplitude and frequency in the X, Y, Z-axis. First is the "Cut" action which occurs most often in the cooking process. Although they are all performed by a knife, they can be quite diverse, and the presentation of the ingredients is also very different. The sub-actions of Cut are Cube, Slice, Strip, Dice and Mince. According to the three amplitude diagrams of video analysis results, we can see these actions in the X-Axis and Y-Axis and the amplitude difference is quite significant. Cube is the highest, and Julienne Mince is the lowest. These differences can also be observed by eyes. Variation of two-point distances can be regarded as the displacement of the utensil movements in the Z-axis, the variation of the action obviously presents regularly decreasing, which means that action is far away from the camera. Also, we used the Fourier Transform to calculate the frequency value of each action in the three axis of the highest frequency. We are able to observe that the frequency of julienne and mince are higher than cube from the action videos and analysis data; however, the precise value of distinction depends on Decision Tree Learning. Discussing the results of machine learning from the result of decision Tree learning, we can separate Cube, Slice, Dice and Julienne precisely. The method of classification is showing in figure 5. First is the Frequency of X-axis, division value is 4.051, >4.051 for Cube and Slice, <4.051 for Dice and Julienne. Cube and slice have greater movements and lower frequency due to the bigger ingredients, while Dice and Julienne have smaller movements and higher frequency due to the smaller ingredients. From the research result, we can find out that Frequency of X-axis will be affected by the altitude of ingredients. Second is slope of Z-axis amplitude, the greater slope value means the bigger movements in the same time. Cube and slice are able to be distinguished by slope value 6.49, >6.49 for Cube, <6.49 for Slice, and the reason is that Cube has thicker ingredients, so as the movements. And Julienne and Dice are able to be distinguished by slope value 10.42. The incorrectly classified precision between Julienne and Mince is very high, so although total precision is 73.8462%, if we take of the Mince action data, total precision will increase to 96.1538%. Because it's very similar in ingredient's size and thickness between Julienne and Mince, so it's hard to define the attribute. The most obvious difference between them is the relationship of time. Julienne is the previous step before Mince; this difference can also be a reference of action recognition in smart kitchen system.

Then, the category of Press action is Crash and Mush, their movement is very similar, but there are only two sub-actions, so it only need one key attribute to distinguish them apart.

In addition to the difference of the amplitude and frequency of three-axis direction can separate the similar actions. Space and time differences are also other clues to help finishing a list of action items with all the actions corresponding to the relationship between the regional and the time listed. Therefore, we can use the system identification process in accordance with these relationships classified. First, the system can detect the location of the camera in the environment, such as near to the stove or countertop. It can first determine whether the next activity is cooking or preparing. Judging, again according to what the user came to the kitchen to use attached to the kitchen on the totem determining what kitchen utensils are used, such as round totem indicating frying, star totem indicating mixing. Finally, use the data threshold of motion element established in this study to determine the different actions performed by the same kind of utensils. With such a judgment process, the system can judge the actions of various dishes with higher precision.

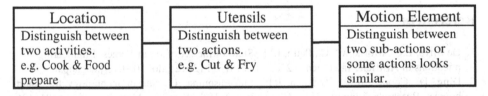

Fig. 5. System recognize process

These results can be used as the foundation for action recognition for smart kitchen systems in order to determine if the user is still running or has finished specific actions.

5   Conclusion

Smart kitchen should focus its development on the actual interaction with the user and the environmental objects, rather than emphasizing on complicated instructions and feedback. Our research's purpose is to analyze user's motion and action in the cooking process and ingredients preparation, and to discover multiple action identification characteristics for the user and cooking utensils. While many differences in cooking actions can be found by observation, how to let the system know user's action is very important for activity recognition system. Our study classified common used actions in various cooking activities.

Since the purpose of this study is to establish a set of identification process, one part of our recognize process is base on the use of different types of patterns on kitchen utensils for judgment, which are not available. This study uses green points for reference in video analysis, in addition to using the color as a reference; we can also change the use of different totems for this study.

The green point tagged on the front and near the end of utensils are to avoid the mask of hands and ingredients, it will have the range limits by using the color as the reference. If using totem for identification, we can use its characteristics of continuity to avoid masking problems. In addition, there is only a side shot with utensils, we use the size difference to analyze the z-axis data. In the future study, we can consider tagging the patterns on the top of utensils, and use two cameras for video recording. This may increase the accuracy of the z-axis data analysis, but may also increase the complication of the system analysis process.

Meanwhile, the research has also built a good database procedure to follow if there are additional actions to add or subdivide the present actions, such as thick slices and thin slices, to make this database more complete.

Acknowledgments. The authors would like to thank the National Science Council of ROC for financially supporting this research under Contract No. NSC100-2221-E-006 -204 -MY3.

References

1. De Silva, L.C., Morikawa, C., Petra, I.M.: State of the art of smart homes. Engineering Applications of Artificial Intelligence 25(7), 1313–1321 (2012), doi:10.1016/j.engappai
2. Ding, D., Cooper, R.A., Pasquina, P.F., Fici-Pasquina, L.: Sensor technology for smart homes. Research Support, U.S. Gov't, Non-P.H.S. Review. Maturitas 69(2), 131–136 (2011), doi:131-136. doi: 10.1016/j.maturitas. 2011.03.016
3. Hashimoto, A., Funatomi, N.M., Yamakata, T., Kakusho, Y., Minoh, K., Smart Kitchen, M.: Smart Kitchen: A User Centric Cooking Support System. Paper presented at the Proceedings IPMU (2008)
4. Borchers, J.: A Pattern Approach to Interaction Design. In: Gill, S. (ed.) Cognition, Communication and Interaction, pp. 114–131. Springer, London (2008)
5. Morioka, S., Ueda, H.: Cooking Support System Utilizing Built-in Cameras and Projectors. Paper presented at the The 12th IAPR Conference on Machine Vision Applications. Nara Centennial Hall, Nara (2011)
6. Miyawaki, K., Sano, M.: A Virtual Agent for a Cooking Navigation System Using Augmented Reality. In: Prendinger, H., Lester, J.C., Ishizuka, M. (eds.) IVA 2008. LNCS (LNAI), vol. 5208, pp. 97–103. Springer, Heidelberg (2008)
7. Chaaraoui, A.A., Climent-Pérez, P., Flórez-Revuelta, F.: A review on vision techniques applied to Human Behaviour Analysis for Ambient-Assisted Living. Expert Systems with Applications 39(12), 10873–10888 (2008), doi:10.1016/j.eswa.2012.03.005
8. Moeslund, T.B., Hilton, A., Krüger, V.: A survey of advances in vision-based human motion capture and analysis. Computer Vision and Image Understanding 104(2-3), 90–126 (2006), doi:10.1016/j.cviu

Understanding Requirements for Textile Input Devices Individually Tailored Interfaces within Home Environments

Martina Ziefle[1], Philipp Brauner[1], Felix Heidrich[1], Christian Möllering[2], Kriz Lee[3], and Claudia Armbrüster[4]

[1] Human-Computer-Interaction Center (HCIC), RWTH Aachen University, Germany
[2] Enervision GmbH, Aachen, Germany
[3] Institute for Textile Engineering (ITA), RWTH Aachen University, Germany
[4] Geometry Global, Berlin, Germany
philipp.brauner@rwth-aachen.de,
{ziefle,heidrich}@comm.rwth-aachen.de,
c.moellering@enervision.de,
Kriz.Lee@ita.rwth-aachen.de, C.Armbruester@argonauteng2.de

Abstract. In the last few years, many countries showed an increased public awareness regarding the consequences of the demographic change, which presents considerable challenges on future health care systems in the next decades. As a framework of the research presented here, we introduce a currently running interdisciplinary research project in which novel textile input devices are to be developed, iteratively designed, and evaluated. In order to learn about the individual requirements for using smart textiles in a home context, we carried out a exploratory questionnaire study in which 72 participants (aged 20-76) evaluated perceived benefits and barriers of smart textiles in the home context. Results show a first insight into user experience and the general willingness to adopt smart textile input devices. Also, the perceived suitability of functions to be controlled by those novel input devices as well as the reported appropriateness of different rooms and general device styles into which smart input devices could be integrated were collected. Results show, overall, a high willingness of participants to use smart textiles as input devices.

Keywords: Smart textiles, technology acceptance, user diversity.

1 Motivation and Related Work

Drastical demographic changes and aspects such as increased life expectancy, improved medical healthcare, or reduced fertility rates, will lead to a growing number of frail older people who will need medical treatments and long-term care provided by public health care systems [1] [2]. In order to master the exigent requirements of an aging society, developments in medical engineering in combination with information and communication technologies are indispensable to offer novel or improved possibilities for older patients to keep mobile and maintain their independence in old age

C. Stephanidis and M. Antona (Eds.): UAHCI/HCII 2014, Part III, LNCS 8515, pp. 587–598, 2014.
© Springer International Publishing Switzerland 2014

[3] [4] [5]. The spectrum of emerging technical applications covers a broad variety of developments, reaching from internal medical technologies (e.g. implants for monitoring physiological signals) over devices integrated into clothes (e.g. smart textiles, wearable technologies) to healthcare robots or smart home technologies that support older people in keeping up their independent life at home [2] [6] [7]. So far, research on medical technology is mostly dominated by technical, medical, and economic disciplines. The same holds true for the development of new medical products, which are in most cases guided by medical necessity, technical feasibility, and economic interest [8]. This exclusively technical and economic focus on technological advancement disregards the actual end-users' motives and possible barriers to the technology from all aspects of the design and development process. However, medical technology – especially in the home-care and rehabilitation sector – can only tap its full potential and benefit graying societies if the people who will need to use the devices help develop them to fit their specific requirements. This includes clearing acceptance barriers of electronic applications [9] [10].

Supporting seniors in maintaining independent lifestyles at home will only be achievable by systems able to monitor and control health-related information. The devices should also be portable and communicable, and fit into the ecology of existing mobile devices as well as into the individual home context of older adults. This is referred to as Ambient Assistant Living [11] [12]. Though the development in mobile technology is impressive, practical experience shows that technical solutions – novel and timely as they may be – do not necessarily guarantee the successful distribution of these innovations. In order to reach a high degree of user acceptance, taking into account only the technical and engineering aspects is not sufficient. The human aspects of these technologies have to be carefully considered as meeting users' wants and needs regarding privacy, dignity, and individual requirements is pivotal for the users' approval of these medical technologies [13] [14]. Thus, the success of (future) technologies at home largely depends on the extent to which technical developments meet the specific needs and demands of users, and on their willingness to use and integrate devices into their personal spaces [15] [16].

As a framework, we introduce a currently running interdisciplinary research project in which novel textile input devices are to be developed, iteratively designed, and evaluated. We report on a first empirical study in which users' attitudes and perceived requirements regarding textile input devices were explored.

2   Smart Textiles

Smart textiles and clothing represent a promising approach within pervasive healthcare systems. Instead of additional mobile devices, which have to be deliberately picked up and packed, the concept of 'wearable computing' envisions computers as integral parts of our everyday clothing [17]. The goal is to have an always-on and networked computational artifact that assists mobile users in a wide range of everyday situations. Smart textiles can collect different vital parameters, which can be delivered by WLAN to patients' smart phone or computer, the doctor, or even central emergency stations that call an ambulance if necessary [18]. In the last years, a considerable number of approaches integrated communication and sensor technologies into clothing such as shirts and belts or jewelry and wristwatches [19] [20]. In the context of smart shirts, the most popular approach is the Vivo Metrics Life Shirt [21], on the market since 1999, which is equipped with sensors that measure heart and pulmonary as well as other vital values. Other approaches focus on user experience and are based on fun and hedonic aspects [22], communication aspects [23], or sports [24].

Beyond the high potential of smart textiles in terms of functionality, ubiquity, and effectiveness [17] [19], the approach to integrate technical devices or technology into materials familiar to all persons opens up a huge field of applications scenarios. Textiles are usually perceived positively, based on inherent characteristics of the tissue – soft, warm, chic, pleasurable, smooth, velvety, colorful – which makes this technology highly plausible and usable for different usage contexts [4] [18]. Many users wish for more than the pure technical functionality and prefer devices with a high social and hedonic value [26] [27] [28]. As smart technical devices will be increasingly used within home environments, these aspects are likely to gain additional importance in the future [29] [30] [31] [32].

This is of special relevance against the background of user diversity and the challenge to meet age-related changes (psychomotor, cognitive), as well as the sensitive tradeoff between assistance and the wish to live independently from technology, which is often found in older users [33] [34] [35]. In this context, it is crucial to understand the users' needs, the perceived benefits and barriers a technical device may bring for them, potential design requirements that must be individually tailored to the users' abilities, but also the interrelation of functional and aesthetic factors and their consequences for the design, use, and acceptance of smart environments.

3   Intuitex – An Interdisciplinary Project

"Intuitex" is a recent project, funded by the German Ministry of Education. It specifically targets the development of a novel technology which adapts to the users' needs (instead of the other way around) and which seamlessly fits into the natural living space of users. This claim includes not only a true understanding of users' acceptance and their wishes for usable designs but also an understanding of the interrelation of the use of such technical devices in context. The overall goal is to develop an individually tailored textile interface that can be used in the home environment. In Figure 1 shows schematic drawings of potential application scenarios.

A specific focus of the project is directed at the diversity of users, that is the older and frail users and their requirements for usable and well-accepted technical products. Specifically, the project directs to the holistic and human-centered design of textile input devices that are (1) intuitively usable and easy to learn, (2) respect requirements and lifestyles at home, (3) fit to age-related difficulties in the manual control of input devices, (4) have an attractive design and rely on familiar soft and warm fabrics, and (5) may be suitable for different usage contexts.

In the course of the project, we will implement users' requirements into the technological cycle and develop prototypes in iterative cycles with users evaluating the usability, the design, the aesthetics, and the functionality in each of these cycles.

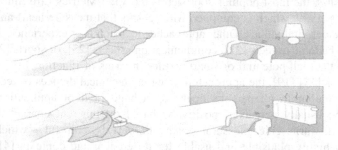

Fig. 1. Schematic drawings of potential applications of smart textiles within the home environment ® Intuitex, RWTH Aachen University

4   Method

Variables and Procedure. Independent variables were the participants' age and gender. In terms of user diversity, both factors might have a distinct effect on the acceptance of smart textiles and the perceived benefits and barriers [4] [8]. In order to collect comprehensive opinions of a broader sample of different ages, we chose the questionnaire-method. The questionnaire was delivered online (completing it took about 20 minutes).

Participants. A total of 72 people participated in the survey (57% female). Their age ranged from 20-76 years (M=29.6, SD=9.8). Participants were reached through the social networks of younger and older adults. They were not remunerated for their efforts, but were keen to learn about innovations in home automation and smart textiles. Only a small fraction (1%) had previous experience with smart textiles, yet about 30% had already heard about the possibility of using smart textiles (mainly from the area of sports).

Structure of the Questionnaire. The questionnaire was arranged into five sections.

1. *Demographic data*. The first part included demographic data regarding participants' age, gender, educational level, and (previous) profession.
2. *Benefits and barriers of smart textiles*. Users were asked to evaluate benefits and barriers of smart fabrics in clothing and furniture (items were the same for both types of textiles to allow a comparison, answered on a 6-point Likert scale.
3. *Requested functions to be controlled by textile input devices*. In a third part, participants were asked to evaluate functions to be controlled by a textile input device. Again, evaluations had to be done on a 6-point Likert scale.

4. *Devices desired as textile input devices.* Participants had to evaluate which possible object or device should be used for the integration of textile input devices.

5. *Home locations in which textile input devices should be integrated.* Participants indicated which rooms at home might be appropriate for the integration of textile input devices.

Questions. The items and answering options were based on previous empirical work in our workgroup in which we collected argumentation patterns as well as user experience of users of a wide age range [36] [37] [38]. In Table 1, items are given.

Table 1. Items and answering options in the relevant sections

Benefits and barriers	Material quality is very important to me • My key criterion is functionality • It is very important that textiles are easy to clean • Material quality is very important to me • I would pay more for a good quality • Durability is important to me • A lower quality is ok if the price is low • Low prize is most important to me • The design is most important to me • High quality is not that important to me • My key criterion is a fashionable look	
Requested functions	• un/look front door • open/close front door • turn on washing machine • set alarm clock • control radiator temperature • draw a bath • water plants • control room temperature • switch TV channel • adjust/change music • set outside lighting • open/close shutters • control interior lighting	
Requested devices	• curtains • carpets • trousers • blankets • table clothes	• pillow • plush toy • kerchief • chair/easy chair
Requested locations	• children's room • bathroom • dinging room • kitchen	• table clothes • office at work • office at home • living room

5   Results

5.1   Evaluation of Smart Textiles (Contrasting Furniture vs. Clothing)

We report on descriptive outcomes, followed by the effects of age and gender on acceptance (M)ANOVA). The level of significance was set at 5%. First, the evaluation of smart textiles in furniture (Figure 2) in contrast to clothing (Figure 3) is described.

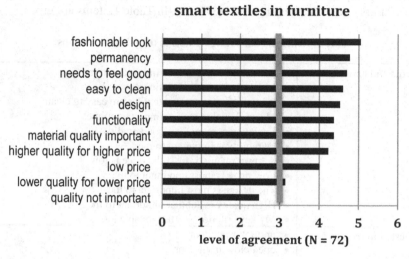

Fig. 2. Level of agreement (means) for the total group regarding requirements of smart textiles implemented in furniture (1 = I do not agree at all, 6 = I completely agree)

When focusing on furniture, we see that the most important dimensions are the "look and feel" and the durability of the material, but also the ease of cleaning and the functionality. Age did not impact the evaluations of smart textiles in furniture. However, there was a significant overall effect of gender ($F(1,42)=2.4$; $p=0.02$), showing that men and women evaluate the use of smart textiles in furniture differently.

A closer look into the single items show that men report to accept more frequently a lower quality to the advantage of a lower price than women do ($F(1,42)=3.8$; $p=0.05$). Furthermore, women report to attach a higher importance to the design of furniture equipped with smart textiles than men ($F(1,42)=3.8$; $p=0.05$). Also, women report to focus much more on the look and feel of smart furniture than men report to do ($F(1,42)=6.4$; $p=0.001$). Interacting effects of age x gender were not observed.

Regarding the evaluations of smart textiles in clothing (Fig. 3), the most important characteristics were the "need to feel good," fashionable looks," "importance of material quality," but also the "durability" of the clothes as well as the "design."

Age did significantly impact the evaluations. The older focused significantly more on the functionality of smart clothing ($F(1,42)=4.9$; $p=0.03$) and attached a higher importance to the "feel good" compared to young adults ($F(1,42)=3.6$; $p=0.05$). Also, gender effects appeared: Durability of smart clothing was more important to men than for women ($F(1,42)=3.7$; $p=0.05$).

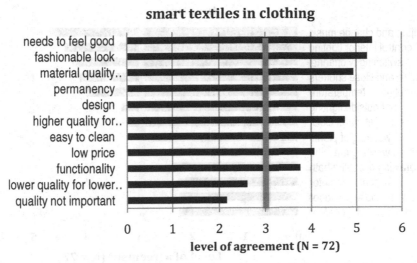

Fig. 3. Requirements of smart clothes (1 = do not agree at all, 6 = completely agree)

5.2   Evaluation of Smart Textiles for Device Types, Functions, and Locations

In addition, it may be important which specific device will be equipped with smart textiles and serve as an input device (Figure 4).

As can be seen, there are clear smart textile "favorites": table clothes, easy chair, outerwear, and kerchiefs were the preferred device types (M = 4.3/6 points). Regarding user diversity, significant age effects for the evaluation of smart textiles in blankets $(F(1,42)=3.4; p=0.05)$, trousers $(F(1,42)=6.3; p=0.02)$, and outerwear $(F(1,42)=3.6; p=0.05)$ were found. Older users evaluated smart blankets (old: M = 3.6; young: M = 2.5), trousers (old: M = 3.5; young: M = 2.2), and outerwear (old: M = 4.3; young: M = 3.3) as more suitable than the younger group did.

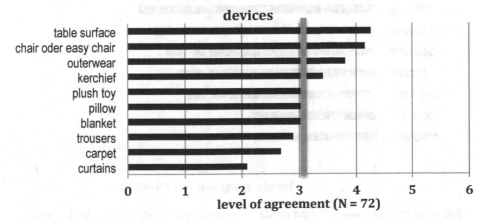

Fig. 4. Perceived usefulness of **device types** (1 = do not agree at all, 6 = completely agree)

The next analysis explored for which functionalities participants perceived smart textile input devices as useful (Figure 5).

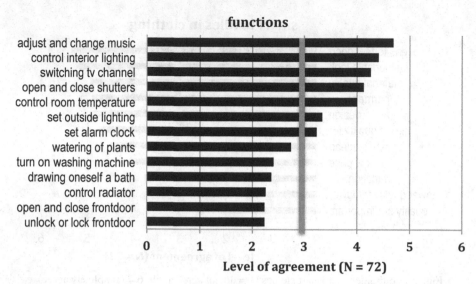

Fig. 5. Perceived usefulness of smart **functions** (1 = do not agree at all, 6 = completely agree)

A final question regarded the evaluation of a suitable location within home and working environments (Figure 6). As can be seen, there are clear preferences. The living room and offices are perceived as most suitable. In contrast, bathroom and children's room are not regarded as appropriate for textile input devices. While both main effects (gender as well as age) did not affect the evaluations differentially, there was a significant interaction effect between gender and age ($F(1,42)=2.9$; $p=0.01$).

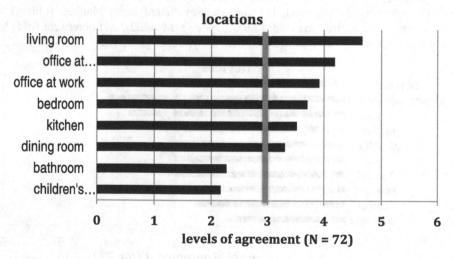

Fig. 6. Suitable **locations** for smart textiles (1 = do not agree at all, 6 = completely agree)

The interaction of age x gender is due to the fact that older men are more positive to use smart textiles in the respective locations than younger men and older women more reluctant than younger women (Figure 7).

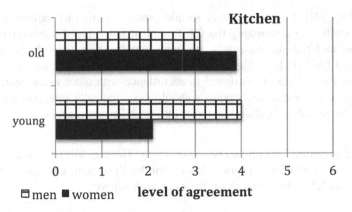

Fig. 7. Interaction of age x gender of smart textile input devices in the kitchen (1 = I do not agree at all, 6 = I completely agree)

6   Discussion and Future Work

In this exploratory paper, we report on the perceived suitability of smart textile input devices integrated into home environments. Overall, there was a high openness to use novel devices in all participants, independent of user diversity. The acceptance of users seems to be higher in familiar objects and not sensitive to usage context. As such, smart textiles integrated in clothes are rated as more suitable than smart furniture, presumably because smart shirts are fairly well known from the sports context and already available on the market [21] [22][23]. Regarding possible functionalities and locations at home, users prefer those settings in which the usage of smart textile input devices is not too intimate (living room and office) and only used for fairly neutral and public functions (e.g., switching TV or music channels). The more sensitive the location and the more security-relevant the function (e.g., bathroom, closing the front door), the lower was the perceived suitability of smart textile input devices.

Even though the reported findings about the acceptance of smart textiles were quite insightful, we should be aware that the questionnaire method applied here allows only a first glimpse into users' attitudes and "what users really feel." As most of the users do not have any experience with the handling of smart textiles, the outcomes presented here lack mostly practical knowledge and factual validity. In the course of the project, therefore, the creation of an experimental space in which potential users can experience and "feel" the technology in order to fairly evaluate it is of pivotal importance [39]. Persons might overemphasize their sensitiveness towards privacy and security violations and their dismissal of novel technology if their judgment only relies on the imagination of using it [40]. This is of particular importance, as potential usage barriers can only be fully understood if users can have a hands-on interaction with the environment and "feel" the impact of natural technology at home.

As a general direction of future technology development, it should be considered that the quality of "good interfaces" relies on more than the exclusive focus on performance aspects (as done in traditional studies dealing with the usability of input devices [33] [34]). Rather, usability should equally focus on traditional pragmatic aspects – attributes emphasizing the fulfillment of individuals' productivity- as well as affective and hedonic aspects – attributes emphasizing individuals' well-being, pleasure, and fun [41] [42]. Especially against the background of an aging society, it is crucial that interfaces are designed in accordance with older users' specificity and diversity [43]. Technical developments should systematically integrate user diversity – age, gender, social and cultural factors – into usability approaches.

Acknowledgements. This project is funded by the German Ministry of Education and Research (No. 16SV6270). Thanks also to Sandra Prautzsch, Chantal Lidynia, Julia van Heek, and Julian Hildebrandt for their research support.

References

1. Ziefle, M., Röcker, C.: Acceptance of Pervasive Healthcare Systems: A Comparison of Different Implementation Concepts. In: 4th ICST Conference on Pervasive Computing Technologies for Healthcare 2010, pp. 1–6 (2010)
2. Leonhardt, S.: Personal Healthcare Devices. In: Mekherjee, S., et al. (eds.) Malware, Hardware Technology Drivers of AI, pp. 349–370. Springer, Dordrecht (2006)
3. Holzinger, A., Searle, G., Auinger, A., Ziefle, M.: Informatics as Semiotics Engineering: Lessons Learned from Design, Development and Evaluation of Ambient Assisted Living Applications for Elderly People. In: Stephanidis, C. (ed.) Universal Access in HCI, Part III, HCII 2011. LNCS, vol. 6767, pp. 183–192. Springer, Heidelberg (2011)
4. Wilkowska, W., Ziefle, M.: User diversity as a challenge for the integration of medical technology into future home environments. In: Ziefle, M., Röcker, C. (eds.) Human-Centred Design of eHealth Technologies. Concepts, Methods and Applications, pp. 95–126. IGI Global, Hershey (2011)
5. Calero Valdez, A., Ziefle, M., Horstmann, A., Herding, D., Schroeder, U.: Mobile Devices Used for Medical Applications. IJDS 2, 337–346 (2011)
6. Park, S., Jayaraman, S.: Enhancing the Quality of Life Through Wearable Technology. The Role of a Personalized Wearable Intelligent Information Infrastructure in Addressing the Challenges of Healthcare 5/6, 41–48 (2003)
7. Schaar, A.K., Ziefle, M.: Smart Cloths: Perceived Benefits vs. Perceived Fears. In: 5th ICST/IEEE Conference on Pervasive Computing Technologies for Healthcare 2011, pp. 601–608 (2011)
8. Ziefle, M., Wilkowska, W.: Technology acceptability for medical assistance. In: 4th ICST Conference Pervasive Computing Technologies for Healthcare, pp. 1–9 (2010)
9. Klack, L., Schmitz-Rode, T., Wilkowska, W., Kasugai, K., Heidrich, F., Ziefle, M.: Integrated Home Monitoring and Compliance Optimization for Patients with Mechanical Circulatory Support Devices. Annals of Biomedical Engineering 39(12), 2911–2921 (2011)
10. Alagöz, F., Ziefle, M., Wilkowska, W., Valdez, A.C.: Openness to accept medical technology - A cultural view. In: Holzinger, A., Simonic, K.-M. (eds.) USAB 2011. LNCS, vol. 7058, pp. 151–170. Springer, Heidelberg (2011)

11. Kasugai, K., Röcker, C., Bongers, B., Plewe, D., Dimmer, C.: Aesthetic Intelligence: Designing Smart and Beautiful Architectural Spaces. In: Keyson, D.V., Maher, M.L., Streitz, N., Cheok, A., Augusto, J.C., Wichert, R., Englebienne, G., Aghajan, H., Kröse, B.J.A., et al. (eds.) AmI 2011. LNCS, vol. 7040, pp. 360–361. Springer, Heidelberg (2011)

12. Kasugai, K., Ziefle, M., Röcker, C., Russell, P.: Creating Spatio-Temporal Contiguities Between Real and Virtual Rooms in an Assistive Living Environment. In: Bonner, J., Smyth, M., O' Neill, S., Mival, O. (eds.) Create 10 Innovative Interactions, pp. 62–67. Elms Court, Loughborough (2010)

13. Ziefle, M., Jakobs, E.-M.: New Challenges in Human Computer Interaction: Strategic Directions and Interdisciplinary Trends. In: 4th International Conference on Competitive Manufacturing Technologies, pp. 389–398. University Stellenbosch, South Africa (2010)

14. Arning, K., Gaul, S., Ziefle, M.: Same Same but Different. How Service Contexts of Mobile Technologies Shape Usage Motives and Barriers. In: Leitner, G., Hitz, M., Holzinger, A. (eds.) USAB 2010. LNCS, vol. 6389, pp. 34–54. Springer, Heidelberg (2010)

15. Gaul, S., Ziefle, M.: Smart Home Technologies: Insights into Generation-Specific Acceptance Motives. In: Holzinger, A., Miesenberger, K. (eds.) USAB 2009. LNCS, vol. 5889, pp. 312–332. Springer, Heidelberg (2009)

16. Ziefle, M., Himmel, S., Wilkowska, W.: When Your Living Space Knows What You Do: Acceptance of Medical Home Monitoring by Different Technologies. In: Holzinger, A., Simonic, K.-M. (eds.) USAB 2011. LNCS, vol. 7058, pp. 607–624. Springer, Heidelberg (2011)

17. Katterfeldt, E.-S., Dittert, N., Schelhowe, H.: Textiles as Ways of Relating Computing Technology to Everyday Life. In: Proc. of the 8th International Conference on Interaction Design and Children, pp. 9–17. ACM Press, New York (2009)

18. Schaar, A.K., Ziefle, M.: Smart Clothes. Perceived Benefits vs. Perceived Fears. In: 5th ICST/IEEE Conference on Pervasive Computing Technologies for Healthcare 2011, pp. 601–608 (2011)

19. Cho, G.: Smart Clothing. Technology&Applications. CRC Press, Boca Raton (2010)

20. Cook, D.J., Das, S.K.: How Smart are our Environments? Journal of Pervasive and Mobile Computing 3, 53–73 (2008)

21. Vivometric: Life-Shirt System, http://www.vivometric.com/

22. Wildshirt, France Telecom, Studio Créatif,
http://www.studiocreatif.com/Vet/Vet02Prototypes05Fr.htm

23. O'Neill: The Hub,
http://www.funktionstextilien.de/content/view/488/122/

24. Falke EKG Shirt,
http://geo-view.eu/index_SPORT_sport-ekg-shirt.php

25. Scheermesser, M., Kosow, H., Rashid, A., Holtmann, C.: User Acceptance of Pervasive Computing in Healthcare. In: Proc. 2nd International Conference on Pervasive Computing Technologies for Healthcare, Tampere, Finland, pp. 205–213 (2008)

26. Hassenzahl, M.: Experience Design – Technology for All the Right Reasons. Morgan & Claypool, San Rafael (2010)

27. Heidrich, F., Golod, I., Russell, P., Ziefle, M.: Device-Free Interaction in Smart Domestic Environments. In: Augmented Human, pp. 65–68. ACM, N.Y. (2013)

28. Heidrich, F., Ziefle, M., Röcker, C., Borchers, J.: Interacting with Smart Walls: A Multi-Dimensional Analysis of Input Technologies for Augmented Environments. In: Proc. of the Augmented Human Conference, pp. 1–8. ACM Press, New York (2011)

29. Aarts, E., Marzano, S.: The New Everyday. Publishers (2003)

30. Weiser, M.: The Computer for the Twenty-First Century. Scientific American 265(3), 94–104 (1991)
31. Mann, W.C. (ed.): Smart Technology for Aging, Disability, and Independence: The State of the Science. John Wiley & Sons (2005)
32. Marti, P.: Bringing Playfulness to Disabilities. In: Proceedings of the 6th Nordic Conference on HCI: Extending Boundaries, pp. 851–856. ACM, New York (2010)
33. Armbrüster, C., Ziefle, M., Sutter, C.: Notebook input devices put to an age test. Ergonomics 50(3), 426–445 (2007)
34. Arning, K., Ziefle, M.: Ask and you will Receive: Training Older Adults to Use a PDA in an Active Learning Environment. Int. J. Hum-Comput. 2, 21–47 (2010)
35. Himmel, S., Ziefle, M., Lidynia, C., Holzinger, A.: Older Users' Wish List for Technology Attributes. In: Cuzzocrea, A., Kittl, C., Simos, D.E., Weippl, E., Xu, L. (eds.) CD-ARES 2013. LNCS, vol. 8127, pp. 16–27. Springer, Heidelberg (2013)
36. Schaar, A.K., Ziefle, M.: What Determines Public Perceptions of Implantable Medical Technology: Insights into Cognitive and Affective Factors. In: Holzinger, A., Simonic, K.-M. (eds.) USAB 2011. LNCS, vol. 7058, pp. 513–531. Springer, Heidelberg (2011)
37. Wilkowska, W., Ziefle, M.: Privacy and Data Security in E-health: Requirements from Users' Perspective. J. Health. Inform. 18, 191–201 (2012)
38. Ziefle, M.: Modelling Mobile Devices for the Elderly. In: Khalid, H., Hedge, A., Ahram, T.Z. (eds.) Advances in Ergonomics Modeling and Usability Evaluation, pp. 280–290. CRC Press, Boca Raton (2010)
39. Woolham, J., Frisby, B.: Building a Local Infrastructure that Supports the Use of Assistive Technology in the Care of People with Dementia. Research Policy and Planning 20(1), 11–24 (2002)
40. Cvrcek, D., Kumpost, M., Matyas, V., Danezis, G.: A Study on the Value of Location Privacy. In: Proceedings of the ACM Workshop on Privacy in the Electronic Society, pp. 109–118. ACM, New York (2006)
41. Bay, S., Brauner, P., Gossler, T., Ziefle, M.: Intuitive Gestures on Multi-touch Displays for Reading Radiological Images. In: Yamamoto, S. (ed.) HCI 2013, Part II. LNCS, vol. 8017, pp. 22–31. Springer, Heidelberg (2013)
42. Golod, I., Heidrich, F., Möllering, C., Ziefle, M.: Design Principles of Hand Gesture Interfaces for Microinteractions. In: Proc. of the 6th Intern. Conference on Designing Pleasurable Products and Interfaces, pp. 11–20. ACM Press, New York (2013)
43. Calero Valdez, A., Kathrin Schaar, A., Ziefle, M.: Personality Influences on Etiquette Requirements for Social Media in the Work Context. In: Holzinger, A., Ziefle, M., Hitz, M., Debevc, M. (eds.) SouthCHI 2013. LNCS, vol. 7946, pp. 427–446. Springer, Heidelberg (2013)

Assistive Robots

Development of a Robot-Based Environment for Training Children with Autism

Emilia I. Barakova[1], Min-Gyu Kim[1], and Tino Lourens[2]

[1] Eindhoven University of Technology P.O. Box 513, Eindhoven, The Netherlands
{e.i.barakova,m.kim}@tue.nl
[2] TiViPE, Kanaaldijk ZW 11, Helmond, The Netherlands
tino@tivipe.com

Abstract. This study is done as a part of design-research processes that aims to co-create technology supported robot centered therapy environment for autistic children. We attempt to evaluate to which extent the therapists who perform behavioral training of children with autism can be supported by robot technology in the process of therapy content creation and training. First, we feature a robot-centered environment that is technically designed to decrease the complexity of programming dynamic, synchronous and parallel interactive robot behavior to a level compatible with content creation. Afterwards, we apply the Cognitive Dimensions Framework (CDF) approach for evaluation of the usability of this environment that is employed to control a robot interacting with children with Autism Spectrum Disorders (ASD). A pilot test with therapists of two clinics followed by a test with adolescents with autism was performed. Participants in the pilot test performed tasks according to the different types of user activity in the CDF, and answered a questionnaire corresponding with the different dimensions. The results show negative attitude towards one particular dimension, but also high scores in other dimensions. As an additional validation of the usability of the environment, 9 adolescents with ASD could also create robot scenarios. We interpret these results as follows. In general, the therapists and autistic adolescents could program relatively simple behavioral scenarios with robots. However, we need to further explore whether assembling and executing of more complex robot scenarios such as programming of dynamic real-life behaviors and task scheduling is possible by end-users.

Keywords: autism spectrum disorder, cognitive dimensions framework, co-creation of contents, robot assisted autism therapy.

1 Introduction

There is increasingly more evidence that robots can be beneficial in behavioral training of autistic children. Robots with different embodiment and level of anthropomorphism have been used to train shared gaze and joint attention abilities [1-13,30]. Attempts have been made to use robots to improve imitation and turn-taking skills [4-9] , to teach facial and body emotions [10] to enhance nonverbal and verbal skills

C. Stephanidis and M. Antona (Eds.): UAHCI/HCII 2014, Part III, LNCS 8515, pp. 601–612, 2014.
© Springer International Publishing Switzerland 2014

27 and initiate social interaction [6], [11-13]. Even though some of these studies are successful, it is challenging to implement the robots in daily training practice. We investigate the problem of how to create a robot-centered learning environment that can be used by therapists/caregivers to support the training of children with autism.

At this stage of deployment of robots in autism research, we consider the experimenters with psychology or clinical background, therapists and caregivers as a primary user of robot technology, who will take active part in creation of robot-mediated training. So we develop training environment to serve primary need of these users. Therefore a robot –centered training environment needs to have first, a sufficient number of robot behaviors that are useful for training, and second, an interface for easy (re-)design, personalization or adaptation of the robot training scenarios and their execution.

The issue of creating a meaningful training sessions with a robot has been addressed previously in [14]. However, in this study the therapist was a knowledge provider and he/she was not meant to create or execute robot scenarios. Robins and colleagues 28 presented a set of ten play scenarios for robot-assisted play for children with special needs; however therapist were not meant to create their own scenarios. The "Therapist-in-the-loop" approach was proposed by Colton and colleagues in [15], in which the authors attempt to engage the child and facilitate social interactions between the child and a team of therapists. We engaged the therapists in a co-creation process for the development of scenarios that they would like to use as an augmentation to their practice. The current research has the far reaching goal to make the therapists able to program, adapt and control the robot in an end-user way, relaying on co-created crucial mass of behaviors and scenarios.

To direct this process, we have chosen a specific training framework. The existing training practices for ASD address specific skills or behaviors like language and communication skills, problem solving skills, daily living skills or socially adaptive behaviors [16], [17] and use huge variety of approaches and underlying theories. We have chosen Applied Behavioral Analysis (ABA) framework, which stimulates desirable actions by children through structural positive reinforcement [18]. Pivotal Response Training (PRT) in particular, as part of ABA, introduces the so called pivotal areas to point out clusters of behaviors which, when targeted during an intervention, also lead to improvements in other behaviors of the children. So far, research has focused on five pivotal areas: responding to multiple cues, motivation, self-management, self-initiations during social interactions and empathy [19], [20]. This therapy requires natural settings. Using a robotic agent to perform different scenarios with a trainer and a child is not a natural circumstance, as is required for PRT. However, we do find these techniques from ABA, and the prompts used in PRT to be a promising course to follow, since they need to be delivered in a consistent and structural manner, which is especially suitable to be done with a robot.

In an attempt to make the robot centered environments a part of the clinical testing and practice, the therapists should be able to use the robot and eventually adapt/personalize scenarios by themselves. Therefore, in addition to our efforts to create useful scenarios, it will be necessary that the therapists can change their scenarios "on the fly", i.e. they need to have robot programming skills. For this purpose we have developed an existing end-user programming environment for the control of a NAO robot and this paper offers a qualitative pilot study of whether the therapists can work with it. The term 'therapists' is used as an umbrella term, covering actual therapists, that perform the training and child psychologists that create the training programs.

In addition, a test has been made to check whether high IQ adolescents with autism could create robot behaviors with this environment.

In this paper, section 2 elaborates on the design of the learning environment that has the affordances of easy creation of interactive and dynamic behaviors by end-users. Section 3 describes the user testing method for the pilot test, section 4 reports the results of testing with both therapists and with adolescents with autism, and section 5 draws conclusions and offers a discussion our findings.

2   Creation of Robot Centered Training Environment

A robot centered learning environment needs to provide possibilities for natural interaction with the robot as well as an interface tools for the therapists/experimenters of this environment to make use these possibilities. In the domains of physical therapy and mental potential development, the so called "dual user" problem exists: a domain specialist that uses the robot as a tool to augment his/her practice, and the client or patient that is traditionally served by the domain specialist and who is now (partially) served by a robot 23. First we need to crate affordances for use by therapists as users that will enable the uptake of robots in therapy.

Therapists cannot be expected to have programming experience, or knowledge on robotics. In addition, only a robot platform is not sufficient to make them use robots. We aim to enable the therapists with a process and a tool that will help them to build naturalistic scenarios quickly; the scenarios should be accurately performed by the robot (errors during the scenario will sabotage the learning moment for the child); in addition, the scenarios has to be fitted to the individual requirements of the child (scenarios should be easy to adapt).

For this purpose we combined a commercially available and affordable robot NAO with the TiViPE graphical programming software integrator platform [21, 23].

2.1   Hardware Platform

NAO robot from Aldebaran robotics is a 58cm tall walking robot, having 25 mechanical degrees of freedom, and has digital cameras, speakers and microphones, different touch sensors and wireless communication capabilities. Using these sensors it can engage in interactive behavior through movement, speech, different LEDs in the face and body, and touch.

Moreover, we do not expect this specific choice of robot to be fixed forever. The TiViPE software platform is set up in such a way that different robots can be fitted to it in the future, as this field is still rapidly progressing, and more robots will become available in the future, a textual robotic language of small sets of meta commands such as (move, say) is being used which have to be adapted to the actuating capabilities of the used robot.

2.2   User-Centered Software Tool

A. Drag and drop interface that incorporates synchronization, parallelism, behavioral dynamics

Graphical programming interfaces are generally known to improve the usability of programming tools. They usually incorporate an easy to use drag and drop interface. The NAO robots are shipped with a graphical programming environment called Choreograph. Commonly the robot manufacturers provide a software environment to control robots, mostly tailored to the specification of the robot (for instance Choreograph and leJOS 29). Besides that these environments are tightly coupled to a specific robot, they lack the ability of more complex control concepts, such as synchronization, parallelism, and creation of dynamic behaviors. We created the TiViPE robot controller, which by design incorporates these concepts. The other advantage of TiViPE is the easy adaptation to any robot, but also the ability to incorporate in the experimental or the training platform another sensors/ devices. This implies that computer or external camera, Kinnect sensor or other sensors can naturally be integrates to the learning environment.

The created robot behaviors are kept up to the environmental changes by a constant flow of sensory information of all robot sensors, they are available to the robot in real-time. The proposed environment uses a box-wire approach to create flowcharts with behavioral sequences. The boxes, which represent behavioral components with different levels of complexity, can be connected to other components, creating a network. Properties of a component can also be modified. Furthermore, networks of components can be merged into new components, which enable users to build complex, interactive and intelligent behaviors. By providing the therapists with a powerful set of components we expect that they can quickly setup a scenario by connecting different components into a network.

B. Textual (string) language for creation and scheduling the priorities of execution of parallel behaviors

The main merit of a textual robot language is that robot actions are described in intuitive to humans terms such as move, LEDs on, etc., and these actions can be executed in a mixture of parallel and serial actions [23]. The complexity of a task such as designing parallel actions (such as speak and move accordingly) is reduced to basic logic (high school arithmetic) using & character for sequential and "|" character for parallel actions. Square brackets are used to bind a set of these textual actions in order to give the priority of their execution where such is needed. Therefore, this textual language has the complexity of learning 10 robot commands and their parameters, and requires understanding of high school arithmetic for scheduling of the robot behaviors. One can easily understand how to schedule commands that come in parallel, or needs to wait until the last of several parallel commands have been completed. Very important feature by this parallel processing is the synchronization between parallel processes (such as bodily expressions and speech).

The advantage of describing actions as a text is that during the execution of the pre-programmed scenario, one can add new actions while training and therefore it is possible to easily personalize or optimize training scenario.

C. Combining the state concept with the flow of constant sensory update for easy creation of dynamic robot behaviors

As previously said, the drawbacks of most graphical programming environments are that they can only deal with rather simple problems. For this purpose in TiViPE within the constant flow of sensory information, a state space concept has been created. The main advantage of using states within a behavior, an active state or a set of states is that state transitions can be set up like solving a tiny task or problem. Once this task is accomplished, the scenario proceeds to the next state or the set of states. The state chart could translate the end-users idea of dynamic behavior (how to go from state to state and back) to a robot dynamic behavior. As a result, the behavior of the robot continues naturally even after unexpected disturbances from the environment occur. The real-time update of the sensory information makes it possible to have a constant feedback on the ongoing robot actions. For instance, when a robot tries to grasp an object it might drop it. The robot will repeat the action of grasping, but since the object has probably fallen at a different position, the robot has to recognize this new position.

In addition, the pace of the sensory and behavioral level of information processing differs a lot. Even the simplest behavior is magnitudes longer than the sensing. In the TiViPE environment the robot sensors are permanently read out and (partly) processed. The sensing takes place in parallel to processing of (textually defined) action commands that are executed on that robot. The sensing is mostly performed on regular update speeds of up to 500 ms and can therefore be one order of magnitude faster than the robot action commands could be executed. This implies that the robot is not always ready to receive a new set of action commands until the previous commands have been executed. To gain an optimal responsiveness, the length of the set of actions should be minimized. The sensing, perceiving, and acting cycle is done therefore in parallel, as recommended in [24, 25]. Constructing behaviors is accomplished by coupling sets of actions by adopting the state chart concept [26], combined with the flow of constantly updating of all the sensory information available to the robot in the graphical flowchart of this behavioral sequence.

D. Hiding Complexity

Once a sequence of behaviors or a state chart of behavioral components is detected to be often used in combination, a simple marking of these components compiles them to a single behavioral block. By the creation of state diagrams, the end-user does not see the sensory flow, only defines the sequences of actions. We are wondering whether such a translation is easy to be automated.

A set of scenarios with specific learning goals was co-developed with the therapists. This is the necessary content for the platform to use during training sessions with the robot and a child.

3   User Testing Method

The therapists play a crucial role in the several design iterations which were performed. This includes designing robot scenarios and behaviors, conducting user tests and evaluations of these and making necessary improvements. We evaluate each iteration phase using the formative evaluation method of the Cognitive Dimensions Framework (CDF). The dimensions that were used and its interpretations taken directly from the manual [22] have the following meaning: The Cognitive Dimension "Abstraction" is interpreted as the types and availability of abstraction mechanisms, "Hidden dependencies" has the meaning that important links between entities are not visible; "Premature commitment " constraints on the order of doing things, "Secondary notation" means extra information (other than formal syntax); "Viscosity" refers to resistance to change; "Visibility" is the ability to view components easily; "Closeness of mapping: is the closeness of representation to domain; "Consistency" means that similar semantics is expressed in similar syntactic forms; "Diffuseness" refers to the verbosity of language; "Error-proneness" notation inventarises mistakes; "Hard mental operations" - high demand on cognitive resources; "Progressive evaluation" means that work-to-date can be checked at any time; "Provisionality" is the degree of commitment to actions or marks; and "Role-expressiveness" denotes that the purpose of a component is readily inferred.

In the formative evaluation we use the cognitive dimensions to give name to difficult to quantify concepts. This makes it easier to compare different concepts and make trade-offs. In this paper, we elaborate on the first evaluation which was a study in two clinics. Five participants from the first clinic and three from the second clinic took part of the experiment.

In the evaluation, the participants were given four different tasks, based on the different types of user activity described in the Cognitive Dimensions Framework, defined as incrementation, modification, transcription and exploratory design. The tasks that we created were respectively: Adding a component, editing a component, adding a new section to the network and making an own contribution to the network. For the tasks, a scenario was provided in flowchart form on paper, and a network representing this scenario was also pre-made. The participants had to complete and use this scenario and network during the four tasks.

In this first evaluation, all participants had their first experience with the programming environment. We described the first task extensively, and each following step with less detail. This gave our subjects the opportunity to quickly become familiar with the functionalities of the program, which gives them the freedom to explore in the final test, where they had to make their own contribution.

The programming environment was not demonstrated beforehand. Instead, a short explanation on paper was provided describing components and how these are connected, along with the task list and flowchart. Participants were asked to think aloud while performing the tasks, and were free to ask questions when they became stuck.

After the tasks the experience of the participants were evaluated with a short questionnaire (in Dutch for our participants). The questionnaire featured 28 statements on their experience with components and network in TiViPE, and 7 statements about how the robot was perceived. There was extra room for comments at the end of the questionnaire. Statements could be answered with a five-point Likert scale (fully don't agree, don't agree, neutral, do agree, fully agree). In this format, it was possible for the participants to quickly give their opinion about their experience. The statements all related to one or more of the cognitive dimensions. We also asked the participants for their experience level with other computer tasks on a five point scale (Basic, below average, average, above average, expert; each level had a description with examples).

The goal of the pilot study was to make sure the questionnaire and tasks were defined properly and was performed with 5 people from different healthcare backgrounds (four female and one male, average age 33, computer skill level was marked from basic to above average). After the pilot, the questionnaire and task list were improved to make the different dimensions in the questionnaire more balanced, and improved the wording.

Three therapists from the second clinic were then invited to go through the tasks and questionnaire. They were all females aged between 24 and 27, and had a higher educational degree than the pilot subjects. They all marked above average on the computer skill level inquiry. The setup with the robot, programming environment and instructions is shown in Figure 1.

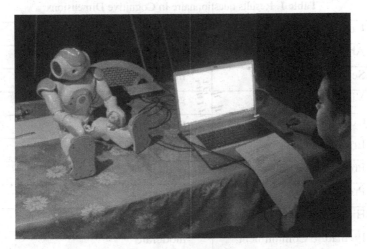

Fig. 1. Experimental setup

4   Results

Results from the questionnaires were compared with the cognitive dimensions each question represented. Together with the qualitative data, statements can then be made about the different dimensions and their trade-offs.

The therapists in the second clinic performed the four tasks faster than the pilot test group (between 15 and 20 minutes compared to 20 to 25 minutes) The difference in training of the therapists from both clinics was that in the first one.

Each participant had a different approach to the final exploratory task. In the group of the second clinic, one subject would add extra components; a second altered the existing components, and a third started looking for other components that were not part of the original scenario.

During both pilot tests, it was observed that the subjects required extra help at the start (first one or two tasks), but quickly managed to use the basic functionalities of the program. There was a need for clear instructions at the start, but each participant was able to do the final task on their own.

The results from the questionnaire were gathered and mapped on the different cognitive dimensions (Table 1). Since a small sample was used, the high scores were marked with good or very good, and neutral scores with moderate. No noticeable negative attitudes towards a specific cognitive dimension were observed. Two dimensions scored noticeably higher than the other ones: role expressiveness (how self-explanatory are the different elements?) and provisionality (how accurately are the user's actions performed?). This means that the users could clearly see how each component of a program relates to the complete robot behavior and that users could with little effort rich accuracy by implementation of the scenario changes and adaptations.

Table 1. Results questionnaire in Cognitive Dimensions

Cognitive Dimension	Score from Questionnaire
Abstraction	good
Secondary Notation	moderate
Viscosity	good
Consistency	good
Error Proneness	moderate
Progressive Evaluation	good
Provisionality	very good
Hidden Dependencies	good
Premature Commitment	moderate
Visibility	good
Hard Mental Operations	moderate
Closeness of Mapping	good
Diffuseness	good
Role-Expressiveness	very good

In both tests the cognitive translation from flowchart to TiViPE network was not straightforward. It took some effort to see the connection between the flowchart model, and the component network. This can be linked to the hard mental operations and abstraction dimensions.

Some mistakes were made with connecting components during the first task, which required precision in clicking sertain areas. This could affect the error proneness, and something that could be improved in the interface. This shortcoming was compensated with different other dimensions, such as provisionality. Decreasing the possibility to make errors can also decrease the speed one can work with the program, or how much control one has while building a scenario.

Within this analysis one has to note that the Cognitive Dimensions framework gives a broad- brush usability profile, intended to provide discussion tools, rather than detailed metrics [20].

Additional usability test with adolescents with autism
As part of a summer camp, two groups of 4 and 5 adolescents (age 16-18, accompanied by their caretakers) visited the robotics lab at the university. We organized an interactive session for them where they got a presentation about the project and the robot, and were then given the opportunity to create a short scenario and perform it together with the robot.

To make sure we would be able to set up a reliable short robot-adolescent interaction within minutes, we used only simple building blocks, i.e. a robot statement and a touch sensor. Still with these blocks two different stories were developed by the two groups. The first one was the robot functioning as a friendly alarm clock. The second was the robot reminding you to take your medication on time.

In both sessions, we asked the adolescents for a volunteer to do the programming in our visual programming environment. We were surprised by how quickly they were able to connect and adapt the different components on their own, which are the two core principles of our program.

5   Conclusion

The results from the evaluation give a positive preliminary results that support our hypothesis that by providing the appropriate design of the user-centered platform and formalizing the process of content creation, high-tech platforms as robots can be used for training children with autism.

The evaluation has been done by utilizing on the flow-chart concept for formalizing robot interaction behaviors only. The therapists were familiar with translating a child learning goal to flow-chart based scenario. Since we aim to introduce more complex and interactive scenarios, it is important how the novel to the therapists and technically more complex concepts are presented, while keeping the interaction with the program simple. The positive results from the cognitive dimensions analysis show that there is a good starting point, and from the qualitative data, we conclude that the participants can handle more complexity.

Creating scenarios that incorporate parallel commands, task scheduling and state concepts are not tested yet. Creating several different scenarios will make possible to formalize elements of the process of scenario creation with the aim to further automate it. In addition, although the programming concepts can be presented in an understandable way within TiViPE and most of the complexity is hidden due to its design, the interface of this tool still appears complex for end users and additional layer if an interface is necessary. We have created simple interface for the control of the robot during therapy sessions, which displays what the robot says and what are the response possibilities of the experimenter or therapist.

We assume that personnel within the clinics are becoming more familiar with computer interfaces. This might further lower the hurdle to work with novel computer interfaces and the upload of training content by non-specialists. Presentation of the information for the participants was important. They mentioned that the handouts with information were very useful, but we can take this a step further, for example with video tutorials.

The sessions with adolescents showed that older adolescents had a keen interest in programming the robot, and were able to contribute in co-designing short scenarios. It may be worth exploring further whether designing social behaviors by autistic adolescents can be beneficial for their development and helpful for the development process of the training program as well since these adolescents understand the thinking patterns of autistic children.

References

1. Giullian, N., Ricks, D., Atherton, A., Colton, M., Goodrich, M., Brinton, B.: Detailed requirements for robots in autism therapy. In: 2010 IEEE International Conference on Systems Man and Cybernetics (SMC), pp. 2595–2602 (2010)
2. Kozima, H., Nakagawa, C.: Interactive Robots as Facilitators of Children ' s Social Development. In: Mobile Robots: Toward New Applications, pp. 269–286 (December 2006)
3. Robins, B., Dickerson, P., Stribling, P., Dautenhahn, K.: Robot-mediated joint attention in children with autism: A case study in robot-human interaction. Interaction Studies 5(2), 161–198 (2004)
4. Bird, G., Leighton, J., Press, C., Heyes, C.: Intact automatic imitation of human and robot actions in autism spectrum disorders. Proceedings of the Biological sciences / The Royal Society 274(1628), 3027–3031 (2007)
5. Brok, J.C.J., Barakova, E.I.: Engaging Autistic Children in Imitation and Turn-Taking Games with Multiagent System of Interactive Lighting Blocks. In: Yang, H.S., Malaka, R., Hoshino, J., Han, J.H. (eds.) ICEC 2010. LNCS, vol. 6243, pp. 115–126. Springer, Heidelberg (2010)
6. Dautenhahn, K., Werry, I.: Towards interactive robots in autism therapy. Pragmatics & Cognition 1(12), 1–35 (2004)
7. Duquette, A., Michaud, F., Mercier, H.: Exploring the use of a mobile robot as an imitation agent with children with low-functioning autism. Autonomous Robots 24(2), 147–157 (2008)

8. Pioggia, G., Igliozzi, R., Sica, M., Ferro, M., Muratori, F.: Exploring emotional and imitational android-based interactions in autistic spectrum disorders. Journal of CyberTherapy & Rehabilitation 1(1), 49–61 (2008)
9. Robins, B., Dautenhahn, K., Te Boekhorst, R., Billard, A.: Robotic assistants in therapy and education of children with autism: can a small humanoid robot help encourage social interaction skills? Universal Access in the Information Society 4(2), 105–120 (2005)
10. Barakova, E.I., Lourens, T.: Expressing and interpreting emotional movements in social games with robots. Personal and Ubiquitous Computing 14, 457–467 (2010)
11. Barakova, E.I., Gillesen, J., Feijs, L.: Social training of autistic children with interactive intelligent agents. Journal of Integrative Neuroscience 8(1), 23–34 (2009)
12. Feil-Seifer, D., Mataric', M.: Robot-assisted therapy for children with autism spectrum disorders. In: Proceedings of the 7th International Conference on Interaction Design and Children, IDC 2008, vol. (2005), p. 49 (2008)
13. Gillesen, J.C.C., Barakova, E.I., Huskens, B.E.B.M., Feijs, L.M.G.: From training to robot behavior: Towards custom scenarios for robotics in training programs for ASD. In: IEEE International Conference on Rehabilitation Robotics, pp. 387–393 (2011)
14. Bernd, T., Gelderblom, G.J., Vanstipelen, S., de Witte, L.: Short term effect evaluation of IROMEC involved therapy for children with intellectual disabilities. In: Ge, S.S., Li, H., Cabibihan, J.-J., Tan, Y.K. (eds.) ICSR 2010. LNCS, vol. 6414, pp. 259–264. Springer, Heidelberg (2010)
15. Colton, M.B., Ricks, D.J., Goodrich, M.A., Dariush, B., Fujimura, K., Fujiki, M.: Toward Therapist-in-the-Loop Assistive Robotics for Children with Autism and Specific Language Impairment. In: AISB New Frontiers in Human-Robot Interaction Symposium, vol. 24, p. 25 (2009)
16. Hume, K., Bellini, S., Pratt, C.: The Usage and Perceived Outcomes of Early Intervention and Early Childhood Programs for Young Children With Autism Spectrum Disorder. Topics in Early Childhood Special Education 25(4), 195–207 (2009)
17. Simpson, R.L.: Evidence-Based Practices and Students With Autism Spectrum Disorders. Focus on Autism and Other Developmental Disabilities 20(3), 140–149 (2005)
18. Harris, S.L., Delmolino, L.: Applied Behavior Analysis: Its application in the Treatment of Autism and Related Disorders in Young Children. Infants & Young Children 14(3), 11–17 (2002)
19. Koegel, R.L., Koegel, L.K.: Pivotal Response Treatments for Autism: Communication, Social and Academic Development, p. 296. Brookes Publishing Co. (2006)
20. Koegel, R.L., Koegel, L.K., McNerney, E.K.: Pivotal areas in intervention for autism. Journal of Clinical Child & Adolescent Psychology 30(1), 19–32 (2001)
21. Lourens, T.: TiViPE—Tino's Visual Programming Environment. In: The 28th Annual International Computer Software & Applications Conference, IEEE COMPSAC, pp. 10–15 (2004)
22. Green, T., Blackwell, A.: Cognitive dimensions of information artefacts: a tutorial. In: BCS HCI Conference (October 1998)
23. Barakova, E.I., Gillesen, J.C.C., Huskens, B.E.B.M., Lourens, T.: End-user programming architecture facilitates the uptake of robots in social therapies. Robotics and Autonomous Systems 61, 704–713 (2013)
24. Gibson, J.: The Senses Considered as Perceptual Systems. Houghton-Mifflin, Boston (1966)
25. Barakova, E.I., Lourens, T.: Mirror neuron framework yields representations for robot interaction. Neurocomputing 72(4-6), 895–900 (2009)

26. http://www.tivipe.com/index.php?option=com_content&view=arti
    cle&id=90:robot-throwing-dice&catid=53:tivipe-use-and-
    applications&Itemid=90
27. Giannopulu, I.: Embedded multimodal nonverbal and verbal interactions between a mobile
    toy robot and autistic children. Presented at the Proceedings of the 8th ACM/IEEE Interna-
    tional Conference on Human-Robot Interaction, Tokyo, Japan (2013)
28. Robins, B., Dautenhahn, K., Ferrari, E., Kronreif, G., Prazak-Aram, B., Marti, P., Iacono,
    I., Gelderblom, G.J., Bernd, T., Caprino, F.: Scenarios of robot-assisted play for children
    with cognitive and physical disabilities. Interaction Studies 13, 189–234 (2012)
29. http://www.idemployee.id.tue.nl/e.i.barakova/

Data Acquisition towards Defining a Multimodal Interaction Model for Human – Assistive Robot Communication

Evita-Stavroula Fotinea[1], Eleni Efthimiou[1], Athanasia-Lida Dimou[1], Theo Goulas[1],
Panayotis Karioris[1], Angelika Peer[2], Petros Maragos[3], Costas Tzafestas[3],
Iasonas Kokkinos[4], Klaus Hauer[5], Katja Mombaur[6],
Ioannis Koumpouros[7], and Bartlomiej Stanczyk[8]

[1] Institute for Language and Speech Processing/ATHENA RC, Athens, Greece
{evita,eleni_e,ndimou,tgoulas,pkarior}@ilsp.gr
[2] Technische Universität München, Munich, Germany
Angelika.Peer@tum.de
[3] Institute of Communication and Computer Systems–NTUA, Athens, Greece
{petros.maragos,ktzaf}@cs.ntua.gr
[4] INRIA–Ecole Centrale Paris, France
iasonas.kokkinos@ecp.fr
[5] Agaplesion Bethanien Hospital/Geriatric Centre at the University of Heideberg, Germany
khauer@bethanien-heidelberg.de
[6] Ruprecht-KarlsUniversität Heidelberg, Germany
kmombaur@uni-hd.de
[7] Diaplasis Rehabilitation Center S.A, Kalamata, Greece
ykoump@teiath.gr
[8] ACCREA Engineering, Lublin, Poland
b.stanczyk@accrea.com

Abstract. We report on the procedures followed in order to acquire a multimodal sensory corpus that will become the primary source of data retrieval, data analysis and testing of mobility assistive robot prototypes in the European project MOBOT. Analysis of the same corpus with respect to all sensorial data will lead to the definition of the multimodal interaction model; gesture and audio data analysis is foreseen to be integrated into the platform in order to facilitate the communication channel between end users and the assistive robot prototypes expected to be the project's outcomes. In order to allow estimation of the whole range of sensorial data acquired, we will refer to the data acquisition scenarios followed in order to obtain the required multisensory data and to the initial post-processing outcomes currently available.

Keywords: assistive robot, natural HRI, multimodal communication model, multisensory data acquisition.

C. Stephanidis and M. Antona (Eds.): UAHCI/HCII 2014, Part III, LNCS 8515, pp. 613–624, 2014.

1   Introduction

Mobility disabilities are prevalent in our ageing society and impede activities important for the independent living of elderly people and their quality of life. The MOBOT project[1] aims at supporting mobility and thus enforcing fitness and vitality by developing intelligent active mobility assistance robots for indoor environments that provide user-centred, context-adaptive and natural support. The driving concept here envisions cognitive robotic assistants that act (a) proactively by realizing an autonomous and context-specific monitoring of human activities and by subsequently reasoning on meaningful user behavioral patterns, as well as (b) adaptively and interactively, by analyzing multi-sensory and physiological signals related to gait and postural stability, and by performing adaptive compliance control for optimal physical support and active fall prevention.

Towards these targets, a multimodal action recognition system is currently under development which needs to monitor, analyze and predict user actions with a high level of accuracy and detail. The main thrust of our approach is the enhancement of computer vision techniques with modalities such as range sensor images, haptic information as well as command-level speech and gesture recognition. In the same framework, data-driven multimodal human behavior analysis will be conducted and behavioral patterns of elderly people will be extracted. Findings will be imported into a multimodal human-robot communication system, involving both verbal and nonverbal communication and will be conceptually and systemically synthesized into mobility assistance models taking into consideration safety critical requirements. All these modules will be incorporated in a behavior-based and context-aware robot control framework aiming at providing situation-adapted optimal assistance to users.

In this framework, end user data become a crucial starting point for the design and implementation of the robotic platforms and also for the definition of the foreseen communication model. The recording sessions for the acquisition of the MOBOT multimodal sensory corpora took place in the rehabilitation centre Agaplesion Bethanien Hospital/ Geriatric Centre at the University of Heidelberg.

In the field of human-action recognition several datasets with rich sets of activities, complex environments representing real-world scenarios have been published. Such datasets that combine video and mocap systems in a systematic way by collecting synchronized and calibrated data include the HumanEva I and II datasets [1]. The creation of HumanEva datasets were motivated mainly by the need for having ground truth that can be used for quantitative evaluation and comparison of both 2D and 3D pose estimation and tracking algorithms. Although the HumanEva datasets have been extensively used in establishing the state-of-the art in human action recognition, their application areas remain limited to evaluation of 2D and 3D motion and pose estimation based on video and mocap data only. There are a number of other multimodal datasets that enhance the standard mocap-video data with additional modalities, such as magnetic sensors or microphones. The TUM Kitchen Dataset [2], which consists of activities in a kitchen setting (i.e., subjects setting a table in different ways), for example includes also RFID tag and magnetic sensor readings in addition to the

---

[1] www.mobot-project.eu/

multi-view video and mocap data. Similarly, the CMU Multimodal Activity (CMU-MMAC) Dataset [3] contains multimodal measures captured from subjects performing tasks such as meal preparation and cooking. The set of modalities utilized in this dataset is rather comprehensive, consisting of video, audio, mocap, internal measurement units (i.e., accelerometers, gyroscopes and magnetometers) and wearable devices (i.e., BodyMedia and eWatch). These two datasets are the first examples of publicly available multimodal datasets with a rich selection of various modalities. Finally, the Berkeley Multimodal Human Action Database (MHAD) is currently the only to-date dataset that systematically combines multiple depth cameras with multi-view video and mocap that are geometrically calibrated and temporally synchronized with other modalities such as accelerometry and sound [4]. The specific dataset consists of multi-view video, depth and color data from multiple Kinect cameras, movement dynamics from wearable accelerometers and the accurate mocap data with the skeleton information. In addition, ambient sound during the action performance was recorded and synchronized to reveal discriminative cues for human motion analysis.

2   MOBOT Database: Sensors Used and Types of Data Collected

The MOBOT database was acquired by means of a sensorised passive rollator (Fig.1) comprising multimodal input from (i) laser range finder sensors, (ii) force/torque sensors, (iii) RGB and RGB-D cameras and (iv) microphones. In addition a motion capture system was used to record human limb movements as well as the rollator and subject's absolute positions in space.

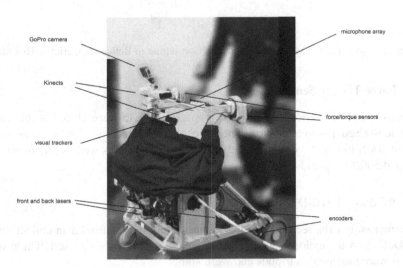

Fig. 1. Instrumented rollator

A diagram of the data acquisition setting implemented during the recording/measurement sessions that took place in Bethanien/Agaplesion Geriatric Hospital is presented in Fig. 2, while details on sensors employed are next provided.

2.1   Laser Range Finders

Two laser range-finder sensors were mounted on the passive rollator platform: One laser scanning range-finder sensor of type Hokuyo UTM-30LX was mounted at the front of the rollator platform facing towards the motion (normal walking) direction, to provide full scanning angle of the walking area. This sensor, also known as Hokuyo Top-URG, provides a 30m and 270° scanning range, and is suitable for robots with high moving speed because of its long range and fast response (~40 scans per second). One laser scanning range-finder sensor of type Hokuyo UBG-04LX-F01 was mounted at the back of the rollator platform facing the user legs, scanning a horizontal plane at the lower limbs (below knee) level, aiming to provide data on the gaiting of the user during typical walking operation with the rollator. This sensor, also known as Hokuyo Rapid-URG, provides a detection range of up to 5m with a 28 msec/scan time, and has a superior accuracy of +-10mm in short range (up to 1m) measurements.

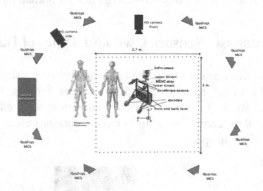

Fig. 2. Diagram of the MOBOT data acquisition setting in Bethanien Geriatric Hospital

2.2   Force/Torque Sensors

Two 6 DOF HR3 force/torque sensors of type JR3 45E15 were placed at the handles of the sensorised passive rollator. They are characterized by a force measurement range of 400N in x and y direction and 800N in z-direction as well as 50Nm around x and y and 500Nm around the z axis.

2.3   RGB and RGB-D Cameras

HD Cameras. For the recording of the scenarios and the required data collection four High Definition technology cameras with sensitive sensors were used. Three of the cameras were mounted on tripods and were static.

The central camera was placed as to record the patient when walking throughout the recording area. The aim was to record the whole body or the largest possible part of it. However, the presence of the rollator in most scenarios has hidden the posture of the torso and legs. So, it was necessary to place another camera in front and at an angle (side) to cover any optical gaps and provide further information of motion and posture of the patient as well as details of maneuvering and possible human interaction with a carer. Moreover, this camera could capture any difficulties in walking or causes in case of stumbling.

An HD camera (GoPro) was mounted on the passive rollator. The main criterion for the choice of this particular camera was the ability to record close and at a constant distance the patient's torso, arms and all its movements and in some cases also the head. Because of its small size and weight and its wide angle lens it was placed on top of the upper Kinect camera (for details see next subsection) mounted on the rollator. Due to the obligatory presence of the expert team in the field of view of the cameras during data capturing, a fourth HD camera was added to avoid or eliminate "visual noise". This camera was always on one side to supplement and give information that was missing or that was not visible from the other cameras. The location was not predefined and its position changed in-between the different scenarios so as to be placed in the optimum position in order to give the best viewing angle.

Kinect Cameras. Before data acquisition, the acquisition team experimented with different sensor choices and sensor placements, with the goal of placing the sensors in a configuration that achieves the broadest possible coverage of the human body, while being at a short distance from it. In particular position constraints did not allow placement of the sensors at a distance larger than 60 centimeters from the typical body position, as this would make the platform difficult to manipulate by elderly users. We therefore focused on solutions that would allow recording the human body from a short distance (Fig.3). We converged on using two Kinect-for-Windows (KFW) sensors, that are equipped with the 'near mode' option, which is absent in the more common Kinect-360 sensors. A considerable amount of effort was invested in order to obtain consistent data streams from the two KFW. We opted for placing the two Kinect sensors to be facing towards complementary directions so as to achieve broad coverage and to avoid interference between the two Kinects. The first sensor is facing horizontally towards the patient, aiming at capturing the area of the torso, waist, hips and the upper part of the limbs. The second sensor is facing downwards, capturing the lower limb motion information, with the aim of enabling the estimation of 3D limb positions and eventually also the analysis of gait abnormalities.

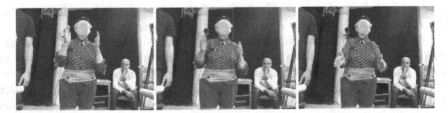

Fig. 3. RGB stream from Kinect

2.4   Microphone Array

As audio capturing device a microphone array has been chosen. Microphone arrays–instead of single sensors– are currently being explored in many different applications, most notably for sound source localization, beam-forming, and far-field speech enhancement and recognition. For data collection purposes, an 8-microphone MEMS array was mounted on the horizontal bar of the MOBOT rollator in a linear configuration (with a 4cm uniform spacing) in front of the user.

2.5   Motion Capture System

For motion capture a Qualisys system[2] was used, with eight cameras mounted on tripods around the recording area. Passive reflective markers were installed on the bodies of patient and carer to measure their human limb movements as depicted in Fig.4. Several limiting factors regarding the informants' population as well as supporting areas on the human body which should stay free of markers were taken into account. Two additional markers were placed on the head of the carer to identify his/her role. Visual markers were also placed onto objects like the door, the door frame, the rollator and the obstacle used in the recordings setting.

3   Multimodal Sensory Corpus Collection

3.1   Introduction: Aims, Scope

Data acquisition sessions were planned and organized to serve the corpus creation goal. In order to secure that the recording sessions would provide all necessary information for the post processing analysis, the scenarios to be recorded were carefully designed and executed. Scenarios include actions, gestures and other close to real life situations such as obstacle avoidance, interaction with other persons, simple everyday life operations (open/close door, switch on/off switch etc.) that needed to be reproduced by the participants in the recordings.

The MOBOT corpus creation was based on the grounds of human action recognition and context-aware robot control. The identified need was for data acquisition that would promote, as much as possible, natural interaction between (elderly) users and mobility aids along with the assistance or not, in some cases, of carers. In order to obtain the multi-sensory recordings, several recording scenarios had to be put in action and tested so that a maximum set of actions and movements would be well represented in the recordings and hence provide significant input from different modalities.

In the recordings, elderly human individuals (of varying age, gender, motor and cognitive abilities) performed a variety of assistance requiring cues in dialogues involving human carers and the passive rollator. Information on the individuals that participated in the recordings, the performed scenarios and their relation to the different modalities and combinations used in natural communication (language-based interaction, gesture-based interaction, multimodal instruction, but also silence in combination with specific body postures) as well as more technical aspects of the recordings such as settings and limitations, is provided in the following sections.

---

[2] http://www.qualisys.com/

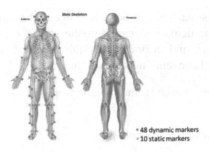

Fig. 4. Used marker set for recordings

3.2   Recording Scenarios

Aims and Scope. The recording scenarios are the outcome of careful design, initially based on an extended pre-described use case list of actions that a user might need to perform in real life situations [5]. The use cases list of actions defines goal-oriented sets of interactions between users and the system. In view of the recording sessions the use case list of actions had to be narrowed down as well as adapted to the recording environment. The envisioned goal was to incite a variety of actions, movements, gestures and functions within the restricted recording setting, in order to obtain enough and representative data as these would set the foundation for the technological development of the assistive device. Previous experience on the design of multimodal corpora [6-7], and multisensory acquisition data [8-9] was proven a valuable background asset, scientifically as well as methodologically.

Use Case Adaptation to the Actually Produced Scenarios. The use case list of actions that defined the goal oriented sets of interactions between users and the system functioned as a super set of real life tasks and/or situations that range from a single-short movement to repetitive long-lasting movements. The idea lying behind this list of action use cases is that mobility-assistants should support moving in different rooms, walking to various spaces as well as to stimulate activity through simplifying and reducing physical and cognitive load. Mainly, these action use cases were based on frequent situations while walking, partly including transfer situations, such as the sit-to-stand movement that is highly frequent. Critical situations or potential barriers due to insecurity, cognitive or physical impairment, as well as the risk of falling – which even though occurs rarely, it is crucial for the importance and usefulness of the device to the user– were taken into account.

A subset of this extensive action use case list [5] was implemented for the scenario creation that would be used in the recording sessions; the chosen action use cases were those that fulfilled all necessary criteria regarding the safety of the informants and were most suitable to technical specifications that the recording environment imposed. In some cases modifications in the course of the scenarios had to be performed leading to simpler acquisition versions of the scenarios than the extremely rich ones originally designed; this was done mainly in order to minimize the fatigue effect of the participants that were of advanced age and hence eliminate to a certain extend the risk of less participation or incomplete sets of recording sessions. For the above mentioned reasons, and in order to acquire data of actions important for all sensorial devices, several conventions were adopted:

1. Three types of variants in each scenario were proposed:

   a. Assisted by a carer
   b. Assisted by the passive rollator only &
   c. Unassisted

2. The number of trials per scenario and per variant presented variation, as there was a minimum set of repetitions required –one or two in most cases– and a maximum set, that was desired and was undertaken only in rare cases, depending on the patient's condition.

In all scenarios performed, data capturing took place from all sensors mounted to the passive rollator. However, in the design of each scenario a specific set of action data was targeted giving priority to different sensors at time. In the descriptions that follow, we focus only on the most important sensorial data with respect to the performed task's goal, while detailed descriptions (scenarios, variants, tasks contained, number of trials etc) can be found in [10].

Scenario 01 was designed to gather information regarding transfers "sit-to-stand" and "stand-to-sit", with or without the use of the sensorised passive rollator, enabling the acquisition of data from the force-torque sensors mounted on the handles of the rollator as well as the capturing data from the Kinect cameras.

Scenario 02 was designed to gather information regarding the gait patterns of the patients while they were walking with the rollator and the force-torque applied to it; the patient used the rollator while walking straight with a constant velocity and then was asked to maneuver while moving back to the start position. Data were captured from the sensors mounted on the handles, the high definition cameras, the Kinect cameras as well as from the infrared cameras placed around the area.

In **Scenario 03** the patient had to perform sit-to-stand transfers and maneuvers in order to avoid an obstacle placed in the testing area, while accelerating and decelerating his/her gait pace. Variants were included to incorporate several audio-gestural commands for communication with the rollator or with the carer, different maneuvering manners, and use or not of the sensorised passive rollator.

Scenario 04 was designed to capture the interaction of the patient while opening, closing a door and passing through a door passage with the use of the rollator. Data were captured by the high definition video cameras and by a camera that was placed on the side of the door to capture the patient's door passing. The total interaction of the patient with the rollator and door were captured by the Kinect cameras as well as the infrared cameras placed around the whole recording area.

Scenario 05 was designed to gather information by closely observing the patient performing a manipulation task that occurs in his daily life, like handling a switch (switching on/off). Data were captured by two separate high definition cameras to have an overview of how the patient behaves in a daily task and how he/she interacts with carer or the environment. The data captured by the Kinect cameras were targeting a. the gait of the patient (lower Kinect) and b. any performed gestures (upper Kinect camera). The microphone array was capturing the verbal commands. For this kind of scenario a manipulation task could only occur if the patient either was using only one hand to grasp the rollator or not holding the rollator at all. In all scenarios, the mounded sensors on the handles of the rollator were capturing force and torques that came from the patients. An indicative example of external and on rollator cameras' views of Scenario 05, can be viewed in Fig. 5.

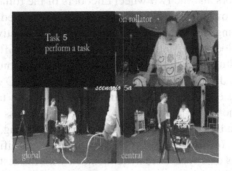

Fig. 5. Scenario Five: Performing a task. Views from external HD cameras and on rollator one.

Scenario 06 was designed to gather information from isolated gestural and verbal commands in order to train a model of human-robot communication. It included audio and gestural commands, uttered simultaneously, repeated a number of times, preferably having the patient in both sitting and standing position.

3.3   Patient-Subjects: Recruitment Strategy and Metadata

As regards patient-subjects' recruitment, the original goal was to recruit at least 10 patients, this being the lowest participation limit, yet opting for at best 15 patients. Due to high commitment and additional recruitment strategy procedures, our final subjects' number was raised to 18 patients. This was the result of a recruitment strategy which consisted into increasing the recruitment potential of the rehabilitation wards by including an associate sport club and by screening patients in acute care geriatric hospital. All participants met the inclusion criteria as all were acute patients in the rehabilitation wards either in the past or will be admitted in the rehabilitation centre in the near future. Inclusion criteria can be found in [5]. In actual figures, altogether 354 persons were screened and contacted within a two week assessment period. The screening process included a personal contact, consulting the patient's charts and contacting care or therapeutic personnel. In case a patient met the inclusion criteria, he/she was informed on the testing and a written consent was asked on his/her behalf, while a personal contact to relatives was also necessary. Participants' metadata consist of information about the gender, age, height, weight and knee height of each subject as well as his/hers cognitive and mobility score (with the aid of the diagnostic tool MMSE

[11-12] and their subsequent classification into a cognitive and mobility category) as detailed in [10]. We briefly report here that both genders have participated in the recordings, 5 male and 12 female subjects, the age range being 74-87 years old.

3.4   Corpus Quantitative Data

Synchronization of multimodal data streams was achieved by recording all the data to a ROS-Robot Operating System[3] bag. For this purpose ROS nodes were programmed for the two laser range finders, the two Kinects and the microphone array. Since the two force/torque sensors and the two wheel encoders of the rollator will be part of the real-time code of the overall control architecture to be realized, and given that low-level drivers for reading these sensor signals from the respective I/O cards were already available as blocks in Matlab/Simulink, a slightly different procedure was adopted for the recording of this type of data: An additional Simulink s-function block was programmed based on roscpp and tlc code to publish ROS topics directly from Simulink after having compiled the diagram using the prt.tlc target implementing a Preempt-RT real-time executable. This allowed seamless integration of the force/torque sensor and encoder data into the overall ROS bag. Motion capture data from Qualisys was recorded in raw format as it requires significant post-processing. Data recordings of this data type were synchronized with the rest of the recordings via a digital synchronization signal output in TTL format from the Qualisys system. In doing so, a cable was used to connect the synchronization output of one of the Qualisys cameras to the I/O card of the rollator. The synchronization signal was read using the respective Simulink block and passed further to the overall ROS bag via the implemented publisher block. Motion capture data will be post-hoc added to the ROS bag as soon as data has been post-processed.

A special launch file was written in ROS to start the different ROS nodes and thus, also the publishing of sensor data. In order to start recording from all the available sensor data topics, a special program was written, which first opens the respective ROS bag, subscribes to the different ROS topics and then waits for a trigger signal to start recording to the ROS bag. This was necessary as opening a ROS bag and subscribing to topics takes several seconds of time, which would have impeded an immediate storage of the data when the trigger signal arrives. The recording was started with a trigger button, which activated the Qualisys recording. As at the same time a synchronization signal was send from Qualisys to the ROS system, also the recording of the ROS bag was triggered and started at the same time.

The amount of ROS bag data collected altogether summarises up to 1.3 TB. The amount of data collected from the two HD cameras and the GoPro camera mounted on top of the passive rollator is approximately 250 GB (437 files), whereas a rough estimation of video data duration is 10 hours for global video duration and 8 hours for useful one (not containing preparations time, meaningless poses etc). Exact quantitative data will be available after post-processing of the acquired corpus, which is required prior to annotation.

---

[3] www.ros.org/

4   Data Post Processing

In order to end up with a corpus of properly annotated video data, the audiovisual materials from the cameras are initially being post-processed to ensure synchronization of video streams from the different capturing devices, prepare data for storage, and also eliminate possible problems or recover defects created during capturing.

Synchronization involves manual video editing to rework the streams and define their common starting point. The streams are being rendered independently and together in a single stream "picture in picture" (PiP) to have all the information accumulated (Fig. 5). Video processing consists mainly in adjusting brightness, especially regarding the camera on rollator and muting noise and external sounds, while amplifying and normalizing useful sounds and speech interactions. There is also an initial need for cleaning the data from visual artifacts due to reflections prior to annotating the markers in Qualisys, followed by the actual post-processing procedure that will allow for the creation of the human biomechanical model in Visual3D. Finally, a common naming convention of the individual files has been adopted to allow for a concise organization of the acquired corpus.

For the annotation process compressed files to mp4 will be used. The annotation of the visual data will be performed in the ELAN environment (ELAN 4.6.2[4]), being an annotation environment specifically designed for the processing of multi-modal resources [13]. Annotation is time aligned; each channel of information will be annotated into a separate annotation tier which may consist of several sub tiers according to the level of fine-grained information that is needed. The output of the annotation procedure is exported into .xml files. A preliminary inspection of the audio-visual data made necessary for the creation of at least 5 different major annotation tiers describing the scenario, the predefined tasks in each scenario, the actually performed actions, information from the audio channel (noise, oral commands), information form the visual channel (noise, gestures, pauses, stumbling etc).

5   Conclusion

Multi-modal sensorial data is a fundamental prerequisite for defining an effective human-robot communication model when developing a multimodal action recognition system. Here we reported on creation of the MOBOT dataset, which enhances the state-of-the art in the field of human-action recognition dataset creation with rich sets of activities in complex environments representing real-world scenarios.

Acknowledgements. The work leading to these results has received funding from the European Union under grant agreement n° 600796. Special thanks to the volunteers Bethanien patients for their participation in the recording sessions and also to the in

---

[4] http://tla.mpi.nl/tools/tla-tools/elan/, Max Planck Institute for Psycholinguistics, The Language Archive, Nijmegen, The Netherlands.

situ recording team, namely Phoebe Kopp-BETHANIEN, Panagiotis Karioris-ATHENA RC, Theodore Goulas-ATHENA RC, Milad Geravand-TUM, Khai-Long Ho Hoang-UHEI, and Davide Corradi-UHEI.

References

1. Sigal, L., Balan, A., Black, M.: HumanEva: Synchronized video and motion capture dataset and baseline algorithm for evaluation of articulated human motion. Int. Journal of Comput. Vis. 87, 4–27 (2010)
2. Tenorth, M., Bandouch, J., Beetz, M.: The TUM Kitchen Data Set of everyday manipulation activities for motion tracking and action recognition. In: IEEE Int. Conf. on Computer Vision Workshops (ICCVW), pp. 1089–1096 (2009)
3. De La Torre, F., Hodgins, J., Montano, J., Valcarcel, S., Forcada, R.: Macey. J.: Guide to the Carnegie Mellon University Multimodal Activity (CMU-MMAC) database. Technical Report CMU-RI-TR-08-22, Robotics Institute, Carnegie Mellon University (2009)
4. Ofli, F., Chaudhry, R., Kurillo, G., Vidal, R., Bajcsy, R.: MHAD: A Comprehensive Multimodal Human Action Database. In: Workshop on the Applications of Computer Vision, pp. 53–60 (2013)
5. MOBOT's Deliverable D5.1- Preliminary report on use cases and user needs
6. Matthes, S., Hanke, T., Regen, A., Storz, J., Worseck, S., Efthimiou, E., Dimou, A.-L., Braffort, A., Glauert, J., Safar, E.: Dicta-Sign – Building a Multilingual Sign Language Corpus. In: Proc. of the 5th Workshop on the Representation and Processing of Sign Languages: Interactions between Corpus and Lexicon (LREC 2012), Istanbul, Turkey (2012)
7. Matthes, S., Hanke, T., Storz, J., Efthimiou, E., Dimou, A.-L., Karioris, P., Braffort, A., Choisier, A., Pelhate, J., Safar, E.: Elicitation Tasks and Materials designed for Dicta-Sign's Multi-lingual Corpus. In: Proc. of the 5th Workshop on the Representation and Processing of Sign Languages: Interactions between Corpus and Lexicon (LREC 2012), Istanbul, Turkey (2012)
8. Wallraven, C., Schultze, M., Mohler, B., Vatakis, A., Pastra, K.: The POETICON enacted scenario corpus - a tool for human and computational experiments on action understanding. In: Proc. 9th IEEE Conference on Automatic Face and Gesture Recognition (2011)
9. Pastra, K., Wallraven, C., Schultze, M., Vatakis, A., Kaulard, K.: The POETICON Corpus: Capturing Language Use and Sensorimotor Experience in Everyday Interaction. In: Proc. of LREC 2010, 7th Int'l Conference on Language Resources and Evaluation (2010)
10. MOBOT's Deliverable D2.1- Data acquisition and multimodal sensory corpora collection
11. Folstein, M.F., Folstein, S.E., McHugh, P.R.: Mini-mental state. A practical method for grading the cognitive state of patients for the clinician. J. Psychiatry Res. 12(3), S.89–S.98 (1975)
12. Woodford, H.J., George, J.: Cognitive assessment in the elderly: a review of clinical methods. Q. J. Med. 100, 469–484 (2007)
13. Brugman, H., Russel, A.: Annotating Multimedia/ Multi-modal resources with ELAN. In: Proc. of LREC 2004, 4th Int'l Conference on Language Resources and Evaluation (2004)

Combining Finite State Machine and Decision-Making Tools for Adaptable Robot Behavior

Michalis Foukarakis[1], Asterios Leonidis[1],
Margherita Antona[1], and Constantine Stephanidis[1,2]

[1] Foundation for Research and Technology – Hellas (FORTH)
Institute of Computer Science
Heraklion, Crete 70013, Greece
[2] University of Crete, Department of Computer Science, Greece
{foukas,leonidis,antona,cs}@ics.forth.gr

Abstract. Modeling robot behavior is a common task in robot software development. However, its difficulty grows exponentially along with system complexity. To facilitate the development of a modular, rather than monolithic, behavior system, proper software tools need to be introduced. This paper proposes combination of a well-known finite state machine and a custom decision-making tool for implementing adaptive robot behaviors. The notion of automatic behavior adaptation reflects the capability of the robot to adapt during runtime based on the individual end-user, as well as the particular context of use, therefore delivering the most appropriate interaction experience. While each tool on its own can be used towards that aim, a unified approach that combines them simplifies the task at hand and distinguishes the roles of designers and programmers. To demonstrate the methods' applicability, a concrete example of their combined use is presented.

Keywords: State Machine, Adaptation, Behavior, Decision-Making.

1   Introduction

Typically, when designing and implementing complex robot behaviors, software developers have to cope with complicated systems with many components that need to efficiently cooperate. Several different technologies and tools can be used for this purpose. Probably the simplest, but the most frequently used one, is a finite state machine [1]. A Finite State Machine (FSM) includes an arbitrary number of states, at any given time only a single state is selected (current state), whereas a change among them is initiated by an event or a condition. They are used in many domains, enabling both hardware and software applications. This paper proposes the use of a tool that complements authoring of hierarchical state machines using an external decision-making mechanism for modeling and creating complex adaptive robot behaviors.

Other approaches towards robot behavior adaptation and decision-making include: (i) cognition-enabled robot control using reasoning mechanisms [2], (ii) generation of behavior networks using finite state machines [3], and (iii) the integration of behavior

C. Stephanidis and M. Antona (Eds.): UAHCI/HCII 2014, Part III, LNCS 8515, pp. 625–635, 2014.
© Springer International Publishing Switzerland 2014

trees [4]. However, FSMs have been selected in this work both for their simplicity and for the fact that many programmers are already familiar with them and can maximize their potential [5-6]. Additionally, the proposed decision-making mechanism can be easily integrated to provide robust behavior structures and to negate some of FMSs' inherent drawbacks, such as limited non-reusable logic.

Both SMACH and DMSL are used in various components of the HOBBIT system [7]. SMACH is used in the development of scripted robot actions (e.g., locating the user), whereas DMSL is used for setting robot initialization parameters and decision-making for HOBBIT's fitness application. However, in the current implementation they are not combined.

Based on the experience acquired in the development of HOBBIT, this paper proposes the augmentation of ROS-compatible [8] finite state machines built using the SMACH library [9] with custom logic rules encoded in a language specifically designed for adaptation oriented decision-making.

2   Creating Robot Behavior with SMACH

The work presented here is based on the use of state machines for describing various robot tasks and actions. This can generally be achieved by mapping high-level tasks (e.g., navigating, planning, scanning the environment) to state machines, which in turn contain other states and state machines for more specific tasks. Building such a system is not trivial and requires careful design of states and state transitions, a robust method of selecting the correct transitions between them, as well as powerful and intuitive implementation tools.

SMACH is a python library that allows the rapid creation of complex robot behavior using state machine concepts. The prerequisite is that all possible states and transitions have to be known in advance and described explicitly, and the scheduling of the tasks has to be sufficiently structured. The advantages of using SMACH for describing robot tasks are many:

- The syntax is python-based, it is suitable for fast prototyping and allows designing complex hierarchical state machines.
- Different modules and tasks are described in a uniform way. State machine containers can describe high-level entities and states can describe actions. State transitions represent the changes in task flow.
- Any relevant data can be easily passed between states.
- State preemption is supported, which can be useful when tasks have to be aborted.
- An introspection tool is included, which doubles as a debugging interface for the state machine execution.
- Many functional states and state machine containers are included in the library and serve different purposes – for example a "Concurrence" state that enables many states to be executed in parallel.
- The library is fully compatible with ROS.

Fig. 1 shows an example state machine for a home robot which might need to locate the user in order to interact with him/her. The robot initially collects information about the current environment and from the user preferences or robot current status.

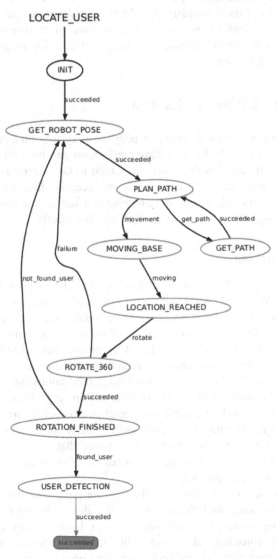

Fig. 1. State machine for the task "locate user". The error states have been omitted to save space.

This information includes current robot pose, last known user position, battery level, user's favorite room, etc. This is done inside states "INIT" and "GET_ROBOT_POSE". Then, the next step is to calculate the path to the next destination, which means that the execution logic transitions to state "PLAN_PATH".

From this point, the robot tries to move to each planned position and rotate in order to detect the user. These actions are described by their corresponding states.

Modeling robot behavior using state machines and state transitions is already a suitable method for implementing robot software. However, this can be improved upon by introducing a more sophisticated decision-making system that can not only select the appropriate transitions, but can also be used to make more complex decisions concerning behavior adaptation. The proposed decision-making mechanism is described in the next section.

3   Decision-Making Mechanism

In order to develop a complete behavior adaptation system and produce consistent behaviors for the robot, a decision-making mechanism can be used to model the different actions and choices that the robot is required to take according to the circumstances. This mechanism should be able to take into account different kinds of parameters that encapsulate the robot, user and environment status, and take the corresponding action according to the behavior rules that have been defined.

3.1   Decision-Making

The notion of automatic behavior adaptation reflects the capability of the robot to adapt during runtime based on the individual end-user, as well as the particular context of use, by delivering the most appropriate interaction experience. The storage location, origin and format of user-oriented information may vary. For example, information may be stored in profiles indexed by unique user identifiers, may be extracted from user-owned cards, may be entered by the user in an initial interaction session, or may be inferred by the system through continuous interaction monitoring and analysis. Additionally, usage-context information, e.g., user location, environment noise, etc., is normally provided by special-purpose equipment, like sensors, or system-level software. In order to support optimal robot behavior adaptation for individual user and usage-context attributes, it is required that for any given robot task or group of robot activities, the implementations of the alternative best-fit behavior actions are appropriately encapsulated.

During runtime, the robot software relies on the particular user, robot and environment profiles to adapt its behavior on the fly, doing the appropriate actions required for the particular end-user and usage-context. In the context of user interfaces, this type of best-fit automatic adaptation, called interface adaptability, was originally introduced in the context of adaptable and adaptive user interface development [10]. In the present work, runtime adaptation-oriented decision-making is engaged so as to select the most appropriate behavior action for the particular user, robot and environment profiles for each distinct part of the robot behavior.

The role of the decision-making component is to effectively drive the behavior adaptation process by deciding which actions or commands need to be selectively executed (or in other words, "activated"). The behavior adaptation process has inherent software engineering implications on the software organization model of the system components. More specifically, as for any component (i.e., part of the inter-face / behavior to support a user activity or task) alternative implemented incarnations may need to coexist, conditionally activated during runtime based on decision-making, the need to accommodate different behaviors arises. In other words, there is a need to organize interface components or robot actions around their particular task contexts, enabling them to be supported through multiple deliveries.

3.2   The Decision Making Specification Language

For implementing decision-making for robot behavior, the Decision Making Specifi-cation Language (DMSL) is proposed. DMSL has been extensively used in the past [11] for user interface adaptation. For the current purposes, DMSL provides a tool for creating complex decision blocks that evaluate decisions for robot behavior.

The main features of the DMSL language are summarized below:

- Supports localized decision blocks for each component.
- Built-in user and context decision parameters with runtime binding of values.
- Can trigger other decision blocks, supporting modular chain evaluations.
- Supports activation and cancellation commands for system components.
- Provides a method for automatic adaptation-design verification.

3.3   Outline of the DMSL Language

The decision-making logic is defined in independent decision blocks, each uniquely associated to a particular component; at most one block per distinct component may be supplied. These components form networks of decision blocks that each corres-pond to a particular system component of the robot

The outcome of a decision session is an activation command, which is directly as-sociated to the component of the initial decision block. For example, when returning to the user after executing a specific task, the robot navigation system could request a decision about which side to approach the user from (left, right, center). The request then enables a specific decision component, which takes into account the appropriate parameters and produces a decision for the navigation system to use. To simplify rule authoring and maintenance, the decision-making logic is defined in independent "if-then-else" decision blocks that add minimal overhead to the robot's execution time. The activate commands return a response that depends on profile attributes at the time of the request. The example in section 4 demonstrates the use of these concepts.

Decision Parameters. The decision parameters are defined as a built-in object whose attributes are syntactically accessible in the form of named attributes. The binding of attribute names to attribute values is always performed at run time.

Each parameter belongs to one of the three profile types: user, robot and environ-ment. This distinction is used for categorization purposes and does not impose any special semantic restrictions or characteristics. The supported parameter types are strings, numbers and true/false values. A description of each profile type follows:

- User profile: The user profile contains personal data associated to a specific user. It includes both static personal data and dynamic data gathered via activity monitoring. Such parameters include (but not limit to):
  — General information; i.e., username, name, surname, age, sex, nationality, preferred language, computer skill, etc.
  — Communication details; i.e., street address, city, postal code, country, e-mail, home telephone number, mobile telephone number, etc.
  — Preferences; i.e., look & feel preference, dialogue mode (guided, simple, normal, advanced), interaction style (touch, manual scanning, automatic scanning, etc.), auditory style, interaction preferences (only visual, only auditory, only gestural, both visual and auditory, etc.), distance during social and not social situations, frequency of spontaneous emotional expressions, frequency of suggestions concerning activities and exercises, frequency of robot initialized interactions, etc.
- Environment profile: The environment profile describes the robot's surroundings to ensure that it adapts its behavior to meet the user's goals within the given context of use. The environment profile includes:
  — Map of the environment used for navigation; i.e., obstacles, pathways, etc.
  — Map of the physical objects; i.e., table, chairs, shelf, etc.
  — Map of the available actuators; i.e., type, name, location, command, etc.
  — Information about the available AAL sensors; i.e., type, name, location and current value, etc.
  — Contextual information resulting from sensor data (e.g. estimated location of user, activity)
- Robot profile: The robot profile describes the internal information of the robot during task execution and social interaction. It defines the current appearance and behavior of the robot as a socially behaving agent at the side of the user. The robot profile includes:
  — General information; i.e., name given to the robot by user, physical dimensions, number and position of sensors, etc.
  — Internal information; i.e., current emotion (e.g., attentive, happy), personality preferred by user (e.g. butler, pet-like), number and status of sensors, energy level and status of battery, position and status of gripper, position and status of tray, etc.
  — Spatial information; i.e., current location, certainty of position, location name, indivisibility with user, direction of movement, direction of sight, etc.

These parameters, apart from settings and preferences, can also describe system statuses and temporary values. For example, the parameter ROBOT.VoiceVolume could have the numerical value that represents the robot voice volume level setting. Another example would be a parameter called ROBOT.CurrentTask, which would indicate what task the robot is executing at a specific time. Finally, sensor data can be very useful for adapting robot behavior, and can also be described by similar parameters.

DMSL "if-then-else" decision blocks include parameters which ultimately define the result of the decision process, influencing robot behavior. The next section describes a detailed example of the way DMSL is used for making a common decision for a home-care robot.

4   Adapting Robot Behavior with Decision-Making

The system considered here includes a robot capable of functioning autonomously and exhibiting variable behavior. Its functions can be divided into tasks and can be explicitly defined. To implement adaptable behavior, different implementations of relevant tasks are included. The objective here is to facilitate robot behavior coordination by providing easy to use tools that separate tasks for programmers and designers and reduce the overall implementation time.

The designers are encouraged to use well-known concepts (state machines) and tools (SMACH) in order to build the initial high-level task architecture for the robot. The process is straightforward and does not require them to dig into complicated code or decide the way to transition from one state to another. They are only concerned with building abstract states, state machines and the possible methods to connect them via state transitions.

The programmers on the other hand use the already designed state machines and their responsibility is to implement the functionalities of each state (for example rotating the robot platform to detect the user requires giving commands to both the platform wheels for the movement and the cameras for detecting). The decision-making procedure is tightly coupled with these actions, since for each action the robot can take (which can also mean transitioning to another state), a decision might be required. The programmers use DMSL decision blocks to encode the logic required by each state for transitioning to the next or for in-state decisions.

In Fig. 2, a simple diagram of how these tools cooperate with the robot's components is shown. At the core of the architecture, SMACH state machines and transitions are responsible for defining high-level tasks and communicate with both the low-level components and the user interface. In addition, the decision-making mechanism interacts with all the other components in different ways. Firstly, the SMACH states will usually require a decision to determine the next state transition. This can be provided by evaluating DMSL rules and getting the desired result back. Secondly, DMSL can provide best-fit user interface alternatives for the robot. Finally, low-level components of the robot may need to set certain profile parameters according to sensor data or system state. These parameters are used by the decision-making mechanism to evaluate DMSL rule patterns and drive the behavior adaptation process.

To demonstrate how to perform decision-making for an autonomous robot using the aforementioned procedures, a concrete example is presented of realistic robot behavior that can be found in a home-care robot: "explore the apartment in order to locate the user and ensure their safety". During movement, the robot is aware of its surroundings due to its internal localization and mapping. However, especially in home environments, objects change places and many obstacles can be found on the

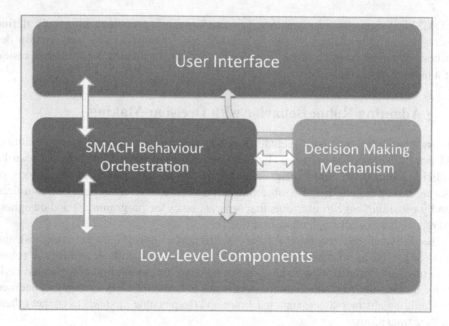

Fig. 2. Communication between SMACH, the decision-making mechanism and robot components

way to the robot's destination. In such a case, the robot has to decide how to overcome that obstacle. For the purposes of this example, it is assumed that two alternative options are available: (i) to call the user to remove the obstacle or (ii) plan an alternative route without bothering the user. The final decision is the based on many different parameters:

- The user might have limited mobility due to advanced age or any kind of disability
- The user might be facing partial or full hearing loss.
- The user might be preoccupied with another activity either unexpectedly or regularly at a given time every day; such cases can be determined through sensors or activity monitoring to identify user habits.
- The user might be unwilling to bond or interact with the robot.
- The user might not like to be disturbed at a certain time, or even at all.
- The robot might not be able to find another path to its destination.
- The robot might determine that the best alternative path is actually the longest one.
- The robot's battery level might be low.
- The robot is at the user's favorite room or the room the user is most likely in, given the time of day.

These are only examples of the possible variations on what can affect the decision to call the user or not. The first five parameters indicate that the robot should not disturb the user, while the rest suggest that the robot should call the user for help. Fig. 3 diagrammatically represents the decision logic for this case.

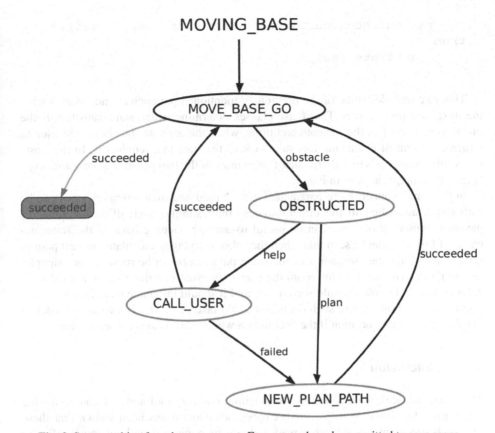

Fig. 3. State machine for robot movement. Error states have been omitted to save space.

The current state is "OBSTRUCTED" and the system needs to determine the next transition. The following DMSL rule is evaluated and the decision determines the next transition:

```
def neutralToBond {0,1,2}
def willingToBond {3,4,5}
def userFreeTimes {10, 11, 12, 13, 17, 18, 19, 20, 21 }

component ObstacleDetected [
  if params.user.hearing = false or
     params.user.age > 80 or
     not params.user.bondlevel in willingToBond or
     params.env.time not in userFreeTimes then
        activate "plan"
  else
    if params.robot.batterylevel < 10 or
       params.env.currentbestpath = false or
```

```
        params.robot.currentroom = params.user.favoriteroom
    then
        activate "help"
]
```

This rule includes some of the previously mentioned parameters and decides what the next state transition is. The if/else clauses determine which state transition is the one that best satisfies the current conditions, while the activate statements are used to return the result of evaluating this rule back to the state that requires it. In this case, the result corresponds exactly to one of the names of the two possible state transitions, "plan" and "help", as seen in Fig. 3.

In the same manner, more parameters can be used and more complex rules can be elaborated, according to the circumstances. Interestingly, a significant number of parameters used in one rule can be useful to another. Getting back to the state machine of Fig. 1, it can be seen that when the robot is trying to calculate the best path to take to search for the user, some of the same parameters can be reused. For example, the user's favorite room or the room the user is in usually at that time is a good indicator of where the robot should search first and it should influence its decisions at that point. Another point where such decisions could take place is when rotating to detect the user, to take into account if the user uses a wheelchair, is usually seated, etc.

5   Conclusion

This paper has described a finite state machine building tool and a decision-making mechanism for implementing complex robot behavior. It has been shown that these two tools complement each other well and can be combined without much effort to produce more advanced behavior systems.

Although the case reported here is restricted to specific parameters (home robot with wheels, user interaction and more), these tools can be used for many more applications that require executing robot tasks and using parameters to define the actions the robot takes.

Acknowledgements. Part of this work has been conducted in the context of the Project ICT-HOBBIT "HOBBIT The Mutual Care Robot", funded by the European Commission under the 7th Framework Programme (Grant Agreement 288146).

References

1. Kent, A., Williams, J.G. (eds.): Encyclopedia of Computer Science and Technology. Applications of Artificial Intelligence to Agriculture and Natural Resource Management to Transaction Machine Architectures, vol. 25(suppl. 10). CRC Press (1991)
2. Beetz, M., Jain, D., Mosenlechner, L., Tenorth, M., Kunze, L., Blodow, N., Pangercic, D.: Cognition-Enabled Autonomous Robot Control for the Realization of Home Chore Task Intelligence. Proceedings of the IEEE 100(8), 2454–2471 (2012)

3. Armbrust, C., Schmidt, D., Berns, K.: Generating Behaviour Networks from Finite-State Machines. In: Proceedings of the German Conference on Robotics (Robotik), Munich, Germany (2012)
4. Bagnell, J.A., Cavalcanti, F., Cui, L., Galluzzo, T., Hebert, M., Kazemi, M., Klingensmith, M., Libby, J., Liu, T.Y., Pollard, N., Pivtoraiko, M., Valois, J.-S., Zhu, R.: An Integrated System for Autonomous Robotics Manipulation. In: International Conference on Intelligent Robots and Systems (IROS), pp. 2955–2962 (2012)
5. Niemüller, T., Ferrein, A., Lakemeyer, G.: A Lua-based Behavior Engine for Controlling the Humanoid Robot Nao. In: Baltes, J., Lagoudakis, M.G., Naruse, T., Ghidary, S.S. (eds.) RoboCup 2009. LNCS, vol. 5949, pp. 240–251. Springer, Heidelberg (2010)
6. Datta, C., Jayawardena, C., Kuo, I.H., MacDonald, B.A.: RoboStudio: A Visual Programming Environment for Rapid Authoring and Customization of Complex Services on a Personal Service Robot. In: International Conference on Intelligent Robots and Systems (IROS), pp. 2352–2357 (2012)
7. Vincze, M.: HOBBIT - Towards a robot for Aging Well. In: ICRA 2013, Workshop on Human Robot Interaction (HRI) for Assistance Robots and Industrial Robots, Karlsruhe, May 6-10 (2013)
8. Quigley, M., Gerkey, B., Conley, K., Faust, J., Foote, T., Leibs, J., Berger, E., Wheeler, R., Ng, A.: ROS: An open-source robot operating system. In: Open-Source Software Workshop Int. Conf. Robotics and Automation, Kobe, Japan (2009)
9. Bohren, J., Cousins, S.: The SMACH High-Level Executive. IEEE Robotics & Automation Magazine 17(4), 18–20 (2010)
10. Stephanidis, C.: The Concept of Unified User Interfaces. In: Stephanidis, C. (ed.) User Interfaces for All - Concepts, Methods, and Tools, pp. 371–388. Lawrence Erlbaum Associates, Mahwah (2001)
11. Savidis, A., Antona, M., Stephanidis, C.: A Decision-Making Specification Language for Verifiable User-Interface Adaptation Logic. Int. J. Soft. Eng. Knowl. Eng. 15, 1063 (2005)

Cooperative Semi-autonomous Robotic Network for Search and Rescue Operations

Garth Herman, Aleksander Milshteyn, Airs Lin, Manuel Garcia, Charles Liu,
Darrell Guillaume, Khosrow Rad, and Helen Boussalis

Structures, Propulsion, and Control Engineering (SPACE) University Research Center
California State University, Los Angeles
5151 State University Drive
Los Angeles, CA 90032 USA
hboussa@calstatela.edu

Abstract. The results presented in this paper prove the viability of developing a robotic network for search and rescue operations. With the capability of peer-to-peer communication, such robots form an ad-hoc network called Cooperative Mobile Network (CMN). All robots in the CMN are semi-autonomous in that each operates in three modes: 1) fully controlled by a human commander; 2) controlled by a human commander for critical operations only; and 3) fully relying on its own intelligence to make decisions for cooperative operations. Due to the constraints of weight and processing power, diverse CMN operations utilize multiple robots with complementing functionalities. This work was performed at the Structures Propulsion And Control Engineering (SPACE) NASA sponsored University Research Center (URC)[1] of excellence at the California State University, Los Angeles.

Keywords: robotic networking, search and rescue, environment-sensing, terrain-exploration, hybrid-routing algorithms, virtual-reality.

1 Introduction

Advances in robotics technology increase the utility of diversely applied platforms. Robots mitigate risk to emergency responders, and facilitate exploration of dangerous environments. Emergency responders may use the device to locate victims of catastrophe. A robotic platform was used to investigate radiation levels after a tsunami decimated a Japanese nuclear reactor on May 11, 2011 [1]. Exploration of Mars depends upon versatile robotic platforms. The Mars Science Laboratory/Curiosity is an automated Mars rover vehicle that propels itself across the surface of Mars, and landed on the Martian surface on August 6th, 2012 [2]. Previously, the Advanced Computation and Communication Team of the Structures Pointing And Control Engineering (SPACE) University Research Center (URC) at California State University of Los Angeles (CSULA) proposed a design of a Hybrid Routing Algorithm Model utilizing semi-autonomous control for the navigation of the mobile robotic platform [3].

---

[1] Acknowledgement to NASA University Research Center Program, Grant # NNX08BA44A.

C. Stephanidis and M. Antona (Eds.): UAHCI/HCII 2014, Part III, LNCS 8515, pp. 636–647, 2014.

This work utilizes a cooperative mode of interaction between several codependent mobile entities which form an ad-hoc network for peer-to-peer communication. The codependent mobile entities include a team of large and small ground robots, an Unmanned Aerial Vehicle (UAV), and a Host Computer Station (HCS) which form the Cooperative Mobile Network (CMN). Each robot communicates with the HCS to acquire optimal paths of movement. Optimal paths are calculated by the HCS based on coarse-scale maps provided from an Unmanned Aerial Vehicle (UAV) [4]. The robots in the CMN are able to autonomously participate in predefined situational task redistribution. Figure 1 depicts a control and communication flow between the UAV, the HCS, and the mobile entities utilizing by the Programmable System on Chip-5 (PSoC-5) microcontroller [5]. Currently, the CMN utilizes two categories of robots, namely the Reconnaissance robots (followers) and the Heavy-Duty robots (leaders). The UAV and the ground robot prototypes are shown in Figure 2.

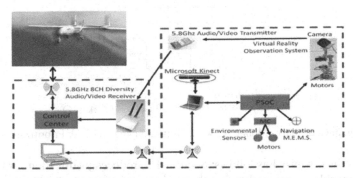

Fig. 1. Robotic Control and Communication with Hybrid Routing Algorithm Model

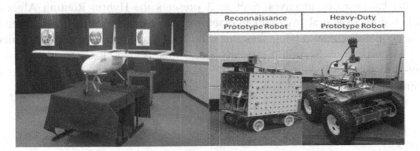

Fig. 2. Cooperative Mobile Network Robot Prototypes

Figure 3 shows a Cooperative Mobile Network scenario with five robotic groups operating within the level 1 area (defined as 1 kilometer by 1 kilometer). Each group consists of four light-weight Reconnaissance robots and one Heavy-Duty robot. The objective of the Reconnaissance robots is to survey the assigned territory for data of interest, such as natural disaster survivors. The Reconnaissance robots operate in their respective level 2 areas (defined as 100 meters by 100 meters). If the Reconnaissance unit detects a survivor in need of immediate medical attention, it communicates through the CMN to the HCS, which in turn assigns this robot's coordinates as a high-priority task. Then the HCS issues an immediate dispatch command to the nearest available Heavy-Duty robot with an Audio/Video (AV) observation system, medical kit, and other situation-specific supplies onboard. On the other hand, the lower priority tasks which do not involve immediate human rescue will be queued until the high-priority tasks are completed. If neighboring Heavy-Duty units are available, they will be dispatched for execution of other low-priority assignments.

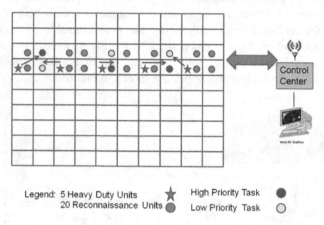

Legend: 5 Heavy Duty Units ★ High Priority Task ●
        20 Reconnaissance Units ● Low Priority Task ○

Fig. 3. Cooperative Mobile Network Unit Grouping and Task Prioritization

This paper is organized as follows: Section 1 introduces justification for the CMN. Section 2 provides a comprehensive discussion of System Architecture, which includes system layers, sensor and actuator interfaces, and interconnections from software and hardware perspectives. Section 3 presents the Hybrid Routing Algorithm Model used for structural environment mapping and semi-autonomous robotic navigation. Section 4 discusses a non-contact method for pulse extraction based on Eulerian Video Magnification. Section 5 presents a real-time Video Observation System for Heavy-Duty robots. Section 6 shows different CMN scenarios including task priority assignment and task redistribution. Section 7 concludes the paper.

2   System Architecture

Semi-Autonomous Mobile Platform architecture is used to facilitate the development of the CMN. It consists of two primary components: 1) the Host Computing Station and 2) the Onboard Embedded Hardware. The HCS is responsible for calculating optimal paths using scale maps created from data provided by a UAV. The embedded hardware facilitates peer-to-peer collaboration, real-time operations, and obstacle avoidance. This hardware consists of three primary layers: the Algorithm, the Platform, and the Driver Layer. The architecture of the robotic platform is shown in Figure 4.

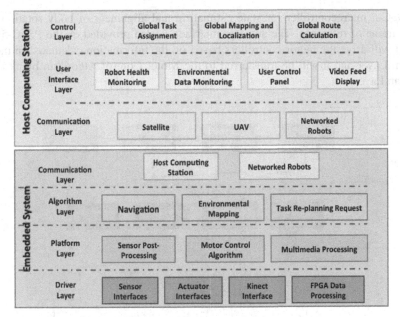

Fig. 4. Robot System Architecture

A prototype of hands-free head-tracking vision control has been implemented to allow human commanders to remotely observe the surrounding environment of a robot. A camera mounted to the robot will move to mirror the motion of the user's head. The goal of the CMN is to perform diverse operations utilizing multiple units with complementing capabilities to overcome constraints in weight and processing power. For example, lighter and faster scouting mobile units only perform environmental surveillance with a set of environmental sensors. This set of environmental instruments includes, but is not limited to, temperature, dust, gas, humidity, altitude IMU, GPS, and IR/Laser obstacle detection sensors. The unit is also equipped with light-weight video camera and an embedded computer that will perform a video magnification process to detect potential survivors either by detecting pulse rate, signs of breath, or subtle body movements. Once any of these signals is validated by the HCS software or its operator, the Heavy-Duty mobile units will be dispatched to the survivor.

Figure 5 shows the data flow between the Algorithm and Platform Layers of the embedded hardware. The motor encoders and the Inertial Measurement Unit (IMU) are responsible for proper mapping and unit localization while the sonar, the IR sensors, and the Kinect depth sensor allow the robot to move autonomously by performing real-time obstacle monitoring. The Driver Layer reveals the sensor interfaces used by the robotic units. The Inter-Integrated Circuit (I2C), Pulse-Width Modulation (PWM) control, Analog-to-Digital Converter (ADC), Universal Asynchronous Receiver/Transmitter (UART), and Serial Peripheral Interface (SPI) are used for interfacing PSoC-5 with the aforementioned sensors. The sensor interface is responsible for acquiring and fusing IMU data from its multiple sensors in order to perform robot mapping and localization. Kalman Filter and Direction Cosine Matrix are implemented on the PSoC-5 microcontroller for state estimation and alignment of body rotation with global frame of reference. The actuator interface is also provided on the PSoC-5 unit, since it will drive the motor controllers based on the information calculated in the Algorithm Layer and it will be transferred to the Motor Control Algorithm block of the Platform Layer.

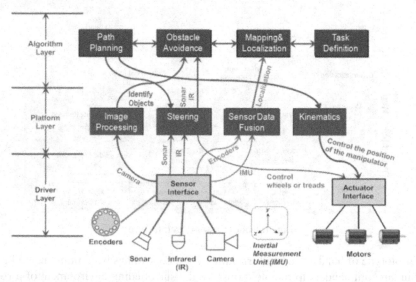

Fig. 5. Control Flow of the Embedded Hardware with Sensor and Actuator Interfaces

3   Hybrid Routing Algorithm Model

A three-level map hierarchy has been defined to efficiently estimate routes by utilizing aerial information obtained from a UAV and transmitted to the HCS for determining level 1(L1) and level 2 (L2) routes. The onboard processor dynamically calculates the optimal level 3 (L3) route to respond to real-time environment changes. Figure 6 shows the three-level map configuration. The A* path finding algorithm is used for determining the shortest route between endpoints [6].

The Kinect system, equipped with multi-array depth sensing capability, has an object detection range from 80 centimeters to 4 meters [7]. It works alongside IR Sharp GP2Y0A21YK0F sensor, which is responsible for 10 - 80 centimeter object detection [8]. The UAV aircraft acquires obstacle data when flying over selected terrain. Ground images are captured and transmitted to a UAV control station. An operator marks appropriate obstacle coordinates (cells on L1 and L2). The left side of Figure 7 shows a prototype application that simulates obstacle-extraction from an aerial view and communication interface between the HCS and the UAV control station. This application converts geospatial coordinates identified by the operator as an obstacle to Euclidian distances. It is performed using an embedded Google-Map applet. The application maps information on the level-specific grid and saves it to a map database in

L1 1 km x 1km

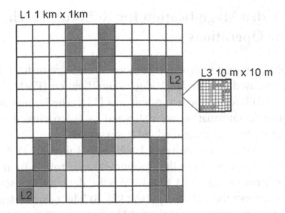

L3 10 m x 10 m

Fig. 6. Three-level Mapping of Hybrid Routing Algorithm Model

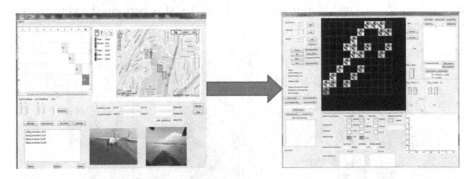

Fig. 7. UAV Control Station Simulation Application and HCS Application

a hierarchical eXtra-Markup Language (XML) format [9]. After receiving a communication acknowledgment request from the HCS, the UAV control station transfers the newly acquired coarse-grain map data.

The HCS is equipped with an implementation of the A* pathfinding algorithm, and is responsible for the pathfinding computations. The right side of Figure 7 shows a default layout of an HCS application. The Open Graphics Library (OpenGL) generated map of an L1 grid is further divided into hundred L2 cells [10]. The L1 grid represents a terrain of 1 kilometer by 1 kilometer, with yellow textures representing L2 obstacles obtained from aerial view (currently simulation). The green texture represents the starting position of the robot within L2 square and the blue texture represents the target destination for the robot. White textures show the calculated optimal path found by the application. The HCS application contains a parser, which recognizes encapsulated aerial information received from the UAV Control Station application and sorts it in the level-specific arrays.

4   Eulerian Video Magnification for Robotic Search and Rescue Operations

The CMN robots are equipped with video cameras which are utilized for human rescue operations. The method of Eulerian Video Magnification (EVM) was discovered and implemented by MIT for medical applications [11]. The human pulse, breathing rate, and other biometric information are extracted as video clips during search and rescue missions to provide immediate medical assessment.

The pulse identification process utilizing EVM is as follows: 1) A facial recognition module shown in Figure 8 allows the Reconnaissance robots to identify the presence of a potential human victim. 2) A real-time pulse detector focuses on the human forehead in order to retrieve the victim's pulse [12]. 3) The nearest Heavy-Duty robot is dispatched to the victim to set up real-time AV communication with the HCS operator. It delivers a medical kit and water to victim(s) who are capable of self-assistance or to people capable of assisting the victim. 4) The original video sequence is recorded for 15-20 seconds and transmitted to the HCS. EVM is performed and the output video is analyzed by the operator.

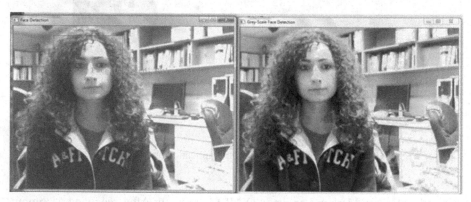

Fig. 8. Face Detection Module for Reconnaissance Robots

EVM applies spatial and temporal filters to an original video sequence and amplifies color and motion to visually represent information that is generally invisible to a human eye. Such information includes blood circulation, breathing, and pulse rate. This information is time critical for rescuing survivors from dangerous areas. The pulse rate is extracted and analyzed immediately, while video sequences of 15-20 seconds is periodically transmitted to the HCS, with an "urgent" tag added to sequences when a human pulse is successfully detected. The non-urgent video sequences are saved on the HCS server and EVM is performed on each video clip. The EVM also amplifies low spatial amplitude motions. For example, if a live human body is trapped under debris, the embedded laptop will not be able to immediately detect and analyze the pulse using EVM. However, it will detect breathing and subtle physical displacement of debris. The EVM detects and amplifies subtle signals

(Figure 9). The HCS database of original and magnified videos will allow operators to review and organize all collected information to aid a rescue mission.

Since the EVM process is sensitive to the temporal characteristics of noise, spatial filtering has to be adjusted to reveal the signal of interest. When analyzing certain signals, the kernel of the separable binomial filter is increased in order to achieve noise suppression. The operator at the HCS has a user interface with the ability to apply various filter settings such as the selection of: 1) spatial and temporal filter types, 2) amplification factor, 3) frequency range, 4) wavelength cutoff, 5) frame rate, 6) attenuation factor, and 7) the radius size of the binomial filter. The side by side display allows the operator to visually compare the original video clip to the magnified output.

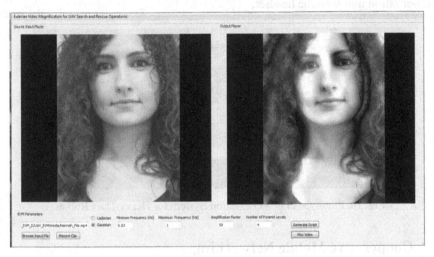

Fig. 9. Eulerian Video Magnification of Original Video Sequence on HCS (Post-Processing)

5   Video Observation System

A user-controlled observation system has been implemented in order to perform real-time remote environment visualization, while maintaining control of the onboard visualization system orientation. A hands-free design allows remote control of an observation system that follows the motion of an operator worn headset.

The observation system is comprised of two modules: a control headset equipped with a video receiver and an onboard observation deck equipped with a video transmitter. The control protocol operates through the main data communication channel between the HCS and the embedded laptop. The control protocol is responsible for controlling the angular displacement of motors with respect to the motion of the headset. Video data is rendered through a dedicated video channel to the HCS and allow the operator to make immediate decisions based on transmission of the real-time visual environment information.

An IMU controlled by a PSoC-5 is attached to the center of iTV-goggles, which are worn by the mission operator [13]. When the unit is operational it collects data from the IMU and estimates the orientation of the headset with respect to a fixed global frame of reference. A Direction Cosine Matrix algorithm transforms rotation coordinates of a moving body (the headset) to a global reference frame. Based on motion with respect to the Earth, PWM signals transmitted to the remote observation system servo motors perform angular displacement of the camera. Video information is transmitted via a 5.8 GHz video transmitter and rendered on the HCS as well as on the iTV ITG-PCX3D device worn by the operator. A prototype of the embedded observation deck, using wired interconnections, is shown on Figure 10. A nested screen provides a snapshot from a real-time video observed by an operator while controlling the observation unit with the headset.

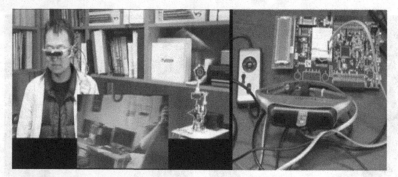

Fig. 10. Prototype of an Observation System for Heavy-Duty Robots

6   Cooperative Mobile Networking

The CMN diversifies operations and utilizes multiple robots with complementing capabilities. Lighter scouting robots, equipped with environmental sensors and a lightweight video camera, utilize EVM to detect potential survivors. If the location of a survivor is verified, the Heavy-Duty robots are dispatched to assist the survivor. The Heavy-Duty robot includes the default aforementioned equipment and houses a powerful 360 degrees observation unit which allows real-time audio and visual communication with the HCS operator. The operator of the HCS observes the environment using the remote observation system and switch responding units from autonomous to manual operation mode if necessary to remotely assist the survivor(s). The Heavy-Duty robot also includes a first-aid medical kit and bottled water in case survivor(s) are capable of assisting themselves either with or without remote supervision.

The CMN can autonomously participate in situational task redistribution. Given situation-specific objectives, the units have the capability of issuing cooperative network commands to adapt with changing environmental conditions. Figure 11 illustrates a CMN firefighting scenario. The robots are initially scouting and mapping unknown territory in a scattered formation. When one of the robotic units detects substantive temperature rise in their current region, it will interrupt the network with an updated CMN objective. It will issue a "Gather Formation" command for Heavy-Duty robots and an "Evacuation" command to units that do not possess firefighting equipment.

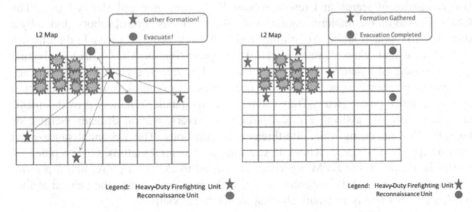

Fig. 11. Cooperative Mobile Network – Gathering Formation and Evacuation

The CMN is also applied to radiation monitoring scenarios. Reconnaissance robots surveying a specific region for hazardous levels of radiation in an initial scattering mode will dispatch other robots after detecting a threshold level of radiation. Responding robots will abandon their scattered search and move towards the location where threshold levels of radiation will be surpassed. This scenario is illustrated on Figure 12. These formation adjustments of the robots will save time and power by switching the CMN to a mission specific mode such as deploying stationary radiation sensors into recently identified areas of interest.

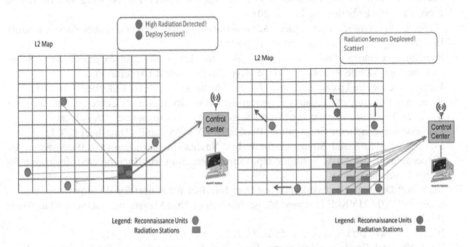

Fig. 12. Cooperative mobile Network – Mission Switching Scenario

7   Conclusion

This paper verifies the concept of a Cooperative Mobile Network (CMN) based on two categories of search and rescue robots: Reconnaissance and Heavy-Duty. The CMN is based on the implementation of semi-autonomous control robots guided by a three-level Hybrid Routing Algorithm Model. A UAV acquires obstacle data for L1 and L2 areas and relays them to the Host Computer Station (HCS). Each individual unit is capable of dynamic navigation within an L3 area. The HCS oversees the ad-hoc communication between the robots. The commander controls a visual observation system installed on the Heavy-Duty robots. The commander remotely provides medical assessment and assistance to catastrophe survivors, natural disaster victims, or humans who are facing other life-threatening situations. The Reconnaissance units provide speedy survivor search while scanning for potential victims. Once a potential victim is identified, the EVM algorithm is utilized to extract a pulse, and a priority level to the rescue task is assigned. In case of high-priority status, the nearest available Heavy-Duty unit is automatically dispatched to the victim.

Future work will focus on complete implementation of the presented CMN. Optimization will be conducted to increase efficacy of the CMN, such as incorporation of different pathfinding algorithms as well as an addition of two-way audio communication between every Reconnaissance robot and the HCS. Robotic classification will be sought to address diverse real-life search and rescue situations.

References

1. Nagatani, K., Kiribayashi, S., Okada, Y., Otake, K., Yoshida, K., Tadokoro, S., Nishimura, T., Yoshida, T., Koyanagi, E., Fukushima, M., Kawatsuma, S.: Emergency response to the nuclear accident at the Fukushima Daiichi Nuclear Power Plants using mobile rescue robots. J. Field Robotics 30, 44–63 (2013)
2. National Aeronautics and Space Administration: Mars Science Laboratory Curiosity Rover, http://mars.jpl.nasa.gov/msl
3. Structures Pointing and Control Engineering University Research Center: Semi-Autonomous Mobile Robots for Cooperative Environmental Exploration,
   http://www.calstatela.edu/orgs/space/sc_MobileRobotics.html
4. Structures Pointing and Control Engineering University Research Center: Unmanned Air Vehicles, http://web.calstatela.edu/orgs/space/sc_UAV.htm
5. Cypress Semiconductor Corporation: PSoC® 5: CY8C55 Family Datasheet (2011)
6. Stentz, A.: Map-Based Strategies for Robot Navigation in Unknown Environments. In: Proceedings of the AAAI Spring Symposium on Planning with Incomplete Information for Robot Problems (1996)
7. Microsoft Developer Network: Natural User Interface for Kinect for Windows
8. Sharp GP2Y0A21YK0F Distance Measuring Sensor Unit Measuring distance: 10 to 80 cm Analog output type,
   http://www.pololu.com/file/0J85/gp2y0a21yk0f.pdf
9. 2008 National Emissions Inventory: Emissions Inventory System Implementation Plan, Section 5 Submitting XML Data to EIS (2008)

10. Wright Jr., R.S., Haemel, N., Sellers, G., Lipchak, B.: OpenGL SuperBible. Comprehensive Tutorial and Reference, 5th edn. Pearson Education, Ann Arbor (2010)
11. Wu, H., Rubinstein, M., Shih, E., Guttag, J., Durand, F., Freeman, W.: Eulerian Video Magnification for Revealing Subtle Changes in the World. SIGGRAPH 31(4) (July 2012)
12. Drennan, B.: Eulerian Video Magnification v0.1 (2011)
13. iTV Goggles-PCX3D,
    http://itvgoggles.com/details.asp?productID=59

Practical Use of a Remote Movable Avatar Robot with an Immersive Interface for Seniors

Masahiko Izumi[1], Tomoya Kikuno[1], Yutaka Tokuda[2], Atsushi Hiyama[1],
Takahiro Miura[1], and Michitaka Hirose[1]

[1] Graduate School of Information Science and Technology, The University of Tokyo,
Hongo 7-3-1, Bunkyo-ku, Tokyo 113-8656, Japan
{masa,kikuno,atsushi,miu,hirose}@cyber.t.u-tokyo.ac.jp
[2] Graduate School of Engineering, The University of Tokyo, 4-6-1 Komaba,
Meguro-ku, Tokyo 153-8904, Japan
ytokuda@cyber.t.u-tokyo.ac.jp

Abstract. Societal aging is an inevitable social problem in many developed countries. In order to manage this issue, it is necessary to drastically change the welfare security and labor system of relevant societies. We have proposed "mosaic-type work" in which a single "virtual worker" is synthesized based on individual workers and seniors through seamless information sharing. In this paper, we specifically focus on the spatial part of the mosaic, namely, the "spatial mosaic," for enabling seniors to work without the burden of movement. Towards the actualization of this concept, we aimed to develop senior-friendly mobile avatar robots that can fit into seniors' daily lives. First, we analyzed problems of seniors' telecommunication with telepresence robots, and two elemental interfaces, the "physically operable interface" and the "acoustic zooming interface." The former is a senior-friendly interface that the seniors can manipulate with their motion, and the latter enables the user to listen to sounds in a specified area that the user can adjust. In order to discuss integrated interface designs, we conducted two exploratory experiments to evaluate the performance of these systems.

Keywords: Mosaic-type work, seniors, information communication technologies (ICT), avatar, interface.

1 Introduction

Population aging is one of the most significant global issues due to decreasing domestic productivity and increasing social security costs. In Japan, seniors accounted for 24.1% of the population in 2013 [1], a number estimated to reach 40.5% by 2055 [2]. The ratio of the young population to the elderly in 2009 was 2.81, which is expected to decline to 1.26 by 2055 [2],thus making it unreasonable to continue the conventional welfare security model, in which multiple young people support one senior. However, 83.6% of all seniors in Japan are healthy enough to not require care [3]. More than half of them are aware of the social contributions they have made and retain a strong desire to work [4]. These

C. Stephanidis and M. Antona (Eds.): UAHCI/HCII 2014, Part III, LNCS 8515, pp. 648–659, 2014.
© Springer International Publishing Switzerland 2014

facts indicate that the present social system needs to be—and can be—changed drastically.

According to a report by Fukushima, seniors have four types of work needs: to work without strenuous effort, to make themselves useful to others, to build personal relationships, and to earn extra money [5]. In particular, ex-white collar workers work for social connections and health enhancement [6]. They have knowledge, experience, and skills that young people do not have. Effective utilization of their ability can gradually change the conventional social system and revitalize work environments. The Silver Human Resource Centers in Japan attempt to meet the various needs of seniors [7]. However, it is difficult to meet all of their needs and effectively allocate seniors to the workforce, because these centers are chronically short-handed and limited to allocating work within their designated area.

Thus, we proposed the concept of a "mosaic-type work" system in which a single "virtual worker" is synthesized from individual work resources using information and communication technologies (ICTs) to supply an autonomous and stable labor force [8,9]. In order to actualize this concept, it is necessary to consider and quantify the workers' time, skills, spatial limitations, and other characteristics, as well as to develop a user-friendly interface for seamless information sharing. In this paper, we specifically describe our development and evaluation of "spatial mosaic" as an adapted model for mosaic-type work in senior employment contexts, with the purpose of exceeding seniors' limitations in daily available work area.

Our paper first discusses concepts pertinent to mosaic-type work and the spatial mosaic system (Section 2), followed by related work regarding telecommunication technologies and their problems (Section 3). Then, we provide an overview of a proposed telecommunication system along with the concepts of social telepresence and acoustic zooming (Section 4). We implemented a prototype interface and conducted two exploratory experiments for these two concepts (Section 5). With these results, we discuss the design of an integrated interface (Section 6).

2 Mosaic-type Work and Spatial Mosaic

2.1 Mosaic-type Work

Mosaic-type work can ensure compatibility between flexible work opportunities for seniors and a stable work force for employers by synthesizing virtual workers from a workforce of seniors. A "mosaic" is defined as a unit of one synthesized worker from multiple workers, as shown in Fig. 1. In this figure, as an example, senior A has expertise in field A, but not enough skill in field B, and also has mild motor and cognitive impairment. Senior B also has motor and cognitive difficulties in addition to insufficient skill in field A, but is highly skilled in field B. A young worker has good motor and cognitive functions, but is poor in fields A and B. Ideally, when their advantages can be synthesized into a virtual worker,

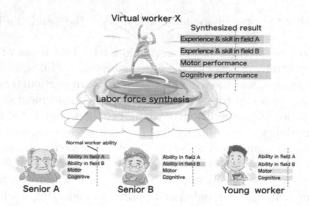

Fig. 1. The concept of "mosaic-type work" that generates a stable virtual worker from a workforce of seniors and young people

this virtual worker can demonstrate stable and superior performance in fields A and B.

In order to actualize this concept, it is necessary to consider and quantify the workers' time, skills, spatial limitations, and other characteristics. In this study, we focused specifically on the generation of a "spatial mosaic."

2.2 Spatial Mosaic

A spatial mosaic involves gathering remote workers in workplaces through ICTs to create a virtual workforce concentration. This concept is illustrated by Fig. 2. In this concept, remote workers can access workplaces in both the virtual and real environments, regardless of the worker's location. In the case of virtual workplaces, as shown in the left part of Fig. 2, various jobs are divided into task elements, and then are allocated to remote workers. This procedure results in co-operative work among a massive number of remote workers. On the other hand, real workplaces, as illustrated in the right part of Fig. 2, are realized by remote systems. In this case, workers remotely access the remote robots installed at the workplaces, and then conduct their activities. Current remote work systems include teleconference systems. We assume that telepresence robots can overcome the movability limitation on remote workplaces and enable remote workers to carry out various business activities. The robots can be useful to smoothly migrate from conventional work styles, in which workers gather in a particular place and work, to the proposed work style. Our concept can also be employed in the workplace using a combination of real and virtual workplaces.

The style of work created by the spatial mosaic enables seniors with movement problems to work more actively. Crowdsourcing is one relevant example that institutes the framework shown in the left part of Fig. 2. Kobayashi et al. reported a crowdsourced proofreading system of digital books for people with visual impairments [10]. In this platform, senior volunteers conducted phrase, ruby, and

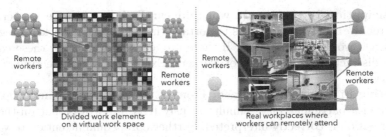

Fig. 2. The concept of a spatial mosaic that overcomes the limitations of real workplaces. [Left]: A workplace is generated in a virtual space. Jobs in the virtual workplace are divided into work elements, and then remote workers complete these tasks in the virtual environment. [Right]: Workplaces are located in real space. Workers can remotely access multiple workplaces in the real environment.

character corrections of the scanned books that were processed through optical character recognition. On the other hand, in order to implement the framework illustrated by the right part of Fig. 2, it is necessary to leverage various support systems for remote workers. Conventional teleconference systems are effective when the participants concentrate on speaking and do not move. The current telepresence robot is useful for moving smoothly in remote real spaces, but remains in the research and development phase. This telepresence robot, released by Double Robotics, is a reasonable robot that can be easily manipulated. However, for seniors, this kind of system should be equipped with an intuitive interface that does not disturb regular communication and creates highly realistic sensations in remote environments for promoting mutual understanding.

The ultimate objective of this study was to develop a support system for enabling seniors to remotely work on the real environment. In this paper, specifically, we focus on a mobile avatar robot telepresence system for remote work, and then propose a manipulation interface for promoting smooth remote communication.

3   Related Work on Telecommunication Technologies

In this section, we discuss relevant work on conventional telecommunication technologies and summarize the problems for implementing the spatial mosaic society-wide.

3.1   Mobility in Telecommunication

In the above section, we discussed the "spatial mosaic" concept, which generates a virtual workforce by gathering remote workers virtually within real and virtual workplaces through ICT. When the spatial mosaic is implemented in our society, the forms of spatial mosaic and its issues are summarized as follows:

1. **Participation in real-world workplaces:** To insert remote workers into the real world using ICT. It is important that the virtual worker integrated into real world appropriately. If there are any abnormalities, these can act as a distraction for on-the-spot workers. Examples: remote lecture, remote interview.
2. **Meeting in a particular space:** From distant locations, many people can meet in a particular place simultaneously It is important that on-the-spot information is correctly interpreted. Furthermore, equal attention to various information is also an important factor. Example: disaster site.
3. **Connect remote spaces in the virtual world:** From distant spaces, many people meet in a virtual world simultaneously. All participants are virtualized; therefore, it is important to create new and appropriate communication methods. Example: remote meeting.

As the first approach to the spatial mosaic, we focused on the participation model, which is the simplest model of telecommunication. Our first step was to insert one remote person into the real world without any abnormalities. Of course, this is a critical factor for telework towards maintaining fluent communication between remote and on-the-spot individuals. For interactions with on-the-spot workers, conventional television conference systems have limitations as an information medium. These technologies can only convey sound and video. They cannot express extensity, which is an important component of face-to-face communication. Therefore, through television conference systems, it is difficult to gauge the physical and psychological distance between on-the-spot workers and remote workers. Thus, proper communication between them is repressed.

If the remote user can move around freely in the remote office, there are benefits of the communication context for the remote user as follows:

- look around the remote space freely
- get up close with on-the-spot workers
- search for static information in the remote space

In addition to these merits for the remote user, there are certain benefits for the on-the-spot worker.

- estimate what the remote user is interested in
- no need to move toward the remote user
- extend presence of the remote user

For these reasons, we focused on avatar robots as a medium of telecommunication. We use "avatar robot" to describe a robot that can freely navigate the real world freely and convey auditory and visual information. In the following section, we discuss communication through avatar robots.

3.2   Telecommunication through Avatar Robots

The telepresence robot is a representation of oneself that enables a user to be anywhere and have an artificial face-to-face conversation with remote people without considering spatiotemporal or economic constraints. Research on telepresence robots began more than ten years ago, and recently, a variety of telepresence robots have been produced by various enterprises [11,12]. Telepresence robots came into widespread use for teleconferences, remote lectures, telemedicine, and so forth [13]. For example, InTouch Health and iRobot developed a telepresence robot RP-VITA for telemedicine [14]. By using RP-VITA, a doctor can ask hospitalized patients detailed questions about their symptoms while sitting in his own home or on a business trip. Thus, telerobotic technology has been rapidly developed. There are currently numerous low-priced products and program libraries for developing telepresence robots.

Under these circumstances, for real-world use—not in controlled conditions— we regard small mobile avatar robots as the most suitable robot for telecommunication. Therefore, we designed a telecommunication method using a mobile avatar robot.

3.3   Problems of Conventional Avatar Robots

Mobile robotics technologies progress daily. There are many considerations involved for using such technology in the real workforce (e.g., remote lectures). We conducted several remote lectures using a mobile avatar robot, named double (double robotics) and extracted the following problems.

- narrow eyesight
- operation complexity
- lack of presence
- difficulty of sound localization
- inviolable area

The narrow eyesight problem will be solved by hardware improvements. Therefore, we will not discuss this problem further. Operation complexity and lack of presence facilitated unsatisfactory social telepresence, which caused ineffective communication. The definition of "social telepresence" is discussed in the following section. Difficulty of sound localization and inviolable area appear to be independent problems, but if we use selective information browsing in remote space, these problems can be solved simultaneously. We call this selective browsing idea 'zooming.' This idea will be discussed further in the next section.

4   Interface Concepts

4.1   Social Telepresence

Social telepresence is defined as the level to which face-to-face communication is simulated. Social telepresence is high when the user feels as though they are in a face-to-face situation. This allows the user to experience more natural talk. Generally speaking, social telepresence become higher with visuals as opposed to sound alone. Returning to the conventional avatar problems, operation complexity is relevant to remote users, whereas lack of presence is relevant to on-the-spot users, which is experienced as a decline in social telepresence. If we can resolve these problems, mobile avatar robots can be the medium to facilitate improved social telepresence over visuals.

First, we discuss operability improvements. A complex operation interface forces users to concentrate exclusively on robot operation, hindering communication with the remote speaker. This issue is akin to putting the cart before the horse. The robot operation interface should be easy to understand and as intuitive as possible. To simplify the operation interface, we propose using body motion as the operation input. With a body motion operation system, in addition to simplifying operation, we believe that users will feel as though their individuality is better projected into the remote avatar robot. This increases the feeling of being in the remote place, which will thereby improve social telepresence.

Second, we describe presence enhancement. In face-to-face communication, nonverbal movement plays an important role in expressing the delicate nuances of thought. For example, eye gaze represents subtle nuances that cannot be expressed by means of language. With these intricate movements, humans infer customer reactions based on their words, movements, and so forth. In other words, customer movements represent the output based on our social input. With a conventional robot operation system, robots do not move unless users operate the robot with intention. Therefore, when remote users become heated in conversations with on-the-spot workers, the user's attention is directed toward speech alone. Attention is directed away from robot operation, such that robots do not show any movement. Under this condition, on-the-spot workers cannot detect any reflection of remote users' true mood, except for sound and visuals. Therefore, it is difficult for on-the-spot workers to know whether remote users can listen to or see on-the-spot information. Communication is reduced by reduced reflection of customer's feelings.

Therefore, we propose an interface that shows the remote user's unconscious movement to on-the-spot workers. By reflecting the operator's subtle movements in the robot's movements, we can simulate nonverbal aspects of communication. We believe that this increases feelings of robot presence among on-the-spot workers, and thus results in the improvement of social telepresence.

4.2   Acoustic Zooming

The word "zoom" means to magnify a section of a picture. Many studies have been conducted to support information understanding based on zooming effects. In this study, the word "zooming" means paying attention to a localized point and thereby understanding its characteristics. In particular, "acoustic zooming" is defined as the zooming of acoustic information.

Fig. 3 illustrates a schematic concept of acoustic zooming and an acoustic cubic volume. In Section 3, we discussed the difficulty of sound localization and inviolable areas as problems of conventional mobile avatar robots. We believe that acoustic zooming can solve these problems simultaneously.

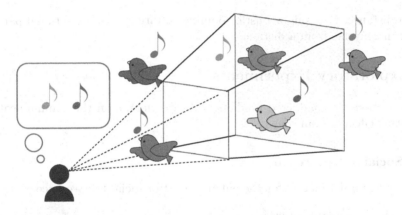

Fig. 3. The concept of acoustic volume. User can only hear sounds within the acoustic volume. In this case, users can hear the voices of orange and blue birds.

First, we discuss the sound localization problem. In the real world, there are many kinds of sound sources. Therefore, the sounds sent to remote users through avatar robots are mixed up with other sounds within the environment. From the perspective of communication, general sound—aside from the customer's voice—is primarily noise, which should be reduced. By targeting the talking partner by way of acoustic zooming, remote users can easily concentrate on talking. Furthermore, acoustic zooming can create a pseudo-cocktail party effect in terms of selective listening. Since the cocktail party effect is a unique effect under the context of face-to-face communication, this effect can enhance feelings of face-to-face communication, thus improving social telepresence.

Second, we discuss the inviolable area problem. In the real world, there are many immobile objects (e.g., posters on the wall and large, heavy monuments). Owing to mobile avatar robots, remote operators can move closer to and observed immobile information. However, the real world is not always suitable for mobile avatar robots. Thus, the area in which robots can move around is limited. For example, using Double [11], a small item in its route can be an obstacle for proper movement. Furthermore, conventional mobile avatar robots aim to enable users to engage in face-to-face-like talk with remote individuals. Thus, the main camera, which primarily streams the partner's face to the remote user, is typically placed level with a human face with a narrow field of view. Therefore, if there is a low-height obstacle, it eludes the avatar's eyesight, which causes the avatar to bump into the obstacle, thereby prohibiting forward movement. Cluttered routes are therefore unsuitable routes for mobile avatar robots. However, there might be intriguing information in the inviolable areas. Under these conditions, users can observe interesting information without any movement using acoustic zooming. This is a natural condition in face-to-face interactions. For example, when users are spoken to from a distance and there are obstacles between the conversational partners, users naturally react to their partner in face-to-face situations. However, with a mobile avatar, it is difficult to converse from a distance. By using acoustic zooming to target a conversational partner, users can converse from a distance.

5 Exploratory Experiments

In this section, we conducted fundamental experiments on the communication-promoting effects of our ideas.

5.1 Social Telepresence

First, we again list factors for the enhancement of social telepresence.

- physically operable interface
- unconscious movement synchronization

We implemented an interface that can have these features for robot operation on a tablet computer. There are two reasons for using a tablet computer. First, tablet computers have sufficiently large monitors to enable experience of authentic audio-visual sensations. Second, tablet computers provide several easy physical operations, such as pinch and rotate operations. These gestures provide more intuitive manipulation and interaction than simple buttons. Holding a tablet computer and wearing headphones, users can explore various objects in the virtual space. The system enables them to experience virtual space as if they were looking through the display.

As a physically operable interface, we introduced the operator's direction into the avatar manipulation interface as shown in Fig. 4. Operators could move the robot by tilting the tablet back and forth, and turn the robot by turning the tablet right and left. The concept of this interface was designed to reflect users' spatial movements into robot movements. In addition to this manipulation method, we implemented a mechanism for reflecting unconscious movements of users. We extracted hand jiggles, which constituted high-frequency data measured by an accelerometer with a high-pass filter. Back-and-forth jiggles were measured for back-and-forth movement, and right and left jiggles were measured for clockwise and counterclockwise turns, respectively. Drastic movements occurred when jiggles induced feelings of strangeness, and thus, we utilized limited threshold gap values.

Using this system, we conducted interface evaluation experiments. Participants were asked to conduct short presentations through the avatar robot. Then, we administered a brief questionnaire on the presenter and listener to understand participants' impressions. Among presenters, feelings of self-projection were enhanced by physically movable operation. This indicates that the feelings of presence in the remote place were also enhanced. Among listeners, presence of presenter was enhanced by the reflection of the presenter's unconscious movements. This fact indicates that listeners paid more attention to presenters when there was unconscious movement projection. Thus, it appears that, under these conditions, social telepresence was enhanced bidirectionally.

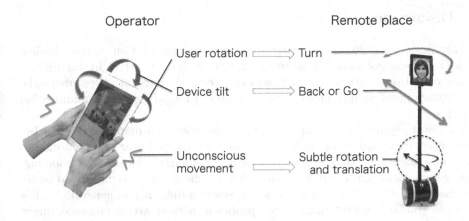

Fig. 4. Design of the physically operable interface. Users can move the avatar robot by tilting the tablet and turn the robot by user rotation. The system senses subtle movements—hand jiggles—and reflects these in the robot as unconscious, nonverbal movements of the operator.

5.2 Acoustic Zooming

Regarding acoustic zooming, we already have conducted a plain experiment [15]. We have also implemented an acoustic zooming system on a tablet computer. With the system, we conducted an experiment to evaluate the efficiency of acoustic zooming. To compare the effect of acoustic zooming with conventional interfaces, we implemented three volume calculation modes, namely, "normal," "direction," and "zooming." Fifteen sound sources—voices of different words— were recorded in advance. These were located within the virtual space, and participants were asked to find specific words.

The zooming mode produced significantly higher performance than the direction mode and significantly more accurate responses than the normal mode. According to the participants' comments, switching functions of the calculation modes and resizable acoustic volumes are important implementations for more effective browsing in various situations.

For these reasons, acoustic zooming is effective as a type of information interaction. Therefore, it is implied that avatar interaction with acoustic zooming can diminish stress related to information seeking in the remote environment. From the perspective of mobile avatar manipulation, it is important that the operation interface provides operation of robot movements and targeting of acoustic zooming, simultaneously. Notwithstanding substantive robots, it is unrealistic to produce fast-moving robots due to safety concerns. If the target is constantly moving, chasing it manually is difficult for these robots. Therefore, when implementing a zooming system into the avatar operation interface, the system should lock and chase the target automatically. This saves the user from unnecessary concentration.

6   Discussion

In this section, we discuss our next steps, namely, integration of the physical UI and acoustic zooming. These two methods are both effective in building an avatar operation interface. Thus, if we can effectively integrate these methods, our avatar operation interface can have enhanced long-distance communication abilities.

The most significant issue in need of consideration is a mapping method between user action and robot motion. This time, we mapped user's body motion to robot movement, and the pinch motion on a tablet surface for acoustic zooming. However, motions that are most suitable for specific robot motions should be researched. In particular, operation preferences might differ across generations. For example, younger generations, who are proficient with smartphone usage, might be accustomed to using a touch display interface. However, older generations are less likely to be accustomed to this. In this case, the young have a mental model for using touch-panel devices, but the elderly do not. The interface should be easy to make using image for the user who have no proper mental model.

The most appropriate interface will change dynamically change across scenes. The purpose of the present study, however, was to evaluate our ideas. Thus, we did not focus on particular work scenes. Hereafter, we will aim to use mobile avatar robots in a daily life context in order to clarify patterns of work using the spatial mosaic method, and design an interface for robot operation in specific scenes.

7   Conclusion

In order to make full use of the strengths of the senior workforce, such as its rich knowledge, experience, and skill, the spatial mosaic formation system and its fundamental technologies were discussed. We discussed the mosaic and spatial mosaic systems as well as conventional avatar robot communication problems. We proposed two interaction concepts to resolve the stated problems: "physically movable operation interface" and "acoustic zooming interface." We conducted an exploratory experiment for each interface. Results verified the efficacy of these interfaces. The physically movable operation interface enhanced social telepresence as experienced by the presenter and felt by the listener. This indicates that body movement is an important factor, as we predicted in Section . The acoustic zooming interface is useful for sound information browsing. We plan to conduct a similar experiment in real-world scenarios. Future studies will integrate these two concepts into one interface for avatar robot operation. Then, using this interface, our research target will be the difference in feelings and proficiency between the young and the aged.

Acknowledgments. This research was supported in part by S-innovation (Strategic Promotion of Innovative Research and Development) funding under Industry Academia Collaborative R&D Programs administered by the Japan Science and Technology Agency (JST).

References

1. Cabinet Office: Annual Report on the Aging Society 2013,
   http://www8.cao.go.jp/kourei/whitepaper/w-2013/gaiyou/s1_1.html
   (in Japanese) (last viewed February 7, 2014)
2. Kaneko, R., Ishikawa, A., Ishii, F., Sasai, T., Iwasawa, M., Mita, F., Moriizumi, R.: Population Projections for Japan: 2006-2055 Outline of results, methods, and assumptions. The Japanese Journal of Population 6(1), 76–114 (2008)
3. Ministry of Health, Labour and Welfare: Change in the number of people who are certified to be in need of long-term care by care category,
   http://www.mhlw.go.jp/seisaku/2009/03/01.html
   (in Japanese) (last viewed February 26, 2013)
4. Cabinet Office: White Paper on the National Lifestyle 2006,
   http://www5.cao.go.jp/seikatsu/whitepaper/h18/06_eng/index.html
   (last viewed February 26, 2013)
5. Fukushima, S.: Analysis of desires to work with elderly people (this translated title was prepared by the authors). Japan Labor Review 558, 19–31 (2007) (in Japanese)
6. Japan Organization for Employment of the Elderly, Persons with Disabilities and Job Seekers: Report of an investigation on the work and life of Japan's baby boomers (this translated title was prepared by the authors),
   http://www.jeed.or.jp/data/elderly/research/dankai22.html
   (in Japanese) (last viewed February 26, 2013)
7. Osada, H., Suzuki, T., Takata, K., Nishishita, A.: Social activity and relevant factors in the elderly: Focus on members of senior manpower center and senior citizen's club. Japanese Journal of Public Health 57(4), 279–290 (2010)
8. Hiyama, A., Sano, M., Kobayashi, M., Hirose, M.: Senior Cloud: ICT platform for improving society by circulating the experience, knowledge, and skills of the elderly. In: Proc. 17th VRSJ 2012, pp. 157–160 (2012) (in Japanese)
9. Nakayama, M., Hiyama, A., Miura, T., Yatomi, N., Hirose, M.: Support system of time-mosaic formation in flexible work styles for seniors. IPSJ Journal 55(1), 177–188 (2014) (in Japanese)
10. Kobayashi, M., Ishihara, T., Itoko, T., Takagi, H., Asakawa, C.: Age-based task specialization for crowdsourced proofreading. In: Stephanidis, C., Antona, M. (eds.) UAHCI 2013, Part II. LNCS, vol. 8010, pp. 104–112. Springer, Heidelberg (2013)
11. http://www.doublerobotics.com/
12. https://www.suitabletech.com/beam-plus/
13. Tsui, K.M., Desai, M., Yanco, H.A., Uhlik, C.: Exploring use cases for telepresence robots. In: 2011 6th ACM/IEEE International Conference on Human-Robot Interaction (HRI), pp. 11–18. IEEE (2011)
14. http://www.intouchhealth.com/products-and-services/products/rp-vita-robot/
15. Izumi, M., Hiyama, A., Miura, T., Tokuda, Y., Hirose, M.: Acoustic information zooming interface. In: Proc. of Asiagraph, vol. 8 (2013)

Meeting Requirements of Older Users?
Robot Prototype Trials in a Home-like Environment

Tobias Körtner[1], Alexandra Schmid[1], Daliah Batko-Klein[1], and Christoph Gisinger[1,2]

[1] Academy for Ageing Research at Haus der Barmherzigkeit, Seeböckg. 30A, Vienna, Austria
{tobias.koertner,alexandra.schmid,daliah.batko-klein,
christoph.gisinger}@hausderbarmherzigkeit.at
[2] Donauuniversität Krems, Dr.-Karl-Dorrek-Straße 30, Krems, Austria

Abstract. A prototype of an assistive robot for older people was tested in three different countries in life-like lab settings. A sample of potential older users with different grades and types of age-related impairments completed a sequence of tasks with the robot. Subsequently, usability issues, user acceptance, and their willingness to pay for such a robot (affordability) were assessed to find out if the robot caters to the needs of the impairment groups. Main results of the data analyses were: ease of use was deemed satisfactory by the majority of participants. Task speed was considered to be rather slow. Additionally, it could be shown that participants were sceptical of buying a robot for their own use, but would be willing to rent one. A significant difference in classifying the robot prototype as helpful for the home was found in participants with mobility impairments compared to participants without mobility impairments.

Keywords: social robotics, human-robot interaction, assistive technology, user requirements, older users, prototype trials.

1 Introduction

In view of the demographic development in Europe [1] with its rising number of older people, Assistive Technology becomes an essential element to improve senior citizens' quality of life. Robotics could contribute to helping senior citizens stay longer at their own homes and feel safe. Solutions in robotic technology, however, not only need to be reliable in terms of task performance, but also have to meet users' acceptance and fulfil their needs. Acceptance is described as "the demonstrable willingness within a user group to employ technology for the task it is designed to support" [2].

Several European projects in the field have attempted to tackle this issue. The most recent examples (among others) are KSERA [3], DOMEO [4], Companionable [5], SRS [6], or Accompany [7].

The HOBBIT-project aims at developing a highly acceptable and affordable socially assistive robot supporting older adults in staying independently at home. To

C. Stephanidis and M. Antona (Eds.): UAHCI/HCII 2014, Part III, LNCS 8515, pp. 660–671, 2014.
© Springer International Publishing Switzerland 2014

become a real benefit for senior persons, such a robotic solution needs to cater to the target-groups needs. As people age, they become more fragile and may become more dependent on other people to accomplish everyday life activities [8]. Especially falls and their consequences are often considered a contributing reason for admission to a nursing home [9, 10]. People decide to move into a care facility, because they do not feel safe in their own home after a fall, or they are in need of more intense care due to the health consequences of a fall. Assistive technology thus should help preventing falls and improve emergency handling.

As Hegel et al. (2007) found [11] the more an application is used in a private context, the higher the intensity of interaction. Accordingly, an everyday benefit needs to assure frequent usage of a robotic assistant. As a consequence, HOBBIT should fulfil tasks at home which reduce risk of falling (i.e. keeping floors clutter-free, searching and bringing objects), and offer further functionalities that focus on user needs. Using HOBBIT on a daily basis will also facilitate its implementation in the household. It has been found that users' expectations are often hard to meet in real interaction [12]. In order to identify such benefits, the analysis of user requirements plays an important role.

The following section briefly describes the findings about user requirements leading to the functionalities of the prototype, section 3 described the prototype used for the trials, and section 4 then described the trial procedure and the most important results. Finally, conclusions are drawn from the trial results (section 5) and the study is discussed with an outlook to future work (section 6).

2   Assessment of User Requirements

In order to guarantee high usability and user acceptance, the conception of HOBBIT followed a user-centred approach. Several iterative pre-studies led to the identification of needs and requirements of older persons that formed the basis of functionalities in the prototype trials. Based on the idea of focus groups [13] four creative workshops were conducted in Austria and Sweden with older participants and   people who had a direct connection to the topic of "age and assistance at home" (medics, therapists or relatives of older people) [14]. These led to first explorative results concerning user expectations and requirements of a robotic helper at home. Requirements mentioned by the workshop participants mainly concerned household tasks (which is in line with findings from literature [15]), emergency detection, and providing/supporting social contacts. Some functions mentioned were beyond technical feasibility, for instance complex or physically demanding household tasks, and thus were not taken further into consideration within the HOBBIT project.

As a next step, a questionnaire, based on this preliminary collection of ideas, was handed out to senior citizens in Austria, Greece and Sweden. Questionnaire items covered feasible, helpful functions identified in the workshops, and design issues to assess acceptance of HOBBIT. 113 potential primary users (PUs) aged 70 or older completed the questionnaire. Results of this survey led to a clearer picture of (technically feasible) functions that were important to older persons, but also what operation mode they would prefer, and basic design preferences.

Finally, 38 potential PUs were interviewed, in order to gain more details about user's needs and ideas regarding the interaction with the robot. In combination with the findings from workshops, interviews, and literature on falls and fall prevention in elderly, the identified user requirements were translated into technically feasible functionalities of a first HOBBIT prototype (PT1).

3   The HOBBIT Prototype

The prototype used in the trials is a mobile platform equipped with a multitude of sensors for navigation and perception purposes. To fulfil the tasks the robot has one light-weight arm with five degrees of freedom. The arm features a gripper based on the FESTO "Finray effect". Thus, a number of small everyday objects can be grasped.

As user requirement assessments have also shown, it is vital to offer different modalities with which to operate the robot. The centre of this approach with HOBBIT is the multi modal interface. It consists of a tiltable touch screen, automatic speech recognition, text to speech functionality and also a gesture recognition interface.

On a 'face screen', HOBBIT displays positive and negative facial expressions as a means to communicate with the user. Altogether, the size of PT1 is approx. 1.20m.

A more detailed description of PT1 components and specifications is given in [16].

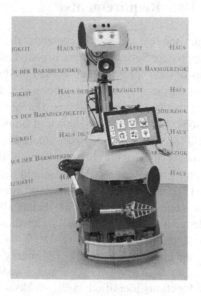

Fig. 1. HOBBIT PT1

4   Trials

The aims of these trials were:

- Assessing if user requirements were met by functionalities of the HOBBIT.
- Gaining an insight into the usability, acceptance and affordability notions of potential older users, and to collect data for improvements to be implemented in a second prototype.
- Analysing if the type of participants' impairments had an influence on their perception of the robot.

4.1   Sample and Setting

Sample. Representative PUs were recruited in Austria, Sweden and Greece. All participants were 70 years or older and had at least moderate, typical age-related impairments. The most common age-related impairments occurring at that age were identified from literature [17, 18, 19, 20]. These are: vision, hearing or mobility impairments. Cognitive impairments were an exclusion criterion for participation in the trials.

In order to assess grade of impairment (from "none" to "severe"), all participants were asked to complete a screening questionnaire before taking part in the trials. The screening questionnaire consisted of 18 items formulated as statements to be answered on a 4-point Likert scale, in order to find out about PUs' difficulties regarding vision, hearing and mobility. Additionally, all participants were asked how often they used a computer and if they had ever fallen at home. It was expected that multi-morbidity would occur in the sample group, i.e. that there would be PUs with several limitations. PUs who had no form of impairment in the screening questionnaire were excluded.

Apart from the impairment grading, PUs had to fulfil the following inclusion criteria for PT1 trials:

- Men and women aged 70+
- Single-living at home (due to considerations that acceptance of an assistive robot among senior couples might be lower than for single-living persons)
- Possibly also receiving (moderate) home care; help in the household
- Sufficient mental capacity to understand the project and ability to give consent
- No pacemaker

The final sample consisted of 49 PUs (between the age of 70 to 88 years; 35 female and 14 male) and 35 accompanying relatives or close contact persons (so-called secondary users; SUs; 24 female and 11 male). In Austria 12 PUs and 9 SUs took part in the study; in Sweden 21 PUs and 11 SUs and in Greece 16 PUs and 15 SUs.

78% in the PU sample had at least one impairment graded as "moderate". 44 PUs (89.8%) had some form of multiple impairment. Six participants had a severe vision impairment (12.2%), four had a severe hearing impairment (8.1%) and three had a severe mobility impairment (6.1%).

Setting. Two pilot trials were carried out with PUs in Austria before, in order to test the wording and comprehensibility of the used questionnaire items and robot dialogue, and length of trials in general.

Trials took place at three sites from March 2013 until May 2013. The setting consisted of two adjacent areas with separation screens and a doorway in between at all three sites (Austria, Greece and Sweden). There was a Briefing Area/Kitchen that consisted of a kitchen corner (sideboard, a small oven/cooker, dishes, dishtowels and cutlery) and an eating area with a table, two chairs and a side table.

The other area was the Main Testing Area, decorated as a living room: a cosy chair for the PU, a small couch table, a chest with drawers, and space in the background for SUs, the observer, and a technician who remained in the background to navigate the robot with remote control and assure that the robot functioned correctly. This semi-autonomous setting allowed for a controlled, yet still realistic test of the robot's functionalities in pre-defined scenarios.

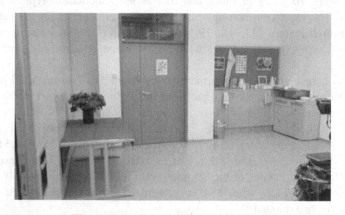

Fig. 2. Kitchen area at trial site in Austria

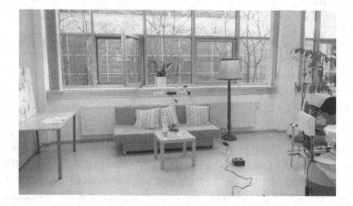

Fig. 3. Living room area at trial site in Austria

Measures and Procedure. After an introduction of the project, signing of informed consents and a short introduction of the robot and how to use it, PUs were seated in a chair in the living room area and given written instructions for each task. After each task, there was a short break for usability questions (based on the NASA Task Load Index [21], plus a few individual items). After the series of tasks, a debriefing questionnaire for PUs (including the System Usability Scale [22]) and SUs, time for questions from the participants and a snack ended the trial. Questions of the debriefing questionnaire, apart from a few open-ended items, had to be answered on a 4-point Likert scale. To obtain a further external assessment of the participant's behaviour and attitude towards the robot during interaction, a structured observation protocol was used by an observer who was present, as well as the SUs.

One trial lasted on average 2.5hours (including introduction and debriefing questionnaire). If wanted, participants could take breaks in between.

Based on the user requirements, the following sequence of tasks was chosen for the trials:

— Call the robot (via a call button from the other room)
— Clear floor (PU commanded the robot to autonomously pick up an unknown object from the floor and put it on its tray)
— Teach an object to the robot (PU taught robot a new pre-defined object by putting it on a turntable that the robot grasped)
— Search and bring (PU commanded robot to search and bring a learned object from the adjacent room)
— Emergency call (a project member simulated a fall which triggered HOBBIT's emergency dialogue. PUs completed a verbal dialogue with HOBBIT finally establishing a demo-emergency call.)

4.2   Analysis

Quantitative data were analysed using SPSS 18. The data from questionnaires were subject to frequency analyses, correlations and non-parametric tests on significance (i.e. Mann-Whitney-U-Test). Additionally, qualitative data from observation forms were analysed descriptively and added interesting information.

4.3   Results

Usability. On the Nasa Task Load Index, the majority of PUs rated the tasks as being "rather" or "very easy". Task-speed of the robot was mostly perceived as being rather slow. Only 18.4% of the PUs found the robot complex, and despite a whole lot of new information in the briefing phase and the new situation of interacting with a robot, only 32.6% felt that they needed to learn a lot beforehand. 91.9% thought HOBBIT was easy to use in general. PUs were also asked to rank which mode of operation they preferred in the debriefing questionnaire. The result showed the following order: voice commands came first (49%), then touch screen (42.9%) and gestures (6.1%).

SUs (n= 35) also chose voice most often as their preferred option (49%), touch screen was in second place (16.3%) and then gestures (2%). This, however, also has to be connected to the fact that only two gestures (yes and no) had been integrated at that point which explains the higher interest in voice and touch screen.

Qualitative data from the observation protocols provided important information: On the whole, the observers noted that most participants were sceptical or insecure in the beginning, but then became more and more confident in the interaction with the robot. Icons and font size were liked by PUs, but a few participants stated that they had problems with recognising them and that the text should be larger. It was furthermore often observed that participants began with speech in a task as the preferred interaction mode and then switched to the touch screen. Speech commands, even though very much appreciated in the user needs assessments before the trials, posed problems for many PUs: participants did not feel at ease or could not remember the speech commands for HOBBIT. Most participants often talked in the natural way one would use when talking to a human being, which often led to speech commands not being understood by HOBBIT.

PUs using a computer more frequently also stated that they would like to use the robot more frequently (r=.44/p=.01). At the same time, a significant negative correlation was observed between the amount of computer use and finding the robot "awkward to use" (r=-.39/p=.02).

Bearing age-related impairments in mind, the question remained, whether HOBBIT catered to requirements of older users. Mann-Whitney-U-Tests showed that hearing impairments had a notable effect on the emergency task: PUs with hearing impairments found accomplishing this task more difficult (p=.048) than the other PUs. Accordingly, PUs with hearing impairments liked using the touch screen significantly more than other PUs (p=.030). No other significant differences between types of impairments were found.

Functions Supporting User Acceptance. The debriefing questionnaire mainly focussed on functionalities that were classified as high priority functions from user requirement assessments and which were also in keeping with the HOBBIT approach of fall prevention. These were tasks that could be subsumed under 'household' and 'care'. Other data that was collected in the questionnaire covered design issues. In the following, the main results are presented.

a) Household. PUs ranked fetching objects from the floor as the most important picking up-function (49% of the sample), followed by fetching objects from a high shelf (32.7%). The same result was found for SUs. 52.2% chose 'picking up objects from floor' as the most important function. 77.6% of the PUs and 53.1% of the SUs furthermore found a transporting functionality important.

The grade of mobility impairment and agreement to this question were significantly correlated (r=.314/p=030), which means that a high grade of mobility impairment was linked to PUs finding it important that the robot could transport objects. What is more, finding it important that the robot transports objects correlated significantly with finding it important to use the robot as a walking stick (r=.285/p=.050), as an aid to stand up from the floor (r=.395/p=.006) and as an aid to stand up from a chair (r=.448/p=.001).

b) Care. Using the robot as a walking aid and as a stand up support, either from the floor or from a sitting position, were identified as possible fall prevention functionalities in the user requirement assessments. PT1 did not feature such functionalities, but the participants were asked how important they would be to them. PUs chose the aid to stand up from the floor most often as the preferred one (55.3%), standing up from a chair was in second place (18.4%), and the walking aid in third place (15.8%). In the same ranking, SUs chose standing up from the floor as the most preferred option (36.7%), walking aid second (16.3%) and then standing up from a chair (14.3%). Asked about the importance of such functionalities in general, 65.8% of the PUs stated, that help in standing up after a fall was "very important" to them. Importance of mobility aids was less distinct among SUs.

Asked about the emergency dialogue in the trials, feedback from PUs was very positive: length of the emergency dialogue was rated as "just right" by 91.8% of the PUs, the speed by 87.8%, and spatial distance between robot and user in the emergency scenario was rated "just right" by 81.6%. When asked whether they found the emergency dialogue calming, 32.7% of the PUs chose "rather" and 53.1% "very much".

57.2% were in general favour of having a robot at home for a longer period, and even more (65.3%) could imagine that HOBBIT takes care of them. 49% found the robot as they experienced it "rather" or "very helpful" at home. SUs were also asked to state how helpful they thought HOBBIT was for their relatives/acquaintance's home. They were slightly more positive than the respective PUs: 42.9% chose "rather" and 10.2% "very much" as answers, which in total makes 53.1% agreeing that such a robot could be helpful.

Again, HOBBIT's functionalities seemed to especially cater to PUs with mobility impairments. There was a significant correlation between mobility impairment and the opinion that the robot could be helpful in one's own home ($r=.372/p=.009$).

Results of U-tests confirmed an expectable difference between persons with a mobility impairment and PUs without. Mobility impaired PUs found it more important to use the robot as a walking aid ($p=.007$) and could also imagine having a robot taking care of them significantly more ($p=.038$). At the same time, they judged the robot to be less useful without an arm ($p=.005$), hinting at the importance of picking up objects for this group once more, and generally found PT1 more helpful for their home than PUs without mobility impairments ($p=.001$). No significant differences were found for other impairment groups.

c) Design. Even though PT1 still possessed a very rudimentary design and thus could not give the impression of a finished product, a few questions regarding design were included in the debriefing questionnaire. PT1's basic design already had been developed with the goal of approaching user requirements assessed beforehand. Those were: anthropomorphic design with head/face and body, an arm, and a moderate height that would not intimidate sitting participants.

PUs were asked how they liked the face and the voice of the robot after they had interacted with PT1 in the trials. 69.4% enjoyed the face design (34.7% each rating it with either "liked it very much" or "rather liked it") and even more (87.8%) enjoyed the voice. On the whole, the female voice was slightly preferred over the male voice: 55.1% of the PUs chose the female voice for interaction in the trials.

SUs were less enthused by the face. Only 16.3% liked it "very much". The voice was generally liked (over 60% giving it positive ratings), but some SUs said they would like a less 'mechanical' and more 'natural' voice.

Another question addressed the robot's size. 51% of the PUs found it the "right size" for being helpful at home, yet 40.8% stated it should be "smaller". From the SUs, 40.8% found the size "right" and 26.5% said it should be "smaller".

Among the SUs, liking the design was significantly correlated with imagining to buy the robot for one's relative ($r=.405/p=.020$) and renting it ($r=.361/p=039$), thus emphasising the influence that design can have on acceptance. No similar correlations were found among the PUs.

Affordability. Asking persons about willingness to buy something they hardly have any experience with and which only exists as a first prototype at the moment of the survey can lead to vague results at best. Nonetheless, we let PUs and SUs reflect on whether they could imagine buying and/or renting a HOBBIT.

The realistic price of the prototype amounted to € 14.000. This was clearly far too costly for the participants. Only 4.1% of the PUs could "rather" imagine purchasing HOBBIT for that price. Nobody agreed "very much" to do so. Buying a HOBBIT in general (without giving a specific price), however, met with slightly more approval. 4.1% could "very much" imagine doing so, and 30.6% could "rather" imagine buying it in general. 49% could "very much" imagine renting a HOBBIT.

The SUs also found the realistic price not acceptable. Still, 2% could "very much" imagine spending € 14,000 and 4.1% opted for "rather". 18.4% could imagine buying a robot for their PU in general. This is still not a very high number, but indicates that SUs are to be seen rather as the marketing target group instead of PUs. Renting the robot was a "very" attractive thought for 22.4% and "rather" conceivable for 26.5%.

Nonparametric correlations showed obvious, yet nonetheless interesting linkages: Those PUs who stated that they would like to use the robot frequently were also more prone to buy a robot in general ($r=.458/p=.001$). Additionally, the more they thought the robot could be helpful in their home ($r=.390/p=.007$) and the more they could imagine having a robot at home for a longer period ($r=.326/.025$), the more they also could imagine buying the robot in general. Hence, only when perceiving the robot as reliable and helpful, buying it can become a realistic option for PUs. Interestingly SUs of PUs with a vision impairment could imagine buying such a robot for their relative significantly more than SUs of participants without a vision impairment ($p=.034$). There were, however, no significant differences among PUs with different types of impairments observable.

5   Conclusions

The trial results presented here generally indicate that user requirements are met by HOBBIT. PUs mostly enjoyed the trial situation, found the tasks easy to accomplish and the operation of HOBBIT clear. As with all prototypes, some definite areas that are in need of improvement, in order to fulfil the target users' needs, could be identified: dialogues and instructions from the robot have to be legible for users and must not contain "loops" which can lead to frustration, if people are asked the same questions repeatedly. In the learning task it was often unclear and complicated for older participants to know what to do with the robot. Speed of the robot might also be something to be improved. The design of the touch screen menu seems usable for PUs. Minor changes are necessary, though, regarding a clearer arrangement of menu icons, and an adaptable font size to better accommodate PUs with vision impairments.

In terms of acceptance, picking up objects from the floor has been singled out as the function within HOBBIT's range that is most important for older users, especially in case of age-related mobility issues. This is followed by picking up objects from a high shelf and a transport function of the robot. A stand-up and a walking aid are highly interesting for the participants in the trial sample.

The design clearly was not a finished one at this stage, which was also clear to the participants. Some helpful conclusions can nonetheless be drawn from participants' replies regarding design issues: robotic voices should try to approach 'natural' human modulation and style. For an improved version of HOBBIT, also several voice options for each gender could be implemented. The size of a social robot for older persons should not be intimidating; 1.20m might already be too much in some cases. At the same time, it needs to be considered that PUs in a home setting will not always be in a sitting position when interacting with HOBBIT.

Finally, results on affordability showed that the prototype price was too expensive for the majority of participants, but feedback often included that a final working model of HOBBIT could be worth the money. From the sample, SUs seemed more likely to be a market target group, purchasing or renting a robot for their older relatives. Apart from financial resources, this also reflects scepticism among older people to use robots as assistants in the near future. A renting model is preferred and might reduce scepticism from PUs.

Differences between impairment groups could be analysed, which show that the functionalities are catered to meet requirements especially of mobility impaired users. Rating of functions indicates HOBBIT's intended helpfulness in terms of fall prevention. The multimodal operation of HOBBIT (screen, voice and gestures) could make up for difficulties certain impairment groups might face in some tasks.

6   Discussion

The findings presented here also must be viewed from a critical point of view as well. PUs generally gave positive feedback on the prototype. This is not unproblematic. Older participants tend to give favourable comments to developers rather than voicing their opinion, thereby being very positive about prototypes they are presented and tending to blame themselves rather than the interaction modalities if not being able to cope with the system [23]. Self-reporting can also be influenced by age-related factors. [24] showed, for example, that there are age differences in the ways in which people respond in self-reports. Hence, findings from the PT1 trials have to be judged as tendencies which have to be confirmed or further looked into in future research.

Another limitation of this kind of trials is the rather small sample size and the difficulty to arrive at a balanced number of women and men. One also has to consider that participants were in a controlled environment and trials followed a clearly structured sequence of tasks. To gain more reliable and in-depth feedback from elderly users' experiences, and to gain insight to specific situations in which the robot is perceived as either helpful or impractical, long-term trials in a natural home environment would be necessary, which leaves room for future scientific work.

The main focus of this paper was on the question if user requirements based on age-related difficulties were met by our prototype. Despite the fact that findings partly did differentiate between impairment groups and it could be shown that mobility impaired participants rated the robot significantly as more helpful than the other groups, screening impairments by means of a self-report questionnaire has certain weaknesses. It was, for instance, observed that some participants rated themselves fitter than they actually appeared when being observed in their movements during the trials. Using a more 'objective' screening method, such as easy medical tests, for instance, might have led to an even more reliable group of potential users. Yet, such methods would have required the assessment of medical experts. Such an approach, however, must be judged from an ethical point of view as well. Subject older participants, who are a 'vulnerable' target group, to medical assessments would turn the participants into the objects of testing and research instead of the robot prototype. This clearly cannot be the aim of a usability study.

To gain more insight into affordability and attitudes of users, it will be necessary to ask them about their own cost ideas and maybe use a different methodology. As PUs and SUs in this project are expected to have little to no experience with robots, open answers about willingness to buy a product that has only been experienced in a controlled environment and in prototype status are to be treated carefully. Again, assessing price details is more plausible in a setting with an already more finished version of HOBBIT (in terms of design, behaviour and functionalities).

It follows that future work will have to concentrate on long-term trials in homes of potential uses with respective age-related impairments. For results on acceptance in real life, it needs to be made sure that assistive robots give (older) users a feeling of helpfulness and safety on a long-term basis.

Acknowledgment. The research leading to these results has received funding from the European Community's Seventh Framework Programme (FP7/2007-2013) under grant agreement No. 288146, Hobbit.

References

1. European Commission–Eurostat: Key figures on Europe 2007/2008 edition. Luxembourg: Office for Official Publications of the European Communities (2008)
2. Dillon, A.: User acceptance of information technology. In: Karwowski, W. (ed.) Encyclopaedia of Human Factors and Ergonomics. Taylor and Francis, London (2001)
3. KSERA. Deliverable D1.1 – Scenarios, Use Cases & Requirements. EU FP7 (2012)

4. Domeo, http://www.aat.tuwien.ac.at/domeo/indexen.html
5. Companionable, http://www.companionable.net
6. SRS, http://srs-project.eu
7. Accompanyproject, http://www.accompanyproject.eu
8. Walker, A., Walker, C.: Ageing and Disability: A Quality of Life Perspective. In: Conference on Ageing and Disability, Graz, June 8-9, European Association of Service Providers for Persons with Disabilities (EASPD) (2006)
9. Dias, N., Kempen, G., Todd, C.: The German version of the Falls Efficacy Scale-International Version (FES-I). Gerontol. Geriatr. 39, 297–300 (2006)
10. Jansenberger, H.: Sturzprävention in Therapie und Training. Thieme, Stuttgart (2011)
11. Hegel, F., Lohse, M., Swadzba, A., Wachsmuth, S., Rohlfing, K., Wrede, B.: Classes of Applications for Social Robots: a User Study. In: 16th IEEE International Conference on Robot & Human Interactive Communication, Korea, pp. 938–943 (2007)
12. Lohse, M.: Bridging the gap between users' expectations and system evaluations. In: ROMAN, pp. 485–490. IEEE Press, New York (2011)
13. Boissy, P., Corriveau, H., Michaud, F., Labonté, D., Royer, M.-P.: A qualitative study of in-home robotic telepresence for home care of community-living elderly subjects. Journal of Telemedicine and Telecare 13, 79–84 (2007)
14. Körtner, T., Schmid, A., Batko-Klein, D., Gisinger, C., Huber, A., Lammer, L., Vincze, M.: How Social Robots Make Older Users Really Feel Well– A Method to Assess Users' Concepts of a Social Robotic Assistant. In: Ge, S.S., Khatib, O., Cabibihan, J.-J., Simmons, R., Williams, M.-A. (eds.) ICSR 2012. LNCS, vol. 7621, pp. 138–147. Springer, Heidelberg (2012)
15. Fausset, C.B., Kelly, A.J., Rogers, W.A., Fisk, A.D.: Challenges to aging in place: Understanding home maintenance difficulties. Journal Housing for the Elderly 25(2), 125–141 (2011)
16. Fischinger, D., Einramhof, P., Wohlkinger, W., Papoutsakis, K., Mayer, P., Panek, P., Koertner, T., Hofmann, S., Argyros, A., Vincze, M., Weiss, A., Gisinger, C.: HOBBIT – The Mutual Care Robot. In: ASROB-2013 in Conjunction with IEEE/RSJ International Conference on Intelligent Robots and Systems (IROS), November 7, Tokyo Big Sight, Japan (2013)
17. Schiller, J.S., Lucas, J.W., Ward, B.W., Peregoy, J.A.: Summary health statistics for U.S. adults: National Health Interview Survey, National Center for Health Statistics. Vital Health Stat. 10 (2010)
18. Brocas, A.M., Dupays, S., Hini, E.: Une approche de l'autonomie chez les adultes et les personnes agées. Études et Resultats 178, 1–8 (2010)
19. Lindenberg, U., Smith, J., Mayer, K.U., Baltes, P.B., Delius, J.: Die Berliner Altersstudie, 3rd edn. Akademie Verlag, Berlin (2010)
20. Bundesministerium für Familie, Senioren, Frauen und Jugend: Altern im Wandel, Berlin (2012)
21. NASA Task Load Index, http://humansystems.arc.nasa.gov/groups/TLX
22. Brooke, J.: System Usability Scale (SUS). Digital Equipment Corporation (1986)
23. Eisma, R., Dickinson, A., Goodman, J., Syme, A., Tiwari, L., Newell, A.: Early user involvement in the development of Information Technology-related products for older people. Universal Access in the Information Society 3(2), 131–140 (2004)
24. Marquié, J.C., Jourdan-Boddaert, L., Huet, N.: Do Older Adults Underestimate their Actual Computer Knowledge? Behaviour and Information Technology 21(4), 273–280 (2002)

Embodiment in Emotional Learning, Decision Making and Behaviour: The 'What' and the 'How' of Action

Robert Lowe

University of Skövde, Interaction Lab, Sweden
robert.lowe@his.se

Abstract. Connectionist and bio-inspired approaches to the study of emotional learning and decision making often emphasize, or imply, an executive role for the brain whilst paying only lip service to the role of the non-neural body. In this short paper I will discuss approaches to modelling emotions that have attempted to take into account, in one form or another, the role of the body in emotional learning and decision making. More specifically, I will argue that the 'how' of behavioural responding and not just the 'what' must be factored into any learning algorithm that purports to be emotional. Furthermore, I will refer to research that has utilized abstract artificial environments designed to explore the relevance of how behaviours are carried out with a view to scaling performance to more complex, including human-based, environments.

Keywords: Emotions, Neural Networks, Homeostatic grounding, Abstract environments.

1   Introduction

Connectionist and bio-inspired approaches to the study of emotional learning and decision making often emphasize, or imply, an executive role for the brain whilst paying only lip service to the role of the non-neural body. In this short paper I will discuss approaches to modelling emotions and emotion-like mechanisms that both in the absence or presence of accounting for bodily variables illuminate the need to consider emotional learning and decision making as inextricably linking the behavioural components of the 'what' (which behaviour is selected) and the 'how' (what degree of energization and also the temporal realization of behaviour). Work that has attempted to take into account, in one form or another, the role of the body, specifically, the internal body, in emotional learning and decision making, is focused on in this article. More specifically, I will argue that the 'how' of behavioural responding and not just the 'what' must be factored into any learning algorithm that purports to be emotional. I refer to research that has utilized abstract artificial environments designed to explore the relevance of how behaviours are carried out with a view to scaling performance to more complex, including human-based, environments.

C. Stephanidis and M. Antona (Eds.): UAHCI/HCII 2014, Part III, LNCS 8515, pp. 672–679, 2014.
© Springer International Publishing Switzerland 2014

2   Connectionism and Emotional Learning

The connectionist approaches to emotional learning and decision making we briefly review can be summarized as follows:

- *Neural-computational*: Typically modelled at a systems (neural-anatomic) level or informational (e.g. reinforcement learning) level of abstraction.
- *Robotic 'embodied' neural models or bio-inspired architectures*: Where neural models and bio-inspired architectures are utilized within robots either to assess the effects that physical activity has on neural/controller activity, or to evaluate the transferability of the neural model to a physically embodied system.

At a systems, or neural-anatomic, level neural computational learning mechanisms have been studied to account for the oft-cited but somewhat opposing emotional learning perspectives of LeDoux (1996) and Rolls (2001, 2005). Armony (2005) tested the dual-route hypothesis, and its neuroanatomical basis, using a computational model with self-organized winner-take all modular dynamics that they proposed captured the fundamental neural-computational features of the purported rat brain fear circuitry. The general finding was that the simulated thalamic-amygdala route was sufficient to produce Pavlovian conditioning to a tone stimulus. Lowe et al. (2009) produced an analysis of the Armony et al. model and made a number of criticisms of the modeling approach. The main limitation of the model was found to be its inability to fail to condition to the conditioned stimulus in spite of lesioning modules of the model – a trivially simple network provided similar results to the dual-route model concerning behavioural output.

The neural-computational model of Balkenius et al. (2001) (and Moren 2002), on the other hand, implements a Rolls-like contextual reinforcement algorithm. Similar to the Armony et al. model, Amygdala and Cortical modules exist. However, the Orbitofrontal Cortex (OFC) module of Balkenius et al. (2001) has a specific function – it affords context – specific inhibition of the learned amygdala output. Balkenius and Moren used a Rescorla-Wagner (1972) based algorithm for learning neutral stimulus – reinforcer stimulus associations. Amygdala units did not unlearn whereas OFC units produced fast learning context-specific activation (omission of reinforcer at stimulus presentation) enabling quick *acquisition* and *reacquisition*. Such learning might be likened to maintaining a fear representation of a snake stimulus that is behaviourally suppressed according to the context of its being in a glass cage. The context specific triggering of learned responses (inhibited or activated) comprise a particular form of affective computation.

The Balkenius and Moren model captures more data relevant to emotional learning than the Armony model and identifies the significance of key mechanisms for learning processes. Furthermore, it has been adapted and embedded within a physical robot platform (Balkenius et al. 2009) – a humanoid robot head – where cortical inputs are filtered through saliency maps based on the work of Itti and Koch (2001), see also Balkenius et al. (2008). This work increases the sense of physical embodiment in the emotional learning by demonstrating the *transferability* of the connectionist model and permits simple decision making by considering abstract motivational states that have an attentional gating effect (in relation to robot salience perception). For a further review of emotional learning neural networks see Roesch et al. (2010).

3   The Role of the Body in the 'What' of Action

The models of Armony et al. and Balkenius et al. are both lacking, from the embodiment point of view, in terms of instrumental control, i.e. which affects how behaviour regulates emotional (or value-based) learning. In particular, the aspect of timing in relation to when a particular event or behaviour can yield a rewarding or punishing outcome is of critical importance to embodied systems. Models exist that have made use of temporal difference (TD) like reinforcement learning algorithms for learning the interval of time between a predictive stimulus and a reinforcing outcome. In the case of work by Alexander and Sporns (2002) a TD-like algorithm was tested in three stages i) a disembodied neural network stage – to compare network performance against animal neurobiological learning profiles (cf. Schultz et al. 1997), ii) a physical transfer stage where the network was embedded into a khepera robot and demonstrated to perform comparably to stage i) in a non-action selection task, iii) an autonomous navigation task where the instrumental behaviour of the robot directly modulated the profile of emotional learning and resulted in emergent nesting behaviour in relation to movable objects within the robot's environment. While the robots evaluated in these cases had a simple pre-programmed behavioural/decision making repertoire concerning avoiding or approaching and then gripping coloured objects – the 'what' of action – the temporal nature of emotional learning which affected how behaviour was carried out led to a macro, or emergent behavioural response – at a different timescale - this was interpreted as a type of nesting/clustering behaviour of the movable objects.

4   The Role of the Body in the 'How' of Action

Another aspect of emotional learning and behaviour that is often ignored is the vigour of behavioural responding. This may be considered a central component of 'how' an action is carried out. While this has been of interest in a computational framework to neural-computational modellers in recent years (e.g. Niv 2009, Boureau and Dayan 2010) it has been less incorporated in connectionist-based emotional learning models embedded within robots. Vigour, when behaviourally manifested, might be interpreted in terms of speed or effort involved in movement. It provides an energizing of behavioural response. An example of an approach that has looked into the effects of energized action includes the bottom-up evolutionary robotics approach of Lowe et al. (2010). In this work a simulated e-puck robot was employed to navigate to one of two objects that represented water or food. The robot's basic motivation to approach either object depended on its artificial metabolic needs, provisioned by a model of a microbial fuel cell stack (cf. Montebelli et al. 2013).   The energetic constraints that the artificial metabolism provided, following evolved configuration of a neural network interface, determined the speed, or vigour of movement. Critically, the robot approach behaviour was a function of its ability to exploit low energy cost active vision ('saccading') in tandem with motor movement. If it moved too fast, or too slow, in relation to its 'anticipatory' active vision, it could not produce viable behaviour – sustained navigation – towards objects. How the robot carried out the behaviour was as important as what behaviour it carried out in regard to satisfying 'emotional' needs. The genetic algorithm-tuned decision making of the robot was thereby grounded in its need to appropriately energize its responses whilst exploiting facets of behaviour (saccading) with low energy constraints. The simple environment and connectionist network used are depicted in figure 1.

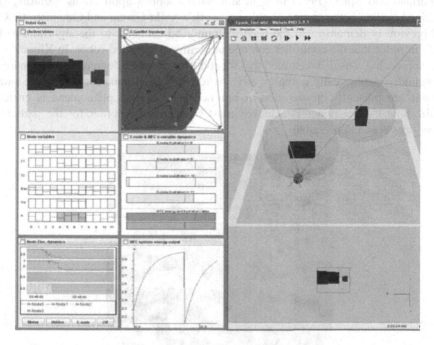

Fig. 1. E-puck *robot with artificial metabolism interfaced with neural network controller (E-GasNet).* The robot's decision making is grounded in its energizing processes – its decision making is a function of how fast it can move relative to its saccading ability. The left-hand side depicts the network dynamics (see Lowe et al. 2010 for details). The right-hand depicts the abstract environment used (in Webots) with 'food' (left) and 'water' (right) objects. Simple environments such as these allow for systematic studies of fundamental agent behaviour and cycling of decision making.

The figure illustrates the simple e-puck robot moving in an abstract artificial environment. The internal dynamics (network activity and artificial metabolism) are also visible. We do not concern ourselves here with the details of the internal dynamics. The purpose of the figure is to demonstrate that with a simple abstract environment it is possible to systematically evaluate the relationship between neural network (brain), the internal body (artificial metabolism dynamics) and the external body (robot behaviour). Identifying how the three interact in decision making can inform designing robots to interact in more complex environments.

Further recent work concerning the invigoration of performance and its effect on basic decision making within a bio-inspired architecture concerns that of Kiryazov et al. (2013a,b). This work again uses abstract environments that objectify the basic need of a robot to cycle between work and refueling activities. Kiryazov et al. demonstrated the importance of adding an arousal component which when tied to energetic constraints was critical to the sustained cycling of behaviours of a humanoid robot (the iCub). This work built on the ethological, simple model – the cue x deficit model – of McFarland and Spier (1997) used in simulated robotics applications requiring the sustained cycling between 'refueling' and 'work'. Avila-Garcia and Canamero (2005) had previously demonstrated the need for minor adjustments to the algorithm to be made in order that the controller can operate within a wheeled robot. In Kiryazov et al.'s approach it was demonstrated that for robots with more degrees of freedom, e.g. humanoids, in physically complex and challenging environments, e.g. where other humans are present, consideration of non-neural embodied phenomena is critical. Again, how the behaviour is achieved must be factored in order for the particular behaviour chosen to be viable.

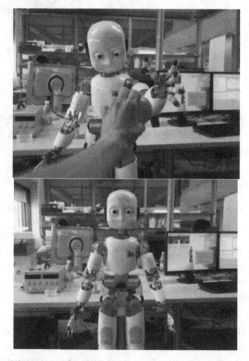

Fig. 2. iCub *robot carrying out a 2-resource action selection problem: when to 'work' (left) and when to 'refuel' (right).* In this case, the robot's 'work' entails tracking a ball moved in space by a human interactor. The faster the ball moves, the faster must the robot moves its arm to track the ball. Refuelling here entails the robot producing an orthogonal behaviour – moving its arms to its side at which point its battery can be recharged. From Kiryazov et al. (2013a,b).

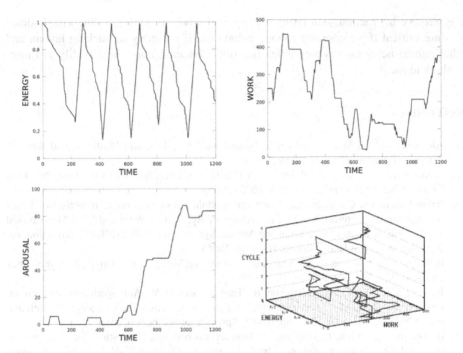

Fig. 3. The *work and fuel performance of the iCub robot (in fig. 2)*. As work performance reduces, arousal (constrained by 'energization', i.e. battery level) increases. This increase enables the robot to improve work performance, i.e. increase ball-tracking speed, and maintain behavioural stability (cf. McFarland and Spier 1997) – see bottom right sub-figure. From Kiryazov et al. (2013a).

Kiryazov et al. (2013b) also implicated 'safety' as a purported third 'resource' affecting decision making and behaviour. Essentially, for any robot to interact in natural environments – e.g. with typical/atypical adults or children – it must factor into the 'how' of its behaviour not just the speed/effort of movement required to complete a task but also how that speed/effort might potentially endanger the human interactant.

5   Grounding the 'What' and the 'How' of Emotional Learning and Decision Making in Abstract Environments

In the examples of the behaviour cycling robots, given in the previous section, using connectionist and bio-inspired models of emotion-motivation, artificial environments have been used to assess the importance of bodily variables to decision making according to an ethological/biological imperative of behaviour cycling. It is suggested that simple environments such as these provide a fundamental tool for apprehending the utility of emotional mechanisms in robots. This provides an important first step in modeling and understanding the relation between learning and decision making on the one hand, and behaviour on the other when scaled to more complex environments that may require interaction with typical or atypical adults or children. Such methodologies are critical if we consider robotic behaviour, if correctly mimicking human and other animal behaviour, is a complex function of neural, non-neural bodily and morphological factors.

References

1. Alexander, W.H., Sporns, O.: An Embodied Model of Learning Plasticity, and Reward. Adaptive Behavior (3-4), 143–159 (2002)
2. Armony, J.L.: Computational Models of Emotion. In: Proceedings of the IEEE Int. Joint Conf. on Neural Networks, pp. 1598–1602 (2005)
3. Avila-Garcia, O., Canamero, L.: Hormonal modulation of perception in motivation-based action selection architectures. In: Proceedings of Agents that Want and Like: Motivational and Emotional Roots of Cognition and Action, Symposium of the AISB05 Convention, pp. 9–17. University of Hertfordshire, Hatfield (2005)
4. Balkenius, C.: Emotional Learning: A Computational Model of the Amygdala. Cybernetics and Syst. 32, 611–636 (2001)
5. Balkenius, C., Förster, A., Johansson, B., Thorsteinsdottir, V.: Anticipation in attention. In: Pezzulo, G., Butz, M.V., Castelfranchi, C., Falcone, R. (eds.) The Challenge of Anticipation. LNCS (LNAI), vol. 5225, pp. 65–83. Springer, Heidelberg (2008)
6. Balkenius, C., Morén, J., Winberg, S.: Interactions between Motivation, Emotion and Attention: From Biology to Robotics. In: Cañamero, L., Oudeyer, P.-Y., Balkenius, C. (eds.) Proceedings of the Ninth International Conference on Epigenetic Robotics, vol. 145. Lund Univeristy Cognitive Studies (2009)
7. Boureau, Y.-L., Dayan, P.: Opponency revisited: competition and cooperation between dopamine and serotonin. Neuropsychopharmacol. Rev. 1, 1–24 (2010)
8. Itti, L., Koch, C.: Feature combination strategies for saliency-based visual attention systems. Journal of Electronic Imaging 10(1), 161–169 (2001)
9. LeDoux, J.E.: The Emotional Brain. Simon & Schuster, NewYork (1996)
10. Kiryazov, K., Lowe, R.: The role of arousal in embodying the cue-deficit model in multi-resource human-robot interaction. In: European Conference of Artificial Life (ECAL) (2013a) (accepted)
11. Kiryazov, K., Lowe, R., Becker-Asano, C., Randazzo, M.: The role of arousal in two resource problem tasks for humanoid service robots. In: 22nd IEEE International Symposium on Robot and Human Interactive Communication (Ro-Man) (2013) (in press)
12. Lowe, R., Humphries, M., Ziemke, T.: The dual-route hypothesis: evaluating a neurocomputational model of fear conditioning in rats. Connection Science 21(1), 15–37 (2009)
13. Lowe, R., Montebelli, A., Ieropoulos, I., Greenman, J., Melhuish, C., Ziemke, T.: Grounding motivation in energy autonomy: a study of artificial metabolism constrained robot dynamics. In: Fellermann, H., Drr, M., Hanczyc, M., Laursen, L., Maurer, S., Merkle, D., Monnard, P.-A., Sty, K., Rasmussen, S. (eds.) Artificial Life XII, pp. 725–732. The MIT Press, Odense (2010)
14. McFarland, D., Spier, E.: Basic cycles, utility and opportunism in self-sufficient robots. Rob. Auton. Syst. 20, 179–190 (1997)
15. Montebelli, A., Lowe, R., Ziemke, T.: Toward Metabolic Robotics: Insights from Modeling Embodied Cognition in a Biomechatronic Symbiont. Artificial Life 19, 299–315 (2013)
16. Morén, J.: LearningandEmotion. Ph.D. thesis, Lund University (2002)

17. Niv, Y.: Reinforcement learning in the brain. J. Math. Psychol. 53, 139–154 (2009)
18. Rescorla, R.A., Wagner, A.R.: A theory of pavloviancon- ditioning: variations in the effectiveness of reinforcement and non- reinforcement. In: Black, A.H., Prokasy, W.F. (eds.) Classical Conditioning II: Current Research and Theory, Appleton- Century-Crofts, New York (1972)
19. Roesch, E.B., Korsten, N.: I, Fragopanagos, J.G, Taylor. Emotions in artificial neural networks. In: Scherer, K.R., Baenziger, T., Roesch, E.B. (eds.) Blueprint for Affective Computing: a Sourcebook. Oxford University Press, Oxford (2010)
20. Rolls, E.: Précis of the brain and emotion. Behavioral and Brain Sciences 23, 177–234 (2001)
21. Rolls, E.T.: Emotion Explained. Oxford University Press, Oxford (2005)
22. Schultz, W., Dayan, P., Montague, P.R.: A neural substrate of prediction and reward. Science 275, 1593–1599 (1997)

Towards a Multi-modal User Interface
for an Affordable Assistive Robot

Peter Mayer and Paul Panek

AAT – Centre for Applied Assistive Technologies, Vienna University of Technology, Austria
{mayer,panek}@fortec.tuwien.ac.at

Abstract. This paper describes the multimodal user interface (UI) of an affordable assistive robot for older persons developed within the FP7 HOBBIT
project. Similar approaches are briefly outlined and discussed to identify similarities and differences with regard to the UI domain. The paper describes how
the developed UI enhances user interaction based on the use of available information and simple principles for a broad range of use. Some results from the
user trials with first prototype in 3 countries and 49 users are outlined. Several
UI related improvements are currently under development. The UI approach so
far seems promising and the consortium is working towards improvements for
the upcoming final HOBBIT prototype and the trials in users' homes.

Keywords: HRI, HCI, AAL, Assistive Robots.

1   Introduction

The rapidly growing area of Ambient Assisted Living (AAL) aims at developing new
services and systems for older persons in order to support their independent life as
long as possible [1]. One of the most innovative topics within AAL is the emerging
research field of assistive robots for older persons.

The Human-Robot Interaction (HRI) for (socially) assistive robotics applications
has developed to an evolving research area on its own driven by the prospects of a
growing-old population [2-6]. HRI is still based on well-established HCI principles
but also adds new challenges [7]. The physical embodiment and the autonomous activity in a shared space with the user open up new dimensions of complexity. On the
communication side, with the often anthropomorphic appearance, natural multi-modal
interaction via speech, gestures and touch but also emotions and physical cues are
called for. The expectations towards an autonomous robot include (social) situated-
ness, adaptive behavior, natural language understanding and reasoning which usually
demand rich sources of information to be collected.

In the FP7 HOBBIT project a prototype of such an assistive service robot for older
persons has been designed and developed. Considering the existing barriers the consortium decided to put the focus on user acceptance, usefulness but also affordability.

The HOBBIT robot provides autonomous navigation, a manipulator with a gripper
and a multi-modal user interface (UI) allowing interaction via speech, gesture and

C. Stephanidis and M. Antona (Eds.): UAHCI/HCII 2014, Part III, LNCS 8515, pp. 680–691, 2014.
© Springer International Publishing Switzerland 2014

touch screen and wireless call buttons [8-9]. The communication between HOBBIT modules is based on ROS [10]. The UI e.g. provides easy and unified access to information in the web, videophone service, serious games, control of robot functions (e.g. the manipulator), emergency call features and control of the AAL environment in an accessible and consistent way [11]. It is also the channel to communicate the status of the robot and ask feedback from the user. Additionally, a small display on top of the robot presents emotions by expression of eyes and mouth.

In this paper the features of the UI developed and the information it makes use of are described. It starts with an overview about the basic features of the HOBBIT robot and the discussion of some similar UI solutions. The underlying Mutual Care paradigm [12] is introduced and its influence on the UI is described and the shared context with the AAL environment is addressed.

The main part of the paper describes the different UI features. First results from user trials are reported and their taking-up in the second prototype of the UI are presented.

2   The HOBBIT Robot

The HOBBIT project aims at an affordable final prototype with limited resources excluding deep research into single aspects, development or use of costly components and substantial adaptations to the environment. Gesture recognition and localization/navigation are done with cheap Kinect-type sensors, speech recognition (ASR) and text to speech (TTS) for the user languages (Greek, Swedish, and German) are based on a commercial product and for the AAL environment a very basic set of devices is optionally foreseen.

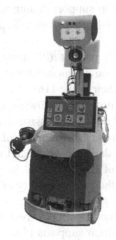

Fig. 1. HOBBIT research prototype 1 as used in first user trials

The HOBBIT robot (Fig .1) can detect with some probability whether a user is present and where by using information provided by its camera and by the distributed AAL sensors but the information is not always available with high probability because of mentioned constraints. Also the ASR and gesture recognition are not always working perfectly over the widely varying interaction distance [13], [14].

3   Similar Attempts

Many socially assistive robots for the support of old persons in the home environment have been developed as research platforms so far (e.g. NurseBot Pearl [15], DOMEO [16], KSERA [6], [17], Cogniron [18], Companionable [19], SRS [20], Care-O-Bot [21], Accompany [22], HERB [23], and many others). Nevertheless, hardly any robot really entered private households besides autonomous vacuum cleaners and lawn mowers. Robots for "real world environments" still are a challenging endeavor tackled mostly in the form of prototype research. There is even little evidence of long term trials at the users' home so far.

However the concrete robot platform has been designed, it needs a user interface (UI) sub system. Below some UI aspects of selected projects are briefly described and discussed.

3.1   Some Robot UI Examples

In the paper [24] an overview of the UI in different assistive robot projects was given including some basic information about project objectives as these also can influence the design of the UI.

- ALIAS Project: The project ALIAS ("Adaptable Ambient Living Assistant") developed a robotic platform able to support "communication and social interaction between the user and his/her social network as well as between the user and the robot platform" [25], [26].
- DOMEO Project: The DOMEO project ("Domestic Robots for Elderly Assistance") aimed to develop a new companion robotic system that allowed cognitive assistance to elderly persons in their home [16].
- KSERA Project: The KSERA project ("Knowledgeable SErvice Robots for Aging") developed a prototype of a socially assistive robot that supports older persons, especially those with Chronic Obstructive Pulmonary Disease (COPD). The aim was to provide support for daily activities and care needs and to offer means for effective self-management of their disease. In this way the independent and self-determined way of life and the overall quality of life can be enhanced [6] [17].
- CompanionAble Project: The project CompanionAble ("Integrated Cognitive Assistive & Domotic Companion Robotic Systems for Ability & Security") developed the robot "Hector" which supports older persons living at home with a specific focus on provision of cognitive support [27].

3.2   UI Similarities and Differences

The "big line" in the architecture of the UI is similar in all of the mentioned projects, e.g. a central module often called "Dialogue Manager" is available in all approaches to control the UI output based on user input and system state and coordinating the different input and output modalities.

Some differences can be attributed to the diverse robotic platforms, e.g. size and appearance of DOMEO's Kompai robot and CompanionAble's Hector robots are quite different to KSERA's small humanoid NAO robot (Fig. 2).

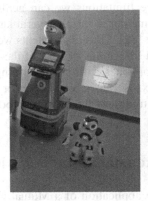 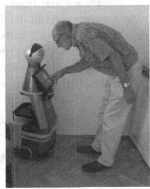

Fig. 2. Robots NAO (from KSERA) [17] and Kompai (from DOMEO) [16]

The mobility aspects of assistive robots foster the use of "hands-free" modalities, as e.g. speech recognition – despite its limited performance in noisy environments – which is useful in cases where the distance between user and robot position does not allow using the touch screen device [26], [28].

A common element in all designs is the use of some form of head, with either movable eyes (ALIAS), eye-like displays (CompanionAble's Hector, HOBBIT) or at least a fixed face (DOMEO). Touchscreens are either mounted in an approximately 45° angle or tiltable to foster the use from sitting or standing position. KSERA makes use of a beamer instead of a touchscreen [29].

When analyzing the implementations of the graphic user interface (GUI) some differences in the GUIs can be noted: while ALIAS provides text and icons (graphics) in a rather balanced way using a large text size, focus on HOBBIT's GUI is on graphics (providing only short corresponding text). In contrast, DOMEO's main menu puts its focus on a graphic only presentation. CompanionAble uses both, only icon buttons and big buttons with only text. More details in [24].

3.3   ASR Challenge

Although many projects and above UIs implement ASR, hardly any results of actual trials can be found in literature. In case of HOBBIT we found that while state of the art ASR technology works well for different applications this is only the case in the near field, i.e. short distance between user's mouth and microphone (as e.g. in case of wearable wireless microphone or a headset). As soon as the microphone is moved farther away from the user the ASR performance drops significantly. The latter case is called distant or far-field ASR and shows a significant drop in performance, which is mainly due to three different types of distortion [30]: (a) background noise, (b) echo and reverberation and (c) other types of distortions, e.g. room modes or the orientation of the speaker's head [31].

The typically needed distance for controlling the robot via voice varies from approx. 0.5 to several meters, up to situations where robot and user are in different rooms. Due to user acceptance and resource limitations we can neither expect the older persons to wear a microphone all the time nor to install several large distributed microphone arrays in the user's private home [32]. Thus experiments were carried out to explore what is possible within the current limitations of state-of-the-art ASR technology and to identify suitable (array) microphones with beam forming capabilities. We found that no off-the-shelf solution exists but acceptable error rates can be achieved for distances up to 3m by careful tuning of the audio components and the ASR engine [13].

4   Mutual Care Paradigm and Adaptability of Behavior

In HOBBIT one of the research goals is the application of a Mutual Care paradigm (robot and user helping each other) including different robot personalities from 'device' to 'butler' and 'companion'-like behavior and an evolving social role of the robot over time of use [12], [33]. As one element of the concept the user can reward the robot and the robot can offer support.

On top of the base functionality additional behavior based on the Mutual Care derived social role of the robot has been implemented. Distances and approach direction and the form of user interaction are modeled according to the intended behavior. HOBBIT is also adjusting other functions like periodically patrolling to remove obstacles from the floor and to look for the user according its social role status. The advanced behavior is derived from the social role by adaptation of certain parameters of the base functionality. In the dialogues with the user the wording and frequency of interaction are automatically adapted to the robot's role. In general, for all texts several versions for each role exist and are applied at random.

The default settings of HOBBIT are a good starting point for most users. To allow for individual adaptation a so-called Initialization Script, which is run upon first introduction of the robot to the user and later on user request, guides the user through a set of questions. The user is asked for preferences on volume and speed as well as gender of the speech output voice; the user is invited to try out speech, gesture, and screen input and can give the robot an individual name it will answer to. The final prototype will also allow configuring the individual behavior settings, such as different robot personalities (more companion-like or more machine-like) and proxemics parameters. The selected values are directly demonstrated during the process to give the user immediate feedback.

5   AAL Environment

The autonomous robot as the mobile element of HOBBIT shares information with the (AAL) environment in which it is operating in order to establish enriched context awareness. Also, the robot can make use of actuators in the environment to extend its capabilities [34], [11].

To facilitate easy calling of the robot to a specific place when user and robot are not in the same room (and therefore the ASR will not work), self-powered (energy harvesting) wireless call buttons are used as part of the AAL environment. Such stationary buttons can be placed e.g. near the bedside, in the kitchen or in the living room wherever the user frequently will be. When the user presses the call button, the robot will directly navigate to the known place of the button so that it brings itself into a closer interaction distance and pose relative to the user which is suitable for touch-screen, speech and gesture operation.

A small set of wireless movement (PIR) and contact sensors can be added to provide location based activity information to the robot in form of accumulated activity status indicators. Actuators can be installed to e.g. control lights during nighttime to reduce the risk of falling.

For the AAL environment tests in an AAL lab [11] with different zones modeled similar to a realistic home environment were performed.

The implemented HOBBIT AAL interface is basically based on a USB transceiver for the EnOcean standard and is prepared for integration of other already in place automation devices via generic interfaces e.g. OpenHAB [35].

6   HOBBIT's User Interface (UI)

In the project a concept for handling limited reliability and sparse information as base for a multi-modal UI without the full functionality yet in place had to be found. Despite its flexibility and the internal handling of some interaction aspects the UI nevertheless shall offer a highly predictable interface to the task execution modules responsible for the navigation and grasping. This requires some autonomy of the UI including independent fusion of modalities and own capabilities for performing sub-dialogues with the user.

As core of the UI the multi-modal dialogues are based on a graphical UI (GUI) with a menu structure of several levels containing buttons with the commands that can be given to the system. This menu structure is handled autonomously by the GUI and many functions (media, information) are handled internally by the GUI. Knowledge from previous successful user centered research projects with older persons has been integrated in the design of the menu structure [36], [37]. Commands related to robot functions are forwarded to the robot control engine via ROS and handled there making use of a UI Dialogue Manager service for dynamic feedback.

The dynamic prompts that are used for reporting status and asking feedback from the user follow a common design with the static GUI menu pages the user can navigate through (Fig. 3). Usability aspects and as far as possible design for all principles have been an important consideration when designing the UI.

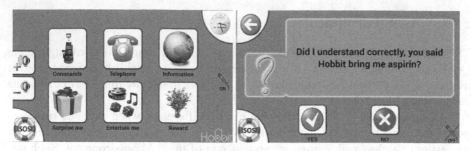

Fig. 3. GUI used for prototype 1 (PT1): static menu and dynamic prompt

Users over time often become annoyed by robot-like i.e. lifeless and stereotypic behavior. The robot therefore shall be able to make use of emotions and variants of formulations when presenting output avoiding saying exactly the same phrase again every day [3, p.687] On the other hand the behavior must not become totally surprising to avoid uneasy feeling towards the dependability of the robot. Most users prefer a robot companion to be predictable, controllable, considerate and polite [3, p.688].

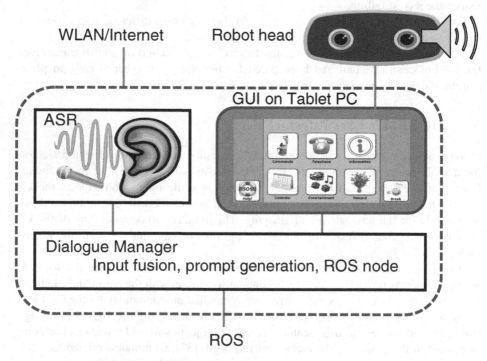

Fig. 4. UI Architecture overview

The finally chosen UI architecture combines the strengths of a basic GUI in the core with dynamic prompts under the control of a dialogue manager for all the input and output modalities. The command options for the user and any output are shown on the GUI and announced by TTS, user input can come from ASR, touchscreen or gesture as chosen by the user and is always followed by consistent multi-modal feedback clearly showing which selection was made and which options are available. For the HOBBIT system the UI appears as one single ROS node handling all user interaction (Fig. 4).

Although not strictly part of the UI, the expressiveness of the UI can optionally be combined and enhanced with a set of emotions shown via the robot's eyes (tired, surprised, concerned...) on the head displays and movements of the robot platform (nervous, happy...). Such behavior is controlled by emotion parameters in the dialog requests and automatically adapted to the current social role of the robot.

Nowadays quite impressive server based ASR solutions exist and have been considered (e.g. Siri, Google), however, for reliability reasons the decision was made to avoid the dependence on an external data link and go for a fully local solution. Also existing local dictation engines (Dragon) have been considered but found to be limited to few languages and depending too much on dictation context for good results. As a result, a local context free command grammar based ASR engine was chosen. The UI handles input by gestures and ASR based on their confidence levels and autonomously asks the user to repeat a command (by any modality) or to confirm (Fig. 3).

As the available ASR solutions are not fully satisfactory, the ASR module was designed as a standalone solution which can easily be replaced in future. For the ASR microphone a small microphone array with beam-forming, noise suppression and echo cancellation post-processing was chosen as the best compromise.

TTS output is provided by a set of SAPI-based male and female voices. Speaker independent ASR and text to speech (TTS) are currently offered in the user site languages (Greek, Swedish, German and English). The language dependent settings (ASR grammar, texts for GUI and TTS) are part of the configuration and allow for easy localization via editable text files.

A set of hand gestures are detected by a specialized HOBBIT ROS module working with Kinect-type camera input [14]. These gestures are combined with other input in the Dialogue Manager and can transparently be used to call for help, point to objects, or answer prompts of the UI.

As conclusion, the interaction with HOBBIT based on distance of the user to HOBBIT can be done either by:

— Wireless call button (far, from other rooms),
— Speech (ASR) and gesture (2-3m),
— Touchscreen (arm length).

6.1 Lessons Learned from first User Trials

First empirical user studies in a controlled laboratory setting with the HOBBIT prototype were carried out in Austria, Greece, and Sweden, with a total of 49 primary participants [38]. The studies were based on six representative tasks that should demonstrate the key behaviors of HOBBIT to the participants and that should enable us to explore the following research questions:

— How do older adults (with representative age impairments) perceive the multimodal interaction possibilities of HOBBIT in terms of usability?
— Do older adults accept HOBBIT as assistive household robot after interacting with it in the laboratory?
— How do older adults perceive the value of HOBBIT as support to enable independent living at home with respect to affordability and willingness to pay for it?

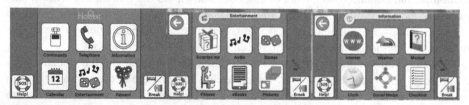

Fig. 5. Early UI prototype for upcoming PT2 considering findings from PT1 trials

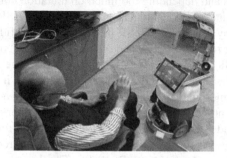

Fig. 6. User interaction test scene

Regarding UI the most important findings were in the usability area: the multimodal user interface based on touch screen, gestures and voice input was found to be useful by the vast majority of users (96%). Voice commands and touch screen were liked best as operation mode by primary users. This and some other lessons learned from PT1 user trials guided the redesign for prototype 2 (PT2):

— The round corner icons of the GUI were not always identified as buttons and therefore were changed to the rectangular design of the other buttons. For the GUI of the PT2 a set of new icons have been designed including those for the new PT2 functions (Fig. 5).
— The extendible UI mounted on a mechanical slider so that it could be pulled towards the user for the most ergonomic position was rarely used although the users were reminded of it. As a consequence, the mounting of the touchscreen in PT2 was changed to a fixed, protruding position.
— Many users did not wait to give voice commands only after the beep indicating that the ASR is listening for commands. In PT2 this restriction was released (Fig. 6).

Another test series was performed to find out the robot's ability to draw user's attention by its behavior [39]. For this test a setup was chosen where a user was busy doing a complex search task. The robot several times approached and offered help (which it could not actually provide) or showed some other behavior. The results indicate that necessary distracting behaviors (e.g. the robot has to remind the user of something) can be designed in a socially normative manner and that a robot not necessarily bothers the user, but only distracts him/her from a primary task [39].

7   Conclusions and Outlook

This paper described the development of an UI in the HOBBIT robot project, how the developed UI architecture enhances user interaction based on the use of available information and simple principles for a broad range of use.

Despite the limitations due to the project's vision of an affordable (low cost) assistive robot the UI approach so far seems promising and the consortium is working towards improvements for the upcoming final HOBBIT prototype and the final trials in users' homes.

Acknowledgements. The research leading to these results has received partial funding from the European Community's FP7 under grant agreement No. 288146. For details on the project see http://hobbit.acin.tuwien.ac.at/.

References

1. van den Broek, G., Cavallo, F., Odetti, L., Wehrmann, C.: Ambient Assisted Living Roadmap. VDI/VDE-IT (2009)
2. Feil-Seifer, D., Mataric, M.J.: Defining socially assistive robotics. In: Intern. Conf. on Rehabilitation Robotics, pp. 465–468 (2005)
3. Dautenhahn, K.: Socially intelligent robots: dimensions of human–robot interaction. Philos. Trans. R. So.c Lond B Biol. Sci. 362(1480), 679–704 (2007)
4. Dautenhahn, K.: Human-Robot Interaction. In: Soegaard, M., Dam, R.F. (eds.) The Encyclopedia of Human-Computer Interaction, 2nd edn. The Interaction Design Foundation, Aarhus (2013),
   http://www.interaction-design.org/encyclopedia/
   human-robot_interaction.html
5. Tapus, A., Mataric, M.J., Scassellati, B.: Socially assistive robotics. IEEE Robotics and Automation Magazine 14(1), 35 (2007)
6. Johnson, D.O., Cuijpers, R., Juola, J.F., Torta, E., Simonov, M., Frisiello, A., Bazzani, M., Yan, W., Weber, C., Wermter, S., Meins, N., Oberzaucher, J., Panek, P., Edelmayer, G., Mayer, P., Beck, C.: Socially Assistive Robots: A comprehensive approach to extending independent living. International Journal of Social Robotics, 1–17, doi:10.1007/s12369-013-0217-8
7. Goodrich, M.A., Schultz, A.C.: Human–Robot Interaction: A Survey 1(3), S.203–S.275 (2007), doi:10.1561/1100000005
8. Fischinger, D., Einramhof, P., Wohlkinger, W., Papoutsakis, K., Mayer, P., Panek, P., Koertner, T., Hofmann, S., Argyros, A., Vincze, M., Weiss, A., Gisinger, C.: HOBBIT - The Mutual Care Robot. To be printed at Assistance and Service Robotics in a Human Environment Workshop in conjunction with IEEE/RSJ International Conference on Intelligent Robots and Systems, Tokyo (November 2013)

9. Zagler, W.L., Mayer, P., Panek, P., Vincze, M., Weiss, A., Bajones, M., Puente, P., Huber, A., Lammer, L., Fischinger, D.: Roboter-Unterstützung zu Hause - Das Projekt HOBBIT (Robotic support at home – The HOBBIT project). In: 7th German AAL Congress, Berlin, Germany (2014)

10. Robot Operating System, http://www.ros.org/

11. Mayer, P., Panek, P.: A Social Assistive Robot in an Intelligent Environment. BioMed. Tech. 58, 1 (2013)

12. Lammer, L., Huber, A., Zagler, W., Vincze, M.: Mutual care: Users will love their imperfect social assistive robots. In: Proc. Intern. Conf. on Social Robotics (ICSR 2011), Amsterdam (2011)

13. Panek, P., Mayer, P.: Challenges in adopting speech control for assistive robots. In: 7th German AAL Congress, Berlin, Germany (January 2014)

14. Papoutsakis, K., Padeleris, P., Ntelidakis, A., Stefanou, S., Zabulis, X., Kosmopoulos, D., Argyros, A.A.: Developing visual competencies for socially assistive robots: the HOBBIT approach. In: To appear in Proceedings of Workshop on Robotics in Assistive Environments (RasEnv 2013), Conjunction with PETRA 2013, Rhodes, Greece, May 28-30 (2013)

15. Pineau, J., Montemerlo, M., Pollack, M., Roy, N., Thrun, S.: Towards robotic assistants in nursing homes: Challenges and results. Robotics and Autonomous Systems 42(3), 271–281 (2003)

16. Project Domeo, http://www.aal-domeo.org/

17. Project KSREA, http://ksera.ieis.tue.nl/

18. Project Cogniron, http://www.cogniron.org/

19. Project Companionable, http://www.companionable.net/

20. Project SRS, http://srs-project.eu/

21. Project Care-o-Bot, http://www.care-o-bot.de/

22. Project Accompany, http://www.accompanyproject.eu/

23. Project Herb, http://www.cmu.edu/herb-robot/

24. Mayer, P., Beck, C., Panek, P.: Examples of multimodal user interfaces for socially assistive robots in Ambient Assisted Living environments. In: 2012 IEEE 3rd International Conference on Cognitive Infocommunications (CogInfoCom), Košice, Slovakia, December 2-5, pp. 401–406 (2012)

25. Rehrl, T., Blume, J., Geiger, J., Bannat, A., Wallhoff, F., Ihsen, S., Jeanrenaud, Y., Merten, M., Schönebeck, B., Glende, S., Nedopil, C.: ALIAS: Der anpassungsfähige Ambient Living Assistent. In: 4th German AAL Congress, Berlin (2011)

26. Goetze, S., Fischer, S., Moritz, N., Appell, J.E., Wallhoff, F.: Multimodal Human-Machine Interaction for Service Robots in Home-Care Environments. In: Proceedings of the 1st Workshop on Speech and Multimodal Interaction in Assistive Environments, Jeju, Republic of Korea, July 8-14, pp. 1–7 (2012)

27. Merten, M., Bley, A., Schröter, C., Gross, H.M.: A mobile robot platform for socially assistive home-care applications. In: Proc. 5th German Conference on Robotics, Munich, Germany, pp. 233–238 (2012)

28. Granata, C., et al.: Voice and graphical -based interfaces for interaction with a robot dedicated to elderly and people with cognitive disorders. In: 2010 IEEE RO-MAN. IEEE (2010)

29. Panek, P., Edelmayer, G., Mayer, P., Beck, C., Zagler, W.L.: Mobile Video Phone Communication Carried by a NAO Robot. In: Ambient Assisted Living, pp. 315–325. Springer, Heidelberg (2014)

30. Wölfel, M., McDonough, J.: Distant Speech Recognition. John Wiley & Sons Ltd., Chichester (2009)

31. Vincent, E., et al.: The second 'CHiME' speech separation and recognition challenge: an overview of challenge systems and outcomes. In: 2013 IEEE Automatic Speech Recognition and Understanding Workshop (2013)
32. Distant-speech Interaction for Robust Home Applications, http://dirha.fbk.eu/
33. Huber, A., Lammer, L., Vincze, M.: Mutual Care in Social Assistive Robotics. In: Proceedings of the International Conference on Cognitive Systems (CogSys 2012) (2012)
34. Cavallo, F., Aquilano, M., Bonaccorsi, M., Limosani, R., Manzi, A., Carrozza, M.C., Dario, P.: On the design, development and experimentation of the ASTRO assistive robot integrated in smart environments. In: 2013 IEEE International Conference on Robotics and Automation (ICRA), pp. 4310–4315. IEEE (May 2013)
35. OpenHAB, http://www.openhab.org
36. Oberzaucher, J., Werner, K., Mairböck, H.P., Beck, C., Panek, P., Hlauschek, W., Zagler, W.L.: A videophone prototype system evaluated by elderly users in the living lab schwechat. In: Holzinger, A., Miesenberger, K. (eds.) USAB 2009. LNCS, vol. 5889, pp. 345–352. Springer, Heidelberg (2009)
37. Werner, K., Oberzaucher, J., Panek, P., Beck, C., Mayer, P.: Development of an assistive home user interface together with older users. In: Everyday Technology for Independence and Care–AAATE 2011. Assistive Technology Research Series, vol. 29, pp. 473–480. IOS Press, Amsterdam (2011)
38. HOBBIT Deliverable D1.4: Report on the results of the PT1 user trials, HOBBIT consortium (May 2013)
39. Weiss, A., Vincze, M., Panek, P., Mayer, P.: Don't Bother Me: Users' Reactions to Different Robot Disturbing Behaviors. In: To be printed in HRI 2014, Bielefeld, Germany (2014)

Advances in Intelligent Mobility Assistance Robot Integrating Multimodal Sensory Processing

Xanthi S. Papageorgiou[1], Costas S. Tzafestas[1], Petros Maragos[1], Georgios Pavlakos[1], Georgia Chalvatzaki[1], George Moustris[1], Iasonas Kokkinos[2], Angelika Peer[3], Bartlomiej Stanczyk[4], Evita-Stavroula Fotinea[5], and Eleni Efthimiou[5]

[1] Inst. of Communication & Computer Systems,
National Technical Univ. of Athens, Greece
{xpapag,gmoustri}@mail.ntua.gr,
{ktzaf,maragos}@cs.ntua.gr,
geopavlakos@gmail.com,
gchal@central.ntua.gr
[2] INRIA Ecole Centrale Paris, France
iasonas.kokkinos@ecp.fr
[3] Technische Universität München, Munich, Germany
Angelika.Peer@tum.de
[4] ACCREA Engineering, Lublin, Poland
b.stanczyk@accrea.com
[5] Institute for Language and Speech Processing,
ATHENA RC, Athens, Greece
{evita,eleni_e}@ilsp.gr

Abstract. Mobility disabilities are prevalent in our ageing society and impede activities important for the independent living of elderly people and their quality of life. The goal of this work is to support human mobility and thus enforce fitness and vitality by developing intelligent robotic platforms designed to provide user-centred and natural support for ambulating in indoor environments. We envision the design of cognitive mobile robotic systems that can monitor and understand specific forms of human activity, in order to deduce what the human needs are, in terms of mobility. The goal is to provide user and context adaptive active support and ambulation assistance to elderly users, and generally to individuals with specific forms of moderate to mild walking impairment.

To achieve such targets, a reliable multimodal action recognition system needs to be developed, that can monitor, analyse and predict the user actions with a high level of accuracy and detail. Different modalities need to be combined into an integrated action recognition system. This paper reports current advances regarding the development and implementation of the first walking assistance robot prototype, which consists of a sensorized and actuated rollator platform. The main thrust of our approach is based on the enhancement of computer vision techniques with modalities that are broadly used in robotics, such as range images and haptic data, as well as on the integration of machine learning and pattern recognition approaches regarding specific verbal and non-verbal (gestural) commands in the envisaged (physical and non-physical) human-robot interaction context.

C. Stephanidis and M. Antona (Eds.): UAHCI/HCII 2014, Part III, LNCS 8515, pp. 692–703, 2014.
© Springer International Publishing Switzerland 2014

1 Introduction

1.1 Motivation

Mobility problems, particularly concerning the elderly population, constitute a major issue in our society. According to recent reports, approximately 20% of people aged 70 years or older, and 50% of people aged 85 and over, report difficulties in basic activities of daily living. Mobility disabilities are common and impede many activities important to independent living, [1], [2]. A significant proportion of older people have serious mobility problems. Furthermore, current demographics show that the elderly population (aged over 65) in industrialized countries shows a constant increase, [3].

Mobility is a crucial activity especially in the elderly since it promotes physical exercise, independence and self-esteem. Robotics seems to fit naturally to the role of assistance since it can incorporate features such as posture support and stability, walking assistance, navigation in indoor and outdoor environments, health monitoring etc. Our motivation in this approach stems from the fact that for an efficient and intelligent robotic assistant, a variety of multimodal interaction and cognitive control functionalities must be embedded, so that the robot can autonomously reason about how to provide optimal support to the user whenever and wherever needed.

1.2 Related Work

Several intelligent robot mobility aids are known, which are divided into two large categories: robotic wheelchairs and robotic walkers, [4]. They are designed to accommodate a normal walking pattern with opposite arm and leg moving together. Most robotic walkers are robotized variations of the typical Rollator frame, which is a standard walking frame attached to wheels, mainly used where balance -rather than weight bearing- is the major problem.

Many robotic walkers have been developed, generally presenting some of the following functionalities: (i) physical support; (ii) sensorial assistance; (iii) cognitive assistance; (iv) health monitoring and (v) advanced human - machine interface, [5]. These platforms largely fall into two categories: passive and active devices, [6]. While passive mobility aids either steer or brake, but cannot move forward without the human applying forces on them, [7]-[9], active devices are equipped with actuators and thus, their motion and interaction behaviour can be actively controlled, [10]-[12].

The research work reported in this paper aims to further extend and enhance the functionalities of such systems, by focusing on the development of robotic mobility aids for indoor environments that provide intelligent and active walking/mobility assistance (standing up, walking, and sitting down) to elderly people (with and without enough strength to support and stabilize themselves), in particular by supporting safe autonomous proactive control (for instance, by incorporating fall prevention features) and adaptive user-robot interaction, through multimodal sensory processing and intuitive human-robot communication.

1.3   Organization and Overview

This paper is organized as follows. In Section 2, the first prototype of the experimental platform is described. The multimodal information processing and action recognition system is discussed in Section 3. The appropriate analysis and identification of human walking motions and classification of specific mobility weaknesses are discussed in Section 4. The design of a context-aware control architecture for an active mobility aid robot is briefly analysed in Section 5. Finally, conclusion and plans for future work are given in Section 6.

2   Experimental Platform

The experimental platform consists of a sensorised passive rollator prototype, as depicted in Fig. 1, which has already been used for the purposes of data collection and recording in a set of predefined typical use-cases and scenarios involving elderly people. The system incorporates multimodal information from laser range finder sensors, force/torque sensors, RGB and RGB-D cameras, encoders, and microphones.

First of all two laser sensors are used on the experimental platform. The first sensor (Hokuyo UTM-30LX) is placed at the front of the platform facing towards the motion direction, to provide full scanning of the walking area. For the purpose of human legs' detection and tracking, a second laser range finder (Hokuyo UBG-04LX-F01 rapid LRF) sensor is mounted at the back of the experimental platform facing the user legs, scanning a horizontal plane at the lower limbs at a height of approximately 40cm from

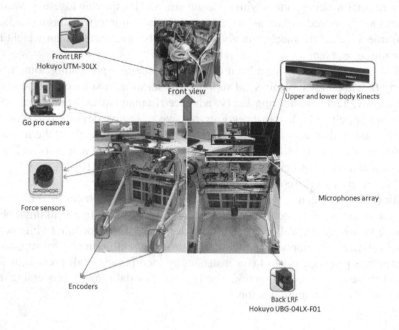

Fig. 1. Experimental platform: first sensorized prototype used for data acquisition and recordings

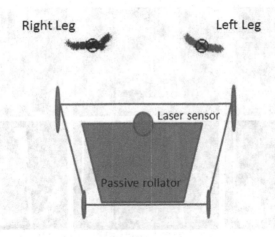

Fig. 2. A snapshot of the detected user's legs along the legs' centers

the ground, in order to take measurements from the users' gaiting performance. An example of the detected subject's legs is depicted in Fig. 2. A rectangular area (a search window) in front of the laser sensor is defined, inside of which we search for the potential user legs. For the detection process, a simple background extraction is used, in which we discard outliers that do not satisfy certain constraints defined for the potential legs, such as the minimum distance between consecutive points in each scanning frame and also the jump distance between neighboring laser groups. Subsquently, a K-means clustering algorithm is implemented to detect the legs' clusters.

Furthermore, two 6 DOF HR3 force/torque sensors (JR3 45E15) are placed at the handles of the experimental rollator in order to measure the applied forces between the patient and the rollator. In addition to the above sensors, an HD small, high performance and versatile video camera (GoPro) is also mounted on the rollator. This device is able to record the patient's head, torso, arms and all his/her movements and it provides necessary information for the subject's condition.

Another set of sensors placed on the rollator consists of two Kinect-for-Windows (KFW) sensors. This set of sensors allows the recording of the human body from a short distance. The first KFW sensor is placed horizontally towards the patient, in order to capture the area of the torso, waist, hips and the upper part of the limbs. The second KFW sensor is facing downwards in complementary direction with the first one, so as to achieve broad coverage and not to interfere with each other. This second sensor is able to capture the lower limb motion information, and therefore to enhance the localisation of limb positions and assist the analysis of gait abnormalities.

In addition to the above, an array of 8-microphone MEMS is also used as audio capturing device, mounted on the horizontal bar of the experimental platform in a linear configuration (with a 4cm uniform spacing) in front of the user (see Fig. 1). An example of a specific audio-gestural command is depicted in Fig. 3 (the captured audio visual data for the command "MOBOT: I want to stand up"). The visual data is obtained from the RGB and depth stream of the Kinect visual sensor while the audio data from the

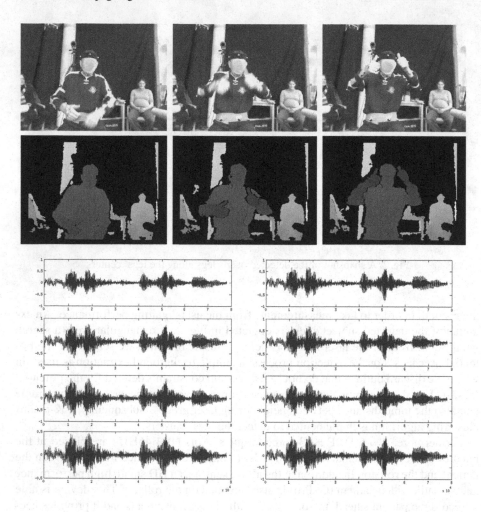

Fig. 3. Multimodal data captured for a specific audio-gestural command ("MOBOT: I want to stand up", "MOBOT: Ich will aufstehen"). Top: RGB data from Kinect, Middle: Depth data from Kinect, and Bottom: Multichannel waveform outputs from MEMS microphone array.

microphone array mounted on the rollator. A distinct waveform for each channel of the MEMS microphone array is presented along with indicative frames of the visual stream.

3   Multimodal Sensory Processing for Human Action Recognition

Different sensory modalities need to be combined into an integrated human action recognition system. The development of robust and effective computer vision techniques are needed in order to achieve the visual processing goals based on multiple cues such as spatio-temporal RGB appearance data as well as depth data from Kinect sensors. The enhancement of computer vision techniques with modalities that are broadly used in robotics, such as range images and haptic data will be introduced. Another major challenge is the integration of recognizing specific verbal and non-verbal (gestural) commands in the considered human-robot interaction context. All the above technical problems and research challenges embody all tasks related to visual, speech, haptic, and physiological data processing for detecting, tracking and recognizing the human actions. Specific objectives include the following:

- detection of human actions rapidly and robustly based on low and high level information,
- classification of human actions by analyzing spatio-temporal video information,
- analysis of walking patterns and detection of abnormalities by tracking human body pose,
- processing of multimodal data (visual, speech, haptic, physiology) originating from different sensors,
- developing of isolated spoken and gestural command recognition capabilities for human-robot communication, and
- ultimately performing human action recognition by multimodal sensory integration.

The approach followed towards this end is divided into several tasks in the current study. The first task focuses on visual processing for human localisation and action classification, based on a set of enhanced visual features and object representations. Another task is related to limb localisation and body pose estimation, combining visual appearance, motion and range data, that is, also exploiting data provided by the Kinects' depth sensors. Results of this task will also be integrated in a system performing isolated gesture recognition, which is currently under development and testing. Preliminary results in this direction are very promising, showing that the combination of multiple modalities enhances specific performance characteristics. Another task focuses on spoken command processing for human-robot communication and is based on HMMs for the recognition of specific spoken commands from distant microphones. Multimodal fusion approaches are also being investigated to achieve human action recognition, integrating cues from various sensorial modalities, including vision (RGB appearance, depth, tracking data) and speech modalities.

4 Human Action Analysis

One of the main goals of our work is to perform analysis and identification of human walking motions and classification of specific walking pathologies and associated mobility weaknesses. The idea is to conceptually and systematically synthesize all the modules performing multimodal recognition and inference regarding human behaviour and user intent, onto generative context-aware mobility assistance models. Towards this end, we investigate a completely non-invasive framework for analyzing a normal human walking gait pattern, which is described in this section.

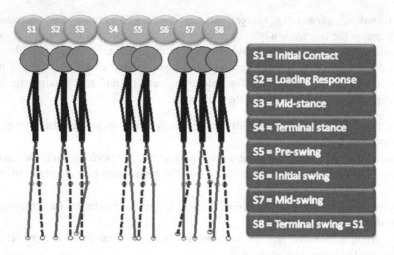

Fig. 4. Internal states of normal gait cycle (Left Leg: blue dashed line, Right Leg: red solid line)

4.1   Normal Human Gait Cycle Description

A well-known fact is that the walking patterns are gaits, that is, cyclic patterns with several consecutive phases. These cyclic motions can be modelled using a set of consecutive and repetitive gait phases. A basic requisite of the act of walking is the periodic movement of each foot from one position of support to the next. This element is necessary for any form of bipedal walking to occur, no matter how distorted the pattern may be by an underlying pathology, [13]. This periodic leg movement is the essence of the cyclic nature of human gait.

There are two main phases in the gait cycle, [14,15]: The **stance phase**, when the foot is on the ground, and the **swing phase** when that same foot is no longer in contact with the ground and is swinging through in preparation for the next foot strike. The stance phase may be subdivided into three separate phases: 1. First double support, when both feet are in contact with the ground, 2. Single limb stance, when only one foot is in ground contact and the other foot is swinging forward, 3. Second double support, when both feet are again in ground contact. The same terminology would be applied for both the left and right side of the body. For a normal person, each side is half a cycle behind (or ahead) of the other side. Thus, first double support for the right side is second double support for the left side, and vice versa. In normal gait there is a natural symmetry between the left and right sides, but in pathological gait an asymmetrical pattern very often exists.

Traditionally the gait cycle has been divided into eight events or periods, five during stance phase and three during swing.

The stance phase events are as follows (see Fig. 4):

1. Heel strike initiates the gait cycle and represents the point at which the body's centre of gravity is at its lowest position.

2. Foot-flat is the time when the plantar surface of the foot touches the ground.
3. Midstance occurs when the swinging (contralateral) foot passes the stance foot and the body's centre of gravity is at its highest position.
4. Heel-off occurs as the heel loses contact with the ground and pushoff is initiated via the triceps surae muscles, which plantar flex the ankle.
5. Toe-off terminates the stance phase as the foot leaves the ground, [16].

The swing phase events are as follows:

6. Acceleration begins as soon as the foot leaves the ground and the subject activates the hip flexor muscles to accelerate the leg forward.
7. Midswing occurs when the foot passes directly beneath the body, coincidental with midstance for the other foot.
8. Deceleration describes the action of the muscles as they slow the leg and stabilize the foot in preparation for the next heel strike.

Thus, there are eight events, but these are sufficiently general to be applied to any type of gait as shown in Table 4.1.

Table 1. Gait Cycle Events, [14]

Gait Phase	% Duration
1. Initial contact - **IC**	(0%)
2. Loading response - **LR**	(0-10%)
3. Midstance - **MS**	(10-30%)
4. Terminal stance - **TS**	(30-50%)
5. Preswing - **PW**	(50-60%)
6. Initial Swing - **IW**	(60-70%)
7. Midswing - **MW**	(70-85%)
8. Terminal swing - **TW**	(85-100%)

4.2   Detection of Gait Cycle Based on Hidden Markov Model

Hidden Markov Models are well suited for gait analysis and recognition because of their statistical properties and their ability to reflect the temporal state-transition nature of gait. An HMM is defined as a doubly embedded stochastic process with an underlying process that is not observable (i.e. it is hidden), but can only be observed through another set of stochastic processes that produce the sequence of observations [17][18]. This means that the states underlying the data generation process are hidden and can only be inferred through observations. HMMs are very common in several applications such as speech recognition [18][19], biological sequence analysis [20], gesture recognition [21], as well as human activity analysis [22].

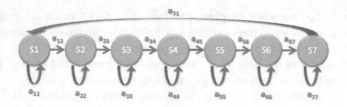

Fig. 5. The topology of the network used for gait analysis and recognition is based on a left-to-right Hidden Markov Model

Based on the analysis of Subsection 4.1, the idea is to build a model that can distinguish between the different gait phases in order to analyze the normal gait cycle. The number of phases used in this study are seven, since the Terminal Swing phase is characterized by heel strike, which is an equivalent trigger as for Initial Contact phase, meaning that these two phases (TW and IC) can be eventually treated as identical. These seven gait phases, thus, correspond to the hidden states of the HMM. As observables, several quantities that represent the motion of the subjects' legs are used. These quantities are estimated using sequential signals from the laser range finder sensor that collects appropriate data (such as relative position w.r.t. the laser, velocities, etc.), while the rollator follows the subject's motion.

Following the HMM notation, the transition probability matrix is defined as

$$A = \{a_{ij}\}, \quad \text{where} \quad a_{ij} = P[s_{t+1} = j | s_t = i], \quad \text{for} \quad 1 \leq i, j \leq N,$$

where N is the number of states, and the (i, j) element of the matrix A represents the transition probability from the ith state, at a given time step t, to the jth state at the following time step (where $t = 1, 2, ..., T$, and T denotes the total time). In the normal gait cycle, the gait phases follow each other sequentially. Thus, this HMM is a left-to-right model. This means that the only feasible transitions from a state i will be either to remain in the same state or to jump to the following adjacent state, as depicted in Fig. 5. The transition probability matrix, as well as the prior probability vector (i.e. the vector of probabilities π_i of the system being at state i at the initial time t_0), are estimated using the standard and well known Baum-Welch algorithm, [18].

Initial results obtained by applying this model in normal human gait data are very promising [23], and demonstrate that this human data analysis scheme has the potential to provide the necessary methodological (modeling, inference, and learning) framework for a cognitive behavior-based robot control system. More specifically, the proposed framework has the potential to be used for the recognition of abnormal gait patterns and the subsequent classification of specific walking pathologies, which is needed for the development of a context-aware robot mobility assistant.

5   Context-Aware Robot Control

All the subsystems and individual signal processing and control modules developed to achieve some of the aforementioned functionalities need to be integrated seamlessly

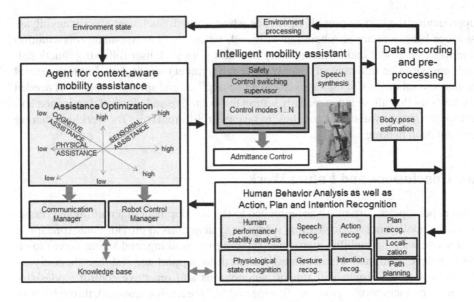

Fig. 6. Context-aware Mobility Assistant Architecture

into a full-scale robot control system. The current form of the overall functional robot control architecture, encompassing all these submodules, is depicted in Fig. 6. One of the most important characteristics of this system is that it must perform context-aware operations, that is, it must reason and adapt its operational behaviour based on the following information:

– environment state,
– user behaviour, physiological state, and action, plan, and intention recognition,
– user-robot interaction context (verbal or non-verbal, vocal or non-vocal, physical or non-contact, etc.).

Two basic modules are currently being integrated and tested on the platform. Firstly, all the methods and algorithms necessary to enable autonomous sensor-based navigation of the mobile robot assistant in an indoor domestic environment are being developed and integrated. These include: map creation and localisation on static or dynamic maps, global path planning (using metric and/or topological map representations), obstacle detection and on-line collision avoidance, and targeted (goal-oriented) motion control supported by realtime path planning. Secondly, all methods and control algorithms for physical user-robot interaction are being developed, Currently, an adaptive admittance controller is being integrated on the platform, providing haptic collision-avoidance assistance to the user. Indeed, the robot walking assistant is equipped with two haptic interaction points (force/torque sensors on the two handles) and is able to apply different assistance policies when physically supporting a user.

Non-physical user-robot interaction modules are also under development, meaning that the mobility assistant does not necessarily have to be in continuous contact with the user, but could accompany him/her while walking from one place to the other, only approaching the user to provide assistance when needed. Such user-accompanying assistance behaviors are also being investigated, where the corresponding robot motion controllers that will endow the mobility assistant with such user following functionalities are based on non-contact (mainly, laser rangefinder) sensor data. In more general terms, several models of user assistance can be applied, and special emphasis is needed on schemes that allow independently setting the cognitive and physical dominance levels for the mobility assistant and thus, to take over different roles for workload sharing and decision making.

6 Conclusions and Future Work

This paper reports current advances related to the development of a multimodal framework for intelligent robotic mobility aids. The system aims to provide context-adaptive and active walking/mobility assistance (standing up, walking, and sitting down) to elderly people (with and without enough strength to support and stabilize themselves). In particular, the system will support autonomous and proactive control modes (for instance, by incorporating user monitoring and fall prevention features), through multimodal sensory processing empowering intuitive human-robot interaction.

For further research, a reliable multimodal action recognition system needs to be enhanced, that will monitor and analyse human actions and predict user intentions with a high level of accuracy and detail. Different modalities will be combined into an integrated action recognition system. The main thrust of our approach is based on the enhancement of computer vision techniques with modalities that are broadly used in robotics, such as range images and haptic data, as well as the integration of pattern recognition modules focusing on specific verbal and non-verbal (gestural) commands in the considered human-robot interaction context. A context-aware robot control architecture will be further developed to synthesize all these multimodal sensory processing and pattern recognition modules into human-adaptive assistance models, aiming to provide optimal physical and/or cognitive support to the user.

Acknowledgment. This work is supported by 7th Framework Program of the European Union, ICT Challenge 2, Cognitive Systems and Robotics, contract "EU-FP7-ICT-2011-9 2.1 - 600796 - MOBOT: Intelligent Active MObility Assistance RoBOT Integrating Multimodal Sensory Processing, Proactive Autonomy and Adaptive Interaction".

References

1. Parkinson Disease Foundation. Statistics for parkinson's disease (2010)
2. Stroke Center. Stroke statistics (2010)
3. USCensus. The elderly population (2010)
4. Machiel Van der Loos, H.F., Reinkensmeyer, D.J.: Rehabilitation and health care robotics. In: Siciliano, B., Khatib, O. (eds.) Springer Handbook of Robotics, pp. 1223–1251. Springer, Heidelberg (2008)

5. Martins, M.M., Santos, C.P., Frizera-Neto, A., Ceres, R.: Assistive mobility devices focusing on smart walkers: Classification and review. Robotics and Autonomous Systems 60(4), 548–562 (2012)
6. Ko, C.-H., Agrawal, S.K.: Walk-assist robot: A novel approach to gain selection of a braking controller using differential flatness. In: American Control Conference (ACC), pp. 2799–2804 (2010)
7. Hirata, Y., Hara, A., Kosuge, K.: Motion control of passive intelligent walker using servo brakes. IEEE Transactions on Robotics 23(5), 981–990 (2007)
8. Kulyukin, V., Kutiyanawala, A., LoPresti, E., Matthews, J., Simpson, R.: Iwalker: Toward a rollator-mounted wayfinding system for the elderly. In: 2008 IEEE International Conference on RFID, pp. 303–311 (2008)
9. Wasson, G., Sheth, P., Alwan, M., Granata, K., Ledoux, A.: Cunjun Huang. User intent in a shared control framework for pedestrian mobility aids. In: Proceedings of the 2003 IEEE/RSJ International Conference on Intelligent Robots and Systems (IROS 2003), vol. 3, pp. 2962–2967 (2003)
10. Lee, G., Jung, E.-J., Ohnuma, T., Chong, N.Y., Yi, B.-J.: Jaist robotic walker control based on a two-layered kalman filter. In: 2011 IEEE International Conference on Robotics and Automation (ICRA), pp. 3682–3687 (2011)
11. Graf, B., Hans, M., Schraft, R.D.: Care-o-bot ii—development of a next generation robotic home assistant. Autonomous Robots 16(2), 193–205 (2004)
12. D'Angelo, L.T., Loercher, A., Lueth, T.C.: A new electrically driven walking frame for both passive and active mobility support. In: 2011 IEEE Conference on Automation Science and Engineering (CASE), pp. 816–821 (2011)
13. Ralston, H.J., Todd, F., Inman, V.T.: Human walking. Williams & Wilkins, Baltimore (1981)
14. Perry, J.: Gait Analysis: Normal and Pathological Function. Slack Incorporated (1992)
15. O'Connor, J.C., Vaughan, C.L., Davis, B.L.: Dynamics of Human Gait. Human Kinetics Publishers (1992)
16. Cochran, G.V.B.: A primer of orthopaedic biomechanics. Churchhill Livingstone, New York (1982)
17. Rabiner, L., Juang, B.: An introduction to hidden markov models. IEEE ASSP Magazine 3(1), 4–16 (1986)
18. Rabiner, L.R.: Readings in speech recognition. chapter A tutorial on hidden Markov models and selected applications in speech recognition, pp. 267–296. Morgan Kaufmann Publishers Inc., San Francisco (1990)
19. Katsamanis, A., Papandreou, G., Maragos, P.: Audiovisual-to-articulatory speech inversion using active appearance models for the face and hidden markov models for the dynamics. In: ICASSP, pp. 2237–2240. IEEE (2008)
20. Yoon, B.-J.: Hidden markov models and their applications in biological sequence analysis. Curr. Genomics 10(6), 402–415 (2009)
21. Theodorakis, S., Katsamanis, A., Maragos, P.: Product-hmms for automatic sign language recognition. In: ICASSP, pp. 1601–1604. IEEE (2009)
22. Turaga, P., Chellappa, R., Subrahmanian, V.S., Udrea, O.: Machine recognition of human activities: A survey. IEEE Transactions on Circuits and Systems for Video Technology 18(11), 1473–1488 (2008)
23. Papageorgiou, X., Chalvatzaki, G., Tzafestas, C., Maragos, P.: Hidden markov modeling of human normal gait using laser range finder for a mobility assistance robot. In: Proceedings of the 2014 IEEE International Conference on Robotics and Automation (ICRA 2014) (2014)

Design of a Low-Cost Social Robot: Towards Personalized Human-Robot Interaction

Christian G. Puehn, Tao Liu, Yixin Feng, Kenneth Hornfeck, and Kiju Lee

Case Western Reserve University
Cleveland, Ohio 44106, USA
kiju.lee@case.edu

Abstract. This paper presents a low-cost social robot, called *Philos*, and human-robot interaction (HRI) design. The system is accompanied with a user interface that allows customization of interactive functions and real-time monitoring. The robot features eight degrees of freedom that can generate various gestures and facial expressions. HRI is realized by two elements, internal characteristics of the robot and external vision/touch inputs provided by the users. Internal characteristics determine the predefined personality of Philos among the five: Friendly, Hyperactive, Shy, Cold, or Sensitive, and set the behavioral control parameters accordingly. Vision-based interaction includes face tracking, face recognition, and motion tracking. Embedded touch sensors detect physical touch-based interaction. Behavioral parameters are updated in real time based on the user inputs, and therefore Philos can engage each user in personalized interaction via uniquely defined behavioral responses. The cost of Philos is estimated to be relatively low compared to other commercially available robots promising a broad range of potential applications for domestic and professional use.

Keywords: Human-Robot Interaction, Social Robot, Face Tracking, Face Recognition, Behavioral Control.

1 Introduction

Social robots are designed to entertain, assist, or provide service to humans though vision, touch, and sound-based interaction. Therefore, human-robot interaction (HRI) often resembles the way humans interact with each other. Recently, social robots have been receiving growing interest for their great potential as a long-term health care solution. For example, a social robot can serve as a companion for older people by helping them maintain independent living [1]. In addition, recent studies have demonstrated potential uses of social robots in behavioral training for children with developmental disabilities [2], [3], [4].

Over the past several decades, a number of socially interactive robots have been developed, covering a range of design and functionality objectives. The Huggable, a robot with the outer appearance of a teddy bear, focuses on implementing a sophisticated touch–sensitive skin, allowing for therapeutic interaction

C. Stephanidis and M. Antona (Eds.): UAHCI/HCII 2014, Part III, LNCS 8515, pp. 704–713, 2014.

through physical touch inputs and responses [5]. Sparky and Feelix are mobile robots with actuated faces, each with 4 degrees of freedom [6], [7]. Kismet is an anthromorphic head with 21 degrees of freedom that can produce complex facial expressions in response to user inputs [8]. Sage is also a social robot that serves as a robotic tour guide while adjusting behavioral parameters over time based on external interaction [9]. Olivia, is another robotic tour guide that can inform and entertain visitors [10]. Targeting one of the public health epidemics, Autom^{TM} demonstrates its use as a weight loss coach [11].

NAO is a commercial robotic platform that is often employed for various research and education applications. For example, some recent studies employed NAO in social training for children with autism spectrum disorders. NAO has a combination of lights, vocal cues, and motions to interact with children. While simple behaviors are autonomously generated, more complex motions were controlled by researchers monitoring the process. In addition, NAO has the capability to record video and detect touches on its head. By utilizing an intuitive graphical user interface (GUI), NAO allows clinicians to interact wirelessly with the users and has shown success in clinical studies involving children with autism spectrum disorders [12]. Paro and NeCoRo are designed to provide companionship to older people [13], [14], [15]. iCat is another commercially available platform that can recognize objects and faces, recognize speech and sound, and generate various facial expressions [16]. Similar to Paro, iCat was also tested for its potential benefits to the elderly population. The results showed that older people are more comfortable and more expressive with a more sociable robot than with a less social one. In the design of iCat, all emotion expressions are enabled through facial movement and voice generation. However, one existing problem is that while interacting with iCat, there will be no direct body contact between iCat and the human user, which may limit the range and type of interaction. While many existing social robots have proven their effectiveness in entertaining, assisting, and providing service to human users, the cost and maintenance of such robots may discourage many from considering the purchase. The commercial price of Paro is about $6,000 and Nao costs over $15,000. Furthermore, personalized HRI is still a challenging problem to be addressed.

This paper presents Philos, a low-cost social robot for use in a broad range of applications that involve personalized human-robot interaction. The estimated commercial price of Philos is less than $3,000, where all associated software can be available for free when used for research or educational purposes. Philos can interact with users via touch, face detection/recognition, and motion detection. Philos is actuated by eight servo motors that can generate various gestures and simple facial expressions using moving eyebrows. The behavioral control of Philos is based on two elements: 1) internal characteristics of the robot and 2) external vision and touch inputs provided by the users. Internal characteristics determine the robot's initial personality and set the behavioral control parameters accordingly. Therefore, Philos can engage each user in personalized interaction via uniquely defined behavioral responses tailored for each user.

2   Hardware and Software Design

2.1   Hardware Design and Control Scheme

Philos is capable of performing a wide range of simple behavioral motions, including nodding or shaking its head, waving, flapping its arms, and moving the eyebrows through actuation of eight servo motors: two for each arm, two servos enabling the head to pan and tilt, and two for eyebrows [17]. Moving eyebrows allow Philos to generate simple facial expressions, representing three emotional statuses: positive, neutral, and negative as shown in Fig 1. The servos are controlled by an mbed ARM® core microcontroller through serial communication. Philos utilizes 14 force-sensitive resistors (FSR) that cover its chest, head, hands, and feet. These FSRs allow Philos to detect where the robot is touched as well as determine whether it is an aggressive or gentle touch. Philos also has a small speaker installed in its body chassis. This speaker is controlled via the mbed device to playback prerecorded sound clips including human voices, music, or penguin sound. The robot also has two cameras on its head for face detection, face recognition, and motion detection. The exterior covering of Philos is designed to resemble a penguin. Inside the plush outer surface, there is a thin plastic shell to protect the inner components of the robot and to attach the FSRs so that they read more accurately.

Philos utilizes two microcontrollers working in tandem. Philos uses an mbed ARM® core microcontroller for behavioral control and voice generation. A Raspberry Pi is used to read the raw image data and to apply the face and motion detection algorithms. These microcontrollers were chosen due to their respective strengths in terms of processing speed and cost. The Raspberry Pi has fairly high processor speed for an embedded controller and uses a Linux based operating system enabling the use of OpenCV. FSRs are low-cost and widely available sensors can effectively detect touch and its magnitude up to 100N. Each sensor has a surface area of 1.5×1.5 inch^2. The mbed controller receives and processes analog data from the FSR clusters and the noise from the circuit is accounted for by implementing a sampling rate to the FSRs. The servos are controlled via pulse-width modulation (PWM) in order to move the eyebrows of Philos to express emotions. The movement of the arms and head of Philos is controlled by six AX-12 servo motors via half-duplex serial communication. This communication protocol allows

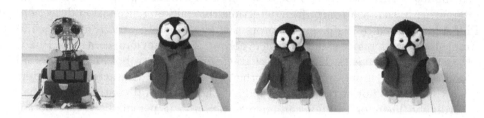

Fig. 1. Internal view of Philos and three emotional statuses (positive, neutral, and negative) represented by the eyebrow angles and hand gestures

the servo motors to be connected in series and for multiple servos to be controlled with a single command. This particular servo greatly reduces the cost of using multiple servos as only two of the GPIO pins must be dedicated to AX-12 control.

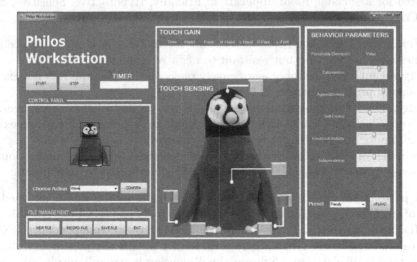

Fig. 2. Philos workstation for programming behavior parameters and real-time monitoring of HRI

2.2   Software Interface

The Graphical User Interface (GUI) allows the user to personalize the robot and monitor real-time interaction data (Fig. 2). The GUI is designed to enable non-technical users to easily reprogram the robot when desired. Real-time monitoring data is also realized in the GUI by displaying current interaction data. In addition to numerical data, a graphical representation of the force applied on different parts of the body is overlaid on a picture of the robot in the main section of the GUI. The data collected during interaction can also be exported to a text document with time stamps if further analysis is desired. Reprogramming, manual control, and data collection are enabled by wireless Zigbee technology using a USB dongle connecting an XBee with the computer.

3   Human-Robot Interaction Design

There are two elements that influence the behavioral characteristics of Philos: 1) the internally defined personality and 2) external inputs provided by human users to Philos. An operator can initially specify a personality type for Philos which will generate a unique set of behavior parameters. Philos behavioral responses are also affected by external user inputs provided through touch-based and vision-based interactions enabled by onboard sensors.

3.1   Generation of Internal Characteristics

Methods: Based on the big five dimensions of human personality as defined by several psychologists [18], we consider five predefined personality types that are adapted for a sociable robot application: Friendly, Hyperactive, Sensitive, Shy, and Cold, as described below:

- **Friendly:** The robot tends to seek out interaction. It is prone to positive increases in behavior, but resistant to negative changes.
- **Hyperactive:** The robot aggressively seeks out interaction. It is not exceptionally prone to changes in behavior.
- **Shy:** The robot avoids interaction and is not prone to behavior changes.
- **Cold:** The robot avoids interaction. It tends to respond negatively to external inputs and is resistant to behavior changes.
- **Sensitive:** The robot neither avoids nor aggressively seeks interaction. It is very prone to behavior changes and is easily affected by user inputs.

Each personality type is classified by a predefined set of values assigned to each of the following personality dimensions: Extraversion (EXT), Agreeableness (AGR), Self-Control (SC), Emotional Stability (ES), and Independence (IND). The values range from 1 to 5 where a value of 1 means the personality dimension is weakly displayed and 5 means the dimension is strongly displayed. These internal characteristics generate the following behavioral parameters of Philos:

- **Room scan frequency** (f_{scan}): The frequency at which the robot will scan the room for faces when it has not recently detected one.
- **Face track probability** (p_{track}): The likelihood that the robot will follow a subjects face after the face has been detected.
- **Frequency of idle state activity** (f_{idle}): The frequency at which the robot considers itself idle during a period of no human interaction, and will exhibit some action to draw attention to itself.
- **Range of idle state activity** (d_{idle}): The number of behaviors the robot may exhibit when it has been idle for a period of time, which is defined by the idle behavior frequency.
- **Level of positive behavioral response** (r_p): A higher value indicates a higher probability that the robot will respond positively to external inputs provided by a user and will be more inclined to seek out interaction.
- **Behavioral change factors** (c_{inc}, c_{dec}): The factors that determine the magnitude that the above parameters will either increase due to positive external inputs or decrease due to negative ones.

Preliminary Testing of the Algorithm: To evaluate the effects of internal parameters on Philos' behavior and user interaction on Philos' behavior, a simple laboratory test was conducted. Behavioral dimension values, (EXT, AGR, SC, ES, IND), for each personality are defined as: Friendly (4, 5, 4, 3, 3), Hyperactive (5, 4, 2, 2, 5), Shy (1, 2, 3, 4, 1), Cold (2, 1, 5, 5, 2), and Sensitive (3, 3, 1, 1, 4). Holding r_p constant, 200 "gentle" and 200 "harsh" touch inputs were provided

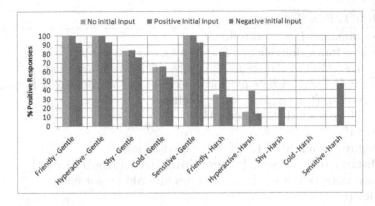

Fig. 3. Percentage of positive and negative responses as affected by user input and programmed personality

based on the predefined threshold for the force sensors. The number of positive responses enacted by Philos was recorded. In order to determine the probability that a positive response would occur after a series of either positive or negative user inputs, we conducted the following test. For each predefined personality, ten touch inputs were provided while r_p was allowed to change. All ten were either "gentle" or "harsh." After the first ten, an additional 200 inputs were given, the first 100 "gentle" and the next 100 "harsh", while r_p was held constant. The results of the tests where the first 10 inputs were positive and the tests where the first 10 inputs were negative are also both plotted in Fig. 3.

The data presented in Fig. 3 shows how Philos' behavior is affected by either positive or negative user input. Personalities with a high value for AGR (i.e. Friendly, Hyperactive) are more significantly affected by positive inputs than negative. The opposite is true for personalities with a low AGR value (i.e. Shy, Cold). Furthermore, the lower the value of ES, the more drastically the behavior will change. This explains why the effects of positive input cause Philos' behavior to change a similar amount for both the Sensitive and Friendly personalities, even though AGR is higher for the Friendly personality type.

3.2   User-Based Interaction

Touch-Based Interaction: Touch based interaction is realized through clusters of FSRs that cover the hard shell of Philos. These clusters are located on the body, the hands, the feet, and the top of the head of Philos. The FSR clusters are created by connecting multiple FSRs in parallel. Touches are first categorized as either being harsh or gentle. The threshold values for gentle and harsh touches can be prespecified or determined by initial parameter training.

Real-Time Face Tracking: Initial face detection uses the AdaBoost Classifier, Haar classifiers, and skin color based algorithm [19], [20], [21]. However, these

---

Algorithm 1. Face Tracking

1: **loop** Command from controller
2:    % Use frame difference to find edges of moving object
3:    $F_{i-1} \leftarrow$ *Capture Frame* at t_{i-1}; $F_i \leftarrow$ *Capture Frame* at t_i
4:    $M_i = F_i - F_{i-1}$ where moving objects in the M frame are white on black
5:    **if** Average(Center(M_i)) != $[0, 0]$ **then**
6:       Move toward the Center(M_i)
7:    **end if**
8:    Preprocessing: RGB to GRAY, Equalization
9:    **Optimize the potential searching area (Algorithm 2)**
10:    Face Detection using Haar cascades and Skin color filter
11: **end loop**

Algorithm 2. Optimize Potential Searching Area

1: **loop** Camera moved to follow the object
2:    $V_i = (P_i - P_{i-1})/\Delta t$
3:    $P_{i+1} = P_i + V_i \times \Delta t$
4:    **if** Face is not found **then**
5:       Increase Searching Area by 10% until the face is found
6:    **else**
7:       Pan Camera Searching
8:    **end if**
9: **end loop**

---

methods are often not suitable for embedded, real-time tracking. To reduce the detection time, two strategies are applied: 1) reducing the searching area within the image and 2) optimizing the potential area by projecting the face location in the future frame. First, the original image in the RGB space is transformed into a gray scale and then smoothened by the equalization process. Secondly, the potential face area that projects the future face location is estimated assuming that the user's face will move without erratically changing direction and speed using the results from face detection in current and previous frames. Typically, a *potential face area* indicating possible face locations in the next time frame is slightly larger than the detected face window. Depending on the speed of face movement, the size of the potential face area is dynamically determined as described in Algorithm 2. For example, if the face moves quickly within the image in two consecutive frames, the potential area for searching is increased accordingly. Otherwise, if the face moves slowly, the potential area is reduced. Increasing the potential area by 20% of the actual face size and decreasing the searching area by 10% ensures that if the face either moves closer or farther from the camera it will not be outside the potential area, and accounts for the face moving left or right in relation to the camera. In this way, we can significantly lower the searching time. Table 1 compares computational times depending on

Table 1. Detection time with various sizes of the searching area applied. PA: Potential Area, SA: Searching Area

Searching area	Original	120% PA & 80% SA	120% PA & 90% SA
50*50	985ms	433ms	376ms
80*80	1303ms	553ms	462ms
160*160	2997ms	739ms	507ms
400*400	7814ms	1190ms	696ms

the size of the searching area. Algorithm 1 and 2 shows our overall face tracking strategies.

Face Recognition: Face recognition is enabled by the Principal Component Analysis (PCA) and adaptive learning algorithm for gradually improved performance presented in [21]. To first obtain a standardized image of a person, the image is rescaled to 320×240 pixels and an ellipse shade is applied to eliminate the hair. Ten images for each person are taken and an average image is calculated. By comparing the difference between a user and these average images it is possible to determine if the person is in the database and if they are not in the database, he or she can be added to it.

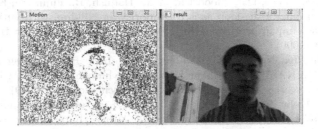

Fig. 4. The processed image and motion detection result

Motion Detection: Motion detection aims at face detection of moving objects/persons at a relatively low resolution. For example, if someone moves toward Philos from a distance, the robot may not be able to obtain images that are suitable for face detection. However, the motions can be detected and tracked. In order to accomplish this, two consecutive frames of the image are compared to calculate the differences between the two frames [22]. The images are first converted into a gray scale to further reduce the processing time and THEN compared for each pixel. If two pixels in two images show the same value, it is marked as 0. If not, it is marked as 1. Then the center of the areas marked with 1's is calculated. Fig. 4 shows this process.

4 Conclusion

In this paper, we presented Philos, a social robot for personalized social interaction. Personalization is realized by predefined internal characteristics of the
robot and HRI based on external user inputs. Data collection and processing
is performed on board. Philos can provide users a low-cost platform for various
education and research applications with its estimated mass-production cost of
about $3,000. Building on the current prototype, we are developing the next
generation of Philos with improved hardware and user interface design. Furthermore, speech recognition is one of the important areas of exploration while it is
omitted in the current version of Philos.

Acknowledgement. This work was supported by the Clinical and Translational Science Collaborative (CTSC) of Cleveland.

References

1. Pearce, A.J., Adair, B., Miller, K., et al.: Robotics to enable older adults to remain
   living at home. J. Aging Res. 2012, 538169 (2012)
2. Robins, B., Dautenhahn, K., te Boekhorst, R., Billard, A.: Robotic assistants in
   therapy and education of children with autism: can a small humanoid robot help
   encourage social interaction skills? Univ. Access Inf. Soc. 4, 105–120 (2005)
3. Colton, M.B., Ricks, D.J., Goodrich, M.A., Dariush, B., Fujimura, K., Fujik, M.:
   Toward therapist-in-the-loop assistive robotics for children with autism and specific language impairment. In: AISB Symposium: New Frontiers in Human-Robot
   Interaction (2009)
4. Dautenhahn, K., Nehaniv, C., Walters, M., Robins, B., Kose-Bagci, H., Mirza,
   N., Blow, M.: KASPAR: a minimally expressive humanoid robot for human-robot
   interaction research. Applied Bionics and Biomechanics 6(3) (2009)
5. Stiehl, W., Lieberman, J., Breazeal, C., Basel, L., Cooper, R., Knight, H., Lalla,
   L., Maymin, A., Purchase, S.: The huggable: A therapeutic robotic companion for
   relational, affective touch. In: Proceedings of the IEEE Consumer Communications
   and Networking Conference, Las Vegas, NV, p. 15 (2006)
6. Ferrari, E., Robins, B., Dautenhahn, K.: Therapeutic and educational objectives in
   Robot Assisted Play for children with autism. In: IEEE International Symposium
   on Robot and Human Interactive Communication, pp. 108–114 (2009)
7. Scheeff, M., Pinto, J., Rahardja, K., Snibbe, S., Tow, R.: Experiences with sparky,
   a social robot. In: Socially Intelligent Agents, pp. 173–180 (2002)
8. Breazeal, C.: Emotion and sociable humanoid robots. International Journal of
   Human-Computer Studies 59(1-2), 119–155 (2003)
9. Nourbakhsh, I.R., Bobenage, J., Grange, S., Lutz, R., Meyer, R., Soto, A.: An
   affective mobile robot educator with a full-time job. Artificial Intelligence 114(1),
   95–124 (1999)
10. Niculescu, A., van Dijk, B., Nijholt, A., Limbu, D.K., Lan See, S., Li, H., Wong,
    A.: Socializing with Olivia, the youngest robot receptionist outside the lab. In: Ge,
    S.S., Li, H., Cabibihan, J.-J., Tan, Y.K. (eds.) ICSR 2010. LNCS, vol. 6414, pp.
    50–62. Springer, Heidelberg (2010)

11. Kidd, C., Breazeal, C.: A robotic weight loss coach. In: Proceedings of the National Conference on Artificial Intelligence, pp. 1985–1986 (2007)
12. Shamsuddin, S., Yussof, H., Ismail, L., Hanapiah, F.A., Mohamed, S., Piah, H.A., Zahari, N.I.: Initial response of autistic children in human-robot interaction therapy with humanoid robot NAO. In: 2012 IEEE 8th International Colloquium on Signal Processing and its Applications (CSPA), pp. 188–193 (2012)
13. Wada, K., Shibata, T.: Social effects of robot therapy in a care house - change of social network of the residents for two months. In: IEEE International Conference on Robotics and Automation, Rome, Italy, pp. 1250–1255 (2007)
14. Kidd, C., Taggart, W., Turkle, S.: A sociable robot to encourage social interaction among the elderly. In: IEEE International Conference on Robotics and Automation, pp. 3972–3976 (2006)
15. Libin, E., Libin, A.: New diagnostic tool for robotic psychology and robotherapy studies. Cyber Psychology and Behavior 6(4), 369–374 (2003)
16. van Breemen, A., Yan, X., Meerbeek, B.: iCat: an animated user-interface robot with personality. In: Proceedings of the fourth International Joint Conference on Autonomous Agents and Multiagent Systems, pp. 143–144 (2005)
17. Hornfeck, K., Zhang, Y., Lee, K.: Philos: A Sociable Robot for Human Robot Interactions and Wireless health Monitoring. In: Symposium on Applied Computing, 2012 (Extended Abstract) (2012)
18. Digman, J.: Personality structure: Emergence of the five-factor model. Annual Review of Psychology 41, 417–440 (1990)
19. Wu, X., Gong, H., Chen, P., Zhi, Z., Xu, Y.: Intelligent household surveillance robot. In: Robotics and Biomimetics, ROBIO 2008, pp. 1734–1739 (2008)
20. Liu, Q., Peng, G.Z.: A robust skin color based face detection algorithm. In: International Asia Conference on Control, Automation and Robotics, pp. 525–528 (March 2010)
21. Zhang, Y., Hornfeck, K., Lee, K.: Adaptive face recognition for low-cost, embedded human-robot interaction. In: Lee, S., Cho, H., Yoon, K.-J., Lee, J. (eds.) Intelligent Autonomous Systems 12. AISC, vol. 193, pp. 863–872. Springer, Heidelberg (2012)
22. Yang, J., Waibel, A.: A real-time face tracker. In: Proceedings of 3rd IEEE Workshop on Applications of Computer Vision, pp. 142–147 (1996)

Mobility, Navigation and Safety

Mobile Navigation through a Science Museum for Users Who Are Blind

Márcia de Borba Campos[1], Jaime Sánchez[2], Anderson Cardoso Martins[1],
Régis Schneider Santana[1], and Matías Espinoza[2]

[1] Faculty of Informatics, Pontifical Catholic University of Rio Grande do Sul,
Porto Alegre, Brazil
marcia.campos@pucrs.br,
{anderson.martins.001,regis.santana}@acad.pucrs.br
[2] Department of Computer Science and Center for Advanced Research in Education (CARE),
University of Chile, Santiago, Chile
{jsanchez,maespino}@dcc.uchile.cl

Abstract. This paper presents the design and implementation of mAbES, a mobile, audio-based environment simulator to assist the development of orientation and mobility skills in people who are blind. The modeling scenario of mAbES was a science and technology museum in Porto Alegre, Brazil. The application was designed for use by people who are blind without the supervision of a facilitator or aid. The mAbES software allows for testing the creation of mental maps when people who are blind navigate through the museum.

Keywords: People who are blind, Mental map, Orientation and mobility, Navigation, Mobile application.

1 Introduction

Lacking vision is not synonymous with having low levels of spatial perception or comprehension. In general, people with visual impairment, when adequately trained, are capable of orienting themselves, and develop a pretty precise mental representation of the environment. This indicates that visual experience is not strictly necessary in order to create mental representations of space, as other senses also provide valuable spatial information [10]. In his research, Millar proposes that vision does influence coding and spatial representation, but that it is not a sole determinant of such abilities [10].

A person with visual impairment must be competent with orientation and mobility (O&M) in order to achieve a solid level of navigation, including moving about safely, efficiently and with agility, as well as independently in both familiar and unfamiliar environments [4]. The learning of O&M skills includes a set of defined techniques that children who are blind, young people and adults (or those with visual impairment) must practice stage by stage. However, learning such skills also involves other aspects such as training and refining systems of perception, and both conceptual and

C. Stephanidis and M. Antona (Eds.): UAHCI/HCII 2014, Part III, LNCS 8515, pp. 717–728, 2014.
© Springer International Publishing Switzerland 2014

motor skills development [4]. Such skills are essential precedents for learning formal O&M techniques [4]. The primary objective of O&M is to achieve independence and to improve the quality of life for people who are blind or who have visual impairments. Instruction in such skills occurs in stages, in which the level of difficulty of the training involved varies according the learner's particular characteristics [4].

For example, mobility when navigating a route does not just require moving from point A to point B, but doing this efficiently and knowing where one is, where one is going, and how to get there [1].

It is important to point out that movement refers to the act and practice of moving, but also to the act of evaluating known facts and places in the environment in order to facilitate effective movement and to exercise one's own capacity for autonomous navigation [11]. This means that when people with visual impairment relate to their environment, they encounter certain "spatial problems". For this reason, they must constantly make "spatial decisions" regarding how to successfully navigate an environment.

From a geographical perspective [3], quality of life for both sighted and people who are blind depends on the individual's ability to infer information and make spatial decisions.

In O&M, the capacity for orientation ideally progresses from a concrete understanding of the principals of mobility, to a more functional plane for applying such principals, and finally arriving at an abstract level through which the learner can function effectively in an unfamiliar environment [4]. In this transition, it can be inferred that psycho-motor, senso-perceptive, conceptual and practical training in the use of O&M techniques and materials, are important tools for being able to generate a representation of space. This is because these tools allow for a learner to practice and test out different methods of movement in context, use memory, and to pick up on and interpret his surroundings.

The cognitive map, as a process of spatial reasoning, provides spatial information that is useful for mobility [12]. For some authors, the function of cognitive maps for an individual is to coordinate adaptive spatial behaviors, or in other words to generate action plans prior to or during the navigation of an environment, and to execute those plans effectively while moving through the environment [1].

Spatial knowledge, made up of simple concepts, complex ideas, locations and relations, is retained in the mind through cognitive images of the surrounding environment, which make up cognitive maps. The basic structure of the images consists of simplified extracts of reality, built by using perceptual and conceptual information [1]. This means that people with visual impairment also form images, which can be quite elaborate, but constructed differently than sighted people. For example, these images could be built based on sensations and movement, memories, textures, sounds, etc.

The study of spatial representation can provide relevant information regarding how people move, what information they need for mobility, and how this information is distributed in a given environment [5].

Support on a perceptual and conceptual level is important for the development of orientation skills and the construction of cognitive maps [7]. The notion of a map speaks of an internalized representation of space, a mixture of objective knowledge and subjective perception. As most of the information needed to form a mental map is collected through the visual channel [7], some authors claim that people who are blind use other sensory channels to compensate this and use alternative methods for exploration in order to construct mental maps [12].

If real-life surroundings are represented through virtual environments, it is possible to create several training applications that allow a user who is blind to interact with the elements in the simulated environment during navigation [13][14].

Videogames, when integrated with virtual training environments, represent an important tool for the development of various abilities, and O&M skills in particular [16][17]. For example, the software AbES [13][14] allows for the creation of videogames, focusing on the mental construction of real and/or fictitious environments by users who are blind navigating through virtual environments, using a computer keyboard in order to execute actions and receive audio feedback, with the aim of supporting the development of O&M.

AbES expands on the concept of using fictitious corridors used in its predecessor AudioDoom [9], in order to generate an audio-based virtual representation of real environments, thus serving as a videogame that allows for O&M training [14]. In addition, the use of audio allows increases the potential for various forms of interaction between the user and the computer.

Another study presented an audio-based virtual reality system that allows the user to explore a virtual environment by using only his sense of hearing [2]. Other authors performed empirical evaluations of various approaches through which spatial information on the environment is transmitted through the use of audio cues [6].

Various virtual environments have been designed in order to train people who are blind, and to assist them with the development of O&M skills [7][9][14]. To navigate through an environment, it is necessary to have access to the information that can be recovered from the environment, in order to then filter useful information in a way that is coherent and comprehensible for whoever needs it.

It is for this reason that in the case of people who are blind, the use of virtual environments and appropriate interfaces allows them to improve their O&M skills [15]. Such interfaces can be, for example, haptic or audio based. Such resources can also be used for recreational purposes. Other studies have researched the use of mobile applications to assist in user navigation of the city [13][14][15].

The purpose of this work is to present the design and implementation of mAbES, a mobile audio based environment simulator to assist the development of orientation and mobility skills in people who are blind. We introduce a model scenario using mAbES together with an application for navigating through a science and technology museum in Porto Alegre, Brazil. The software mAbES was designed based on a previous model of AbES.

2   AbES, Audio-Based Environments Simulator

AbES represents a real, familiar or unfamiliar environment to be navigated by a person who is blind. The virtual environment is made up of different elements and objects (walls, stairways, doors, toilets or elevators) through which the user can discover and become familiar with his location. It is possible to interact with doors, which can be opened and closed. Regarding the rest of the objects, it is possible for the user to identify them and their location in the environment. The idea is for the user to be able to move about independently and to mentally map the entire environment.

The simulator is capable of representing any real environment by using a system of cells through which the user moves [17]. The user receives audio feedback from the left, center and right side channels, and all actions are carried out through the use of a traditional keyboard, where a set of keys have different associated actions. All of the actions in the virtual environment have a particular sound associated to them. In addition to this audio feedback, there are also spoken audio cues that provide information regarding the various objects and the user's orientation in the environment. Orientation is provided by identifying the room in which the user is located and the direction in which he is facing, according to the cardinal compass points (east, west, north and south).

Stereo sound is used to achieve the user's immersion by providing information on the location of different objects, walls and doors in the virtual environment. In this way, the user is able create a mental model of the spatial dimensions of the environment. While navigating, the user can interact with each of the previously mentioned elements, and each of these elements provides different kinds of feedback that help the user become oriented in the environment. AbES includes three modes of interaction: Free Navigation, Path Navigation and Game Mode.

The free navigation mode provides the user who is blind with the possibility of exploring a building freely in order to become familiar with it. The facilitator can choose whether the user begins in a particular starting room, or let the AbES software randomly choose the starting point. Path navigation provides the user who is blind with the task of finding a particular room by first choosing an initial and destination room, and selecting the number of routes to be taken.

The game mode provides blind users with the task of searching for "jewels" placed in the building. The purpose of the game is to explore the rooms and find all the jewels, bringing them outside one at a time and then going back into the building to continue exploring. Enemies are randomly placed in the building, and try to steal the user's jewels and hide them elsewhere.

Different versions of AbES have been developed in order to simulate various real life, closed spaces. One of these versions corresponds to the St. Paul's building at the Carroll Center for the Blind in Newton, MA, USA. Later, other versions were developed to simulate the Santa Lucia School and Hellen Keller School, both located in Santiago, Chile. In the version for the St. Paul's building the entire environment could be navigated freely (see Fig. 1). The design and development of AbES was carried out by considering the ways in which blind users interact, and how audio can help them to increment certain spatial navigation skills and facilitate their cognitive development.

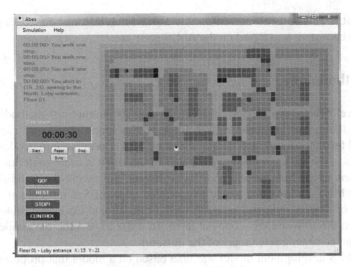

Fig. 1. A screenshot of AbES

3   Museum of Science and Technology

The application introduced here, mAbES, represents the actual physical environment of the Museum of Science and Technology, of the Pontifical Catholic University of Rio Grande do Sul, Porto Alegre, Brazil (MCT-PUCRS). This museum is one of the largest interactive natural science museums in Latin America. Its mission is to generate, preserve and disseminate knowledge through its collections and exhibitions.

It has an area of over ten thousand square meters dedicated to public exhibitions, and about 700 interactive apparatuses that can be used by visitors. The interactive nature of the many experimental sites provides for playful experiences that facilitate the understanding of scientific concepts and theories for all ages in a creative environment.

Among the scientific exhibitions, the most impressive are related to the areas of Zoology, Botany, Paleontology and Archaeology, which are utilized by researchers and some graduate and post-graduate student of PUCRS, as well as other national and foreign institutions.

Despite the fact that the MCT is designed as a space of learning and information, there are still limitations regarding the active and autonomous participation of people with certain disabilities. There are structural accessibility and information related problems for people who use wheelchairs, people who are deaf, people who are blind, or people with cognitive disabilities. In order to facilitate the construction of a more inclusive society that recognizes the diversity of people with disabilities and the importance of their individual autonomy and independence, the MCT has formed partnerships for the development of activities that promote accessibility to the physical environment, education and information for people with disabilities.

In this context, the need emerged for the development of a software application to support the navigation (orientation and mobility) of people who are blind that visit the

MCT-PUCRS. This software was named mAbES (mobile Audio-based Environment Simulator), because it was based on the AbES software.

4   Methodology

For the development of mAbES, an XP (eXtreme Programming) methodology was utilized, including weekly technical meetings with a specialized team from the museum, rapid feedback loops, and the provision of weekly programming codes.

Members of the museum team participated in meetings in order to define the scope and to prioritize the functionalities of the software. Following the definition of the areas of the MCT-PUCRS that would be included in mAbES, a museum architect and a professor of physics, who are also part of the Educational Coordination team of the MCT, joined the software development team. In order to develop the application, the team went on constant guided tours of the museum.

The mAbES development model was also based on a model that proposes an iterative development process for mobile videogame-based software in order to improve the orientation and mobility skills of blind users [16][17]. This process includes the following phases: 1. Definition of the cognitive skills needed for navigation; 2. The software engineering process for the design and development of the applications; and 3. A validation process for the tools that are developed.

The mAbES software application was developed by using Unity, a platform for videogame development. In addition, the following were also utilized:

- Google Translate: used to convert texts of up to 101 characters into MP3 audio. The mAbES was used to generate the audio cues for the users. For example, if the user crashes into a wall, mAbES informs him: "This is a wall". This audio was produced based on: http://translate.google.com/translate_tts?tl=pt&q=this is a wall.
- Soar MP3: Utilized to turn text conversations with over 101 characters into audio. Was used to generate an audio description of the selected MCT-PUCRS experiments.
- AutoCAD: Used to manipulate the floor plans of MCT/PUCRS in order to export them for use with Unity.
- Google Sketchup: Utilized to create 3D objects based on MCT-PUCRS, which were then exported for use with Unity.
- AutoDesk 3DS Max Design: Used to convert the museum's floor plan files, which had been generated using AutoCAD, to a file format compatible with Unity.
- JavaScript: Optimal programming language for the Unity environment.

5   Results

The mAbES software was designed in stages, based on the decisions made regarding the specific experiments to be mapped. These choices were made according to the museum's demands. The first phase involved the experiments in the energy section. This choice was based mainly on the following issues: the experiments were among those that had the longest shelf life in the museum, and those that represent areas of knowledge that people generally have difficulty understanding. The posterior phases will continue to map related experiments within the energy section.

In the first phase, 3 experiments were chosen: Nuclear Power Station, Energy Train, and Cool House, located on the third floor of the museum. In mAbES, these experiments are represented with 3D graphics, and information on them is available in audio format. This paper describes the results of one of these experiments.

5.1   Interfaces

The mAbES software presents information regarding the physical space of the MCT-PUCRS, the selected experiments, and also responds to the user's movements through the museum. The physical space of the museum and the experiments are represented through 3D graphics, allowing for its use by people with visual disabilities, low-level vision and sighted people as well. The interaction between mAbES and the user occurs mainly through an audio interface, while the user communicates with the software by interacting with a smartphone screen, which utilizes an array of points of the Braille system (see Figures 2 and 3).

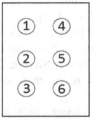

Fig. 2. Matrix of Braille points

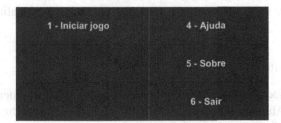

Fig. 3. Startup screen of mAbES

In following the AbES model [16][17], the user's movement using mAbES occurs in three different ways: forward, right and left. The user's movement through the museum is achieved by using the forward button, which represents the user's individual steps. The right and left buttons are used when the user turns in either direction.

The transition between floors in the MCT-PUCRS is achieved through the use of escalators (Figure 4), in which it is possible to observe the areas involved in the user's interaction when moving forward, turning right or turning left. When the user reaches an escalator, mAbES provides an audio-description about its physical appearance, functioning and how the user who is blind should use the escalator in the real context of the Museum.

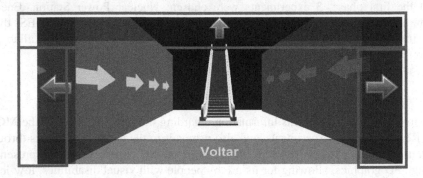

Fig. 4. Transitions between floors of the MCT-PUCRS

Information on the museum or the experiments is available to the user in audio format. The options for hearing the audio cues are: 1 – Play, 2 – Pause, 3 – Increase speed, 4 – Go back, 5 – Go forward, 6 – Help.

When the user arrives at the third floor, which is the purpose of phase 1, mAbES presents the experiments that are mapped so that the user can choose which one he wants to interact with: 1 – Nuclear Power Station, 2 – Energy Train, 3 – Cool House, 4 – Explore the space freely, 5 – More information, 6 – Exit, according to the Braille matrix.

When the user crashes into any object (wall, pillar, or escalator, for example) or comes upon any experiment (Nuclear Power Station, Energy Train, Cool House), mAbES informs the user by naming the object or experiment, and the options that are available to the user. In addition, the device's vibration functionality is utilized for each collision.

5.2   Experiments

In the following section, one of the experiments is described in order to illustrate the application of mAbES in a general area of the MCT-PUCRS, regarding the specific issue of Energy.

In the MCT-PUCRS, the Nuclear Power Station experiment simulates the production of nuclear energy, based on a mechanical interaction between the user and the technological devices involved in a nuclear power station. When a user comes upon this experiment, mAbES presents 5 different options for interaction: Challenges (options 1, 2 and 3), audio-description of the experiment (option 4), and information for exiting the Nuclear Power Station experiment (option 6). Figure 5a illustrates the nuclear power station interaction screen, while Figure 5b shows the options for interaction that are available to the user.

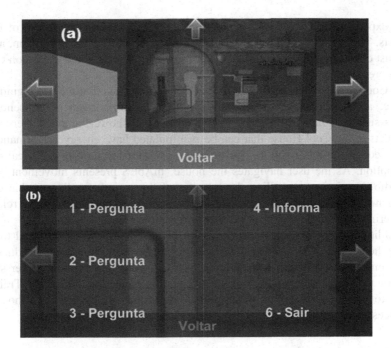

Fig. 5. (a) Nuclear Power Station, (b) Interaction options

The options 1, 2 and 3 present questions related to a nuclear power station as well as response options. Option 1 presents the challenge: "In the first stage of energy production, what happens to the water? Click 1 if you think that the water turns into fuel. Click 2 if you think that the water turns to steam. Click 3 if you think the water goes into the holding tank in liquid form". The options are presented using the Braille matrix. If the user chooses option 2, mAbES informs the user that the answer is correct. Otherwise, the software states that the answer is wrong.

For Option 2, the user must answer the challenge, "What is the function of the electric generator in a nuclear power station? Click 1 if you think that it is to transform the energy trapped in the movement of the water vapor into electrical energy. Click 2 if you think that it is to turn water into steam. Click 3 if you think that it is to reduce the maximum number of fission reactions". If the user chooses option 1, mAbES informs the user that the answer is correct. Otherwise, it states that the answer is wrong.

Option 3 involves the following challenge: "What happens to the steam after it makes the turbine move? Click 1 if when the steam exits the turbine, it ends up producing energy. Click 2 if the steam comes into direct contact with the seawater in order to restart the cycle. Click 3 if the steam is cooled by the seawater, turning it into a net-liquid state so that the process of energy production can be resumed". If the user chooses option 3, mAbES informs the user that the answer is correct. Otherwise, it states that the answer is wrong.

Starting at the Nuclear Power Station experiment, in following the virtual hallway represented on mAbES forward, the user will come upon the Energy Train and Cool

House experiments. The Energy Train is made up of cartoon characters of energy scientists. The mAbES application provides information on each one of them, and the user must choose the correct name of the corresponding scientist. The cartoon characters are presented as the user moves along the train.

The Cool House is one of the MCT-PUCRS experiments that require a guided experience, as it includes activities that involve the manipulation of household appliances such as a hair dryer, iron, stove, bathtub and shower, among others. All of the objects in the Cool House that can be manipulated have energy performance meters. Based on this information, questions are presented regarding electrical energy consumption. As the user navigates the house, mAbES presents movement options and audio descriptions regarding the location of the various appliances that can be manipulated. When exiting the Cool House, the software presents questions related to the experiments that the user now has the information needed to respond.

In addition, mAbES presents some questions that the user must respond to when visiting the MCT-PUCRS, such as those related to the use of fuel in the production of nuclear energy, how electrical generation turbines work in a nuclear power station, regarding the physical appearance of the scientists presented at the Energy Train, and related to electrical energy consumption when using certain kinds of household appliances.

6   Discussion and Conclusions

This study presents the design and implementation of mAbES, a mobile audio based environment simulator to assist in the development of orientation and mobility skills for people who are blind. We also introduce a model scenario for using mAbES together with an application for navigating through a science and technology museum in Porto Alegre, Brazil. This application was focused on a specific topic area, pertaining to the concept of energy and other related topics.

We present and describe the main interfaces of mAbES including both audio and graphic design, and explain the different modes of user interaction. The mAbES software was designed for use by people with visual impairment, but without excluding the possibility that sighted people can also use the application, in order to promote social inclusion.

The mAbES software supports navigation through the museum by a group with both visually impaired and sighted visitors. In this way, a blind visitor and a sighted visitor can share the use of a smartphone and earphones, and create collaborative experiences as a result of using and interacting with mAbES. This may help to avoid people with visual impairment being isolated while visiting the museum. The issue of user isolation when using a mobile museum guide is mentioned in some studies as a disadvantage [8].

Finally, future work will involve the implementation of a full usability evaluation of mAbES, with both visually impaired and sighted users. Such work would also imply the design and implementation of an impact evaluation study focusing on orientation and mobility skills. In this sense, measuring the impact of the use of mAbES on the development and practice of navigation skills is the priority for future work.

Acknowledgements. This report was funded by the Chilean National Fund of Science and Technology, Fondecyt #1120330, and Project CIE-05 Program Center Education PBCT-Conicyt. It was also supported by the Program STIC-AmSud-CAPES/CONICYT/MAEE, Project KIGB-Knowing and Interacting while Gaming for the Blind, 2014.

References

1. Carreiras, M., Codina, B.: Cognición espacial, orientación y movilidad, consideraciones sobre la ceguera. Integración (11), 5–15 (1993)
2. Frauenberger, C., Noisternig, M.: 3D audio interfaces for the blind. In: Proceedings of the 2003 International Conference on Auditory Display, Boston, MA, USA, July 6-9, pp. 1–4 (2003)
3. Golledge, R.: Geography and the disabled. A survey with special reference to vision impaired and blind populations. Transactions of the Institute of British Geographers, New Series 18(1), 63–85 (1993)
4. Hill, E., Ponder, P.: Orientación y técnicas de Movilidad, Una guía para el practicante. Comité internacional pro-ciegos, México (1981)
5. Jacobson, R.D.: Cognitive mapping without sight: four preliminary studies of spatial learning. Journal of Environmental Psychology (18), 289–305 (1998)
6. Jain, S.: Assessment of audio interfaces for use in smartphone based spatial learning systems for the blind. Master of Science Thesis in Spatial Information Science and Engineering. University of Maine (2012)
7. Lahav, O., Mioduser, D.: Haptic-feedback support for cognitive mapping of unknown spaces by people who are blind. International Journal of Human-Computer Studies 66(1), 23–35 (2008)
8. Lanir, J., Kuflik, T., Dim, E., Wecker, A.J., Stock, O.: The influence of location-aware mobile guide on Museum visitors'behavior. Interacting with Computers 25(6), 443–460 (2013)
9. Lumbreras, M., Sánchez, J.: Interactive 3D sound hyperstories for blind children. In: Proceedings of the SIGCHI Conference on Human Factors in Computing Systems: the CHI Is the Limit, CHI 1999, Pittsburgh, Pennsylvania, United States, May 15-20, pp. 318–325 (1999)
10. Millar, S.: La comprensión y la representación del espacio, Teoría y evidencia a partir de estudios con niños ciegos y videntes, 406 págs. ONCE, Madrid (1997)
11. ONCE, Organización Nacional de Ciegos Españoles: Glosario de Términos de Rehabilitación Básica de las Personas Ciegas y Deficientes Visuales, Entre Dos Mundos, Revista de traducción sobre discapacidad visual (1998)
12. Sanabria, L.: Mapeo cognitivo y exploración háptica para comprender la disposición del espacio de videntes e invidentes. Tecné, Episteme y Didaxis: Revista de la Facultad de Ciencia y Tecnología 21, 45–65 (2007)
13. Sánchez, J., Maureira, E.: Subway Mobility Assistance Tools for Blind Users. In: Stephanidis, C., Pieper, M. (eds.) ERCIM Ws UI4ALL 2006. LNCS, vol. 4397, pp. 386–404. Springer, Heidelberg (2007)
14. Sánchez, J., Oyarzún, C.: Mobile Audio Assistance in Bus Transportation for the Blind. International Journal on Disability and Human Development (IJDHD) 10(4), 365–371 (2011)

15. Sánchez, J., de la Torre, N.: Autonomous navigation through the city for the blind. In: Proceedings of the 12th international ACM SIGACCESS Conference on Computers and Accessibility (ASSETS 2010), pp. 195–202. ACM, New York (2010)
16. Sánchez, J., Sáenz, M., Pascual-Leone, A., Merabet, L.: Enhancing navigation skills through audio gaming. In: Ext. Abstracts CHI 2010, pp. 3991–3996. ACM Press (2010)
17. Sánchez, J., Tadres, A., Pascual-Leone, A., Merabet, L.: Blind Children Navigation through Gaming and Associated Brain Plasticity. In: Proc. of the Virtual Rehabilitation 2009 International Conference, Haifa, Israel, pp. 29–36. IEEE (2009)

Evaluating Tactile-Acoustic Devices for Enhanced Driver Awareness and Safety: An Exploration of Tactile Perception and Response Time to Emergency Vehicle Sirens

Maria Karam

Kings College London, Strand, London, WC2R 2LS, UK
maria.karam@kcl.ac.uk

Abstract. A feasibility study was conducted to determine if real-time emergency vehicle sirens can be detected when presented to a driver using a tactile display device. Public usability methods were employed to evaluate the tactile-perceptibility of siren sounds when a driver's hearing ability is impaired, due to temporary deafness that is induced when listening to loud music, road noise, or by active noise cancelling systems installed in automobiles. The study evaluates siren detection rates and response times of drivers who are artificially deafened by loud music using tactile-only stimuli as an alert system. Results of the study suggest that the use of an ambient tactile display can provide persistent access to siren sounds for drivers who are deafened in both low and high stress conditions. Details of the experiments are presented, along with a discussion on next steps, which includes recommendations for integrating the tactile displays into driving simulators as an alternative form to haptic displays that can improve driver awareness of and response to emergency vehicle signals.

Keywords: Tactile acoustic devices, primary and secondary attention, cognitive processing, hearing loss, driving simulation, emergency vehicle response, automotive safety.

1 Introduction

Sensory overload is a rapidly growing problem for drivers aiming to keep their eyes and ears focused on the road despite the rampant digital information that is being increasingly made available from our mobile phones, onboard computer systems, and information systems. Demand on visual and auditory attention for vehicle operators is increasingly expanding the cognitive load drivers must manage, while maintaining attention and safety on the road. In addition, drivers often experience a form of temporary hearing loss caused by many factors including loud music, road and engine noise, active noise cancellation, or phone and passenger conversations, which can drastically reduce the ability to recognize and respond to emergency vehicle signals (EVS).

C. Stephanidis and M. Antona (Eds.): UAHCI/HCII 2014, Part III, LNCS 8515, pp. 729–740, 2014.
© Springer International Publishing Switzerland 2014

Tactile devices are an effective way to increase driver awareness of their surroundings even when hearing is obstructed. To assess siren sounds from the environment as a source of tactile stimuli, a feasibility study was conducted using a tactile-acoustic device that was developed to assist deaf and hard of hearing people in accessing sound from movies and music. The study explores low and high stress scenarios, where participants are artificially deafened using loud music, and asked to respond when they detect tactile siren signals. In the low stress condition, participants focus on trying to detect the vibrations while relaxing and listening to music. For the high stress condition, participants are placed in a driving simulator and asked to race a car while signaling when they can feel the sirens. Using the public usability methodology, the study focuses on gaining a preliminary understanding of the perceptibility of siren signals when directly presented to the body as tactile vibrations. Details of the study are presented, along with recommendations for implementing tactile-audio devices into automobiles as an ambient sensory augmentation technology for increasing awareness and safety for vehicle operators.

1.1 Background

Eyes are the primary sensory organ used for driving, but hearing provides early warning signals that can improve awareness, reduce accidents and increase safety [8]. Because hearing is critical for detecting emergency vehicles in advance of their approach, ensuring drivers have access to the early warning signals from oncoming ambulance or fire trucks can lead to increased safety and awareness of surroundings. All drivers, even those who are not deaf or hard of hearing, can experience some form of hearing loss while driving, often due to masking from engine sounds, road noise, loud music, or conversations. Additional mechanisms that also cause temporary hearing loss include temporary threshold shift (TTS), and noise-induced hearing loss (NIHL), often prevalent in commercial motor vehicle operators [8].

1.2 Temporary Hearing Loss

TTS can occur when noise levels drivers experience tend to fluctuate between high and low frequencies, which can cause perceptual distortion of sounds, or lead to low signal reception levels [8]. Aging is another factor that can lead to a decrease in hearing ability, and older adults often lose some or all hearing ability in the high frequency range. Further, some hearing aids may produce a whistling sound or completely cancel out the high frequency signals that are so common in sirens, further reducing access to emergency vehicle signals. Hearing aids may also lead to deafening of a driver to the sounds of sirens as they may whistle when detecting high frequencies, and lead to noise cancellation of the high frequency signals like sirens. Missing early warning signals and sounds from sirens, railway crossings, and other cars can be disruptive and dangerous for drivers when audio signals cannot be detected, potentially compromising safety and awareness.

1.3   Tactile Alert Systems in Automobiles

Haptic display technologies represent one method used to increase safety and awareness in drivers. However, haptic systems are typically used to provide spatial information that can help alert drivers to lane departures, objects coming in close proximity to the vehicle, or to provide tactile messages about road conditions [3]. Motors, piezoelectric devices, or transducers used in haptic devices represent an excellent method of ensuring a driver is effectively alerted to the indicators that a haptic device delivers [2]. Signals and messages are predominantly presented by the spatial location or coded pattern presented to the vibrators as physical icons or 'tactons' [1]. Current haptic systems that are being included in 2014 automotive models may adopt a simple set of signals designed to inform drivers of lane departures or approaching objects by leveraging the spatial location of vibrators to the left or right side of the drivers seat. But as the number of signals and notifications increase, haptic systems may also contribute to sensory overload in drivers, who must learn and properly identify haptic messages while maintaining primary attention on the critical task of driving.

1.4   Ambient Tactile Displays

An alternative system that can alleviate some of the learning requirements and potential information overload related to haptics involves the use of a persistent audio signal to deliver tactile signals to the driver, and is referred to as a tactile-acoustic device (TAD) [6]. TADs offer a different form of tactile information to the body, one that is based on the delivery of real time sounds to the body in a tactile format. Providing drivers with persistent access to ambient sounds from the environment could improve EVS detection by vehicle operators when hearing is reduced.

2   Tactile-Acoustic Devices (TADs)

TADs are systems that deliver a form of sensory augmentation of sound to the skin, which can increase the entertainment value of movies and music for people who are deaf or hard of hearing. Emotion and intentionality expressed through sound such as musical timbre, and voice qualities can be easily identified and associated to the source audio even by people who may never have heard sound before [9,5]. For critical applications, where increased access to sounds can improve safety and awareness of one's surroundings, automotive seats represent a natural application for augmenting sound with vibrations. Sensory augmentation of sound through vibrations may provide drivers with an ability to detect sirens and other warning signals even when their hearing is impaired. The sense of touch has strong implications as an information channel for drivers to use in addition to hearing and sight. Most of the research on tactile devices focuses on haptic systems, and the structured patterns and directional information that vibrations can communicate to the body. Tactons, which represent a type of tactile signal often associated with haptics, use vibration patterns to convey messages to the skin, analagous to icons meant to be seen, and earcons meant to be heard [1].

2.1 Ambient Tactile Awareness

Using the TAD system, which was originally developed to augment hearing in the Emoti-Chair [6], drivers may experience improved and persistent access to emergency vehicle signals, resulting in increased awareness towards reducing accidents. Tactile-acoustic signals can be sampled directly from the environment and used as ambient information presented to the body through a tactile device. Although siren signals are much higher than what is recommend for optimal tactile stimulation, ranging from approximately 700 - 1500 Hz, the TAD system works by including the entire sound spectrum in the display, distributing along the body to maximize the information that can potentially be interpreted by the user. Although the vibrations tend to be subtle, tactile-acoustic signals can communicate complex information from sound to the body, including emotional content, intentionality, and prosody.

2.2 Exploring Sound as Vibrations

One of the challenges of using sounds as tactile stimuli relates to the frequency range of sirens, which tend to be higher than the optimal tactile detection range of skin, which lies roughly between 250 and 500Hz. Audio signals that are used in haptic systems must be manipulated, transformed, modified, or otherwise interpreted into sensations or vibrations within the optimal tactile detection range. This type of signal is limited to conveying tactons or other pattern-based vibrational messages. Sound however, contains complex frequency patterns that cannot be easily captured by a motor or single vibration level and presents challenges that are beyond what haptic system can communicate. Tactile acoustics provides additional sound information to enhance what we should be hearing, with vibrations created by sounds, to provide a more complex and rich signal to a user, serving as an alternative sensory modality to hearing.

3 Feasibility Study

This research considers the feasibility of using emergency vehicle signals as real time input to a tactile acoustic device designed to convey sounds to people with limited or no access to sounds. A public usability study was conducted in a cafe, [4], where patrons of the cafe were asked to take part in a short evaluation of a new technology designed to provide tactile access to emergency vehicle signals (EVS). This is an agile method for collecting user feedback on a system when considering new application domains, or other aspects of usability in the tactile or haptic domain and will be proposed as a contribution to the development of a framework for standardizing haptic and tactile device evaluations [10].

3.1 Approach

The TAD considered in this work is designed to deliver sound to the body in a format that can be recognized and processes by the user with little or no advanced training.

This study considers three fundamental principles of computing as the framework for this evaluation: input, processing, and output. Each of these factors can be changed, while maintaining the same experimental protocol. For example, in this study, we examine EVS (input), standard TAD frequency split (processing) and the 4-channel TAD (output). With this perspective, different signals, different processing algorithms, and different tactile devices can be assessed for the same application. In this way, subsequent data collected from experiments conducted using this method can be compared with other experiments using a common set of measurements. Variables explored include detectability of EVS vibrations, their just noticeable difference (JND) and efficacy as an alert for distracted drivers, listed in table 1.

Table 1. Summary of variables, files, and conditions used in this study. 0dB = source signal level at 60-65dB

Factor	File	Samples	Condition
Detectibility	Recog.wav	4 EVS x 5 repetitions	Cafe
Efficacy	Race.wav	4 EVS x 2 repetitions	Racing
JND	JND.wav	-20dB, -15dB, -10dB, -05dB, 0dB	Cafe /Racing

Detectability and JND are considered in the cafe study, which is presented as the first phase of the feasibility study. The driving simulation test is conducted as a case study and evaluates JND and efficacy. The variables in table 1 are evaluated based on the context of the system and the interaction it provides. To generalize an approach to the different components that can be assessed using this method, the system is evaluated for the different types of audio signals that can be used for vibrations. The manipulations the system can perform on the signals is the processor, and the type of display used to provide the vibrations is the output. This provides a framework that supports extended studies on multiple components over time that can be compared with current results or to evaluate other systems. A summary is provided in table 2.

Table 2. Summary of approach applied to this series of studies

Component	Current Configuration	Manipulations
Input	EVS	Tactons, music, speech
Processing	Signal split and pass through	Pitch shift, wave modification, filters
Output	4 channel pairs	8 channel pairs, 16 channels

The TAD system provides a variety of settings that can be configured to modify the audio signal in many ways.

Frequency bands, intensity levels, filtering, q-factor, and individual channel control are possible for each of the transucers. The default setting of the system is used in this study, which processes signals between 100Hz and 1500Hz and distributes them to the 8 channels. The portable device used in the cafe study includes signals from 500Hz to 1500Hz split onto 4 channels to encompass the range of the EVS samples. The driving simulator includes the full range spread across 8 channels, to include the engine sounds in the vibrations.

Signals. EVS were chosen to represent the local emergency sounds, which were based on Toronto fire, police and ambulance sirens. EVS samples were sourced from the website of a siren manufacturing company who supplies the sirens used by local emergency vehicles [7]. Four signal samples were used in each stage of the study: wail, yelp, horn, and manual wail. Signals were presented in audio files that arranged the four samples together to make up the different versions of the trials presented to users.

3.2 Experimental Setup

A TAD 4-channel system built into a leather seat cushion was used for this study. The pad was placed on a bench at the CoffeeLab. Intensity levels for vibrations are set at a default level, roughly approximating 65dB. Each participant sits on the pad, and wears a pair of BOSE Quiet Comfort noise cancelling headphones and listens to music at a level that is loud enough to block out most sounds from the environment. EVS signals are presented on the TAD, and the participants are asked to indicate when they detect siren vibrations by saying siren or tapping on the table. Eight samples are presented in the JND test, and 20 in the recognition test. Responses are recorded, noting time of detection, false positives and false negatives detection. Default levels were set for the signal output, which was approximately 60-65dB based on a standard noise meter reading, which is significantly lower than the roughly 90dB level that sirens output, but serves to create the in-the-distance effect of advance warnings.

10 Participants were recruited from the cafe, and each participant received a coffee or tea for their time. Amplitude levels for the music and the EVS were independently controlled, maintaining the 65Hz level for the vibrations, and allowing the participant to adjust the volume of the music to a level that was comfortable, but loud enough to block most of the sounds from the sirens that could be heard through the TAD. Interviews were conducted with each participant to gather additional information about their experience and opinion of the system and the experiment. Because of the public usability design, the study is designed to be quick and fun for participants, and intended to reveal different characteristics of the interaction that may not otherwise be noticed in more controlled settings.

3.3 Results

The cafe study uses a hybrid ethnography-empirical approach to gathering a broad range of feedback and data from users. The first four participants recognized all 20 samples presented to them in the Recog.wav file, while wearing headphones and being seated on the portable TAD. Sample durations and participants timed response are shown in figure 1.

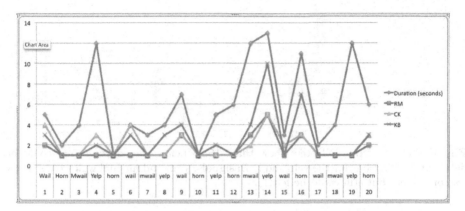

Fig. 1. EVS Samples and durations presented in the study

Timed results from four of the participants who completed the 20-file test were recorded, and are shown in figure 2. These four participants recognized all 20 of the samples, and were timed, showing a standard deviation of 0 - 1 for most of the samples, with trials 14 (sd=2.9) and 16 (sd=2.3) having the greatest deviation. The results of participant response times for each sample are displayed in figure 2.

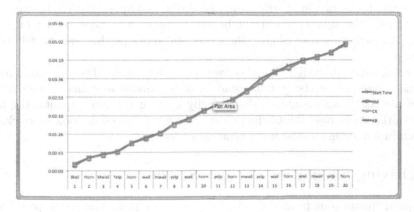

Fig. 2. Cafe response times were very close. Durations along the y-axis.

Five participants took part in the JND test, also suggesting that tactile EVS can certainly be detected as vibrations in a low stress environment like the cafe, when users are relaxing and paying attention to the signals. The table of results for the JND are presented in figure 3.

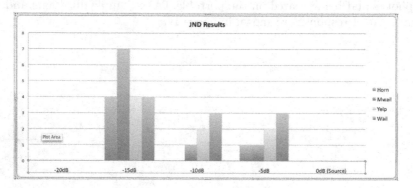

Fig. 3. Results of the JND test show that -15dB below the source signal could be detected as vibrations for the yelp and horn signals. Wail and manual wail were slightly less prominent but still could be felt.

3.4 Discussion

Seven participants completed the 20 sample evaluation, one had to leave early, and two were distracted by activities in the cafe and did not complete both tests. Participants reported being able to clearly detect the siren vibrations, but even with the headphones on and the music, some of the signals could be heard from the vibrations.

Variance in the music may have contributed to the moments of silence that corresponded with some of the signals, but the preliminary results suggest that there are some tactile elements coming through the vibrations that can obviously be detected by users. One participant who did not complete the study expressed concern that the signals would not be strong enough to be detected in a real driving scenario, because of the vibrations and motions that can be felt while driving.

Overall, participants felt that there would be the potential to use this in a car, and most agreed that the system could serve to provide feedback while driving. But while the signals could be detected by each of the participants, the next phase of the study moved into the Lounge Lab where we could look more closely at EVS in a driving simulator scenario in a case study.

4   Driving Simulation: 2 Case Studies

Two participants (one from the cafe study, and one first time participant) took part in the driving simulation test to evaluate a more stressful driving scenario to test the EVS signals for their efficacy at attracting driver attention while engaged in the cognitively demanding task of racing. The driving simulation system includes a TAD 8-channel system, a 42 inch Samsung LCD screen, and the Sony Playstation 3 running Gran Turismo 6, and the Thrustmaster Ferrari GT Cockpit 430 Scuderia Racing Controller. The study took place at the Lounge Lab, which is in a private home next to the Cafe, where a gaming and theatre environment is maintained for other public usability studies.

4.1 Evaluations

Two participants agreed to be case studies for this project. Each participant was already familiar with the driving simulator, and with the TAD system. This was the first time the siren experiment was conducted in this environment, which is typically used to evaluate games and movies for tactile content in the TAD seat. Each driver raced an intense race, and was asked to say 'siren' when they could feel the vibrations. The conditions explored EVS in the tactile system, with and without including the sounds of the car on the speakers, as vibrations, or both. Music was played over the speakers in the room, and the EVS were presented either as vibrations, audio signals, or both. Drivers raced the Chevy Camaro using the advanced races in the game. The same samples were used in this study for the JND test, with an audio file with eight samples of EVS: 2 x 4 EVS samples at five seconds each, over a three minute period.

4.2 Results

This part of the feasibility study revealed several interesting factors about the tactile stimuli, showing the conditions, and the response times for each participant in figure 4. The high stress involved racing, which led to a few false positive

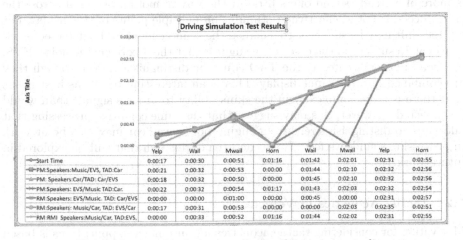

Fig. 4. Racing simulation results for the two case studies

and false negative response, which did not happen in the low stress condition at the care. Interesting results show EVS responses were comparable to the audio EVS, even while game sounds were included in the TAD, suggesting that users can distinguish different signals through the combined vibrations. Drivers could also hear some of the signals during the trials, but overall, most of the EVS tactile signals were accessible during stressful conditions.

5   Discussion and Future Work

Results of this feasibility study suggest that real time audio signals from EVS could serve as input to a tactile display without any modifications to the signal as they appear to provide enough energy to convey information to the user while driving. Based on the first study, where participants were only listening to music, the signals appear to be highly tactile. Two of the participants expressed concern that the signal may not be strong enough to get their attention in a driving situation where they were focusing on the road.

5.1   EVS as Tactile Acoustic Vibrations

Although participants from the case study found the EVS vibrations to be detectible, even when mixed in with the engine vibrations, there are some modifications that can be performed on the signal, which could help to enhance the vibrations. For example, applying a pitch shift to the EVS would drop the frequency range of the signals closer to the optimal tactile range, making the vibrations stronger. Another modification to the signal could be to distribute the frequency ranges of the system to better highlight the signal. In the yelp signal, there is a significant fluctuation in the frequencies, which is effectively reflected in the movement across the transducers of the TAD. The wail, which is more of a steady sound offers little in the way of motion of signal across the transducers, is not as effective at stimulating multiple points of the display, but a pitch shift may be sufficient to enhance the sound enough to be detected as vibrations. Results from the case study suggest that the mix of engine noise, EVS, and road noise presented in the TAD could be distinguished, even though they are combined into the same display. This is an interesting result, as it suggests that there is more complexity in the skins ability to process signals than would be expected. However, this may suggest that the same cognitive processing that allows us to distinguish sirens from engine noises we hear may also be at work in processing sounds we feel. This is an area of research that will be explored in future work.

5.2   Tactile Acoustics in Vehicles

Motivation for considering tactile acoustics for automotive applications is based on the inherent success of haptic devices, which have now been adopted by at least one major automotive manufacturer [3]. Tactile acoustics represents a natural form of stimuli that can be used as a complimentary system to the haptic devices to provide ambient tactile signals to drivers. While haptic systems are very effective at providing drivers with vibrational feedback for lane departures and collision warnings, they are not intended to provide constant information to the user about the environment, and they rely on visual input, which can easily map onto the spatial configuration of the vibrators. Haptics are being considered as a way to warn drivers about numerous dangers on the road, including bad weather, road conditions, phone messages, or GPS directions for example. However, with an increase in the number of haptic messages users have to memorize and recognize, comes an increase in the cognitive load placed on the driver, which defeats the original intention of using haptics in automotive applications. Tactile acoustics can provide additional access to the environment as tactile signals without requiring the driver to first learn to identify the signals, provided that they are constrained to sirens and other EMS. However, in order to better understand the system, an in-situ experiment is underway, using the TAD portable device in a real car, where we will be able to test the system in more realistic scenarios, simulating siren sounds and creating a noisy environment with music playing.

6 Conclusions

Results from this feasibility provides some evidence to suggest that EVS awareness could be increased by including tactile acoustic signals to assist drivers whose hearing is obstructed permanently, or temporarily. Although EVS signals tend to be in the high frequency ranges, they can create perceptible tactile vibrations without being modified. But lowering the pitch or increasing variation in the signal through system or device manipulations could improve tactile-perception of real time EVS. While the signals were detected by participants, there are additional factors that must be considered for actual use in a car: road noise, engine noise, fluctuations in the signal, and gaining access to real time sounds from the environment influence how the system could be implemented. The results of combining tactile signals from both the engine, and the sirens showed promise in providing drivers with a sense of an approaching EVS, even when the acoustiv vibrations are occluded by noise introduced into the vibration signal. Integration into existing haptic systems can be potentially advantageous to drivers want to maintain ambient awareness of their surroundings without using their eyes or ears. Further studies will install TADs into a prototype vehicle for validation in an actual driving scenario, towards improving driver safety, awareness, and access to information while driving.

Acknowledgements. With great appreciation to all the participants who took part in the study, the Sideshow cafe, and WM Perry and RM Indrigo for their continued support in making this research possible.

References

1. Brewster, S., Brown, L.M.: Tactons: Structured tactile messages for non-visual information display. In: Proceedings of the Fifth Conference on Australasian User Interface, AUIC 2004, vol. 28, pp. 15–23. Australian Computer Society, Inc., Darlinghurst (2004)
2. Cao, Y., van der Sluis, F., Theune, M., op den Akker, R., Nijholt, A.: Evaluating informative auditory and tactile cues for in-vehicle information systems. In: Proceedings of the 2nd International Conference on Automotive User Interfaces and Interactive Vehicular Applications, AutomotiveUI 2010, pp. 102–109. ACM, New York (2010)
3. Hogema, J.H., De Vries, S.C., Van Erp, J.B.F., Kiefer, R.J.: A tactile seat for direction coding in car driving: Field evaluation. EEE Trans. Haptics 2(4), 181–188 (2009)
4. Karam, M.: The coffee lab: developing a public usability space. In: CHI 2010 Extended Abstracts on Human Factors in Computing Systems, CHI EA 2010, pp. 2671–2680. ACM, New York (2010)
5. Karam, M., Nespoli, G., Russo, F., Fels, D.I.: Modelling perceptual elements of music in a vibrotactile display for deaf users: A field study. In: Proceedings of the 2009 Second International Conferences on Advances in Computer-Human Interactions, ACHI 2009, pp. 249–254. IEEE Computer Society, Washington, DC (2009)
6. Karam, M., Russo, F.A., Fels, D.I.: Designing the model human cochlea: An ambient crossmodal audio-tactile display. EEE Trans. Haptics 2(3), 160–169 (2009)
7. C. S. Manufacturers. Sa classic 400 sirens
8. Palmer, C.V., Talbott, E., Lave, L.B., LaPorte, R.E., Songer, T.J.: Hearing disorders and commercial motor vehicle drivers (revised). Technical report, Pittsburgh Univ., PA. Dept. of Epidemiology (1993)
9. Russo, F.A., Ammirante, P., Fels, D.I.: Vibrotactile discrimination of musical timbre. Journal of Experimental Psychology-Human Perception and Performance 38, 822–826 (2012)
10. Sinclair, I., Carter, J., Kassner, S., van Erp, J., Weber, G., Elliott, L., Andrew, I.: Towards a standard on evaluation of tactile/Haptic interactions. In: Isokoski, P., Springare, J. (eds.) EuroHaptics 2012, Part I. LNCS, vol. 7282, pp. 528–539. Springer, Heidelberg (2012)

TActile Glasses (TAG) for Obstacle Avoidance

Georgios Korres[1], Ahmad El Issawi[2], and Mohamad Eid[1]

[1] Applied Interactive Multimedia Lab, Division of Engineering,
New York University Abu Dhabi, United Arab Emirates
{george.korres,mohamad.eid}@nyu.edu
[2] Lebanese University, Nabatieh, Lebanon
ahmadissawi@email.com

Abstract. In this paper, we present a wearable tactile device called TAG (TActile Glasses) to help visually impaired individuals navigate through complex environments. The TAG device provides vibrotactile feedback whenever an obstacle is detected in front of the user. The prototype is composed of – in addition to the eyeglasses – an infrared proximity sensor, an ATMEGA128 microprocessor, a rechargeable battery, and a vibrotactile actuator attached to the right temple tip of the glasses. The TAG system is designed to be highly portable, fashionable yet cost effective, and intuitive to use. Experimental study showed that the TAG system can help visually impaired individuals to navigate unfamiliar lab environment using vibrotactile feedback, and without any previous training. Participants reported that the system is intuitive to use, quick to learn, and helpful.

Keywords: Haptic user interface, Interaction Design, Tangible user interfaces, user support systems.

1   Introduction

The World Health Organization (WHO) estimated in October 2013 that about 285 million people are visually impaired worldwide, with 90% living in developing countries (around 15% blind and 85% with low vision) [1]. Although 80% can be cured through clinical treatment, the remaining 20% rely on modern technology and innovation to enhance awareness of their surroundings.

Traditional mobility assistance techniques such as walking stick or trained dogs suffer from several limitations [2]. For instance, walking sticks are not efficient and result in undesirable heavy cognitive load whereas trained dogs are too expensive and require extensive training. Advanced technologies for mobility assistance seem a promising approach to complement (or maybe replace) traditional approaches using other modalities such as touch and audio.

There are two categories of multimedia aides for the visually impaired: audio feedback and haptic feedback [3]. Auditory feedback has few limitations such as cognitive obtrusiveness since it hinders the user's ability to hear background auditory cues (speech, traffic, etc.). Moreover, auditory cues require significant training to interpret

C. Stephanidis and M. Antona (Eds.): UAHCI/HCII 2014, Part III, LNCS 8515, pp. 741–749, 2014.
© Springer International Publishing Switzerland 2014

the sound-scape in order to de-multiplex the temporal data into spatial cues. On the other hand, although individuals who loose vision have difficulty maintaining their independence and mobility, they become more acquainted with tactile interaction than people with normal vision [4]. Consequently, several haptic interfaces have been developed to convert visual cues to tactile stimuli on different parts of the body such as on the head, chest, arms, and fingertip [5].

One fundamental need for the visually impaired individual is safe navigation through collision avoidance. Geometry-to-tactile translation systems have been utilized in the literature where ultrasonic transceiver behaves like a 'cane' and translates geometry information (such as the size and the depth of an obstacle) into a tactile cue that is displayed using tactile interface [3][6]. However, current tactile display approaches for spatial information are challenged by relatively low space resolution, poor recognition rate, and cognitive obtrusiveness [7].

The motivation behind this work is to seize the hardships faced by visually impaired individuals in dealing with their daily navigation activities. The proposed system, embedded in fashionable eyeglasses with circuitry in the grip, detects obstacles in front of the user and alerts her/him via vibration. The vibration intensity increases nonlinearly as the user approaches a physical barrier. Despite its simplicity, the integrated hardware solution improves safe mobility.

The remainder of the paper is organized as follows. Section 2 introduces state-of-the-art related work and highlights existing limitations and potential challenges. Section 3 introduces the hardware and software design of the TAG device. In section 4 the experimental setup and procedure, along with the obtained results, are presented. Finally, section 5 summarizes the merits of the paper and provides perspectives for future work.

2   Related Work

Existing research on tactile-visual sensory substitution for the blind or the visually impaired adopts two major approaches. One consists of imitating the concept of the cane for the blind and converting the sensed distance-to-obstacle to vibrotactile cue on the hand [8-9]. The distance is measured using ultrasound, infrared, or laser range-finders. The other approach uses imaging devices, such as a camera, to drive a two-dimensional haptic display placed on the user's skin [10-11]. Both approaches have experienced limitations related to intuitive cognition [12].

An early study has confirmed the feasibility of using a haptic display for navigation guidance [13]. A wearable navigation system based on tactile display embedded in the back of a vest, with infrared sensors and a predefined map to locate the user, provided route planning [13]. Another example is the Intelligent Glasses System (IGS) – a travel aid system that grants visually impaired users a simplified representation of the 3D environment [14]. A 2D map is displayed using an Air Mass Flow (AMF) actuator that stimulates tactile sensations.

A remote robot provided visual-to-tactile substitution for visually impaired in the field of obstacle detection and avoidance [15]. The authors presented a visual-to-tactile mapping strategy and experimental results with visually impaired subjects. Subjects have shown increased navigational abilities when provided with spatial information through the tactile modality. A similar system used a smart phone with Catadioptric stereo imaging to acquire spatial data and display vibrotactile sensations using an interface comprised of an 8x8 matrix of coin vibration motors [16].

A multimodal interaction device, named Tyflos [18], provided reading and navigating assistance for visually impaired users [19]. The device integrated two cameras to capture the surroundings and a 2D vibration vest to display 2D depth image. A similar prototype provided a sense of position and motion by inducing rotational skin stretch on the skin at the elbow [17]. Experimental results showed that rotational skin stretch is effective for proprioceptive feedback myoelectric prostheses.

Experimental results in previous works show that the users need to learn a large number of tactile patterns and map them to spatial properties, which results in an undesirable heavy cognitive load and excessive training. This paper presents the work towards an easy to use and learn tactile interface that provides visually impaired users with obstacle avoidance assistance. The TAG prototype implements a mapping algorithm to translate range of obstacles into intensity of vibration.

3   TAG System Design and Implementation

We are designing the TAG system to allow users perceive range distance to an obstacle using vibrotactile stimuli, much like a 'haptic radar'. An infrared sensor is capable of sensing obstacles, measuring the distance to the obstacle, and displaying this information as a vibrotactile cue using the vibrotactile motor attached to the tip of the right temple of the glasses. A snapshot of the TAG prototype is shown in Figure 1.

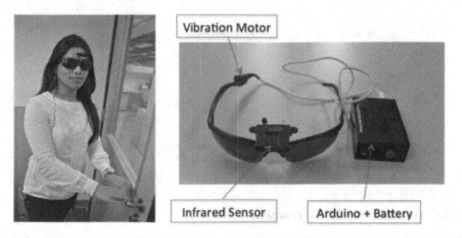

Fig. 1. TAG prototype as a wearable device

3.1   Hardware Design

The TAG system is composed of the Sharp GP2Y0A02 infrared range sensor, the Atmel microprocessor (ATMEGA128), a chargeable battery, and the Pico-Vibe Precision Microdrives vibrotactile motor (Figure 1). The microprocessor and the chargeable battery are packed in a small box that can be placed in the user's pocket. The microprocessor receives signal from the Sharp GP2Y0A02 sensor, determines the distance to the obstacle, and generate Pulse Width Modulation (PWM) signal to control the vibrotactile motor. The infrared sensor and vibration motor are selected based on distinguished features, namely low cost, high availability, and efficient power consumption.

The infrared range sensor (Sharp GP2Y0A02) is characterized by a spatial awareness range of 20cm to 150cm. The Pico-Vibe Precision Microdrives vibration motor is an off-weight coin motor that rotates at 13500 RPM. Since the vibration motor's speed and frequency of vibration are proportional to the voltage applied to the motor, we apply PWM signal to control precisely the intensity and frequency of vibrotactile stimulation.

3.2   Software Architecture for the TAG System

The software architecture for the TAG system is shown in Figure 2. The Obstacle Detection component processes the infrared signal and determines whether an obstacle is in front of the user. Once an obstacle is detected, the infrared sensor data is transmitted to the Geometry Estimation component to compute the distance to the obstacle. The distance to the obstacle is transmitted to the Geometry-to-Tactile Translation component to generate the corresponding tactile stimulus (intensity and duration of vibration). The Actuator Driver component generates a PWM signal and supports sufficient current to drive the vibrotactile motor to vibrate at the desired frequency and intensity.

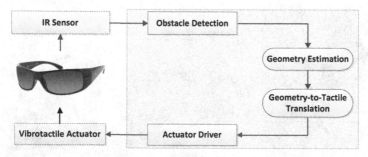

Fig. 2. Software architecture for the TAG system

3.3   Geometry-to-Tactile Translation

Vibrotactile cues were designed to convey range and size of the obstacle. The intensity of vibration is inversely proportional to the distance to the obstacle. Note that the sensor is not capable of distinguishing multiple obstacles and thus we assume one obstacle scenario. Equation 1 shows the intensity to distance mapping where a_0 is the maximum displayable intensity and $\propto_0$ is the vibration adaptation coefficient. Obstacles that are closer to the subject produce higher intensity of vibration. The frequency of vibration is proportional to the size of the obstacle. Equation 2 describes the mapping between size and frequency of vibration where a_1 is the maximum displayable frequency and $\propto_1$ is the frequency adaptation coefficient).

$$I = a_0\, e^{-\propto_0 d} \tag{1}$$

$$F = a_1\, e^{-\propto_1/s} \tag{2}$$

Note that the constants $\propto_0$ and $\propto_1$ can be used to fine-tune the vibrotactile stimulation cues to meet specific application requirements or personal user's preferences. A usability study can be conducted to find the optimal values for these parameters. In the current prototype, the range-to-intensity of vibration mapping (equation 1) is been utilized whereas the size-to-frequency mapping (equation 2) will be implemented in future work.

4   Experimental Study

A pilot experimental study was conducted to investigate the effectiveness of the TAG device to help visually impaired individuals perceive the range of obstacles and actively avoid them. The objective of the experiment was to evaluate the experience of subjects performing a real world navigation task, designed particularly for this experiment.

4.1   Experiment Test-Bed

A total of fourteen participants took part in this experiment, aged between 22 and 44 (three of them were female). All the participants were well-experienced computer users and half of them were using eyeglasses. All of the participants reported normal visual and haptic abilities. The experiment took about 15 minutes on average per subject. The performance metric was defined in terms of the following parameters: the Task Completion Time (TCT) and the Obstacle Avoidance Rate (OAR).

4.2   Method

After a brief practice session of less than 5 minutes, twelve blindfolded participants were asked to use the TAG device to navigate a route designed particularly for the experiment in the engineering lab of New York University Abu Dhabi (Figure 3). Ten obstacles were used in the simulated route. All subjects performed the same activity. As the subject traversed the course, a test moderator was counting the number of obstacles actively avoided and the number of obstacles hit by the subject; he also recorded the time it took to complete the task. At the end of the course, the subject was debriefed for feedback and comments.

In order to evaluate the learnability of the TAG device, two additional subjects were asked to perform the navigation task 12 times and observed the improvement in performance over iterations. Note that the obstacles locations were changed randomly for each trial to avoid any biases from subjects learning the navigation path and the obstacles locations.

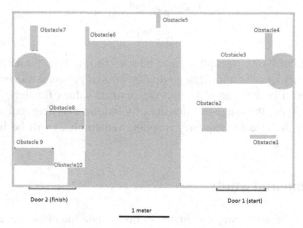

Fig. 3. Navigation task with 10 obstacles

4.3   Experiment Results

Table 1 shows the average and standard deviation for the two quality parameters TCT and OAR. During the experiment, participants were able to avoid obstacles and navigate comfortably without any previous training (about 70% of obstacles were actively avoided using the TAG device, with a standard deviation is 8.28%). This is promising as it demonstrates that the TAG device can be used intuitively. However, a relatively higher variance was observed in the task completion time (standard deviation of 2.15 minutes). Finally, participants also reported the TAG device as intuitive to use, quick to learn, and helpful.

Table 1. TCT and OAR for 12 participants

Parameter	Average	Standard Deviation
Task Completion Time (TCT)	4.28 (minutes)	2.15 (minutes)
Obstacle Avoidance rate (OAR)	70.0 (%)	8.28 (%)

Figure 4 shows that subjects have learned very quickly (only after 3 iterations) how to use the system and actively avoid obstacles. Figure 5 demonstrates a similar trend in terms of task completion time (the time to complete the task has significantly dropped from around 7.2 minutes at the first iteration to around 2 minutes at the ninth iteration).

Figure 4 and Figure 5 clearly show that the overall performance of both subjects has significantly improved (both, in terms of obstacle avoidance rate and task completion time) with less than 10 trials. Note that Figure 4 and Figure 5 are based on the average data for the two subjects.

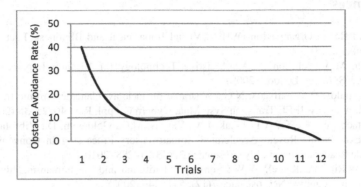

Fig. 4. Obstacle Avoidance Rate (OAR) over iterations

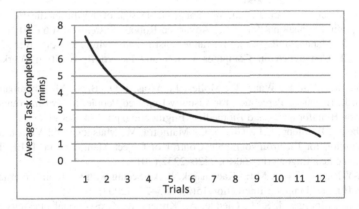

Fig. 5. Task Completion Time (TCT) over iterations

5 Conclusion

In this paper, we presented the TAG device to assist individuals with visual impairments to actively avoid obstacles in unknown environments using vibrotactile feedback. The experimental study demonstrated how intuitive it was to use the system for the first time (70% of the obstacles were actively avoided using the TAG device). However, few subjects expressed interest in receiving hints regarding the direction to take to reach a particular target while avoiding the obstacle.

In future work, we plan to investigate a way to capture more information about the geometry of the obstacle so the TAG device would provide guidance on how to get around obstacles and reach safely a particular target. Another important functionality that we plan to explore is the ability to detect small obstacles such as small steps and stairs to help the user navigate safely along a path. We will consider means to increase the coverage range and precision to detect smaller obstacles.

References

1. World Health Organization (WHO), Visual Impairment and Blindness. Fact Sheet (282) (October 2013)
2. Hersh, M.A., Johnson, M.A.: Assistive Technology for Visually Impaired and Blind People. Springer, London (2008)
3. Dakopoulos, D., Bourbakis, N.G.: Wearable obstacle avoidance electronic travel aids for blind: A survey. IEEE Trans. on Syst. Man. Cybern C Appl. Rev. 40, 25–35 (2010)
4. Bhattacharjee, A., Ye, A.J., Lisak, J.A., Vargas, M.G., Goldreich, D.: Vibrotactile Masking Experiments Reveal Accelerated Somatosensory Processing in Congenitally Blind Braille Readers. Journal of Neuroscience 30(43), 14288 (2010)
5. Bach-y-Rita, P., Kercel, W.W.: Sensory substitution and the human-machine interface. Trends in Cognitive Neuroscience 7(12), 541–546 (2003)
6. Visell, Y.: Tactile sensory substitution: Models for enaction in HCI. Interacting with Computers 21(1-2), 38–53 (2009)
7. Wu, J., Zhang, J., Yan, J., Liu, W., Song, G.: Design of a Vibrotactile Vest for Contour Perception. International Journal of Advanced Robotic Systems 9, 166 (2012)
8. Yuan, D., Manduchi, R.: A tool for range sensing and environment discovery for the blind. In: IEEE Conference on Computer Vision and Pattern Recognition Workshop, p. 39 (2004)
9. Moller, K., Toth, F., Wang, L., Moller, J., Arras, K.O., Bach, M., Schumann, S., Guttmann, J.: Enhanced Perception for Visually Impaired People. In: 3rd International Conference on Bioinformatics and Biomedical Engineering, pp. 1–4 (2009)
10. Rombokas, E., Stepp, C.E., Chang, C., Malhotra, M., Matsuoka, Y.: Vibrotactile Sensory Substitution for Electromyographic Control of Object Manipulation. IEEE Transactions on Biomedical Engineering 60(8), 2226–2232 (2013)
11. Bach-Y-Rita, P., Tyler, M.E., Kaczmarek, K.A.: Seeing with the brain. International Journal of Human Computer Interaction 15(2), 285–295 (2003)
12. Ptito, M., Moesgaard, S.M., Gjedde, A., Kupers, R.: Cross-modal plasticity revealed by electrotactile stimulation of the tongue in the congenitally blind. Brain 128, 606–614 (2005)
13. Ertan, S., Lee, C., Willets, A., Tan, H., Pentland, A.: A wearable haptic navigation guidance system. In: Second International Symposium on Wearable Computers, pp. 164–165 (1998)
14. Pissaloux, E.E., Velazquez, R., Maingreaud, F.: On 3D world perception: towards a definition of a cognitive map based electronic travel aid. In: 26th Annual International Conference of the IEEE Engineering in Medicine and Biology Society, pp. 107–109 (2004)
15. Zelek, J.S., Asmar, D.: A robot's spatial perception communicated via human touch. In: IEEE International Conference on Systems, Man and Cybernetics, vol. 1, pp. 454–461 (2003)
16. Akhter, S., Mirsalahuddin, J., Marquina, F.B., Islam, S., Sareen, S.: A Smartphone-based Haptic Vision Substitution system for the blind. In: IEEE 37th Annual Northeast Bioengineering Conference (NEBEC), pp. 1–3 (2011)

17. Wheeler, J., Bark, K., Savall, J., Cutkosky, M.: Investigation of Rotational Skin Stretch for Proprioceptive Feedback With Application to Myoelectric Systems. IEEE Transactions on Neural Systems and Rehabilitation Engineering 18(1), 58–66 (2010)
18. Bourbakis, N., Keefer, R., Dakopoulos, D., Esposito, A.: A Multimodal Interaction Scheme between a Blind User and the Tyflos Assistive Prototype. In: 20th IEEE International Conference on Tools with Artificial Intelligence, pp. 487–494 (2008)
19. Dakopoulos, D., Bourbakis, N.: Towards a 2D tactile vocabulary for navigation of blind and visually impaired. In: IEEE International Conference on Systems, Man and Cybernetics, pp. 45–51 (2009)

Driving Assistance with Conversation Robot
for Elderly Drivers

Yoshinori Nakagawa[1], Kaechang Park[2], Hirotada Ueda[3], and Hiroshi Ono[4]

[1] Kochi University of Technology, Kami City, Japan
nakagawa.yoshinori@kochi-tech.ac.jp
[2] Kochi Kenshin Clinic, Kochi City, Japan
park@kenshin.or.jp
[3] Kyoto Sangyo University, Kyoto City, Japan
ueda@cc.kyoto-su.ac.jp
[4] HondaHonda R&D Co.,Ltd, Tokyo, Japan
hiroshi_B_Ono@hm.honda.co.jp

Abstract. On the one hand, mobility of elderly people is critical for their quality of lives and welfare. On the other hand, older drivers have higher crash rates per vehicle-mile of travel. In order to achieve the two conflicting goals, driving safety and mobility of the elderly, the present paper aims to discuss the possibility that intelligent artifacts can play a role of reducing crash risk of elderly drivers. A research design for obtaining empirical evidence on the effectiveness of robot presence in vehicles is also discussed.

Keywords: Driving, Crash risk, Passenger presence, and Conversation robot.

1 Introduction

Mobility of elderly people is critical for their quality of lives and welfare. According to summaries by Stutts and Wilkins [1] and the authors, loss of mobility among the elderly may lead to loss of identity and increased dependency; physical and mental problems such as increased depression, heart disease, fractures, and stroke; and decreased social integration, as measured by the number and frequency of social contacts. Therefore, it is important for elderly people to continue driving as long as possible.

A problem arises here, because older drivers have higher crash rates per vehicle-mile of travel [2] due to factors such as the decline in their driving abilities. Therefore, significant motivation exists to explore measures that would compensate for these deficiencies [3].

This motivation is gradually becoming stronger because the number of patients with dementia is expected to increase rapidly over the next few decades in many countries, including Japan. In Japan, according to [4], there were 1.49 million patients with dementia in 2002, and this number is estimated to increase to 3.85 million in 2040. Although dementia can impair driving and increase crash risk, the reality is that

C. Stephanidis and M. Antona (Eds.): UAHCI/HCII 2014, Part III, LNCS 8515, pp. 750–761, 2014.
© Springer International Publishing Switzerland 2014

around one-third of drivers with dementia continue to drive [5]. Therefore, measures for reducing the risks of these drivers are strongly required.

It is often discussed that encouraging passengers to accompany elderly drivers in vehicles appears to be one of the most promising measures to compensate for the decline in their driving ability. As described in greater depth in the following section, earlier studies have consistently found that passenger presence has a protective effect for older drivers.

However, it seems too optimistic to believe that promoting elderly drivers to accompany their family members will be a dominant approach for crash risk reduction, because the family members do not necessarily have time to be with their elderly family members. Thus, it is meaningful to consider the possibility that intelligent artifacts can play the role of human passengers and reduce crash risks of elderly drivers, in place of human passengers.

Thus, on the bases of the earlier empirical findings of the authors, the present paper aims to discuss this possibility. The structure of the present paper is as follows. In section 2, findings of earlier studies of the authors are presented regarding the psychological influences of passenger presence on drivers. In section 3, ethnographic and experimental findings of the authors are presented regarding the attachment and other feelings of human toward intelligent artifact. Taking into account the contents of these two sections, section 4 discusses how robots are likely to play the supportive roles in vehicles as passengers. Section 5 considers research designs required to investigate whether and under what conditions the supportive roles of robots emerge.

2   Influences of Human Passengers on Drivers

Earlier studies have consistently found that passenger presence has a protective effect for older drivers. For example, Hing, Stamatiadis, and Aultman-Hall [6] found that the presence of two or more passengers negatively affected the probability of drivers aged 75 years or older being at fault in crashes. Lee and Abdel-Aty [7] found that drivers aged 60 years or older generally displayed safe driving behavior when accompanied by passengers and having more passengers reduced their crash risk. Engström, Gregersen, Granström, and Nyberg [8] also found that crash risk was higher for those who drove alone, regardless of their age, and that the protective effect increased with every extra passenger (up to eight). Rueda-Domingo et al. [9] found that the protective effect of passengers was higher for drivers aged more than 45 years and lower for drivers aged 23 years or less.

It is also known that passenger presence can be a risk factor for drivers in specific circumstances, especially when young (teenage) drivers are accompanied by passengers of the same generation [10].

Although the above mentioned influence of passenger presence on drivers is important, the psychological mechanisms underlying these effects on drivers are yet to be sufficiently understood. Many researchers have speculated on how these effects emerge, in order to account for the observed increase or decrease in crash risk with regards to the presence of passengers in specific circumstances. For example,

Rueda-Domingo et al.[9] considered the possibility that decreased crash risk in the presence of passengers younger than 15 years is the result of a more defensive driving behavior by parents. They also considered that the protective effect of female passengers on male drivers is attributable to the active role of women in trying to modify male drivers' style towards safer practices. Hing, Stamatiadis, and Aultman-Hall [6] suggested that passengers pose a distraction to older drivers and enhance crash rates if the level of the distraction exceeds a certain point. Simons-Morton, Lerner, and Singer [11] considered that teen passengers cause distractions to the driver by various actions, such as talking, fiddling with the radio or CD player, moving about, or touching the driver. They also considered that teenage drivers are inclined to drive in a more reckless manner (e.g., drive faster, catch up with, and pass another vehicle) when accompanied by teenage passengers because the drivers perceive that the latter view such driving behavior as desirable or expected. Vollrath, Meilinger, and Krüger [12] considered the following possibilities: passengers help drivers in detecting critical situations; the presence of passengers leads to a more responsible driving behavior; and conversations with passengers draw drivers' attention away from driving-related tasks. Lam, Norton, Woodward, Conner, and Ameratunga [13] considered that passenger presence may be a distraction to drivers, because of the greater verbal interaction, music playing or even physical interactions with drivers. They also considered that passenger presence distracts drivers and impairs their ability to detect changes in the surrounding environment.

Not only after comprehensively identifying dimensions in reference to these earlier studies but also after adding new ones after brainstorming by the authors, the present paper considered the following as a tentative list of dimensions: (1) calmness, (2) distraction, (3) flattery, (4) overdependence, (5) pique, (6) direct pressure, (7) indirect pressure, (8) relaxation, (9) relief, (10) responsibility, (11) slackness, (12) shrinkage, and (13) vanity. Possible feelings of drivers are shown below that are associated with each dimension either positively or negatively.

1. Calmness

— With him/her as a passenger, I am less frustrated in traffic congestion.
— With him/her as a passenger, I can make decisions calmly.
— I appreciate him/her as a passenger because he also gets angry when I encounter dangerous drivers or when I am bothered by very slow drivers.

2. Distraction

— I want him/her to keep quiet while I drive.
— His/her wrong sense of direction makes me frustrated.
— With him/her as a passenger, I get frustrated because we do not have the same taste in music (or radio programs)

3. Flattery

— When signals change from blue to yellow, I accelerate over the cross sections in order to comply with his/her intent.

— I exceed the speed limit in order to comply with his/her intent.
— I reduce the following distance in order to comply with his/her intent.

4. Overdependence

— While entering main roads from restaurants or shop parking lots, I assume that he/she should be looking out for cars in the direction I am not looking.
— While turning right[1] at cross sections, I assume that he/she should be looking out for pedestrians and bicycles crossing the road that I am going to enter.
— While changing lanes, I assume that he/she should be looking out for cars approaching from behind in the new lane.

5. Pique

— When he/she gives me driving suggestions, I feel that my driving skills are underestimated.
— With him/her as a passenger, his/her suggestion hurts my self-esteem.

6. Direct pressure

— He/she pressures me by urging me to exceed the speed limit.
— He/she pressures me by urging me to reduce the following distance.

7. Indirect pressure

— I would like to follow his/her request to reduce the following distance.
— I would like to follow his/her request to drive faster.

8. Relaxation

— With him/her as a passenger, I cannot feel relaxed while driving.
— With him/her as a passenger, I can enjoy driving.
— With him/her as a passenger, I get less bored in traffic congestion.

9. Relief

— While entering main roads from restaurants or shop parking lots, I appreciate his/her advice on when to start the car.
— While entering main roads from restaurants or shop parking lots, I appreciate that he/she looks out for cars in the direction I am not looking.
— While turning right at cross sections, I appreciate that he/she looks out for pedestrians and bicycles crossing the road that I am going to enter.

10. Responsibility

— With him/her as a passenger, I feel that I do not want him/her to be injured by crashing while I am driving.

---

[1] Right-hand side traffic is adopted in Japan.

— With him/her as a passenger, I feel that I have his/her life in my hands while I am driving.
— With him/her as a passenger, I keep a longer distance between the car ahead in order to ensure safety.

11. Slackness

— With him/her as a passenger, I become big-hearted.
— With him/her as a passenger, I do not strongly feel that I have to follow the speed limit.
— With him/her as a passenger, I do not strongly feel that I have to fasten my seat belt.

12. Shrinkage

— With him/her as a passenger, I am afraid he/she will scold me if I make a mistake while driving.
— With him/her as a passenger, I am afraid he/she will scold me if I have difficulty in timely starting the car when turning right at intersections with heavy traffic or when turning left onto main roads.

13. Vanity

— With him/her as a passenger, I do not want to appear to be unskilled at driving.
— With him/her as a passenger, I want to show him/her that I am skilled at overtaking.
— With him/her as a passenger, I feel ashamed if I cannot smoothly park in parking lots.

These thirteen dimensions can obviously be classified into two groups according to whether they help drivers to concentrate on driving (dimensions 1, 8, 9, and 10) or they prevent drivers to do so (dimensions 2, 3, 4, 5, 6, 7, 11, 12 and 13). Although there is no empirical evidence in the literature, it is likely that dimensions in the former group are associated with reduced crash risks of drivers.

3   Psychological Effects of Robots on Human

Nowadays, we can see various forms of communication between human and intelligent artificial things such as toys with autonomy, communication robots, and nursing robots. Whether these robots can really play a role of human passengers and reduce crash risk is our greatest concern.

The authors have conducted two preliminary studies for identifying psychological effects of robots on human. This section reviews of the findings of these studies.

3.1   Study 1: Robot in Ubiquitous Home [14]

Within robotic engineering, there are several experimental efforts underway to bring the robot into people's daily life. Kanda et al. put a robot in the elementary school over 18 days with the purpose of examining the interaction between children and robots. The children became tired of interacting with the robots by the beginning of the second week, while they actively interacted during the first week [15]. Another experiment showed that users maintained long-term interaction with robots in their daily lives. Matsumoto et al. investigated the cognitive activities of residents who lived in the Ubiquitous Home with task-oriented robots. Interviews with the residents showed that the residents gradually came to consider the robot to be an artifact and they also see it as a cohabitant at the same time, although they had no affection for the robot in the early stage [16].

The objective of this study was to examine an unprecedented phenomenon in communication between human and intelligent artifacts within the home environment over the course of a 16 day-long experiment.

Experimental Design. The robot in the Ubiquitous Home is called "Phyno1." Phyno is being designed as a visible-type robot for the Ubiquitous Home. It provides the owner with multiple services such as TV program recommendations (at living room), providing recipes (at living room and kitchen), and a reminder service (entrance room). In addition, the robot is able to turn on/off the light, TV, an alarm clock, and air conditioner. In the Ubiquitous Home, there are five robots in total at each room (entrance, living room, kitchen, bedroom, and study room). All robots have voice recognition and synthesis systems based on Julius2. The voice recognition result is preserved in the text data.

The subjects who resided in the Ubiquitous Home are a couple composed of a 64-year-old male and a 60- year-old female. Both have no contact with robots in daily life. Subjects resided in the home for 16 days from 14 to 29 January 2006. Subjects were asked to live an ordinary life at the Ubiquitous Home. The instruction was as follows: 1) The purpose of this experiment is a data collection of an ordinary life at the home of the future. 2) Please have as natural a life as possible, and talk to the robot freely. 3) Please turn on/off the light, TV, and air conditioner through the robot. Subjects read an easy manual for instructions on how to request tasks of the robot before the experiment.

Method of Analysis. The recorded voices of the subjects were transcribed and were classified into four categories: task request (e.g., "Turn on the light"), conversation with the robot ("Thank you"), evaluation of the robot (e.g., "Brilliant"), and description (e.g., "Phyno said something") and direct action (e.g., touching, patting, hitting). Then it was analyzed how the frequency of voices in each category changed throughout the 16 days. This analysis was conducted by dividing the 16 days into three phases and comparing the frequencies in these phases.

Results and Discussions. From results of time-series analysis that utterance frequencies in the first term occupies about half (44.6%) (Table 1), it is interpreted that utterance frequencies decreases because users get accustomed to the intelligent artifacts, while they have strong interests in it in the early stage. In the utterance contents, the category "task request" does not have a significant difference within three phases (Figure 1). Users follow the instruction and use the robot consistently to request any tasks. The category "conversation", "description", and "direct action" were significantly different in each phase. The category "description" and "direct action" has a significant difference in plus in the first phase, gradually decreased in the middle phase, and again increased in the last phase. This may also indicate that users have contact to the intelligent artifacts with strong interests at first, and then gradually they get familiar with the robots. On the other hand, in the category "conversation" the ratio increased in the second phase (Figure 1). It is reported that people frequently talk to the object (cf. pet, toy, pet robot) which they have attachment emotions. In our research, the ratio of conclude that users' attachment for the intelligent artifacts had gradually grown.

Table 1. Utterance frequencies in three phases

The 1st phase	The 2nd phase	The 3rd phase
959 (44.6%)	572 (26.6%)	618 (28.8%)

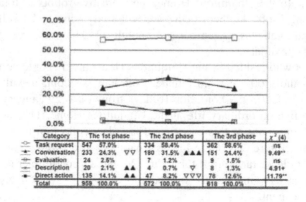

Category	The 1st phase			The 2nd phase			The 3rd phase		χ^2 (4)
Task request	547	57.0%		334	58.4%		362	58.6%	ns
Conversation	233	24.3%	▽▽	180	31.5%	▲▲▲	151	24.4%	9.49**
Evaluation	24	2.5%		7	1.2%		9	1.5%	ns
Description	20	2.1%	▲▲	4	0.7%	▽	8	1.3%	4.91+
Direct action	135	14.1%	▲▲	47	8.2%	▽▽▽	78	12.6%	11.79**
Total	959	100.0%		572	100.0%		618	100.0%	

Fig. 1. Cognitive differences in time-series change

The results indicate that (a) users get accustomed over time to the intelligent artifact and attachment emotions are elicited gradually with the passage of time.

3.2   Study 2: Cooking Support Robot [17]

The next study aimed to examine the influences of the conversational robot in the cooking support system. Though many systems to support cooking activities have been developed [18,19], cooks have to cook solely in most of them. Solitary cooking makes cooks bored and tired. In addition, inexperienced cooks cannot sometimes carry on cooking because they have little motivation. A cooking support system should maintain their motivation for cooking by provision of not only pleasure but also motivator. Therefore, we developed a cooking support system with a conversational robot in our previous research [20]. This is because we hypothesized the robot in the cooking support system can cover the shortcomings of existing systems.

Experimental Design. The cooking support system instructs a cook by images, speeches and the robot. In our previous research, we used images and speeches originally used in PTC. After running PTC on the game machine, we captured images on the screen and speeches from the speaker. In the previous research participants complained of robot's speeches of the cooking instructions. Therefore we decided to change the original speeches into human voices. This could solve their complaints and provide them with a comfortable cooking environment. To create high-quality and profluent speech data, an announcer in our university's broadcasting station who has clear voice help us. We created high-quality speech data by recording and editing his speeches that he read aloud lines. In addition, an agent character appeared in PTC images was erased from the captured so as not to have effects on the result of the experiment. The captured image is shown on the cooking table by the projector installed in the ceiling. The speech is outputted from the speaker on the cooking table. The position and size of the image and the position and volume of the speaker were calibrated in advance so as not to interrupt the cook's activities.

The experiment is conducted by Wizard of Oz (WOZ) method. A microphone and camera are put to enable the experimenter to see what the participants are doing. The experimenter was in the bedroom, and controlled the timing of changing a cooking step and the robot's actions by monitoring the kitchen through the camera and microphone. We chose "Dashi rolled egg omelet" as a recipe for the experiment. This is because the participants can cook Dashi rolled egg omelet in a short time. In addition, Dashi rolled egg omelet is moderately difficult for cooking novices but they can develop their cooking skill by repeated practices. Two tasks are used in the experiment. One is a task using only the cooking support system (abbr. non-robot task), and the other is a task using the cooking support system with the conversational robot (abbr. robot task). In non-robot task, the participants cook according to an image projected on the cooking table and a speech from the speaker. On the other hand, in robot task, they cook according to a gesture of the robot in addition to the image and the speech.

We measured a cook's pleasure and motivation for cooking because we hypothesized that the effects includes improvements of the pleasure and motivation. The pleasure has two types; that caused by enjoyment and immersion. A decrease of the motivation arises cook' s tired and annoyed feeling. Therefore, the questionnaire includes four questions: "Did you enjoy the cooking?" and "Did you immerse yourself in the cooking?" for measuring pleasure, and "Did not you get tired of the cooking?" and "Did not you get annoyed with the cooking?" for measuring motivation.

The participants were twenty one males and five females. To minimize variability of the level of cooking, we had a questionnaire about the experience of cooking before starting the experiment. The result showed that eight participants have lots of experience and eighteen participants lack experience. Therefore, we assigned four experienced people and nine non-experienced people to non-robot task and robot task respectively.

The participants conducted one task either non-robot task or robot task. Ingredients and tools are prepared by the experimenter and put on the cooking table in advance. The experimenter provided the participants with prior explanation before starting the experiment. The prior explanation included how to use the cooking support system and ingredients. After finishing a task, the participants answered a questionnaire about the system. Here, if there are remaining tasks, they conducted the cooking and answered the questionnaire again. When the participants performed the task three times, the experiment was finished.

Results and Discussions. The results (enjoyed, immersed, not tired and not annoyed) are illustrated in Figure 2. It shows the mean value and standard deviation of each trial. The higher the value is, the higher evaluation is. As a result of t-test between the non-robot task and robot task, no significant differences were found, in spite of our expectation that robots would enhance the evaluation.

Then we evolved this system more sophisticated. The voice of the robot was changed into recorded voice of man from the synthesized speech. Speech of the robot was improved to vary de pending on the situation properly between courtesy and brevity. As a result of them, it was found that fine-grained control of the speech of the robot had a significant effect. It was also revealed that the effect acquired by adding a dialog robot to a cooking supporting system serves as the maximum to cooking beginners.

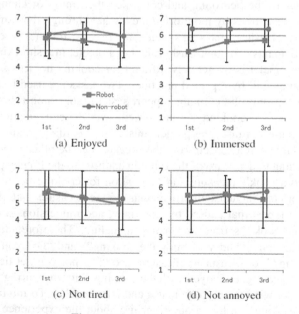

(a) Enjoyed   (b) Immersed

(c) Not tired   (d) Not annoyed

Fig. 2. Results of an experiment

4   Expected Effects of Robots as Passengers on Drivers

Section 3 revealed that human passenger presence can have influence on drivers. Taken together with the findings in Section 4, it is not too optimistic to believe that robots can have protective effects on drivers in place of human passengers. Furthermore, taking into account the fact that human passenger presence does not always influence drivers positively, it may be possible to design passenger robots so that they can have higher net protective effects on drivers than human passengers do. In this section, it is discussed what kind of empirical evidence will be necessary to come up with such a design.

4.1   Generating Positive Effects of Robot Passengers on Drivers

Among the thirteen dimensions on the psychological effects of human passenger presence on drivers, there were four dimensions that obviously have protective effects on drivers: (1) calmness, (8) relaxation, (9) relief, and (10) responsibility. Among these four, it seems that dimension (10), responsibility, can be generated by robots. In fact, if drivers feel attachment toward robot passengers, it is likely that drivers feel as if they are living creatures and have a sense of responsibility. Likewise, drivers can feel (1) calmness with such robot passengers.

The effects of (8) relief might also be generated by robots, but the mechanism of the emergence of this dimension should be different from that of dimension (10) responsibility. Drivers feel relief with human passengers if and only if they trust the passengers' ability to give useful information to them. This would be possible if robots provide vocal assistance through a safe-driving navigation system. Taking into account the findings of study 1 in Section 3, fine-grained control of the speech of such a system is critical for generating the sense of (8).

To summarize, emergence of some dimensions of positive effects depends on the presence of robots and the extent to which drivers feel attachment toward them, and emergence of other dimensions depends on how and what the robots speak.

4.2   Minimizing Negative Effects of Robot Passengers on Drivers

In order to enhance the net protective effects of robot passengers, it is also important to minimize negative effects of robot presence. In study 1 of section 3, semi-structured interview was also conducted after the experiment. The subjects had some complains on the function of the home robot such as "my voice is not easily recognized" and "I want the robot not to answer by mistake. In vehicles, drivers may well have similar feelings, and feel the sense of (2) distraction. It is an essential requirement to find how to minimize this effect is

5   Future Tasks for Designing Driving Assistance Robots

According to Vollrath, Meilinger, and Krüger [12] and other authors, the emergence of the protective effect of human passengers might depend on (i) characteristics of the situations under which driving is performed (e.g., location, weather, road surface, time of day, visual conditions, type of road, traffic density, and day of week), (ii) driver characteristics (e.g., gender, age, and familiarity with the region), and (iii) passenger characteristics (e.g., gender and age). Also, the authors previously suggested that whether the protective effect emerges for elderly drivers depends on the cognitive levels of the drivers.

Similarly, in order to design driving assistance robots, it is an essential requirement to identify conditions under which protective effects dominate negative ones. One promising measure of identifying these conditions is to conduct experiments using driving simulators, especially when we would like to identify personal characteristics (rather than situational factors such as weather) that moderate the association between robot presence and driving performance.

By doing so, we can efficiently collect data on the driving performance of treatment group (i.e., drivers accompanied by robots) and control group (i.e., drivers driving alone). All we have to do is to find conditions of personal characteristics under which driving performance of these two groups differs more. The candidates of such personal characteristics include demographic characteristics such as gender and age, personality characteristics measured by various psychological instruments, results of brain diagnosis using brain imaging, scores of cognitive tests, driving skills, and so on.

References

1. Stutts, J.C., Wilkins, J.W.: On-road driving evaluations: A potential tool for helping older adults drive safely longer. Journal of Safety Research 34, 431–439 (2003)
2. McGwin, G., Brown, D.B.: Characteristics of traffic accidents among young, middle-aged, and older drivers. Accident Analysis and Prevention 31, 181–198 (1999)
3. Hing, J.Y.C., Stamatiadis, N., Aultman-Hall, L.: Evaluating the impact of passengers on the safety of older drivers. Journal of Safety Research 34, 343–351 (2003)
4. Ministry of Health, Labor, and Welfare. Annual Report on Health, Labour and Welfare 2007-2008. Ministry of Health, Labor, and Welfare, Japan (2008) (in Japanese)
5. Silverstein, N.M.: When life exceeds safe driving expectancy: Implications for gerontology and geriatrics education. Gerontology and Geriatrics Education 29(4), 305–309 (2008)
6. Hing, J.Y.C., Stamatiadis, N., Aultman-Hall, L.: Evaluating the impact of passengers on the safety of older drivers. Journal of Safety Research 34, 343–351 (2003)
7. Lee, C., Abdel-Aty, M.: Presence of passengers: Does it increase or reduce driver's crash potential? Accident Analysis and Prevention 40(5), 1703–1712 (2008)
8. Engström, I., Gregersen, N.P., Granström, K., Nyberg, A.: Young drivers—reduced crash risk with passengers in the vehicle. Accident Analysis and Prevention 40(1), 341–348 (2008)

9. Rueda-Domingo, T., Lardelli-Claret, P., Luna-del-Castillo, J.D., Jiménez-Moleón, J.J., García-Martín, M., Bueno-Cavanillas, A.: The influence of passengers on the risk of the driver causing a car collision in Spain: Analysis of collisions from 1990 to 1999. Accident Analysis and Prevention 36(3), 481–489 (2004)
10. Cooper, D., Atkins, F., Gillen, D.: Measuring the impact of passenger restrictions on new teenage drivers. Accident Analysis and Prevention 37(1), 19–23 (2005)
11. Simons-Morton, B., Lerner, N., Singer, J.: The observed effects of teenage passengers on the risky driving behavior of teenage drivers. Accident Analysis and Prevention 37(6), 973–982 (2005)
12. Vollrath, M., Meilinger, T., Krüger, H.P.: How the presence of passengers influences the risk of a collision with another vehicle. Accident Analysis and Prevention 34(5), 649–654 (2002)
13. Lam, L.T., Norton, R., Woodward, M., Connor, J., Ameratunga, S.: Passenger carriage and car crash injury: A comparison between younger and older drivers. Accident Analysis and Prevention 35(6), 861–867 (2003)
14. Matsumoto, M., Yamazaki, T., Tokusumi, A., Ueda, H.: An Intelligent Artifact as a Cohabitant: An Analysis of a Home Robot_s Conversation Log. In: Proceeding of Second International Conference on Innovative Computing, Information and Control (2007)
15. Kanda, T., Hirano, T., Eaton, D., Ishiguro, H.: A Practical Experiment with Interactive Humanoid Robots in a Human Society. In: Third IEEE International Conference
16. Matsumoto, N., Ueda, H., Yamazaki, T., Tokosumi, A.: The Cognitive Characteristics of Communication with Artificial Agents. In: Joint Third International Conference on Soft Computing and Intelligent Systems and Seventh International Symposium on Advanced Intelligent Systems (SCIS & ISIS 2006), CD-ROM, pp. 1269–1273 (2006)
17. Suzuki, Y., Shinkou, H., Ueda, H.: Influences of a robot's presence and speeches in a cooking support system. In: CEA 2012 Proceedings of the ACM Multimedia 2012 Workshop on Multimedia for Cooking and Eating Activities, pp. 31–36 (2012)
18. Ide, I., Ueda, M., Mase, K., Ueda, H., Tsuchiya, S., Kobayashi, A.: Planning a menu(<special section>media processing for daily life: The science of cooking activities). The Journal of The Institute of Electronics, Information and Communication Engineers 93(1), 33–38 (2010)
19. Yamakata, Y., Funatomi, T., Ueda, H., Tsuji, H., Minoh, M., Nakauchi, Y., Miyawaki, K., Nakamura, Y., Siio, I.: Cooking(<special section>media processing for daily life: The science of cooking activities). The Journal of The Institute of Electronics, Information and Communication Engineers 93(1), 39–47 (2010)
20. Nanbu, S., Shinkou, H., Ueda, H.: Effectiveness of a conversational robot in a cooking support system - cases of tako-yaki and dashi-maki-. IEICE Technical Report. MVE, pp. 75–80 (2011)

Developing Iconographic Driven Applications for Nonverbal Communication: A Roadside Assistance App for the Deaf

Hugo Paredes[1,2], Benjamim Fonseca[1,2], and João Barroso[1,2]

[1] INESC Technology and Science – INESC TEC
Rua Doutor Roberto Frias 378, Porto, Portugal
[2] Universidade de Trás-os-Montes e Alto Douro – UTAD
Quinta de Prados, Vila Real, Portugal
{hparedes,benjaf,jbarroso}@utad.pt

Abstract. Touchscreens allow interaction with icons and buttons for executing applications or selecting information. This can be used for non-verbal communication, enabling the deaf to communicate without the need for sign language translation and with a richer context than just using text. This paper explores the development process of iconographic driven applications for nonverbal communication following a user centered design approach. MyCarMobile, a mobile application intended to facilitate the communication of the deaf with roadside assistance services, is introduced as a case study. The application follows the iconographic driven interaction model allowing users to describe an occurrence, through the interaction with icons and buttons in a touchscreen device. Based on the implementation of the case study application and previous work a set of guidelines for implementing iconographic driven applications is proposed.

Keywords: deaf, mobile application, roadside assistance, iconographic interface, nonverbal communication.

1 Introduction

Information and communication technologies (ICT) can be perceived from the perspective of filling human needs [1]. Nowadays, ICT are ubiquitous in daily life, providing access to basic services and ensuring the satisfaction of basic human needs. However, ICT are not available to everyone. The access to ICT and their services are often exclusive to standard users. Therefore, the usage of technologies and access to services by people with special needs is usually restricted or closed off.

One of the obstacles is associated with the communication, namely, the communication channels used to access the services. Some of the services are available through a phone call, making them inaccessible to deaf and hearing impaired people. The aging of the population and the increase of hearing problems as they age heighten this problem. A possible solution for the problem is to provide an alternative nonverbal channel of communication for these people, as a short messaging service (SMS) line.

C. Stephanidis and M. Antona (Eds.): UAHCI/HCII 2014, Part III, LNCS 8515, pp. 762–771, 2014.

If on the one hand this would be a solution for elderly, on the other hand semantic communication problems arise when it is applied to deaf and hearing impaired people. In order to address this problem and provide a universal access solution for emergency services, the usage of iconographic interfaces was previously proposed [2]. The experiments revealed many benefits of this approach, and encouraged the development of a generic model for its usage.

The purpose of this paper is to explore the possibility of applying the iconographic interfaces to other situations and discuss their impact. Such an approach intents to be a starting point for the construction of a generic solution to enable access to a set of services for a population that was until now restricted from doing so. This work relies on a user centered design methodology in order to select and specify a case study application that can fill a gap in deaf' autonomy. Interviews with experts and a survey were conducted. A functional prototype of a mobile application for roadside assistance was developed: MyCarMobile. A discussion of the development process and a set of guidelines for developing iconographic driven applications for nonverbal communication are proposed and constitute the major contribution of this work.

The paper is structured as follows: to present the motivation for the research behind this study, we start by describing the current technological environment for deaf communication, providing a state of the art. This is followed by a discussion of the research methods applied, including the description of the survey presented to members of a deaf association. The empirical findings and the design space of MyCarMobile application are presented in the following sections. A discussion of our findings ensues.

2   Research Settings

Communication barriers often restrict access to basic services to the deaf. Reports[1][11] state that the deaf have difficulties to access daily life services as healthcare, education or even security. The difficulties are related to the provision of most services through verbalized channels, which have to be adapted regarding its usage by the deaf and people with hearing limitations. Consequently sign language, lip reading and text is common used by deaf to communicate with other people. There are several technological solutions trying to help break that face-to-face communication barrier. One such tool is HelpTalk[2] a mobile application that allows verbalizing particular situations, using iconographic representations. Another example is the Vox4All[3], a solution for alternative and augmentative communication. Other solutions, more traditional, rely on services of communication mediation, normally with sign language interpreters.

---

[1] http://www.population-health.manchester.ac.uk/primarycare/
npcrdc-archive/Publications/GP%20D.access.pdf
[2] http://www.helptalk.mobi/en/
[3] http://www.imagina.pt/produtos/educacao-especial/
auxiliares-de-comunicacao/vox4all/

The barrier becomes more obvious when the services are offered remotely, usually through a dedicated telephone line. Examples of such services are emergency, medical appointments, roadside assistance and information services. Some of these services refer to basic needs of citizens. Therefore, specific telecommunications channels are made available for the deaf, filling the audio restrictions through video calls with sign language [6, 7, 8, 9, 10] and text messages [3, 4, 5]. However, these two approaches have some flaws. Video calls commonly rely on mediation of communication for the translation into sign language, which depends on the availability of service and represents an additional cost, as sign language is a skill possessed by a few people other than deaf. Moreover, telecommunicating requires a data connection for video transmission, which is an expensive resource and often unavailable while travelling. Text messages are slow and intermittent, requiring several interactions that can interfere with conversation. The message delivery is not guaranteed and imposes technological restrictions due to the asynchronous nature of the service. In other cases, in order to overcome the voice communication limitation, services are available in multichannel platforms, allowing access via the web or mobile applications such as, for example, the case of banking services.

An approach to overcome the communication ineffectiveness of text and video in mobile devices is the use of interactive icons and buttons in smartphones with touchscreen. MyAXA app[4] is an application from an insurance company that allows users to report an incident. However the application falls back on the voice channel when extra information is needed and establishes a voice call with the company call center. In Spain, Telesor[5] is using a mobile application for generic accessible communication. The application enables real time communication through a mediation service for deaf and hard of hearing people. The service aims to ensure customer support for people with special needs in public institutions and businesses. Another sample application is Red Panic Button application[6] that ensures to its users a mechanism for sending emergency alerts using SMS, email or social networks. Within this scope the ubilert project[7], exploits mobile technologies to allow a simple and effective way of asking for help in an emergency situation (health, civil, criminal).

Previously, our research team has developed SOSPhone [2], a prototype of a mobile application that enables users to make emergency calls using an iconographic interface running in a touchscreen mobile device. The prototype implements the client-side of the application and was demonstrated and evaluated by a large number of users, including people without any disability, emergency services professionals and deaf people. Based on the experience gained in the development of this application, and the results obtained in the tests with users, it became clear the need of experimentation in other areas and the generalization of the concept.

---

[4] http://www.axa.pt/axa-mobile.aspx
[5] http://www.telesor.es/
[6] http://www.redpanicbutton.com/
[7] http://ubilert.pt.to/

3   Research Methods

Software development requires a more user-centered approach, but this does not prevent the products from having an excessive amount of features. It is essential that the users who indeed need the features and who want to, can actually use the software in an effective manner [12]. Among the various existing methodologies in human computer interaction, participatory design and user centered design following stand out as being based on a user-centered philosophy that seeks the users' engagement throughout the development process. Therefore, the development team is able to get a better understanding of the needs and goals of users, building a more appropriate solution [13]. Given the foregoing and the previous experience in developing universal design solutions using user centered design [14], this methodology was chosen for the development of this project. This decision also took into account the number of potential users who could actively participate in the development process and provide input.

The main purpose of this study lies in the generalization of the development process of iconographic driven applications for nonverbal communication. The first research stage of the study requires the selection of a case study, different from previous work. The process assessed the potential needs of users. The strategy underwent interviews with expert addressing the daily difficulties of the deaf. These interviews were held with two deaf users. During these interviews there was no need for interpreter services since the interviewed had the ability to read lips and could verbalize, which facilitated direct communication. Of the interviews carried out, several hypotheses of services that are only available thought voice channels have been presented. Among those, the highlights services were: scheduling of medical appointments; pharmacy medication request; and roadside assistance provided by an insurance company. The analysis of each of these hypotheses was made with each of the interviewees. The choice of roadside assistance service was consensual. The main reasons associated with such a choice are related with the context in which prospective users may require assistance. In such situations, users can stand alone, without the possibility of requesting help while on the other scenarios they are usually accompanied. Thereby, this application is an asset to the autonomy of the deaf, contrasted with the remaining options examined.

Based on this output, and once the case study was selected, a survey with the objective of understanding and knowing which are the major obstacles that the deaf face when communicating with roadside assistance services. The survey, entitled "survey on the calling of roadside assistance services by deaf citizens", consists of nine multiple selection questions. The questions and possible answers were carefully prepared in order to be concise, simple, using careful and noticeable language. This care and the option of multiple choice questions in detriment of open response is associated with the limitations of people with hearing problems and their undeveloped level of literacy. Besides this care, deaf experts who cooperated in interviews reviewed the survey. The survey follows a traditional structure: a first section for user characterization and a second part with the survey questions. For their characterization users are not asked to provide personal information, ensuring their privacy and anonymity.

However, these data are important for the statistical treatment. The disclosure of the survey was performed through the Internet, for the Portuguese Deaf community.

In the following section the data obtained in the surveys is presented and analyzed.

4   Empirical Findings

The survey was presented to 27 deaf and hearing impaired users from the Portuguese federation of deaf associations through Google Docs survey platform. The surveyed were selected in order to represent a sample from the potential users' universe of the application. From the 27 surveyed, 25 have replied to the survey of which 14 male and 11 female. Respondents are in the range between 20 and 55 years old. As for schooling, this varies between secondary and higher education. About 56% of the respondents have a degree of profound deafness and 32% degree of severe deafness.

The first question of the survey was related with the entitlement to drive of the respondents: 80% said they had entitlement to drive and 20% indicated they did not. The results reveals in the second question that 36% of the users have already had problems with the vehicle, and 64% not. However, 44% declared that they had problems with the roadside assistance, and 56% not. According to the answers to question 4, the users have used several contact methods: 55% sent and SMS to a friend or relative; and 30% have asked another driver or passenger to make the call. Other options with residual choice were: contacted a sign language interpreter, sent SMS to the police, and contacted a deaf association through videoconference. The difficulty to communicate with the operator of the roadside assistance was evaluated in question 5 to which 56% replied that they had difficulties, 8% not, and 36% did not answer. From these, 20% had difficulties sending information to the operator and 40% receiving information from the service. Considering the difficulties, 40% of the respondents said that they did not have assistance due to communication problems and 48% were assisted. In order to solve the problems, 36% had asked a friend or relative for help and 40% did not answer. Finally, from the users inquired about support services for communicating with deaf and people with low hearing, 64% agree that they did not present any support services for communication, while a proportion of 32% did not agree.

The analysis of these inconsistent results can reveal that most respondents present qualification for driving, even though most of them have not had any kind of problems with their vehicle. However, when they needed to contact roadside assistance, and they always resorted to help from others, not directly from the support services due to communication problems. According to the answers given, we may conclude that insurance companies had not presented the most appropriate solutions to solve such problems, and many people are still not assisted because of the communications barriers.

These results confirmed the relevance of the application and the existing perception of the problem, encouraging the development of the alternative solution preconized for MyCarMobile. The combination of the results obtained was used to design and create a prototype of the application, as described in the next section.

5   Design Space

The needs identified by users were the foundation for the design of the application. Therefore, the need to communicate without resorting to the voice channel was taken into consideration as well as the use of a language tailored to their needs. One of the critical non-functional requirements for the application was the low literacy of the majority of the deaf population. Moreover, the context in which aid applications emerge was evaluated: abnormal situations in which individuals may be limited to their skills, to deal with it.

From the functional perspective, the objective of the application was to ensure a basic level of service provided by roadside assistance. Thus, two main situations were considered: accidents and breakdowns. These two situations were complemented with a set of complementary situations, categorized as "other situations". For the characterization of an accident, the accident report declaration used and regulated in Portugal by the standard "7/2006-r, august 30"[8] served as a basis for defining the requirements. Notice that in accident situations the application only intends to report material damage of the vehicle to the insurance company. Breakdowns are typically associated with one or more components of the vehicle. Thereby, blocks were considered as representative parts of the vehicle where the breakdown occurs, so that it is reported for the roadside assistance services. Additional details that could be provided upon the roadside assistance needs across a text conversation channel (live chat) were defined and included in the specification.

The application flow followed the requirements for the characterization of the situation, being divided into the above options. Based on the identified non-functional requisites, the icons were defined by searching for images that characterize each of the situations identified in functional requirements, and which guarantee easy identification to ensure recognition even when the reading of the written explanation is restricted. This approach enhances the need for easier access to the application by the population with hearing disability and its low literacy.

This specification has been implemented in a functional prototype: the MyCarMobile.

6   System Prototype

The MyCarMobile uses interactive graphical information such as icons, diagrams and buttons to allow users to describe problems with the car and report it to a roadside assistance service.

In the first phase, data are collected through various activities implemented in an Android app which originated a simple interface allowing the user to simply interact with the application through touching the screen buttons, describing the situation

---

[8] http://www.isp.pt/NR/exeres/
8C7A83FE-4D1B-431D-90AF-29A7289EBCAD.htm
(in Portuguese).

occurred with some detail. As specified, each occurrence can be classified into three types: breakdown, accident or other situations. In case of a breakdown, it is possible to select through illustrations the location of breakdown in the vehicle. In case of accidents, the same strategy applies to identify the damaged areas of the vehicle and the severity of the damage. In case of another situations is available a list of other situations that may have occurred (Fig. 1). Once all desired options are selected, a summary of the event description is displayed on the screen, giving the user an opportunity to review it. The navigation into the several steps of the description flow is available through a slide menu.

During the process of collecting information (ie, as the user selects the options, and menus are being covered) the values are stored in strings that are accessed by various application activities. After all options have been selected, a global string is obtained containing all the necessary information for describing the occurrence in an encoded format. At that same string are automatically attached the GPS coordinates of the location of the occurrence, available by accessing the location information of the device. When the description is complete, an SMS is sent to the operator. To help in collecting further information that might be needed, the application has a live chat functionality that keeps the user and the roadside assistance service connected with each other.

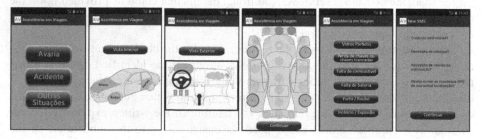

Fig. 1. Some interfaces of the MyCarMobile prototype (only in Portuguese, for now). The leftmost interface is the first screen, where the user can select one of 3 buttons corresponding to 3 basic situations: breakdown ("Avaria"), accident ("Acidente") and other situations ("Outras Situações"). If the first option is selected, the interface changes to the second one, which allows specifying the location of the breakdown: engine ("motor"), doors ("Portas"), inside view ("Vista interior") and wheels ("Rodas"). The third interface shows the inside view, and the fourth is the one for the case of accident, enabling to specify the damaged areas. The fifth and sixth interfaces show refinements in the description of the problem, such as reporting broken glasses, requesting hauling or sending GPS coordinates.

7   Discussion

The use of iconographic interfaces can represent a solution to solve some of the current problems of non-verbal communication, but face challenges in their design.

User preferences reveal the need to use technology they know to communicate, including SMS and videoconference. Moreover, the presented study, like previous studies, highlights the precariousness of solutions as well as the need for technologies that enhance access to basic services. Often this access is closed off since the services make abusively use of verbal communication channels. Clearly the benchmarking analysis set that mobile applications are increasingly a wager of enterprises to create a closer relationship with their customers. This massification could increase new audiences and provide economies of scale in solutions that were addressed to small groups of the population. In this sense, the effort in the development of applications should follow good practice and ensure usability and accessibility solutions for a wide range of the population.

The results presented in the development of MyCarMobile as well as prior experience, give some guidelines for the development of such applications:

- Icon selection: the icons should be intuitive and represent the situation that is intended to describe / abstracting. The representation of objects is simple and direct. However the choice of icons to represent states of mind, actions and other everyday situations is often complex and dependent on the cultural context of the individual.
- Creation of interaction patterns: each situation can be a standardized set of graphic elements, which together represent it. Commonly, graphics are icons. In some situations there may be a need for other elements (eg in the case of a location on a freeway where it is necessary intuitively indicate the direction of movement to rectify the GPS information and mitigate the potential error).
- Application flow definition: the application requirements must be depicted as a flow of information that can be directly mapped to the application flow. The flow should be as close to the reality of their users and their habits in performing the tasks. Combining well-known interaction patterns can carry out the implementation of the application flow.
- Integration with traditional communication models and multimodal interaction options.

8   Final Remarks

This paper presented the development process of a functional prototype of MyCarMobile, a mobile application that allows deaf to contact roadside assistance. The development followed a user centered design approach and intended to collect guidelines for the development of iconographic driven applications for nonverbal communication. This kind of applications follow an interaction pattern, previously presented, that exploits the usage of touchscreens for interaction with icons and select the appropriate information to describe a situation.

The development process started with interviews with experts and selected a case study for the application of the interaction pattern. Following, a survey was conducted with deaf to help in the specification process, and confirmed the relevance interaction pattern. The prototype that was implemented used interaction with icons and buttons to describe the situation to be reported. A discussion of the lessons learned with the development process of this application was carried out. From this process resulted a set of guidelines for the development of iconographic driven applications for nonverbal communication that were presented.

A formal specification of the development process and its application to other case studies will contribute to the validation of the discussed guidelines. This process will require a deeper analysis, reveal possible errors and inconsistencies usual in informal specification, and allow the improvement of the solution [15]. Tools and frameworks for enhancing and scaling up the development of universal access mobile applications that follow the iconographic driven pattern can also be explored using the proposed guidelines and the preliminary results of the work presented.

Acknowledgments. We would like to thank to the UTAD students Beatriz Baptista and Diogo Soares, who supported us in the development of the prototype.

This work is funded (or part-funded) by the ERDF – European Regional Development Fund through the COMPETE Programme (operational programme for competitiveness) and by National Funds through the FCT – Fundação para a Ciência e Tecnologia (Portuguese Foundation for Science and Technology) within project «FCOMP - 01-0124-FEDER-022701».

References

1. Shneiderman, B.: Leonardo's laptop: human needs and the new computing technologies. The MIT Press (2003)
2. Paredes, H., Fonseca, B., Cabo, M., Pereira, T., Fernandes, F.: SOSPhone: a mobile application for emergency calls. Universal Access in the Information Society 13(3) (2013)
3. Power, M.R., Power, D.: Everyone Here Speaks TXT: Deaf People Using SMS in Australia and the Rest of the World. Journal of Deaf Studies and Deaf Education 9(3), 333–343 (2004)
4. Pilling, D., Barrett, P.: Text Communication Preferences of Deaf People in the United Kingdom. Journal of Deaf Studies and Deaf Education 13(1), 92–103 (2008)
5. Henderson, V., Grinter, R.E., Starner, T.: Electronic Communication by Deaf Teenagers. Technical Report GIT-GVU-05-34, Georgia Institute of Technology (2005)
6. Abascal, J., Civit, A.: Mobile Communication for People with Disabilities and Older People: New Opportunities for Autonomous Life. In: 6th ERCIM Workshop, User Interfaces for All (2000)
7. Cherniavsky, N., Chon, J., Wobbrock, J.O., Ladner, R.E., Riskin, E.A.: Activity analysis enabling real- time video communication on mobile phones for deaf users. In: UIST 2009, pp. 79–88 (2009)
8. Ghaziasgar, M., Connan, J.: Investigating the feasibility factors of synthetic sign language visualization methods on mobile phones. In: SAICSIT 2010, pp. 86–92 (2010)
9. Harkins, J.E., Bakke, M.: Technologies for communication. In: Oxford Handbook of Deaf Studies, Language, and Education, vol. 1, pp. 406–419 (2003)
10. Buttussi, F., Chittaro, L., Carchietti, E., Coppo, M.: Using mobile devices to support communication between emergency medical responders and deaf people. In: MobileHCI 2010, pp. 7–16 (2010)
11. França, A., Ono, M.: Interação de Pessoas Surdas Mediada por Sistemas de Produtos e Serviços de Comunicação. Cadernos Gestão Pública e Cidadania, Brasil (2011)

12. Rozanski, E.P., Haake, A.R.: The Many Facets of HCI. In: Proceeding of the 4th Conference on Information Technology Education, CITC 2003, pp. 180–185. ACM Press, New York (2003)
13. Preece, J., Rogers, Y., Sharp, H.: Interaction Design: Beyond Human-Computer Interaction. John Wiley & Sons (2007)
14. Norman, D.: The Design of Everyday Things, 1st edn. MIT Press (1998)
15. Sommerville, I.: Software Engineering, 9th edn. Addison Wesley Longman Publishing Co., Inc., Redwood City (2010)

Barriers Survey: A Tool to Support Data Collection for Inclusive Mobility

Federico Prandi, Michele Andreolli, Matteo Eccher,
Umberto di Staso, and Raffaele De Amicis

Fondazione Graphitech, Via alla cascata 56c, 38123 Trento, Italy
federico.prandi@graphitech.it
http://www.graphitech.it

Abstract. In this paper we describe the potential for using the Volunteered Geographic Information (VGI), and large crowd-sourced survey, in disable people mobility computing applications The challenge is to make these two concepts talking together exploiting the technologies in order to increase the public participation, and to move towards sustainable development. Our goal is to investigate how participative and people-centric data collection can be used to create a low-cost, open platform to survey, annotate and localise pedestrian mobility features and architectural barriers as it is perceived by the citizen themselves. The core of the project consists into the development and deployment of a mobile application and a web platform, which allow the users to collect and manage the information surveyed.

Keywords: Volunteered Geographic Information, Mobile Application, Pedestrian mobility, Smart cities.

1 Introduction

Cities are the part of the world where there are the highest concentration of population. The United Nations estimates that at some time between 2008 and 2009, the worlds urban and rural populations became equal. And beginning of 2019, it is expected that more people will live in cities than in rural areas.

This implies a lot of opportunities but even, a big challenge for administrator, scientists and citizen improving the quality of life within cities. An efficient city administration that provides services to its citizens and fosters businesses, is essential to todays service-based economy. The emerging trend is going towards a unified urban-scale ICT platform transforming a City into an open innovation platform called Smart-City. Smart cities promise to capitalize on new economic opportunities and social benefits. A core component of this approach is using communication and collaboration technologies to manage city information. However cities are a very complex system and, in several cases, it is difficult to collect and maintain this information without expensive surveys and instruments.

One of the big challenges faced on within Smart Cities is how to improve access to city space for wheelchair users and other disabled people. Indeed their

C. Stephanidis and M. Antona (Eds.): UAHCI/HCII 2014, Part III, LNCS 8515, pp. 772–779, 2014.

mobility can be easily affected by environmental barriers and individuals with mobility impairments such as wheelchair users are often a disadvantage when traveling to a new place even for a short trip.

It is quite obiouvs how, nowadays, Mobile phones can provide navigation instructions in real-time, accessing wireless the Internet. Positioning methods like Global Positioning System (GPS) or Global System for Mobile telecommunication (GSM) are used for pedestrian navigation services using pedestrians location for updating the path the user is guided. However, content and granularity of the information requested by pedestrians is not quite clear and needs to be investigated. Furthermore, in this case, pedestrians need a specific set of features to represent the environment and other information including barriers, sidewalks accessibility along the way, points of interest, and even services for disabled people.

Unfortunately providers of these services are not traditional mapping companies and navigation system providers, therefore there is a lack on this data from digital city maps, yellow pages and travel information data sets. Furthermore the collection of this kind of information is extremely expensive and time consuming so municipalities and public body typically avoid to insert they into the survey and map updating.

With terms Volunteered Geographic Information (VGI), or geospatial crowdsourcing, they are indefied all those activities where citizens (volunteers) contribute data and information about the earth and environment that is explicitly or implicitly georeferenced and then disseminated via collaborative projects.

This paper will explore the potential for the Volunteered Geographic Information (VGI) community to improve data access and management in the field of disable pedestrian mobility computing.

The work described in this paper consists on the development and deployment of a mobile application to collect geometrical features supporting routing services for pedestrian deisable people, in order to overcome the abovementioned information lack. The research contributions of this paper are as follows:

1) We outline the features needed to support disabled people mobility, how they are modelled, and their use in routing systems;

2) We outline the OpenStreetMap project, which is the most popular VGI project on the Internet, and show the specific emphasis in OSM on mobility information;

3) We outline how the design of the user interface of the application is fundamental for the VGI survey campaing, specially in this complex case;

4) We outline ways in which VGI could be integrated into rotuing services applications and services;

5) We provide an overview of the challenges and issues that must be considered when VGI is used to support data collection in such complex applications and services.

1.1 Related Works

Several reseaches report application of GPS and GIS to developing navigation maps for individuals with disabilities (see [1] and [2]). However these systems have limited capabilities to provide real time routing information or they are tailored on specific barriers free paths.

Although this effort spent in developing navigation systems for pedestrians, many users with special needs are mostly excluded due to a lack of appropriate geographical data such as landmarks, waypoints, or obstacles. Indeed this kind of information is often very time consuming and expensive to be collected by the municipalities and the result is that there is a lack into pedestrian mobility information at the city level. However in the last years new technologies have created opportunities for citizens to interact with each other, form collaborative groups, collect and disseminate information about their social networks and the world around them, in realtime [3]. This new trend became popular under the term Volunteered Geographic Information (VGI) [4], or crowd-sourced geodata. The work will explore the potential for the VGI community to improve data access and management in the field of disabled mobility services through a specific mobile application to collect pedestrian features and barriers information. One of the most popular and most manifold projects for VGI is the OpenStreetMap (OSM) project [5]. The classic approach is to collect data with a GPS receiver, which afterwards can be edited with one of the various freely available editors, such as Potlatch or JOSM. This approach could not allow high accuracy, specially in dense urban city centre where GPS signal is not good. Our improvement is to add to the classic GPS based approach the capability to draw directly on field the features collected on a mobile device.

Spatial data collection is not immune to user and measurement errors, and it poses concerns regarding accuracy and loss of detail [7]. A variety of web based VGI projects in the fields of assets and inventory mapping, site programming, preference studies and design evaluation have been deployed. For instance The information is acceptable only if the participant is local to the community the data is collected. This can be validated by a qualifier like the zip code or the number of years he or she has lived in the locality.

The system that we present in this paper try to start for these experience in order to improve the quality of data collected, providing a mix of these techniques in order to avoid errors or missing information.

2 Technology Model

A technology model helps to identify and build the necessary technical resources in order to meet the requirements and to answer the research questions. Some of the questions could be How would User Interface forms be rendered?, What technology is used to access data from remote databases? and How do the needs of the final users drive the capabilities built in? It contains within it the development model, and therefore focuses on component development and reusing development resources including source code.

The project in the context of this paper is a system for data collection that is carried out in on a particular features category. The model provides a mobile application to manage the multiple collection while preserving the context of each separate user. It also helps to manage multiple collection within the centralized database.

2.1 System Design

The overall system proposed in this thesis is as shown in Figure 1. The system design includes smart phone application, web services, and a OSM open source map editor. In a typical scenario several information representing the properties of the features should be collected on field. Also geometries can be mapped like barriers, parking and sidewalks. A single mobile application is used for data collection. Users can access their new survey and if the connection is available save the information collected direclty on the Database repository for further editing and deployment.

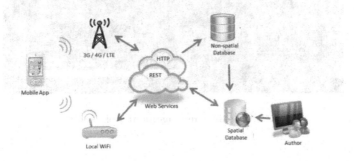

Fig. 1. System Design

The mobile application needs to be installed on a tablet device because, due to the varierty and complexity of the data acquired, a more wide display is needed. It facilitate, direclty on field, the collection of geometries and attributes of the mobility pedestrian features. It enables users to add new features and edit features they added earlier. The app uses Wi-Fi where a wireless access point is available; in the field it uses mobile data access through 3G or 4G provided by the service provider. Web Services enable interaction between the smart phone and other components in the model. Web Map services (WMS) is consumed by the mobile app to display the OSM as background map. HTTP web service is used for user authentication, to send non-spatial attributes to the central repository. The non-spatial Database contains the information collected including images and info about the users. From this database it is possible to export the information already in the format needed for editing into OSM editors. After the editing for routing purpose the information can be loaded on the OSM spatial Database and retrieved by whole community.

2.2   Web Authoring System

The Web Authoring System enables new data collection creation. Only registered users can start a new survey and store information on the database. Each user can further access to his data via web and select two different typologies of export (Figure 3). The first into OSM format in order to be edit for routing purpose and added to the global OSM repository, the latter in .csv format for other different and personal purposes.

The administrator can access to the whole database and disable an unappropriate user or even download data for specific editing purpose.

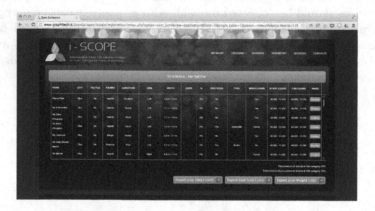

Fig. 2. User data management web interface

2.3   Software Framework

The software framework for the whole system is shown in Figure 3. The main components include the mobile smart phone application and the web data manager. Each component has more modules. The components are loosely coupled. Modules within each component generally interact with one other with high dependencies. The modules in the smart phone app are implemented through iOS Unity framework and are programmed using C-Sharp.

3   Design of Mobile Application

The mobile application for smart phones is the core part of the work presented in this paper. The implementation is currently done for iOS tablet platforms. The components include a local database and three modules: management module, mapping module and form module. Figure 3 on the right side shows the component diagram of the mobile application.

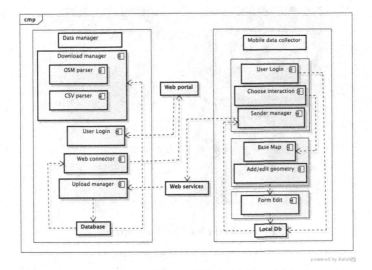

Fig. 3. System Framework

The requirements of the applications were related the possibility to collect several detailed information about the features which influence the pedestrian mobility, in particular of the disabled people. Within this categories we have several geografic features such as sidewalks, zebras, underpass and barriers which are not typically surveied by the typical mapping agencies. So the application should provide to the surveyors the tools to collect all the needed information to set up a routing services for pedestrian people.

This information are not limited to the geometric features but include numerous additional attributes which can affect the accessibility of a particular path such as: the condition of the pavments, the slope, the with or the presence or not of curbs. All this data have to be collected and related to the specific geographic elment that will be a component of the base graph of the routing service.

In a first step, an ontology for datasets is defined as a formal specification of the data model which is applied exemplary on the digital map of the city of Vienna and Cles (province of Trento). The ontology is based on the OSM tagging schema, which is increasingly being developed into a complex taxonomy of real-world feature classes and objects, this is a core part of the OSM initiative and is community-driven. Any member of the community can contribute to and update the schema by proposing new key=value pairs.

Then, based on this data model, the forms for the data collection has been designed (Figure 4).

A central part of the application consists on the interface for georeferencing the features. In a first design phase this was made automatically using the GPS coordinates retrieved by the mobile device. However this approach didn't allow an enought accuracy due to the lack in positioning caused for instance by the bad signal on dense urban areas.

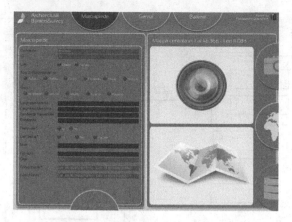

Fig. 4. Form for the data entry

To overcome these errors the mapping modules include functionalities to draw the features directly on the map within the mobile application (figure 5). The coordinates are then saved on the databes. Nevertheless the drawing funcionalities are vey limited (for instance a sidewalks is represented only by the start and ending point); this is related to the fact that even if we teoretically we can draw more complex features; a further post-processing editing is needed in order to prepare the graph for routing purpose. Indeed the route graph needs the connection between node and arcs and it would be impossible to use snap and very complex editing funcionalities on field using mobile devices. So, for convenience, the draw functions are limited on mobile devices in order to make easy and speed up the on field work.

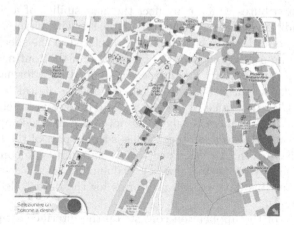

Fig. 5. Particular of the map context with the insertion of a sidewalk feature. The feature is represented by its start and end point visualized using a blu and violet flags.

4   Conclusion

In this paper we present a system to support the design a routing service for disabled pedestrian people based on OSM ontology. The system is splitted into two componets the abovementioned mobile application and a web site for the mananagement of the collected information.The main part of the system is a mobile application designed for the on field data collection, indeed the main issue related to the services implementation is a lack into detailed information to set up the rotuing algorithm.

Due to the nature of the data to be collected, the number of the informtion that have to be surveyed is very high, furthermore it is neeeded to collect also the coordinate of the feature in order to draw the routing graph. For this reason a detailed study of the application design has been carried out in order to preserve the quality of the collected data and a simple user interface useful during on field operations.

Nevertheless even if the application is designed for VGI and Crowd source data collection the user should have some competencies on the disabled pedestrian mobility issues.

Acknowledgement.   The project I-SCOPE has received funding from the EC, and it has been co-funded by the CIP-Pilot actions as part of the Competitiveness and innovation Framework Programme. The author is solely responsible this work which does not represent the opinion of the EC. The EC is not responsible for any use that might be made of information contained in this paper.

References

1. Sobek, A., Miller, D., U-Access, H.J.: a web-based system for routing pedestrians of differing abilities. Journal of Geograph. Syst. 8, 269–287 (2006)
2. Matthews, H., Beale, L., Picton, P., Briggs, D.: Modelling access with GIS in urban systems (MAGUS): capturing the experiences of wheelchair users. Area 35, 34–45 (2003)
3. Mooney, P., Corcoran, P., Ciepluch, B.: The potential for using volunteered geographic information in pervasive health computing applications. J. Ambient Intell. Human. Comput. (2012), doi:10.1007/s12652-012-0149-4
4. Goodchild, M.F.: Citizens as sensors: The world of volunteered geography. GeoJournal 69, 211–221 (2007)
5. Neis, P., Zielstra, D., Zipf, A.: The street network evolution of crowd-sourced maps: OpenStreetMap in Germany 2007-2011. Future Internet 4, 1–21 (2012)
6. Reddy, Y.: Pervasive computing: Implications, opportunities
7. Zhang, J., Goodchild, M.F.: Uncertainty in geographical information. Taylor and Francis, London (2002)

Place Meaning and the Visually Impaired: The Impact of Sound Parameters on Place Attachment and Identity

Charalampos Rizopoulos[1,2], Angeliki Gazi[1], and Yannis Christidis[1]

[1] Department of Communication and Internet Studies, Cyprus University of Technology,
Limassol, Cyprus
{c.rizopoulos,angeliki.gazi,yannis.christidis}@cut.ac.cy
[2] Department of Communication and Media Studies,
National and Kapodistrian University of Athens, Greece
c_rizopoulos@media.uoa.gr

Abstract. This paper outlines some theoretical considerations regarding the concept of place meaning as applied to populations of visually impaired users of mobile location-based applications. The concept of place meaning and its constituent elements, place attachment and place identity, are explored in detail and a research design on place meaning for visually impaired smartphone users is outlined as a first step toward the systematic investigation of the differences in the creation of place attachment and place identity between sighted and visually impaired individuals as a result of auditory stimuli emerging from the urban soundscape.

Keywords: Place meaning, affect, soundscape, location-aware applications.

1 Introduction

The perception of the urban environment is a multidimensional construct comprising sensory, cognitive, symbolic, and social aspects which contribute towards the generation of place meaning. While the term 'space' often refers to the invariant properties of the physical environment (e.g. geometry, color, lighting etc.) as perceived by the subject's sensory subsystems, the term 'place' is reserved for the interpretation of spatial properties with respect to subjective values, norms, attitudes, and predispositions. Place meaning is deeply subjective and is responsible for the wide variety of responses toward parts of the urban environment by the inhabitants of a city.

The generation of place meaning requires active involvement with a particular space. In the case of urban environments, this translates to navigating through various parts of the city, often for a significant amount of time. This process may be considerably difficult to some user groups with special needs, such as the visually impaired. For these users, the act of moving around in the city can be inherently dangerous due to their inability to perceive visual information. This inability also renders the environmental experience of visually impaired users radically different than the experience of sighted individuals. As such, it is expected that the parameters which account

C. Stephanidis and M. Antona (Eds.): UAHCI/HCII 2014, Part III, LNCS 8515, pp. 780–790, 2014.
© Springer International Publishing Switzerland 2014

for the generation of place meaning and the creation of the affective bond with the urban environment will be different for visually impaired users. Due to the lack of vision, audition becomes the most important source of information from the environment [1-2], possibly supplemented by tactile (e.g. the feeling of the ground and the detection of obstacles via distal perception) and, to a lesser degree, olfactory feedback.

This paper attempts to formulate a conceptualization of place meaning generation by visually impaired smartphone users in the city; more specifically, this paper deals with the affective and emotional impact of various characteristics of sound in the perception of the character of various parts of the city by visually impaired smartphone users. Essential sonic events which incorporate various types of categorized sound characteristics influence the type and intensity of one's affective response to places, as well as the extent of social activity that occurs therein. Smartphones are ideal for such a task due to their proliferation and the constant increase in their technical specifications.

Additionally, this paper describes an Android application, currently under development, that allows blind users to provide geolocated affective information. By means of this application, the meaning of place will be approached through practical research aimed at eliciting relevant affective responses by the users. Visually impaired and sighted individuals will be participating in the procedure so as to allow a direct comparison of the parameters that contribute to the generation of place meaning for these two categories of users.

The outline of this paper is as follows: first, "place meaning" and related concepts are outlined. Subsequently, the chosen methodology is explained and its merits and flaws compared to other methodologies are discussed, followed by a description of the application currently under development. Finally, the design of the experimental activity is described in detail.

2   The Concept of Place Meaning

2.1   Place and Identity

While the term "space" is primarily used to describe the objectively perceptible characteristics of an environment, the term "place" essentially refers to spaces endowed with value and/or subjective meaning, i.e. spaces of personal significance [3-8][1]. Place meaning comprises place attachment, an affective bond between the subject and the environment, and place identity, the reflection of a place's importance and congruence with one's self-identity. The most important component of the concept of place is the affective bond between the subject and a specific location [9].

Whether individually or collectively driven, the generation of place meaning necessitates a process of appropriation [9] whereby a place becomes integrated in a

---

[1] These spaces need not be physical; various spatial configurations or locations that do not have a physical manifestation can attain place status, as evident in the game studies literature (e.g. [10-11]).

person's or a collective's identity [12]. At the individual level, indicative of this position is the view that places can be thought of as "extensions of the self", or as integral parts of one's self-concept and self-identity [7]. At the collective level, McCullough's [13] observation that cities function as "repositories of civilization", and the observation by Lentini & Decortis [14] that places can be accompanied by related social cues, thus functioning as a type of social affordances, are also in accordance with this process. Appropriation allows one to adapt a place to one's specific needs and goals [15], and effectively "dwell" in it. In a more ecological (as per [16]) approach, Droseltis & Vignoles [7] mention the notion of "environmental fit" as an undercurrent in the process of place meaning generation. Additionally, the concept of place could potentially be interpreted in evolutionary terms as a result of a process of environmental appraisal or preference [17].

All the above point to the fact that any given spatial configuration may be appropriated by different persons or groups at different times, and thus attain different types of place status. Thus, the concept of place indirectly obtains a temporal dimension [4]. In light of the above, the stability of place meaning is not a given. To put it somewhat differently, a way of testing meaning stability or mutability as a function of physical elements is to systematically vary the configuration of physical environmental elements and determine whether place meaning remains the same or not [18].

It should be noted that spaces may fail to transform to places on account of not being related to subjective or sociocultural values and norms. In that case, that particular space has no distinguishing elements, whether tangible or intangible, and a state of "placelessness" ensues [19].

2.2   Place and the Concepts of Attachment and Belongingness

It should be stressed that sense of place does not ensue exclusively as a result of positive affective connotations; it is possible for a space to be evaluated negatively in terms of affect, but still be given place status. This type of place is exemplified by sites such as concentration camps or locations in which unpleasant events occurred, either at the individual or the collective level. According to Relph [19], the sense of insideness is what denotes a place with which the subject can be identified. Relph regards insideness as a continuum that ranges from existential outsideness to existential insideness:

- *Existential outsideness:* a conscious lack of identification with a place and any elements related to it.
- *Objective outsideness:* the voluntary dissociation between the subject and the place, during which the former views the latter in a more objective manner, essentially as "collections" of persons, objects, or other elements.
- *Incidental outsideness:* the involuntary perception of a space as neutral or devoid of meaning – essentially placelessness.
- *Vicarious insideness:* an indirect perception of a place (e.g. through narrative).

- *Behavioral insideness:* an objective conception of space and the activities performed therein without the dissociation that is present in the case of objective outsideness.
- *Empathetic insideness:* being emotionally invested in what transpires within a place.
- *Existential insideness:* a sense of total belongingness to a place, accompanied by the intuitive perception of the meanings with which it has been endowed.

In combination with other methods, the above categorization could be used for ascertaining the affective impact of a place and the extent of its compatibility with the subject's self-image.

Although places are not necessarily perceived as sources of positive affect, the concept of place attachment seems to imply the experience of positive affective reactions. Scannell & Gifford [8] propose a tripartite model of place attachment, according to which place attachment can be analyzed into three constituent elements: the individual, the place itself, and the psychological processes through which attachment is expressed. At a purely individual level, place attachment signifies the positively evaluated affective bond between the subject and the environment fostered as a result of events of high personal significance. The psychological processes that are involved in place attachment are affective, cognitive, and behavioral. It is clear from the use of the term "attachment" that the role of affective processes is the most important one. In other words, there is a clear tendency toward positive affect, which is the primary element that differentiates place "attachment" from place "meaning". In an investigation on the way the affective bond between children and space is formed, Morgan [20] concluded that this process is related to five affective states which can be seen as components of place attachment: pleasure (of various subtypes), security, love, grief, and identity. With the exception of grief, all other states are positively valenced, and even grief is described by Morgan in a way that emphasizes its positive aspects (i.e. when experiencing grief, the subject is thought to remember a more positive previous condition).

On a behavioral level, place attachment is manifest as a desire to approach a particular place, and entails certain aspects of territorial behavior; however, in contrast to true territorial behavior, the subject approaches a place not to defend or claim it, but to express and explore their identification with it [8]. Additionally, subjects tends to attempt to reproduce elements of the place they are attached to in other environments. This is one of the reasons for ensuring than an environment is malleable, i.e. the ability of the environment to change according to the needs and goals of its denizens. From a functional perspective, the desired degree of malleability for a given space partly depends on the number of functions this space will have to provide or support.

2.3   Categorizing Affective Behaviors and Responses

There are two main types of approaches to categorizing emotion and affect: categorical and dimensional [21]. Categorical approaches propose sets of "basic" emotions, which are thought to be expressed similarly across various cultural contexts. The most prominent advocate of this approach is Paul Ekman, who has proposed a number of basic emotions, the most widely adopted being sadness, disgust, anger, fear, surprise, and happiness [22]. Dimensional approaches, on the other hand, seek to break down discrete emotions into easily identifiable and quantifiable components. The most influential dimensional model of depicting emotional and affective responses is Russell's circumplex model of affect [23-24]. This model classifies emotion along two axes, arousal (activation level) and valence (essentially pleasure derived from a stimulus)[2].

Categorical and dimensional approaches are not necessarily at odds; discrete categories of emotion can be mapped onto a dimensional model of affect, as shown in fig. 1, which depicts the circumplex model subdivided into eight zones.

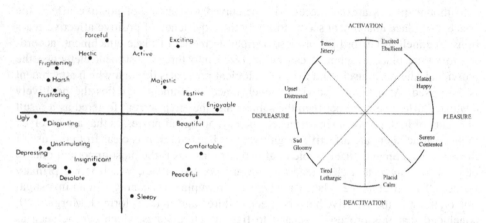

Fig. 1. The circumplex model of affect, with descriptive terms (left) or clusters / zones (right) around the primary axes of deactivation – activation (arousal) and displeasure – pleasure (valence) ([24], p. 312 and [23], p. 148 respectively)

An advantage of dimensional approaches is their analytical character, which results in a more manageable set of quantities to be measured or identified. The circumplex model of affect has been used for the classification of affective responses to places in the application described in another section.

3   Sound and the Urban Environment

3.1   The Importance of Sound in the Perception of the Urban Environment

An important distinction in the literature on sound is the one between listening and hearing [25]. Truax has defined hearing as 'sensitivity to both the detail of physical

---

[2] The PAD (Pleasure – Arousal – Dominance) model, a three-dimensional conceptualization of emotion that is the precursor to the circumplex, also featured the dimension of dominance (the degree of control one can exert on the manifestation of affect), but Russell excluded it from the circumplex because it accounted for only a small percentage of the total variance observed [24] (p. 313).

vibration within an environment and its physical orientation as revealed through its modification of those vibrations' [25] (pp. 15-16). Along with the definition, he has claimed that hearing is able to make someone comprehend, although with not many details, his/her entire environment in all directions at the same time. Indeed, the sense of hearing helps people to evaluate their environment, and adapt themselves into it. However the main concern of hearing remains the actual physical interaction between the human ear and the sound waves, while the process of listening concerns a completely different, more composite concept of communication.

The Soundscape. The term soundscape refers to the acoustic field that is defined taking the position of the listener into account, and its examination should include all interactions between him/her and the sound. Every sonic event that happens and exists in one's audible area is part of a space where a soundscape creates the sound field and involves multi-leveled interactions. Schafer [26] had introduced this notion in the middle of 70s in an effort to raise the world's attention towards the acoustic environment, and also raise awareness, as industrialization was resulting in noisier ambiences and a dangerously rising loud way of life. Thus, it has been important that even if the sound environment acquires compositional properties and is likewise approached as being independent from our actions, we listeners should pay more attention to our behavior regarding sounds – both the ones we produce and the ones we receive. All these lead to a reconsideration of the way people connect to the urban environment through the soundscape. The term 'soundscape' was coined so to describe a sound environment, exactly as 'landscape' describes a visual environment. Other scholars or researchers have broadened its meaning. Regarding one's relationship with the soundscape, Truax indicates 'a tacit knowledge that people have about the structure of environmental sound, knowledge that manifests itself in behavior that interprets such sound and acts upon it' [25] (p. 50). In a contemporary urban environment, the soundscape has been characterized as 'urban soundscape', and its characteristics have been similar throughout the short history of the soundscape studies.

The Urban Soundscape. 'Urban soundscape planning and design' has quickly become an issue of a great importance for a city environment. Areas such as parks, churches, avenues, noisy or quiet streets, playgrounds or alleys create a unique sound environment in cities, although with similar elements to other contemporary cities' identity.

The urban soundscape is a sound environment that includes a lot of information that is also rich in sound variety and acquires a strong 'urban' identity. Already, from the cities from the past, every city had its distinctive sounds: certain animals, the quality of the roads and its crossers, peoples' voices (quarrels or laughs), language, or water crossing the area would be an important element (what later has been called 'sound signals') of a city's soundscape. Also musical and industrial sounds used to be present in such places, and its qualities were different enough to separate the one area from another: 'The shared experience of local 'soundmarks' created what Barry Truax had called an 'acoustic community'. In an urban environment it created overlapping acoustic communities in the same way that visual landmarks and local interaction helped to define overlapping neighborhood communities. Those who belonged to a particular neighborhood recognized its sounds and responded in ways that outsiders did not. Any interruption to the normal local sounds immediately put them on the alert, even if they were not consciously listening: a sudden silence, the clash of swords, or the tramp of marching feet brought everyone to their windows' [27] (p. 10). In modern cities, the inhabitants sound their own unique way: existing in a place where natural sound sources are suppressed or rarely present, people are used to mechanical and/or technological sounds in an impressive way: If an urban inhabitant would be challenged to recall the first sounds that come to his/her mind when thinking of the 'city's aural environment', 'cars' or 'noise' would have been amongst the first responses – and noise would be the sound that was meaningless and/or undesirable. These kinds of sound characterize the urban soundscape to a great extent, as they often dominate it.

Space, Place and the Soundscape. The relative direction from where a sound comes can 'change' in the listener's perception by turning his/her head. Soundscapes create spatial impressions: they have the ability to deliver a sense of size (volume) and distance and due to this function they can define the auditory space, and consequently place. In space, the volume of spaciousness is determined by the senses and thus it becomes evident that 'sound dramatizes spatial experience' [28] (p. 16).

According to Schafer [26] (p. 214), the acoustic space of a sounding object is that volume of space in which the sound can be heard. A variety of qualities of acoustic spaces has been observed, however a basic separation in two levels can facilitate the study of the factors related to the acoustic space.

- On a first level, a house is a concrete acoustic space that deteriorates the sounds coming from the inner space with its walls and prevents them to be heard outside, while at the same time the same walls prevent a considerable amount of sound to enter the house and be audible to the people that live in there. Complex interactions evolve there, as the limits of the acoustic and visual space are set by human construction.

- A second level is the outdoor space, where the conditions of sound existence change. Sound is free to expand in a greater space, where it acquires the potential to be noticed in a large scale; both natural and mechanical sounds that are loud enough to be able to dominate vast outdoor acoustic spaces exist.

The sound environment of outdoor spaces has been, and still is, the principal field of soundscape studies. These sounds, as they flow in the acoustic space, are always dependent on each space's physical characteristics. Acoustic boundaries should be the ones to define the soundscape, placing the listener and his/her subjectivity a primary role. Thus, the trajectory of soundscape differs from the property lines of landscape. Also, sound travels and defines its own acoustic space. However, the physical environment always inevitably defines the form in which sound will reach to the human ear, and space affects sound not only in a physical way, but it can also affect the characteristics of sound production [26]. Thus, the quality of the soundscape also depends on architectural characteristics.

Truax [29] has defined acoustic space as 'the perceived area encompassed by a soundscape, either an actual environment, or an imagined one' to focus on the relationship between sound and space in terms of information exchange: 'every sound brings with it information about the space in which it occurs (for environmental sound) or is thought to occur (as with synthesized sound). With environmental sound, loudness and the quality of reverberation mainly determine the kind of space that is perceived, enclosed or open, large or small'.

According to Blesser and Salter [2] (p. 2), 'a real environment, such as an urban street, a concert hall, or a dense jungle, is sonically far more complex than a single wall'. This is obvious, as sound objects and sound sources are constantly present, and keep changing: Along with them, the sonic field and the listener's soundscape change too. Continuing this thought, the writers support that 'the composite of numerous surfaces, objects, and geometries in a complicated environment creates an aural architecture.' [2] (p. 2). Objects or surfaces clearly create a particular resonance of the existing sounds in the area; but also aural architecture acquires a social meaning. Cultural and social functions are determined by the nature of a sonic experience in a certain place. Also, concerning the cultural context, one must study the acoustic parameters that are involved. The listener, the conditions of his/her situation, the purposes and the meanings are parameters that define the relationship between the listener and the sound object in this context. It is also through the architectural structures, aural and visual, that people can develop cognitive procedures towards a place. 'Visual and aural meanings often align and reinforce each other. For example, the visual vastness of a cathedral communicates through the eyes, while its enveloping reverberation communicates through the ears. For those with ardent religious beliefs, both senses create a feeling of being in the earthly home of their deity' [2] (p. 3).

4   Research Design

4.1   Description of the Application

An Android application that will assist the measurement of the users' affective response to places is currently under development. This application will also be providing navigation assistance functionality to visually impaired users.

Affective Response Logging. Users will be given the option to record their affective state at various points along their route. Sighted users will manipulate two sliders perpendicular to each other, one for each dimension of Russell's circumplex model. Visually impaired users will be entering this information by sliding across the screen, horizontally for one dimension and vertically for the other. Each dimension will comprise a 3-point or 5-point scale.

Trajectory Logging, Audio Recording, and Geolocation. The user's movement will be tracked throughout the activity and their aggregated affective impact ratings will be displayed on a map in numerical or color form. Thus, a mapping of place meaning for various parts of the city of Limassol will be produced. In addition, users will be able to provide short (< 7.5 sec.) voice annotations anywhere along the route. This will result in additional, unstructured content to be subjected to qualitative analysis in order to complement quantitative data analysis.

4.2   Description of the Application

A mixed methods approach will be adopted, employing both quantitative and qualitative methods, chief among them being the soundwalk method. A soundwalk proposes a way of exploring the surrounding acoustic space by careful listening while walking, and a manner of being exposed to detailed sounds, especially the ones that people are not aware of during their everyday activities. The fact that the experience of sound-walking is so subjective is expected to appear useful, as individual discussions and conclusions will evolve regarding the place and its meaning by the participants. Also the flexibility of the method, as it can be done in various hours and days of the week will provide safer information regarding the interactions that happen between the users and the place. Respectively, a variation of the method of the soundwalk is used in this case:

The participants will follow a route specified in advance while carrying a smartphone running the application described in the previous section. At specific, predetermined locations, the participants will stop and be prompted to indicate the affective impact of sounds directed towards them, providing quantitative data by means of the application. The prompt will be either visual (in the case of sighted users) or auditory (in the case of visually impaired users). Even if soundwalk as a method requires a continuous and silent – on behalf of the participant – walk, it will be necessary for the objectives of the research to pause the procedure so that data in situ are obtained. Qualitative data will also be gathered so as to supplement quantitative data analysis. Qualitative data will be obtained primarily through semi-structured interviews featuring questions about the meaning of the experience of the soundwalk as a whole, the emotions participants experienced during the walk, and the relative importance of the locations in which participants provided feedback via the application.

4.3   Summary and Future Work

In this paper, a research design with the objective of ascertaining the affective impact of auditory cues originating from the environment for sighted and visually impaired users was outlined, accompanied by the description of an Android application to be used for that purpose. As evident from the theoretical discussion presented herein, the concept of place meaning is a multidimensional and inherently subjective process that rests on parameters pertaining to the environment, to the user, and the system. Despite its somewhat rigid nature, the soundwalk methodology, if properly implemented, is useful in highlighting the parameters of sound that influence the process of place meaning generation. In the immediate future, the experimental investigation described in this paper will take place, and a concrete theoretical framework of the role of auditory stimuli in the production of place meaning in urban settings will be synthesized.

References

1. Augoyard, J.-F., Torgue, H.: Sonic Experience: A Guide to Everyday Sounds. McGill-Queen's University Press, Quebec (2005)
2. Blesser, B., Salter, L.-R.: Spaces speak, are you listening? MIT Press, Cambridge (2007)
3. Low, S.M., Altman, I.: Place Attachment: A Conceptual Inquiry. In: Altman, I., Low, S.M. (eds.) Place Attachment, pp. 1–12. Plenum Press, New York (1991)
4. Harrison, S., Dourish, P.: Re-Place-ing Space: The Roles of Place and Space in Collaborative Systems. In: Proc. Computer-Supported Cooperative Work (CSCW), pp. 67–76. ACM Press, Cambridge (1996)
5. Dourish, P.: Where the Action Is: The Foundations of Embodied Interaction. MIT Press, Cambridge (2001)
6. Graumann, C.F.: The Phenomenological Approach to People-Environment Studies. In: Bechtel, R.B., Churchman, A. (eds.) Handbook of Environmental Psychology, 2nd edn., pp. 95–113. John Wiley & Sons, New York (2002)
7. Droseltis, O., Vignoles, V.L.: Towards an Integrative Model of Place Identification: Dimensionality and Predictors of Intrapersonal-Level Place Preferences. Journal of Environmental Psychology 30, 23–34 (2010)
8. Scannell, L., Gifford, R.: Defining Place Attachment: A Tripartite Organizing Framework. Journal of Environmental Psychology 30, 1–10 (2010)
9. Sime, J.: Creating Places or Designing Spaces? Journal of Environmental Psychology 6, 49–63 (1986)
10. Nitsche, M.: Video Game Spaces: Image, Play, and Structure in 3D Worlds. MIT Press, Cambridge (2008)
11. Calleja, G.: In-game: From Immersion to Incorporation. MIT Press, Cambridge (2011)
12. Moser, G., Uzzell, D.: Environmental Psychology. In: Millon, T., Lerner, M.J. (eds.) Handbook of Psychology: Personality and Social Psychology, vol. 5, pp. 419–445. John Wiley & Sons, Hoboken (2003)
13. McCullough, M.: Digital Ground: Architecture, Pervasive Computing, and Environmental Knowing. MIT Press, Cambridge (2004)
14. Lentini, L., Decortis, F.: Space and Places: When Interacting With and In Physical Space becomes a Meaningful Experience. Personal and Ubiquitous Computing 14, 407–415 (2010)
15. Lynch, K.: The Image of the City. MIT Press, Cambridge (1960)
16. Gibson, J.J.: The Ecological Approach to Visual Perception. Lawrence Erlbaum Associates, Hillsdale (1986)
17. Kopec, D.: Environmental Psychology for Design. Fairchild Publications, New York (2006)
18. Stedman, R.C.: Is It Really Just a Social Construction? The Contribution of the Physical Environment to Sense of Place. Society and Natural Resources 16, 671–685 (2003)
19. Relph, E.: Place and Placelessness. Pion Limited, London (1976)
20. Morgan, P.: Towards a Developmental Theory of Place Attachment. Journal of Environmental Psychology 30, 11–22 (2010)

21. André, E.: Experimental methodology in Emotion-Oriented Computing. IEEE Pervasive Computing 10, 54–56 (2011)
22. Ekman, P.: Basic Emotions. In: Dalgleish, T., Power, M. (eds.) Handbook of Cognition and Emotion, pp. 45–60. John Wiley and Sons, Sussex (1999)
23. Russell, J.A.: Core Affect and the Psychological Construction of Emotion. Psychological Review 110, 145–172 (2003)
24. Russell, J.A., Pratt, G.: A Description of the Affective Quality Attributed to Environments. Journal of Personality and Social Psychology 38, 311–322 (1980)
25. Truax, B.: Acoustic Communication. Alex Publishing Corporation, New Jersey (1984)
26. Schafer, R.M.: The Soundscape. Our Sonic Environment and the Tuning of the World. Destiny Books, Vermont (1977)
27. Garrioch, D.: Sounds of the city: the soundscape of early modern European towns. Urban History 30, 1–25 (2003)
28. Tuan, Y.-F.: Space and Place. University of Minnesota Press, Minnesota (1977)
29. Truax, B.: Handbook for Acoustic Ecology (1999), http://www.sfu.ca/sonic-studio/handbook/Sound_Signal.html (April 24, 2012) (retrieved)

A Pedestrian Support System by Presenting Implicit/Explicit Human Information

Tsutomu Terada

Graduate School of Engineering, Kobe University, Japan
PRESTO, Japan Science and Technology Agency

Abstract. In crowded places like busy shopping complexes, there are many accidents such as bumping between walkers. One of the reasons for troubles is that it is difficult for each person to recognize the behaviors of other people perfectly. Here, cars implicitly communicate with others by presenting their contexts using their equipment such as signals or the horn, or drive obeying the traffic rules indicated by road signs or road painting. In this paper, we introduce a walking support system using the traffic rules and the information presentation mechanism in cars. The proposed system solves the problems by *presenting the user's context against surrounding people* and *presenting surrounding information to the system user*. Using these two information presentation methods, the proposed system realizes safe and smooth walking. The evaluation results with our prototype system confirmed that our method visually and intuitively presented the user context.

1 Introduction

In crowded places like busy shopping complexes, there are many accidents such as bumping between walkers. For example, to suddenly stop walking sometimes causes bumping into a person from behind, or a stream of pedestrians interfering with a person who wants to go to the other side. It is especially difficult for elderly people or handicapped people to adapt to such a fast stream of people. Moreover, in the situation where two walkers get in the way of each other on an even less crowded street, they may become panic-stricken. One of the reasons for these troubles is that it is difficult for each person to recognize the behaviors of other people perfectly.

In addition to this, there is a problem on recognizing the behaviors of surrounding walkers. For example, there are implicit rules on wide walkways such as people should walk left-hand side of the walkway while pedestrians are required to walk on the right-hand side of the road from a legal standpoint. The people who do not know the rule may walk against the flow of the other people and it makes dangerous situations.

On the other hand, forms of transportation, such as trains and cars, implicitly communicate with others by presenting their contexts using their equipment such as signals or the horn, or drive obeying the traffic rules indicated by road signs or road painting. In particular, although a car does not have a centralized

C. Stephanidis and M. Antona (Eds.): UAHCI/HCII 2014, Part III, LNCS 8515, pp. 791–802, 2014.
© Springer International Publishing Switzerland 2014

facility to regulate traffic like a control room, they present their behaviors to the surrounding cars and people implicitly and intuitively. The reason why people can intuitively understand car behaviors is that we have implicit knowledge of the context presentation methods of cars.

In this paper, focusing on wearable computing technologies, we propose a walking support system using the traffic rules and the information presentation mechanism in cars. The proposed system solves the problems by *presenting the user's context against surrounding people* and *presenting surrounding information to the system user.* The former prevents bumps among walkers by visualizing the user behavior by using information presentation methods based on those found in cars, such as wearing LEDs as brake lights. The latter prevents troubles among walkers by controlling the user behaviors with the traffic rules shown with Augmented Reality (AR) technologies. In the latter system, it indicates the traffic rules based on the surrounding environment recognized by front camera. Using these two information presentation methods, the proposed system realizes safe and smooth walking.

We also evaluate our prototype on the viewpoint of intuitiveness of presenting user contexts, and the visibility effects of changing the mounting position of the wearable devices. Moreover, we evaluate our prototype if it can visualize surrounding walking rules by using image recognition and accumulated recognition data.

2   Related Works

Various systems that visualize human activities have been proposed. Eco-MAME [1] promotes environmentally conscious activities in local communities. The system accumulates the user activities via the Internet and shows the activities of other users who are in a similar environment such as people living in similar neighborhoods. Since this system aims to present the feeling of cooperation and competition by visualizing the activities, it differs from our system, which visualizes the activities of walkers in real-time. On the other hand, there is the application *Sprocket* [2] for the iPad that is used as a method for visualizing the behaviors of a bicycle rider. A rider uses this application while carrying an iPad on their back. The application displays four pictograms such as an arrow and a pointing finger that are used to signal turning right, turning left, going straight, and slowing down. However, since the pictograms are originally made, it is difficult for surrounding people to intuitively recognize their meanings. In addition, the system does not resolve the problems for walkers mentioned in the previous section because it displays information after the completion of a user's activity.

The proposed system visualizes user contexts and helps to alter the behaviors of the surrounding people. Previously, various walking control methods have been proposed such as a system that controls walking based on the congestion reduction in public facilities or a navigation system that guides a user in the right direction. "CabBoots" [3] is a guidance system using a device that inclines the

Table 1. Information presentation methods for cars

Presentation method	Meaning
Brake light	Slowing down, Stop
Turn signals	Turning, Changing lanes, Pulling over
Hazard lights	Stop, Presenting emergency
Reversing lights	backing up
Passing lamps	Caution
Horn	Caution
Clearance lamps	Presence of car
Caution sound	Presence of car

soles of shoes. The system navigates users implicitly by controlling the user orientation using the devices on the soles. Moreover, Yoshikawa propose a pedestrian traffic control method using the Auditory Stimulation on Optokinetic Vection [4]. The vection is controlled by a lenticular lens placed on a floor that has an effect on the visual stimulus. In these systems, the system devices need to be placed on the floor or at the feet of those who are receiving guidance. Therefore, the system does not suit the usage environment of the proposed system in which the place where the system is used and the target who receives the information are unspecified.

3   Design of the System

In this section, we describe the sub systems that are a system for presenting user context to surrounding people and an AR system for presenting implicit rules to the user separately.

3.1   Visualization of Walker Context

The proposed system visualizes user behaviors based on the visualization methods used in cars to inform surrounding people of the context of the user. To do this, the user wears sensors and actuators such as LEDs and accelerometers. Table 1 lists examples of information presentation methods for cars, such as informing about turning or stopping using turn signals or brake lights. Most people can intuitively recognize such meanings since they are familiar with the presentation methods for cars in their daily lives and they have implicit knowledge of these methods.

Figure 1 illustrates a user wearing a *Jacket Type* prototype. The system receives user context from wearable sensors and wearable input interfaces, and it shows the context to surrounding people with output devices such as the LEDs or a speaker.

The proposed system has the following visualizing functions:

Brake Light: When the button on the input device is pushed or the sensors detect the user is slowing down or stopping, the red LEDs on the back illuminate,

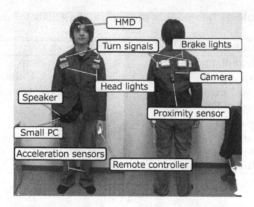

Fig. 1. Snapshot of user wearing prototype

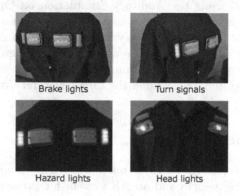

Fig. 2. Presentation examples of prototype

as shown in the upper left photo in Figure 2, to present the intention of slowing down or stopping.

Blinker: When the button on the input device is pushed, yellow LEDs on the back blink, as shown in the upper right photo in Figure 2, to present the intention of turning, changing lanes, or pulling over.

Hazard Lights: When the button on the input device is pushed, both yellow LEDs on the back blink, as shown in the lower left photo in Figure 2 to present the user's presence.

Head Lamps: When the button on the input device is pushed, white LEDs on the chest illuminate, as shown in the lower right photo in Figure 2 to present the user's presence. Moreover, blinking head lamps will draws the attention of the surrounding walkers.

Engine Sound: The system outputs engine sounds using a speaker to present the user's presence based on the walking speed.

Table 2. Example of road signs

Sign	Meaning
Yellow center line	a car cannot pass through another car, with/without running over the line
White center line	a car cannot pass through, with running over the line
White dotted center-line	a car can pass through another car
Halt sign	a car must come to a full stop
Yellow blinking traffic-signal	a car can go while paying attention to other traffic

Horn: When the button on the input device is pushed, the system outputs a horn sound from a speaker, and draws the attention of the surrounding walkers.

The system correctly recognizes the user context for visualizing user behaviors because presentation of incorrect information would cause an accident such as bumping between walkers. On the other hand, we assume that the system will be used in daily life, so that complex operations or unnatural actions are not practical as input methods for the visualization. Therefore, the proposed system recognizes user behaviors using wearable sensors [5]. The contexts that can be recognized by using wearable sensors do not need any input from the user. On the other hand, there are several contexts that are difficult to recognize by using wearable sensors, such as turning right, which should be recognized before the actual turning. For such contexts, the user informs the system of the context using simple operations such as pushing a button on the input device.

3.2 Visualization of Implicit Traffic Rules

This subsystem shows implicit walking rules for surrounding situation as well-known road signs as shown in Table 2. The user of proposed system wears a PC, an HMD (Head Mounted Display), and a camera to acquire the eyeshot of user. The system analyzes the acquired images of the eyeshot and recognizes the flow of pedestrians. Based on the recognition, the system presents traffic signs on HMD to navigate the user correctly.

The proposed system has the following visualizing functions:

Center Line: The system presents yellow center-line and white arrows that indicate the flow of pedestrians as shown in Figure 3. It helps the user to grasp the surrounding situations and to avoid troubles happened by the aberration from the flow of surrounding people.

Halt Sign: The system presents a halt sign on HMD. It calls the user attention to surroundings before happening an accident such as entering crowded area and crossing the flow of pedestrians.

No Entry Sign: The system presents a No-entry sign on HMD when the user walks against the flow of pedestrians.

The system analyses the behaviors of surrounding pedestrians by calculating optical flow of input images from a wearable camera[6]. In addition to this,

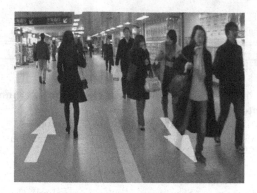

Fig. 3. Yellow line and white arrows

analysis results are stored on Internet and shared with other users. It helps to improve the accuracy of implicit-rule recognition. Concretely, when the system recognizes the behaviors of surrounding pedestrians, it stores and uploads the result with latitude, longitude, and direction of the user. Using this database, the system can present implicit rules to the user even if there is no pedestrian around.

4   Implementation

We have implemented the prototype of a system for visualizing pedestrian behaviors.

4.1   Visualization of Walker Context Subsystem

In this system, a user uses a Nintendo Wii remote controller as the input device, and wireless accelerometers (WAA-006) by Wireless Technology on the user's feet are used to recognize the user walking states and speed contexts by calculating the variances of the velocity. We use a Single-eye HMD Shimadzu DataGlass3/A, a Microsoft LifeCam RLA-00007 as a rear view camera, and a Distance Measuring Sensor SHARP GP2D12 as a backup sensor. We developed the system software using Microsoft VisualC# 2008.

We implemented the following four types of visualization devices.

Jacket Type (Figure 1): It has lamps, a sensor, and a camera on the front and back of a jacket. A user uses the system by wearing it.

Movable Type (Figure 4 left): It consists of a rear unit including turn signals and brake lights, and two front units including turn signals. A user uses the system by attaching these units anywhere such as their backpack, bag, or belt.

Bracelet Type (Figure 4 center): It consists of turn signal rings that works as turn signals and brake light rings that work as brake lights. A user uses the system by wearing the rings on his/her wrists.

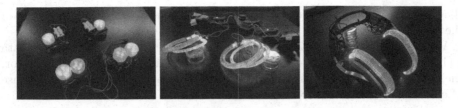

Fig. 4. Snapshots of prototype

Headphone Type (Figure 4 right): It has turn signal lights and brake lights on a set of headphones. The structure of the lamps is almost the same as that of the Bracelet type. A user uses the system by putting on the headphones.

The Jacket type controls the light of the LEDs using a microcomputer called *Gainer* connected to a wearable PC via a USB cable, and the others control the LEDs using *Arduino* with *xBee* wireless unit.

4.2   Visualization of Implicit Traffic Rules Subsystem

We implemented an application that presents implicit traffic rules on HMD as shown in Figure 3. Figure 5 shows a snapshot of the application with optical flow information. Optical flows are calculated from the equally spaced points as shown in the figure. Among the vectors obtained by the analysis, if (1) an extension of a vector runs near the vanishing point of the background, (2) the direction of the vector aims at outside, and (3) the length of the vector is larger than that of moving speed of the user, the system recognizes that the vector represents the flow of pedestrians in opposite direction to the user. The image acquired from the wearable camera is divided into 6 x 4 areas and the context of each area is decided by the ratio of vectors represent these pedestrians. Based on the information, the system draws a yellow center-line and white arrows as

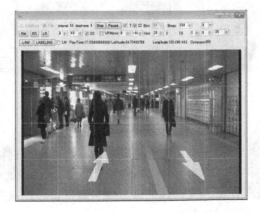

Fig. 5. Snapshot of prototype with optical flow information

shown in the figure. The red square in the figure means the boundary area of the flow of pedestrians.

We also implemented a simulator that can handle movie file with meta-data including latitude, longitude, and direction of the user. Using this simulator, the system can learn implicit rules from a large amount of stored data. We use Microsoft Visual C# to implement the simulator.

5   Evaluation

5.1   Visualization of Walker Context

We made subjects watch videos in which the system is being used in a real environment and answer a questionnaire to evaluate the effectiveness of the proposed system. There were 16 male subjects ranging from 21 to 24 years old, and they evaluated the five videos recorded in a busy shopping complex and around an elevator. The screenshots from video No. 2 and No. 3 are shown in Figures 6 and 7. Each video contains a scene in which a system user presents his/her next action using lighting or blinking lamps, and the video was finished before the user actually does the next action. Table 3 lists the contents and examples of the correct answers for each video. The subjects were shown these videos in random order and answered the forecast of his/her next action on the basis of the system functions in the videos. We showed each video only once to the subjects. Whether the answer is correct or not is decided based on the example answers in the table. For example, in video No. 4, *He will pass on my right side.* or *He will go leftward.* are correct answers. However, *He is greeting.* is not a correct answer.

Table 4 lists the number of people giving correct answers and examples of incorrect answers for each video. As a result, we believe that the proposed system plainly showed the user contexts in the four videos except for in video No. 3.

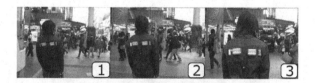

Fig. 6. Screenshots of video No. 2

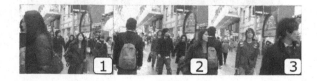

Fig. 7. Screenshots of video No. 3

Table 3. Content of each video

No.	Scene	Used function	Camera viewpoint	Example answer
1	Walking in mall	brake lights	Following user	Slowing down
2	Walking in mall	Left blinker	Following user	Turning left
3	Walking in mall	Right blinker	Passing on his right side	Turning right
4	Getting off elevator	Left blinker	Waiting for elevator	Passing on my right side
5	Walking in mall	Hazard lights	Approaching the user	Standing still

Table 4. Experimental results from actual environments

Correct / all	Example of incorrect answer
14/16	Turning left. Having passed.
16/16	–
4/16	No idea. He is greeting acquaintance. He will step to right side.
14/16	He greeted person who suddenly appeared.
15/16	No idea.

However, only 4 out of 16 subjects answered correctly to video No. 3. One of the reasons for this result is that this video showed the user wearing the system for very short time since he/she suddenly appears from the stream of other walkers. That is, there is a possibility that even the proposed system cannot correctly show the presentation when the surrounding people glance at it.

Although the number of people choosing the correct answer is minimal for the above mentioned reason in video No. 3, we confirmed that the presented information from the proposed system in a real environment was effective throughout the experiment.

Next, our proposed system visualizes user context using the presenting information methods of cars. The reason why we selected these methods is that we believe the surrounding people swiftly and exactly understand the user context based on their implicit knowledge about the context visualizing methods of real cars. To confirm the hypothesis, we conducted comparative evaluations of four situations: with the proposed method, with two other information presenting methods, and without visualization. We prepared the comparative methods using figures (pictograms) and words (in Japanese), moreover, we used 7-inch displays on the front and back of a user as the presenting information device for these methods. Figure 8 shows the presentation examples of comparative system. The subjects watched the four videos for each situation and answered the questionnaire. Each video is composed of two scenes: a user starts turning left and finishes doing it, and a user standing still. There were 16 male subjects ranging from 21 to 24 years old.

The subjects evaluated the easiness of recognizing the meaning or intention and the easiness of seeing the presentation in each situation based on 5 levels from 5 points (easy) to 1 point (hard).

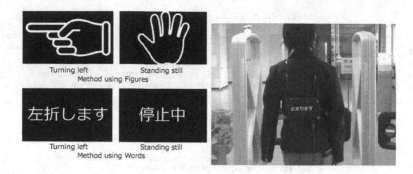

Fig. 8. Presentation examples of comparative systems

Table 5. Average score for each situation

	Turning left		Standing still	
	Content recognition	Recognition distance	Content recognition	Recognition distance
No system	2.1 (Points)	-	1.6	-
System with figures	4.1	4.4	2.1	4.1
System with words	4.9	2.1	4.7	2.1
Proposed system	4.4	4.8	4.1	4.9

Table 5 lists the result. As a result of the multiple comparisons for Steel Duwas analysis, there are significant differences between the scores of the proposed system and those of the system using figures for the easiness of recognizing the meaning for Turning left (p<0.01), and between the scores of the proposed system and those of the system using words for the easiness of seeing presentation in both scenes (Turning left: p<0.01, Standing still: p<0.01). In addition, there were also significant differences between the scores of the proposed system and no visualization (Turning left: p<0.01, Standing still: p<0.01). From these results, we confirmed that the context of walkers was barely understood without visualization.

When we took into consideration items in which significant differences were found, moreover, we confirmed that the system using figures could not exactly convey the meaning of the presentation in the standing scene. This may be because people sometimes mistakenly recognize an illustration of a hand as a command for them (not as the information of the system user), while a presentation itself is conspicuous. Even if other illustration are used, the same problem will happen. On the other hand, for the system using words, the scores of the easiness of seeing the presentation were low because the system presents information only in characters, which cannot be seen at a distance. The system is perfectly conveys the information, but it requires more time for surrounding people to know the contents the system presented. Accordingly, we confirmed that our proposed system had advantages over the comparative methods.

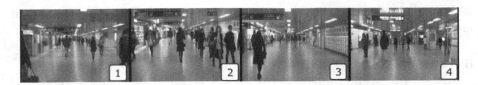

Fig. 9. Screenshots of video No. 1

5.2   Visualization of Implicit Traffic Rules

We evaluate the accuracy of showing implicit rules that is the position of yellow center-line in this study. We recorded four videos (No. 1 – No. 4) on walking through premises of a train terminal. The width and length of the walk space are 10m and 100m, respectively. Examples of snapshot are shown in Figure 9. In that video, the user walked for approximately 35 seconds with passing by 16 pedestrians. We labeled the ground truth to all videos by hand.

Table 6 shows the result. By investigating the video and the evaluation results, we found that the system was correctly able to detect the pedestrians near the user but failed to recognize far from the user. Optical flows made by pedestrians far from the user were not so strong and they were frequently canceled by the movement of camera since the user was walking.

Next, we evaluate the accuracy in the case where the system has database. We made three types of databases using the information from video No. 2, video No.2 + No. 3, and video No. 2 + No. 3 + No. 4. For each dataset, video No. 1 is used for evaluating the accuracy. Table 7 shows the result. Since we did not use the dataset to cancel showing the center line but to show it, the precision dropped as the dataset increased. However, comparing the result of no dataset and that of dataset No. 2, our method achieved greatly advancement in the recall

Table 6. Accuracy of presenting implicit rules

	Precision	Recall
Video No. 1	65.0(%)	73.6
Video No. 2	55.4	60.6
Video No. 3	62.4	57.8
Video No. 4	60.5	69.0

Table 7. Accuracy with database

Dataset	Precision	Recall
Nothing	65.0	73.6
No. 2	62.2	89.6
No. 2 + No. 3	55.3	94.0
No. 2 + No. 3 + No. 4	51.9	98.4

with minor degradation in the precision. It suggests that there is a possibility of improvement in accuracy by selecting the dataset appropriately.

6   Conclusion

We proposed a pedestrian support system using the traffic rules and the information presentation mechanism in cars. The proposed system solves the problems by "presenting the user's context against surrounding people" and "presenting surrounding information to the system user". Using these two information presentation methods, the proposed system realizes safe and smooth walking. Our prototype system visualizes the user behavior such as turning left or stopping, using car-metaphors such as wearing LEDs as brake lights and turn signals. In addition our prototype shows traffic signs to the user by capturing surrounding situations using wearable camera.

The evaluation results with our prototype system confirmed that our method visually and intuitively presented the user context since the presentation method based on implicit knowledge is superior to the methods using objects that can present the dual meanings such as a pictogram. Moreover, we found that our prototype could visualize surrounding walking rules by using image recognition and accumulated recognition data.

In future, we will add more implicit rules to be shown on HMD, and develop more effective system to communicate among pedestrians in the real world.

Acknowledgments. This research was supported in part by a Grant in aid for Precursory Research for Embryonic Science and Technology (PRESTO) from the Japan Science and Technology Agency.

References

1. Tanaka, R., Doi, S., Konishi, T., Yoshinaga, N., Itaya, S., Yamada, K.: Eco-MAME: Ecology Activity Promotion System Based on Human Psychological Characteristics. In: Datta, A., Shulman, S., Zheng, B., Lin, S.-D., Sun, A., Lim, E.-P. (eds.) SocInfo 2011. LNCS, vol. 6984, pp. 324–327. Springer, Heidelberg (2011)
2. Sprocket, http://www.maya.com/sprocket/
3. Cabboots, http://www.freymartin.de/en/projects/cabboots
4. Yoshikawa, H., Hachisu, T., Fukushima, S., Fukukawa, M., Kajimoto, H.: Vection Field for Pedestrian Traffic Control. In: Proc. of the 38th International Conference and Exhibition on Computer Graphics and Interactive techniques (SIGGRAPH 2011), p. 1 (2011)
5. Murao, K., Terada, T., Nishio, S.: Toward Construction of Wearable Sensing Environments. In: Hara, T., Zadorozhny, V.I., Buchmann, E. (eds.) Wireless Sensor Network Technologies for the Information Explosion Era. SCI, vol. 278, pp. 207–230. Springer, Heidelberg (2010)
6. Braillon, C., Pradalier, C., Crowley, J.L., Laugier, C.: Real-time moving obstacle detection using optical flow models. In: Proc. of IEEE Intelligent Vehicles Symposium 2006, pp. 466–471 (2006)

Virtual Walking Stick: Mobile Application to Assist Visually Impaired People to Walking Safely

Thomas Akira Ueda and Luciano Vieira de Araújo

Information System, School of Arts, Sciences and Humanities, University of São Paulo, Brazil
akirajin.usp@gmail.com, lvaraujo@usp.br

Abstract. People affected by temporary visual limitations or early permanent limitations have the challenge of adapting the way to perform their daily tasks. In particular, the activity of walking without support of others not only requires extensive adaptation but also can expose individuals to the risk. For instance, if an object is not identified during the walk, serious accidents may happen. Therefore, assist blind people to walk independently and safely is an important challenge for computational area. With the popularity of smartphones, cameras and new sensors are available at affordable prices and can be used to develop software to help visually impaired people to walk more independently and safely. This paper presents the development of a mobile application to help visually impaired people to walk independently, using the smartphone's camera to alert them about obstacles on the way.

Keywords: impaired vision, walking stick, indoor navigation, safe walk.

1   Introduction

Reports of the WHO (World Health Organization) in 2010 show that about 285 billion people in the world have some type of visual problem. The visual limitations can range from simple cases that can be solved with the use of glasses, by going through cases where the field of vision is reduced, until the more severe cases that include complete blindness. Besides the variation in severity, the visual limitations can be permanent or temporary. People affected by temporary visual limitations or early permanent limitations have the challenge of adapting the way to perform their daily tasks. A special challenge is to avoid object or obstacles during the walking.

In particular, the activity of walking without support of others not only requires extensive adaptation but also can expose individuals to the risk. For instance, if an object is not identified during the walk, serious accidents may happen. Therefore, assist people with visual limitations to walk independently and safely is an important challenge for computational area. The HCI (Human-Computer Interaction) research area has made several contributions to assist people with visual limitations, such as: Interfaces with varying colors and contrasts, text readers, audio messages, voice command

C. Stephanidis and M. Antona (Eds.): UAHCI/HCII 2014, Part III, LNCS 8515, pp. 803–813, 2014.

systems and so on. However, the popularity of smartphones has brought new challenges to establishing appropriate functionality for users with visual limitations, such as the touch screens and the increasing number of apps. In recent years, smartphones have tended design where physical buttons are replaced by virtual icons that increase the amount of features on smartphones. However, the lack or reduction of physical buttons on smartphones limit the use of touch to identify shortcuts to specific applications. Some applications still use the few buttons or labels available references such as the edges of the screen to activate a limited set of applications. The second challenge is the increasing number of applications installed on a smartphone and the need to navigate through screens to locate the desired application. On the other hand, smartphones provide a set of sensors that can be used to create smart shortcuts. This scenario shows the need for creating applications that not only assist in daily activities such as walking independently but also be user-friendly applications for visually impaired.

This paper presents the development of a mobile app to assist visually impaired to identify and avoid obstacles along the way.

2   Related Work

Several works have been developed to create devices and software to assist visually impaired people to walk independently and safely. These works can be classified into indoor and outdoor solutions walking. In general, the solutions to outdoor walks [1] use GPS to guide the user. However, the use of GPS limits the use of these solutions to outdoor locations. This limitation has motivated the search for solutions that guide the user in locations without GPS signal. Typically, solutions for indoor walking are based on some kind of infrastructure to guide the walk. As the use of RFID [2-5] tags, Wifi [6,7] or visual paths based on maps [8] or marked [9,10] paths. These solutions produce specific solutions, such as assisting users to find a way out of a building. However, the generalization of these solutions is not a trivial task. Even its reproduction on a large scale is limited by the cost of deployment of the infrastructure needed, such as installing landmarks or sensors [11].

3   Methodology

The application was developed for Android platform using the SDK API 19. In order to offer an affordable solution, this app was created to only use smartphone built in sensors/device such as autofocus camera and accelerometer. The interface was designed to follow recommendations of NCAM – National Center for Accessible Media. In special, the VWS do not depend of visual interface. All functions are available using gesture command or tactile buttons. Also, there are features to save energy.

The tests were performed using the Samsung Galaxy S4 phones with Android 4.4 and LG Nexus 4 with 4.4.2 android smartphone.

4   The Virtual Walking Stick App

In our work, we develop a mobile app called VWS - Virtual Walking Stick. In order to achieve the proposed objective, the VWS app uses the smartphone's camera to identify objects and people ahead of the camera. In such cases, audible or vibrating alerts are emitted to indicate the object approaching or peoples in front of the user. The distance of the object or the amount of people in front of the user is indicated by the variation of intensity of alerts.

Considering the amount of applications installed on a smartphone, its mobility and its limitations of battery and interface, the application needs to go beyond the main goal, to alert the user to obstacles and people, and offer other usability features for people with limitations visual. In this sense, the VWS app addresses three important usability issues. The first is how to run the application without the use of visual icons. For this case, the VWS app can be activated by shaking the smartphone until an alert be emitted. The second issue is how to find the phone if it falls during use. Using the accelerometer, VWS identifies the fall and smartphone beeps to help locate it. The last point is to allow extended use of the application, without quickly draining the phone battery. Since much of the energy consumption of mobile phones is related to the operation of the screen, the application turns off the display to save power.

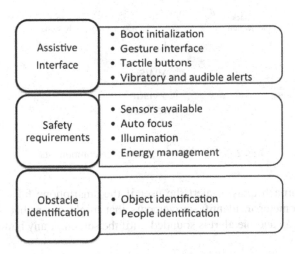

Fig. 1. VWS modules

As shown in Figure 1, the VWS is composed of 3 modules designed to provide the core functionality of the application, as described below.

4.1   Assistive Interface

Since the VWS was developed to assist visually impaired, their functionality and interface are designed to meet the needs of these users. Therefore, the VWS propose a non-visual interface, where gestures or tactile buttons can activate features. The application provides both vibration or sound/voice alerts.

Figure 2 shows the six approaches used by VWS to provide a non-visual interface. The first approach is to *Boot initialization*. It prevents the user from having to find a specific icon to launch the application. Once in memory, the selection between active apps is not an easy task. To simplify this task, we developed the *Shack Activation* function that allows the activation of VWS just shaking the smartphone. When activated, the VWS emits a voice message warning of its activation. The same happens when the application is minimized or closed. The third approach is related to the Vibratoty Alerts, they are used as discrete alerts that are not suppressed by surrounding sounds. The fourth approach is the *Audible alerts*. They allow the transmission of a larger amount of information to the user. The VWS always offers vibration or audible alerts. The selection of the type of alert to be emitted is made using Tactile Buttons. The VWS redefines the function of the volume adjustment buttons. Case these buttons remain pressed for more than 2 seconds; the audible messages are enabled or disabled according to your current status.

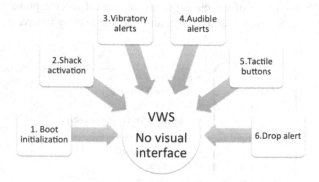

Fig. 2. VWS - No visual interface components

The sixth approach aims to alert the user if the smartphone falls. The drop alert uses the accelerometer to identify movements that might mean that the smartphone fell. In this case, an audible alert is sounded until the screen or any button is touched.

4.2   Safety Requirements

To ensure user safety, the VWS checks if the sensors are available and working properly on your smartphone. For example, although the vast majority of smartphones have built in cameras, not all make it possible to use the autofocus function of Android. In such cases, the application will not function properly and the user needs to be warned. Another limitation related to the smartphone camera is its ability to focus on objects. Figure 2 shows two examples where it is not possible to focus on objects. In figure presents two screenshots of the evaluation of the application interface, since the application does not require a GUI and as a way to save energy.

The screenshot to the left was captured in a situation of absence of light, so the screen is dark and shows the message - Unable to focus. The example on the right, a bright light prevents the focus. In this case, the display appears white and displays the same message - Unable to focus. These limitations have been reduced with the quality evolution of smartphone cameras. More and more cameras feature great capacity light compensation and tend to offer even night vision.

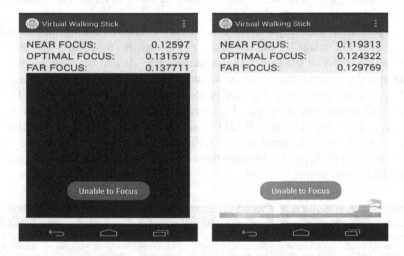

Fig. 3. Example of situation that the camera can not focus on object

Another safety issue is the power management of your smartphone. Despite the VWS reduce energy consumption by simulating the turning off the smartphone screen, the user needs to be alerted about the amount of energy available for your smartphone. Thus, situations where the battery runs out can be avoided.

4.3 Obstatacle Identification

The module of identification of obstacles is responsible for the identification of objects and people in front of camera. The distance between an object and the user is inferred using the focal distance of the object. This value is obtained by using the android method - `getFocusDistance`. This function provides values of 3 variables: Near Focus, Optimal Focus and Far Focus.

To reduce the amount of information to be transmitted to the user, we define three distance values: Near, Medium and Far. These values are based on values of Optimal Focus variable, as follow.

- Near - Optimal Focus ≤ 0.225194
- Medium - $0.225194 <$ Optimal Focus ≤ 0.304033
- Far - $0.304033 <$ Optimal Focus

Thus, an object is considered Near, when the value of the variable Optimal Focus is less than or equal to 0.225194. The object is considered Far, when Optimal Focus is greater than 0.304033. Values between 0.225194 and 0.304033 indicate that the object is at a Medium distance.

The vibrational frequency of alerts depends on the distance of the object. The more closely the object, the more intense is the vibrating alert. In turn, voice messages inform one of three distances for the object.

The Figure 4 shows a sequence of 3 screenshots captured during indoor walking toward a wall. The image on the left presents Optimal Focus value = 0.538894 and displays at the center of the screen the message - Far. At that moment a voice message informs the user that the object is far and vibrating alert has low frequency. The central screenshot shows that the user is closer to the wall with Optimal Focus = 0.251161 and displays the message - Medium. The screenshot at right shows the wall right near, Optimal Focus value = 0.225194 and the message - Near. In situations like this, the vibrating alert is issued at high frequency. Continuously, alerts are emitted when the distance is changed. The same behavior occurs when the user moves toward a closed door or any object.

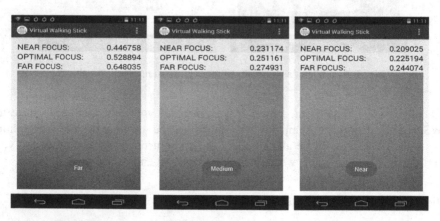

Fig. 4. Indoor walking – Sequence of screenshots of wall approaching

Figure 5 also shows a sequence of 3 screenshots. This time were obtained in a outdoor walk toward a tree. Similarly, as the value of the variable Focus Optimal increases, the messages and the vibrating frequency change.

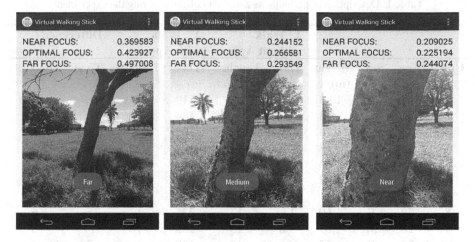

Fig. 5. Outdoor walking – Sequence of Screenshot of tree approaching

5   User Evaluation

For initial evaluation of VWS a qualitative study was conducted to analyse the opinion of individuals with normal vision when performing a walk on a circuit with obstacles and blindfolded to simulate a recent or temporary visual impairment. Therefore, such individuals have no training to use other sensory references as guidance for walking.

The experiment consisted of two walks in circuit with obstacles, always blindfolded and 5-minutes break between them. The circuit was formed by obstacles, walls, people, open and closed doors. The obstacles were chosen to simulate everyday situations. Soft and light barriers were used to prevent risk of injury to participants or fall. In addition, participants were closely monitored throughout the walk. The circuit remained the same for all individuals and walking. Each participant was instructed to walk at a comfortable pace, as if he/she were inside a home or office. It was also recommended to avoid collisions with obstacles. The first walk was performed without the aid of a cane or application. For the second walk, participant received a smartphone with VWS installed. Then he/she was asked to shake the smartphone and start the walk after to hear the message that the app was activated. At the end of the second walk, the participant was guided to an area with padded floor, where he was asked to leave smartphone fall to the ground and then try to locate it. All participants used the same smartphone. We selected 10 participants, 6 men and 4 women, aged between 25 and 35 years old, height ranging from 1.57 m to 1.78 m.

Table 1 shows the obtained results. For each walking, we recorded the time spent to complete the circuit and the amount of touches an obstacle, doors or walls.

Table 1. Description of participants and data collected during the experiment

User	Age	Sex	Height (m)	1st Walk without App		2nd Walk with App		Difference	
				Time (s)	Touches	Time (s)	Touches	Time (s)	Touches
1	27	F	1,63	52	8	119	9	67	1
2	32	M	1,73	82	7	134	9	52	2
3	33	M	1,78	77	13	108	8	31	-5
4	35	M	1,67	74	14	148	13	74	-1
5	35	M	1,66	80	14	165	10	85	-4
6	31	F	1,62	95	13	162	11	67	-2
7	31	M	1,71	102	18	178	12	76	-6
8	29	F	1,60	179	17	235	11	56	-6
9	28	M	1,69	86	13	235	10	149	-3
10	27	F	1,57	66	13	138	10	72	-3

Table 1 shows the Id of the participant, in sequential order of participation, age, sex, height, time taken to complete the task and number of touches on walls, doors and objects, on the both walks without and with the use of the VWS App, respectively. The column with difference of time between walks was calculated using the formula: 2nd Walk Time − 1st Walk Time. Therefore, positive values represent an increase in walking time using the VWS. The difference between obstacle touches was calculated with the formula: 2nd Walk Touches − 1st Walk Touches. Thus, positive values represent an increase in the number of obstacle touches when using VWS app.

The difference in time to complete the circuit showed that all participants needed more time used as the VWS. This increase in time can be explained, since participants started the walk more slowly to understand the relationship between the frequency of vibration and distance of objects. In some cases, the participant waited for a change in the frequency of prompts to continue the walk. Furthermore, we observed an increase in the pace of the walk at the end of the circuit. Regarding touches on obstacles, the comparison between the amounts of touches performed during walks, showed that only two participants increased the number of touches when using the VWS. Most of touches was a type of confirmation of the object presence and we could notice that as the participant felt more comfortable with the use of VWS, he tried to walk without touching the walls and obstacles, as initially oriented. Another examples of touches are the collisions caused by small changes in directions that did not avoid the collision with object.

After the completion of two walks, participants answered six questions such with open answers, as shown in Table 2.

Table 2. List of question used to evalute the use of VWS app

Id	Question
Q1	Compare your feelings/sensations during each walk.
Q2	Was the VWS app useful to identify and avoid obstacles?
Q3	Could you identify people during the app-assisted walk?
Q4	It was easy to find the smartphone after dropping it?
Q5	Did you use the audible alert to find your smartphone?
Q6	What are your suggestions for improvements to App?

Table 3 presents a summary of the responses to the 6 questions. As a strategy for the creation of Table 3, we seek to highlight the criticisms or comments that could assist in the development of the application.

Table 3. Resumo das respostas dissertativas

User	Q1	Q2	Q3	Q4	Q5	Q6
1	More safety	Yes	Yes	Yes	Yes	More/faster alerts
2	More safety	Yes	Yes	Yes	Yes	More/faster alerts
3	More safety with better results	Yes	Yes	No	Didn't work	Sharper alerts
4	Helpful	Yes	Yes	No	Didn't work	More/faster alerts
5	More safety	Yes	Yes	Yes	Yes	Continuous alert
6	Felt confused	Yes	Yes	No	Didn't work	Sharper alerts
7	More safety	Yes	Yes	No	Didn't work	Develop a smartphone's support
8	More safety	Yes	Yes	Yes	Yes	Increase vibration intensity
9	More safety	Yes	Yes	Yes	Yes	Sharper alerts
10	More safety	Yes	Yes	Yes	Yes	Allow

Evaluation of responses showed that users felt more secure through the use of VWS. Only the number 6 volunteer reported that she felt confused by the vibrating alerts. Despite this observation, all participants agreed that the application helped during walking. The identification of people addressed by Question 3, it worked in all cases. However, the drop alert, questions 4 and 5, failed 4 times. Users, who experienced this failure of the function, also reported difficulties in finding the smartphone. When the drop alert worked, the volunteers reported that the smartphone has been found easily. The combination of the answers to Questions 4 and 5 can be interpreted as an indication of the importance of the drop alert. Suggestions for improvements obtained with question 6 show that vibrating alerts may initially cause confusion, since we are not accustomed to using vibrations to guide us. However, despite the participants remember the feeling of confusion when suggesting improvements, they evaluated the application as useful and felt safer when using the VWS. This point will be evaluated more broadly with blind users who already have training to use different kinds of information to guide the walk.

6   Discussion

The VWS was developed for use native solutions of smartphones as cameras and accelerometer or face recognition functions. This approach allows the development of cost-effective and accessible apps for the user. Just install and use the application, without requiring externals devices or processes. A disadvantage of VWS is the need for smartphones with cameras sophistic. However, the evolution of smartphones shows that the prices of smartphone are reduced after a few months of its launch. Especially, when new competitors emerge in the market. The current version of VWS depends on the ability to focus of smartphone camera. Which does not occur in dark environments or lack of contrast, cases where the user is alerted. However, these limitations have been reduced with cameras with great capacity for light compensation.

7   Conclusion and Future Work

The VWS App makes use of sensors and processing power of modern smartphones to assist visual impaired people to identify and to avoid obstacles during the walking. Once, VWS only use smartphone camera to identify objects and peoples, it is ready to use, immediately after installation. None extra devises or infrastructure is required. Thus, it can be used to help walking at any place. Moreover, once the smartphone are become popular, this approach offers a low cost solution and easy to be scaled.

Furthermore, this paper contributes with a one of the main challenges of usability for visually impaired people presenting the development of an app with non-visual interface.

Our ongoing work aims to incorporate functionalities to identify known people, to recognition of voice commands, to describe objects and to guide long walks using GPS.

Acknowledgements. This work was supported by FAPESP (São Paulo State Research Foundation) grant numbers 2011/24114-0.

References

1. Holland, S., Morse, D.R., Gedenryd, H.: Audiogps: Spatial audio navigation with a minimal attention interface. Personal Ubiquitous Computing 6, 253–259 (2002)
2. Ganz, A., Gandhi, S.R., Schafer, J., Singh, T., et al.: Percept: Indoor navigation for the blind and visually impaired. In: EMBC 2011, pp. 856–859. IEEE (2011)
3. Chumkamon, S., Tuvaphanthaphiphat, P., Keeratiwintakorn, P.: A blind navigation system using rfid for indoor environments. In: ECTI-CON 2008, vol. 2, pp. 765–768. IEEE (2008)
4. Kulyukin, V., Gharpure, C., Nicholson, J., Pavithran, S.: Rfid in robot-assisted indoor navigation for the visually impaired. In: Proc. IROS 2004, vol. 2, pp. 1979–1984. IEEE (2004)
5. Willis, S., Helal, S.: RFID information grid and wearable computing solution to the problem of wayfinding for the blind user in a campus environment. In: IEEE International Symposium on Wearable Computers (ISWC 2005) (2005)
6. Rajamäki, J., Viinikainen, P., Tuomisto, J., Sederholm, T., Säämänen, M.: Laureapop indoor navigation service for the visually impaired in a wlan environment. In: Proc. EHAC 2007, pp. 96–101. WSEAS (2007)
7. Riehle, T., Lichter, P., Giudice, N.: An indoor navigation system to support the visually impaired. In: EMBS 2008, pp. 4435–4438. IEEE (2008)
8. Arikawa, M., Konomi, S., Ohnishi, K.: Navitime: Supporting pedestrian navigation in the real world. In: IEEE Pervasive Computing, vol. 6, pp. 21–29 (2007)
9. Gallo, P., Tinnirello, I., Giarre, L., Garlisi, D., Croce, D.: ARIANNA: pAth Recognition for Indoor Assisted NavigatioN with Augmented perception - DEIM, viale delle Scienze building 9, Universita' di Palermo, 90128 Palermo – Italy. In: eprint arXiv:1312.3724, http://arxiv.org/abs/1312.3724
10. Fallah, N., Apostolopoulos, I., Bekris, K., Folmer, E.: The User as a Sensor: Navigating Users with Visual Impairments in Indoor Spaces using Tactile Landmarks. In: Proceedings of the 2012 ACM annual conference on Human Factors in Computing Systems (CHI 2012), Austin, Texas, pp. 425–432 (May 2012)
11. Fallah, N., Apostolopoulos, I., Bekris, K., Folmer, E.: Indoor Human Navigation Systems; A survey, Interacting with Computers. Oxford Journals 25(1), 21–33 (2013)

Author Index

Printed in the United States
By Bookmasters